The Epilepsies

Butterworths International Medical Reviews

Neurology

Published titles

1 **Clinical Neurophysiology**
Erik Stålberg and Robert R. Young

2 **Movement Disorders**
C. David Marsden and Stanley Fahn

3 **Cerebral Vascular Disease**
Michael J. G. Harrison and Mark L. Dyken

3 **Peripheral Nerve Disorders**
Arthur K. Asbury and R. W. Gilliatt

Next title

Multiple Sclerosis
W. I. McDonald and D. H. Silberberg

The Epilepsies

Edited by

Roger J. Porter, MD
Chief, Medical Neurology Branch, National Institute of Neurological and Communicative Disorders and Stroke, National Institutes of Health; and Clinical Professor of Neurology, Adjunct Professor of Pharmacology, Uniformed Services University of the Health Sciences; and Consultant-Lecturer in Neurology, National Naval Medical Center, Bethesda, Maryland, USA

and

Paolo L. Morselli, MD
Director, Clinical Research, Laboratoire d'Études et de Recherche Synthelabo, Paris, France

Butterworths
London Boston Durban Singapore Sydney Toronto Wellington

First published 1985

British Library Cataloguing in Publication Data

The Epilepsies.—(Neurology, ISSN 0260-0137; 5).—
(Butterworths international medical reviews)
1. Epilepsy
I. Porter, Roger J. II. Morselli, Paolo L.
III. Series
616.8′53 RC372

ISBN 0-407-02298-8

Photoset by Butterworths Litho Preparation Department
Printed and bound in England by Robert Hartnoll Ltd., Bodmin, Cornwall

Foreword

For almost a quarter of a century (1951–1975), subjects of topical interest were written about in the periodic volumes of our predecessor, *Modern Trends in Neurology*. Although both that series and its highly regarded editor, Dr Denis Williams, are now retired, the legacy continues in the present Butterworths series in Neurology. As was the case with *Modern Trends*, the current volumes are intended for use by physicians who grapple with the problems of neurological disorder on a daily basis, be they neurologists, neurologists in training, or those in related fields such as neurosurgery, internal medicine, psychiatry, and rehabilitation medicine.

Our purpose is to produce annually a monograph on a topic in clinical neurology in which progress through research has brought about new concepts of patient management. The subject of each monograph is selected by the Series Editors using two criteria: first, that there has been significant advance in knowledge in that area; and second, that such advances have been incorporated into new ways of managing patients with the disorders in question.

This has been the guiding spirit behind each volume, and we expect it to continue. In effect we emphasize research, both in the clinic and in the experimental laboratory, but principally to the extent that it changes our collective attitudes and practices in caring for those who are neurologically afflicted.

C. D. Marsden
A. K. Asbury
Series Editors

Preface

This fifth volume in the Neurology series of Butterworths International Medical Reviews continues the tradition of forwarding the latest developments in a particular neurological discipline, emphasizing those advances which have clinical relevance. In no other area of neurology have recent clinical and laboratory investigations yielded more significant changes than in the management of epilepsy. Extraordinary strides have been made: from new understandings of the GABA receptor to better empirical classifications of seizures; and from drugs designed with knowledge of their mechanism of action to the role of positron emission tomography in the surgical evaluation of the patient with partial seizures. This volume provides a detailed look at these new developments, offers a framework for their application in clinical practice, and predicts how the care of patients with seizures might soon be changing.

The volume begins with four chapters that explain our basic understanding of this heterogeneous disorder and show how we are designing better strategies to enable us to grasp the fundamental mechanisms, while using both rational and empirical approaches to new therapies. Chapters 5 through 16 are concerned with the proper classification and diagnosis of seizures and their appropriate treatment. More emphasis than usual has been placed on surgical evaluation and treatment, a remarkably underutilized approach to the difficult patient with epilepsy. The focus throughout the volume has been on new developments and techniques which are of clinical relevance to the practitioner. As the day-by-day management of patients with epilepsy must go beyond diagnosis and therapy and address the difficulties confronting the epileptic patient in society, the concluding chapters of this volume delineate the latest research on the psychiatric and psychosocial aspects of this complex disorder.

We are grateful to the series editors and to Butterworths for their assistance in the preparation of this volume and for their timely advice. We are also deeply indebted to the international panel of chapter authors, whose expertise and diligence made this book possible.

Roger J. Porter
Paolo L. Morselli

Contributors

Jean Aicardi, MD
INSERM U12, Hôpital des Enfants-Malades, Paris, France

Jean Bancaud, DrM
Directeur de Recherche INSERM; Directeur U97 INSERM, Service de Neurochirurgie, Hôpital Ste. Anne, Paris, France

Leslie D. Cahan, MD
Assistant Professor, Division of Neurosurgery, UCLA School of Medicine, Los Angeles, California, USA

Paul H. Crandall, MD
Professor of Surgery and Neurology, UCLA School of Medicine, Los Angeles, California, USA

Dudley S. Dinner, MD
Section of Epilepsy and Clinical Neurophysiology, Department of Neurology, Cleveland Clinic Foundation, Cleveland, Ohio, USA

Fritz E. Dreifuss, MB, FRCP, FRACP
Professor of Neurology, School of Medicine, University of Virginia, Charlottesville, Virginia, USA

Jerome Engel, Jr, MD, PhD
Professor of Neurology and Anatomy, Reed Neurological Research Center, Laboratory of Nuclear Medicine and Brain Research Institute, UCLA School of Medicine, Los Angeles, California, USA

Ruggero G. Fariello, MD
Professor of Neurology and Pharmacology; Vice Chairman, Department of Neurology, Jefferson Medical College, Philadelphia; Chief of Neurology, Veterans Administration Medical Center, Coatesville, Pennsylvania, USA

Eli S. Goldensohn, MD
Professor, Department of Neurology, Albert Einstein College of Medicine, Bronx, New York, USA

Kenneth G. Lloyd, PhD
Laboratoires d'Etudes et de Recherche Synthelabo, Paris, France

Contributors

Hans Lüders, MD, PhD
Section of Epilepsy and Clinical Neurophysiology, Department of Neurology, Cleveland Clinic Foundation, Cleveland, Ohio, USA

R. L. Masland, MD
H. Houston Merritt Professor of Neurology, Emeritus, Columbia University, New York, New York, USA

Paolo L. Morselli, MD
Director, Clinical Research, Laboratoires d'Etudes et de Recherche Synthelabo, Paris, France

Claudio Munari, DrM
Chargé de Recherches INSERM, Neurochirurgien, INSERM U97, Service de Neurochirurgie B, Hôpital Ste Anne, Paris, France

Roger J. Porter, MD
Chief, Medical Neurology Branch, National Institute of Neurological and Communicative Disorders and Stroke, National Institutes of Health; Clinical Professor of Neurology, Adjunct Professor of Pharmacology, Uniformed Services University of the Health Sciences; Consultant-Lecturer in Neurology, National Naval Medical Center, Bethesda, Maryland, USA

Rebecca Rausch, PhD
Assistant Professor, Psychiatry and Neurology, Reed Neurological Research Center, UCLA Medical Center, Los Angeles, California, USA

Susumu Sato, MD
Neurologist, Epilepsy Branch, National Institute of Neurological and Communicative Disorders and Stroke, National Institutes of Health, Bethesda, Maryland, USA

Dieter Schmidt, MD
Department of Neurology, Charlottenburg Clinic, Free University of Berlin, Berlin, GFR

Bruce S. Schoenberg, MD, DrPH, FACP
Chief, Neuroepidemiology Branch, Intramural Research Program, National Institutes of Health, Bethesda, Maryland; Clinical Professor of Neurology, Georgetown University School of Medicine, Washington, DC, USA

William Sutherling, MD
Assistant Professor of Neurology, Reed Neurological Research Center, UCLA Medical Center, Los Angeles, California, USA

Michael R. Trimble, MPhil., MRCP, FRCPsych.
Consultant Physician and Senior Lecturer, National Hospital and Institute of Neurology, London, UK

Peter Wolf, MD
Professor, Department of Neurology, Charlottenburg Clinic, Free University of Berlin, Berlin, GFR

Contents

1
Biochemical approaches to seizure mechanisms: the GABA and glutamate systems

Ruggero G. Fariello

INTRODUCTION

Epileptiform phenomena have been ascribed to 'a sudden paroxysmal excessive neuronal discharge' (Jackson, 1890). It seems logical to postulate that such abnormal discharges are generated either by potentiation of excitatory mechanisms or by a failure of intrinsic cerebral inhibitory systems as Gowers (1881) intuitively proposed a century ago. Obviously the two hypothetical mechanisms are not mutually exclusive and may synergistically coexist to produce the abnormalities underlying seizure discharges. Excitation and inhibition in the mammalian brain are mediated by many neurotransmitters (Krnjevič, 1974; Snyder, 1984), but the gamma-aminobutyric acid (GABA) and the glutamate–aspartate systems are the most widely represented transmitters in the neuraxis which are involved in inhibition and excitation respectively; recent biochemical investigations into the basic mechanisms of the epilepsies have been more involved with these systems than with any of the others available for study.

Historically the interest in GABA deficit as a possible pathogenic mechanism of seizures has preceded the speculation that glutamate–aspartate abnormalities might cause epileptiform phenomena. Since the discovery of GABA's depressant action by Hayashi (1959) a plethora of reports have stressed the link between GABA's dysfunction and seizure disorders – particularly as far as experimental models of epilepsy are concerned (Meldrum, 1975, 1978). However, until recently the evidence of GABA involvement in human epilepsies, even though much more impressive than for other neurotransmitters, has been circumstantial at best. The only clinical epileptic condition that has been definitely linked to lack of synaptically available GABA is the syndrome of pyridoxine-dependent seizures in infants (Coursin, 1954; Hunt *et al.*, 1954). More recent data, although controversial, suggests an impairment of GABA-mediated inhibition in some patients with medically untreatable partial complex seizures. In addition, newly aroused interest in excitatory mechanisms of seizures has brought forth the suggestion, in some forms of primary generalized corticoreticular epilepsy, that the dicarboxylic-amino acid excitation may be a contributing factor in the appearance of the electroclinical abnormalities.

In view of the importance of the GABA and glutamate systems in the biochemical aspects of the epileptic seizure, this chapter will review the essential data linking the alteration of each of these systems to seizures and will also discuss the rationale for developing compounds that exert antiepileptic action through interference with these two neurotransmitters.

GAMMA-AMINOBUTYRIC ACID

GABA function in the mammalian brain

The actions of GABA in the central nervous system of the mammalian brain are complicated and only partly understood. After release into the synaptic cleft, GABA binds to a complex membrane structure which is known as the GABA receptor site (*Figure 1.1*).

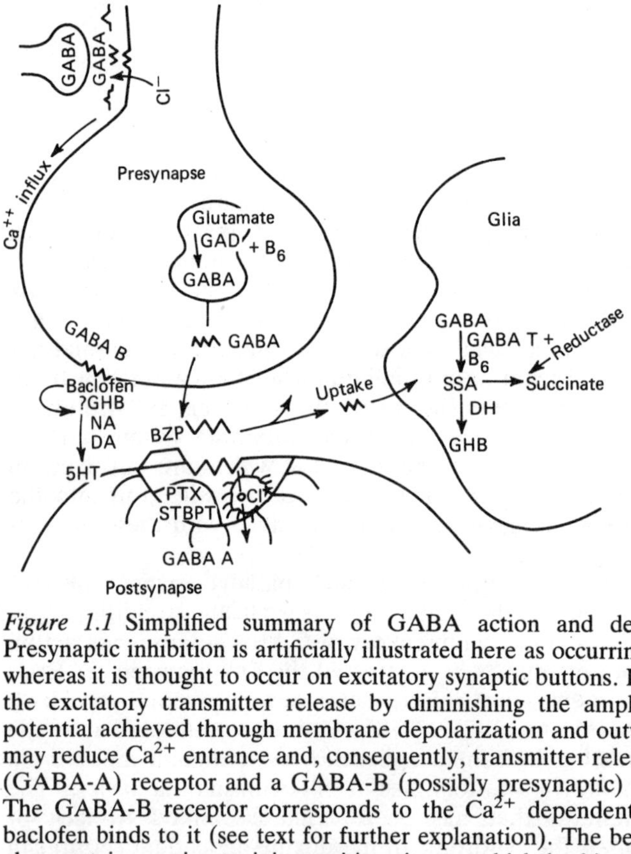

Figure 1.1 Simplified summary of GABA action and destiny at the synaptic cleft. Presynaptic inhibition is artificially illustrated here as occurring on a GABAergic terminal, whereas it is thought to occur on excitatory synaptic buttons. Presynaptic inhibition reduces the excitatory transmitter release by diminishing the amplitude of the arriving action potential achieved through membrane depolarization and outward movement of Cl−. This may reduce Ca^{2+} entrance and, consequently, transmitter release. A benzodiazepine-linked (GABA-A) receptor and a GABA-B (possibly presynaptic) receptor are illustrated here. The GABA-B receptor corresponds to the Ca^{2+} dependent, bicuculline-insensitive site: baclofen binds to it (see text for further explanation). The benzodiazepine-linked receptor also contains a picrotoxinin-sensitive site on which barbiturates are thought to act. The benzodiazepine site, the picrotoxinin site, and the GABA recognition sites all interact to control the permeability of the Cl-ionophore. The metabolism of GABA has been illustrated only within a glial cell for illustrative purposes, but it is known to occur also in neurons. BZP: benzodiazepine; DA: dopamine; DH: dehydrogenase; 5HT: serotonin; GABA-T: GABA transaminase; GAD: glutamic acid decarboxylase; GHB: γ-hydroxybutyrate; NA: norepinephrine; PTX: picrotoxinin; SSA: succinic semialdehyde; STBPT; [35S] *t*-butylbicyclophosphorothionate

The end point of GABA action consists in increasing membrane conductance to chloride ions (Cl^-). Cl^- will flow through the membrane in a direction determined mostly by gradient concentration and electrostatic forces. Negatively charged Cl^- will change the membrane state of polarization – hyperpolarizing it when moving inward, depolarizing it when moving outward. The electrophysiological effects of GABA at the synaptic level have been described in detail. Activation of the benzodiazepine (BZP) linked receptor results in a postsynaptic inhibitory potential (IPSP) associated with membrane hyperpolarization. Depolarization of the membrane has been noticed in the terminals of the primary sensory afferent fibers (Feltz and Rasminsky, 1974), in the olfactory bulb (Brown and Galvan, 1979), in autonomic ganglia (Bowery and Brown, 1979; Brown and Constanti, 1978) as well as in the dendritic receptors in the paleocortex (Algers and Nicoll, 1982). In other instances GABA may activate a separate receptor (GABA-B, Bowery *et al.*, 1980) unrelated to the Cl^- ionophore. Evidence is now accumulating suggesting that the stimulation of this receptor in the CNS activates K^+ conductance in the CNS (Newberry and Nicoll, 1984) whereas in the periphery it blocks the inward Ca^{2+} current that activates the K^+ conductance (Cherubini and North, 1984).

It has become evident that a multiplicity of GABA receptors exist within the nervous system. In a simplified way GABA receptors can be characterized anatomically according to their location, and biochemically according to their affinity for various ligands, their binding characteristic and the complexity of their structural apparatus (Enna and Gallagher, 1983; Snyder, 1984).

Anatomically several sites of receptor location can be identified. Thus we have presynaptic, postsynaptic, somatic, dendritic and possibly axonal (Arenson and Nistri, 1983) receptors.

Pharmacobiochemically we recognize a benzodiazepine-linked low affinity sodium-dependent receptor, a high affinity sodium-independent and a calcium-dependent baclofen sensitive (GABA-B) receptor. The development of various agonists and antagonists to GABA receptors is an important step for their characterization into various subtypes since it may allow the identification of a subpopulation of receptors involved in the epileptogenic process, thus promoting the development of highly selective and targeted agents which would leave unaffected other components of the GABA systems.

It must be emphasized that *in vivo* GABA synapses are part of neuronal chains in which activation of the GABA link might result in excitation (through a disinhibition mechanism) of the terminal chain output. However, 2-deoxyglucose (2DG) studies have demonstrated that systemic administration of GABA agonists results in rather uniform depression of all cerebral structures (Kelly and McCullouch, 1982a and b; Palacios *et al.*, 1982), suggesting (but not proving) that their predominant and global effect in the mammalian cerebrum is in fact inhibitory. Such metabolic depression was seen even when administration of GABA agonists had induced EEG epileptic discharges that could have been explained by a disinhibition mechanism (Fariello *et al.*, 1984).

In conclusion, GABA function in the brain is predominantly inhibitory, but both hyperpolarization and depolarization have been described. GABA's action is mediated by activation of several types of receptors, each one of them having specific pharmacobiochemical characteristics. Most of the data on receptor pharmacology comes from *in vitro* studies and may not reflect the *in vivo* situation, so caution must be exercised when laboratory data is extrapolated for clinical use. It is believed that the low affinity benzodiazepine-linked receptor is physiologically active *in vivo*. Metabolic studies with 2DG indicate that disinhibition probably does not occur after systemic administration of GABA agonists.

Evidence linking GABA function to seizures

Indirect evidence

EXPERIMENTAL DATA

Most of the indirect evidence supporting a relationship between GABA dysfunction and seizures is based on experiments showing that reduction of synaptically available GABA or prevention of its physiological ligation to the receptor site are effective means of inducing epileptic phenomena. Such evidence has been the object of several reviews in the past years (Krnjevič, 1983; Maynert, Marczynski and Browning, 1975; Meldrum, 1975, 1978; Snead, 1983; Tower, 1976) and will not be given further emphasis in this chapter. Studies in the late 1970s, taking advantage of recent refinements in biochemical analytical techniques, have demonstrated that the decrease or increase of GABA which are associated with seizure-like events, or conversely with anticonvulsant properties, are not a generalized metabolic phenomenon but occur in the synaptosomal fraction of the neuronal elements (Geddes and Wood, 1984; Iadarola and Gale, 1979, 1981). Since the synaptosomal fraction is likely to be a measure of synaptically available transmitter this data adds further weight to the hypothesis of a link between GABA changes and seizure susceptibility.

Perturbation of any one of the three major components of the GABA receptor complex results in changes of seizure susceptibility. Convulsant and anticonvulsant barbiturates and picrotoxin interact with the *t*-butylbicyclophosphorothionate (TBPT) sensitive site (*Figure 1.1*); convulsant and anticonvulsant benzodiazepine with the GABA modulin component; bicuculline, 3APS, muscimol, progabide and THIP with the GABA recognition site.

GABA-AGONISTIC PROPERTIES OF ANTICONVULSANTS

Another line of indirect evidence comes from studies that have shown that most of the currently used anticonvulsants share, as a common pharmacological property, some GABAmimetic effects (Barker and Ransom, 1978; Deisz and Lux, 1977; Geller, Taylor and Hoffer, 1978; Hayashi and Negishi, 1979; Macdonald and Bergey, 1979; Möhler and Okada, 1977; Nicoll *et al.*, 1975; Simmonds, 1981; Tallman *et al.*, 1980; Ticku and Davis, 1981; Ticku and Olsen, 1978). For most anticonvulsants it has not been demonstrated that such GABAmimetic properties are essential or even relevant to their anticonvulsant effect. However, recent studies *in vitro* demonstrate the existence of GABA-potentiating effects at concentrations similar to that exerting therapeutic effects in the clinical condition (Macdonald and McLean, 1984). Thus, GABA-agonism is a common denominator of most clinically useful anticonvulsants.

IMPLICATION OF GABA DYSFUNCTION IN SEVERAL (IF NOT ALL) THE STEPS OF EPILEPTOGENESIS

The clinical seizure is often the result of an ingravescent progression of epileptiform abnormalities which start from changes in neuronal membrane properties (Prince and Schwartzkroin, 1978; Schwartzkroin and Wyler, 1980), then include abnormality in synaptic transmission (Ayala *et al.*, 1973, Schwartzkroin and Prince, 1980), altered interaggregate influences and eventually culminate in the recruitment of normal neurons (at time of the entire cerebrum) into the epileptic discharge. Local or systemic administration of GABA agonists may suppress epileptic spikes (Fariello, 1979; Lloyd *et al.*, 1983), may suppress recruiting afterdischarges (ADs) following the spike (that is, the possible seizure initiating event (Fariello *et al.*, 1984), may stop ADs (Krnjevič, Reiffenstein and Silver, 1970), may suppress intrinsic excitatory mechanisms (McNamara, *et al.*, 1984) and may prevent status epilepticus (Ben Ari *et al.*, 1979; Fariello, Golden and Pisa, 1982). GABA agonists can also prevent status epilepticus even in cases where the seizures are induced by agents not acting through the GABA system (Ben Ari *et al.*, 1979a and b; Fariello, Golden and Pisa, 1983; Fariello *et al.*, 1984).

In conclusion, the initial suggestion of a correlation between changes in brain GABA content and seizure susceptibility has been corroborated by the demonstration that such changes occurred in the neuronal region where the machinery for neurotransmission is located. Furthermore, several levels of epileptogenicity are amenable to correction through reinforcement of the GABA system. Altogether the data on GABA changes in relation to seizure susceptibility are rather uniform, and provide strong, although indirect, evidence of a link between the two phenomena.

More direct evidence

Early studies provided conflicting reports on changes in GABA levels during convulsions (Kamrin and Kamrin 1961; Stone, Tews and Mitchell, 1960; Sytinsky and Thinh, 1964), probably due to variable assay sensitivity and difference in time elapsed between tissue removal and analysis. In a systematic longitudinal analysis of amino acid abnormalities in cobalt-induced seizures in the cat's cortex, Koyama (1972) reported on initial increase in glutamate and a decrease in GABA levels which was maximal at the period of behavioral convulsion and tended to return towards baseline values in the weeks following the postconvulsive period when only EEG spikes were evident. The decrease in GABA was not limited to the area of application of cobalt but was detected throughout the brain.

Those initial studies provided the impulse for more sophisticated neurochemical analysis of epileptic tissue. The most extensively investigated experimental model of partial seizures has been cobalt-induced epilepsy. Substantial evidence has been accumulated demonstrating that the GABA system is significantly and, at times, selectively compromised in this model (Craig and Hartman, 1973; Dodd and Bradford, 1976, Dodd *et al.*, 1980). Unfortunately, in several studies (Emson and Joseph, 1975; Ross and Craig, 1981a and b) electrographic or even behavioral data on the presence of seizures were not assessed or at least not reported. Also, with few exceptions (Koyama, 1972; Mutani *et al.*, 1977) the fact that cobalt epilepsy is shortlived has not been exploited to investigate whether the changes in GABA,

GAD and GABA-transaminase (GABA-T) persist or recover after disappearance of the epileptic phenomena, nor has a systematic comparison of the biochemical effect of cobalt in those animals which did not develop epilepsy been performed. In absence of such data a reasonable doubt must persist about the pathogenic importance of GABA variations in this model.

More recently an elegant confirmation of the deficiency of the GABA system in partial seizure was provided in the alumina-cream model in primates (Bakay and Harris, 1981). The changes reported were analogous to the ones found in the cobalt-treated rats. Furthermore, an immunocytochemical study provided morphological demonstration of a selective depletion of GAD-containing buttons in those areas where the EEG epileptic activity was confined (Ribak *et al.*, 1979).

In conclusion, in at least two chronic models of partial epilepsy there is sound evidence of an impairment of the GABA system. The confirmation of similar neurochemical abnormalities in the alumina-cream model and their matching with morphological alterations lends credibility to the data derived from studies of cobalt epilepsy and indicate that GABA impairment may be a widespread phenomenon associated with focal epileptogenesis.

Human epilepsies

Anecdotal reports (Tower, 1960, 1976) described the dramatic response of a few patients to GABA treatment, but this is exceptional. Also, administration of amino-oxyacetic acid (AOAA), which at a certain dose may act as indirect GABA agonist, improved seizure control in nine out of 23 children treated for a 3–6 month period (Tibble and McGreal, 1963).

Recent neurochemical studies by Lloyd *et al.* (1983, 1984) performed on cerebral tissue surgically removed from epileptic patients undergoing stereotaxic implantation of electrodes and surgical ablation, found that the epileptic zone (Lloyd *et al.*, 1983) shows decreased GAD and GABA receptors with normal GABA-T activity in about 50% of patients when compared to the non-epileptic tissue removed from the same group of patients. These data have not been confirmed by Sherwin (1984) and Sherwin and Van Gelder (1984) who have analyzed tissue from *en bloc* resection of the temporal lobes, and compared the spiking versus the non-spiking areas.

Summary of the evidence linking GABA to seizures

Altogether several studies in both experimental models and human epilepsies indicate that an impaired GABA-mediated function is found selectively in some epilepsy-prone areas. Partial seizures with or without secondary generalization are the commonest but certainly not the only form of human epilepsy. In several other conditions such as primary generalized tonic-clonic epilepsy, myoclonic syndromes, tonic seizures, photosensitive epilepsy, the Lennox–Gastaut syndromes and corticoreticular epilepsy of petit mal type, data on a specific deficit of GABA is lacking. Actually in corticoreticular epilepsy all the information from experimental animal studies has consistently demonstrated that administration of GABA agonists enhances the electroclinical phenomena (Fariello, Golden and Black, 1981; Gloor, Pellegrini and Kostopoulos, 1979; King, 1979; Myslobodsky, Ackerman and Engel, 1979; Pedley, Horton and Meldrum, 1979). Moreover, some direct GABA agonists such as THIP and muscimol can induce spike and wave discharges in naive animals (Fariello and Golden, 1984). Thus, considering all the clinical and experimenal data, the best direct evidence pointing to a GABA deficiency as a pathogenic factor in epilepsy is available for animal models and possibly for some cases of human partial seizures. However, this finding is not universal, stressing the fact that different biochemical defects may underlie epileptic conditions. Strong indirect evidence suggests a link between GABA and seizure susceptibility in general. The exact role of GABA in many other clinical epilepsies is uncertain. Based on experimental data, GABA hyperfunction may actually be a pathogenic and/or seizure-triggering component in some forms of corticoreticular epilepsy.

How can GABA agonists correct epileptiform abnormalities?

Administration of compounds that strengthen GABA function in the CNS may ameliorate epilepsy through four mechanisms of action.

(1) Replenishment function

This can be expected to occur in those cases in which a specific depletion of GABA pools exists. In those instances GABAmimetics will act similarly to L-dopa (the dopamine precursor) in Parkinson's disease. In such a case the correction of the biochemical defect is expected to be accompanied by resolution of clinical symptoms as well as of the underlying electrophysiological abnormalities.

(2) A non-specific depressant effect

Most mammalian neurons are inhibited by GABA and related compounds. It is uncertain if epileptic neurons that are generating paroxysmal depolarizing shifts (PDSs) maintain their sensitivity to the action of neurotransmitters. Experimental data suggests that systemic administration of GABA agonists can suppress the activity of spike generating neurons (Fariello, 1979; Fariello and Lalley, 1981; Krnjevič, Reiffenstein and Silver, 1970) whereas iontophoretic application of inhibitory substances fails to modify their firing pattern (Macon and King, 1979; Puil, Reiffenstein and Triggle, 1974). Whether clinically active or inactive on epileptic neurons, GABAmimetics may prevent the recruitment of non-epileptic aggregates into the epileptic discharge during the spread of seizures, thus exerting another important therapeutic effect.

(3) Activation of intrinsic inhibitory structures

The substantia nigra (SN) is an area of intense GABAergic activity (Gale and Casu, 1981). A descending GABAergic nigrostriatal pathway feeds back into the pars reticularis of the substantia nigra (Kim *et al.*, 1971). Lesions in the substantia nigra are associated with increased metrazol threshold (Fariello and Hornykiewicz, 1979) and pharmacological bilateral inactivation of the substantia nigra by injection of muscimol prevents various types of seizures (Gale, 1984; McNamara *et al.*, 1984). GABA agonists may therefore suppress this powerful seizure facilitating system.

The cerebellar output is essentially GABAergic. In certain experimental conditions activation of cerebellar hemispheric output has been associated with suppression of neocortical and limbic seizure discharges (Babb, Mitchell and Crandall, 1974; Mutani, Bergamini and Doriguzzi, 1969). It could be speculated that GABAmimetic activity can also enhance this intrinsic inhibitory mechanism to suppress seizures in specific foci.

(4) Glutamate–aspartate (GLUT–ASP) antagonism

As it will be discussed in further detail in the following paragraphs, glutamate–aspartate may contribute to the onset and dissemination of epileptic activity. At the neuronal level glut–asp excitation are easily blocked by iontophoretic release of GABA. Independently from a possible pathogenic role of GLUT–ASP in epileptogenesis, such GABA action may counteract the dicarboxylic acid induced excitation and thus reduce the spread of excitatory phenomena.

The combination of the above mechanisms of action offer a powerful multifaceted strategy for the treatment of a wide variety of seizure disorders.

Available strategies for GABA therapy

Prodrug

A prodrug is a component that must be used to bypass a step that would prevent the therapeutic action of the intended drug. The prodrug would then turn into the active compound. In the case of GABA one of the greatest hampering factors is its impermeability through the blood–brain barrier (BBB). To achieve the desired effect a GABA prodrug must also bypass the glutamate step, since glutamate excess has been implicated in the pathogenesis of some form of epilepsies (see paragraph below). The only GABA prodrug presently available is progabide, which meets both the above criteria.

GABA metabolism inhibitors

When a sufficient amount of GABA is available for neurotransmission its action can be enhanced by blocking the inactivating mechanism in the synapse (uptake and/or metabolism, *see Figure 1.1*). Valproic acid is a widely used anticonvulsant believed to fall into this category.

A particular category of drugs has been recently discovered. These are the suicidal substrates. Such substrates activate the specific enzymatic system responsible for their destruction (for detailed review of this subject *see* Metcalf, 1979; Palfreyman *et al.*, 1981). Suicidal substrates of GABA-T are gamma-vinyl GABA and gamma-acetylenic GABA. The former is being studied as a potential anticonvulsant.

Direct GABA receptor agonists

Compounds that bind with high affinity to the GABA-A receptor and activate the chloride channel exert the same inhibitory action of GABA. Their potency would also depend on the presence of specific uptake and/or catabolizing mechanisms which will terminate their action. In such a category, Progabide and THIP are under active clinical experimentation.

Drugs that interact with the other components of the GABA receptor complex

Barbiturates seem to interact with the picrotoxin and TBTP-sensitive site to facilitate the effect of GABA. The recent development of more precise pharmacological characterization of this allosteric component of the GABA receptor complex (Ticku, and Maksay, 1983; Ramanjaneyulu and Ticku, 1984) may allow the development of new compounds of potential clinical usefulness. Benzodiazepines (BZP) act at the BZP component of the GABA receptor complex to facilitate the action of GABA. Triazolo-benzodiazepines have shown a very interesting anticonvulsant spectrum in animals and they may be developed for clinical use in the future. However, presently clonazepam and nitrazepam are the only benzodiazepines clinically used for chronic treatments.

Caveats

Several areas deserve careful evaluation when chronic treatment with GABA agonists is used. Some negative factors influencing clinical responses in long-term care may be anticipated on the basis of similarity with L-dopa treatment in Parkinson's disease. As it happens for the majority of Parkinsonians, after a few years of treatment a loss of efficacy might also occur in epileptics. This could be related to the development of desensitization of the receptor system after prolonged pharmacological stimulation. However, Ticku, Fariello and Golden (1983) in a pilot study have observed only variable and minimal changes in the number of receptors after chronic treatment with various GABA agonists in rats. Furthermore, at variance with the Parkinson's disease situation, in most epileptic conditions there is no evidence of any underlying progressive degenerative process which may play an important role in the decay of treatment efficacy.

Another area of concern for several direct and indirect GABA agonists is their capability of inducing in many species frank epileptiform abnormalities: gamma-vinyl GABA, beta-hydroxybutyrate, muscimol, and THIP may elicit bilaterally synchronous spike and wave discharges and at higher doses burst-suppression on the EEG. Fariello and Ticku (1983) have speculated on the possible mechanisms for this paradoxical effect but the reason remains unknown. It is known that proconvulsant effects of benzodiazepines have been occasionally observed upon acute administration (Prior *et al.*, 1972; Tassinari *et al.*, 1972), particularly in cases of secondary generalized epilepsy with bilaterally synchronous spike and wave discharges. It may therefore be expected that at least in an occasional patient a worsening of the epileptic condition might occur after administration of GABA agonists.

Finally, attention should be paid to the broad spectrum of possible side-effects deriving from the indiscriminate activation of all GABA systems in both the central and autonomic nervous system. Motor, sensory, psychic, higher intellectual, autonomic, and endocrine functions as well as the sleep–awake pattern can be all directly or indirectly regulated and/or influenced by the level of GABAergic activity. The possibility of side-effects on all those activities should be carefully monitored in the years to come. On the other hand, the present available evidence based on the clinical experiment of Progabide, the GABA agonist with the longest, although still short, history of clinical investigation, has not revealed major drawbacks related to the above expressed concerns, casting some doubt on their clinical relevance.

GLUTAMATE–ASPARTATE

The importance of glutamate in cerebral metabolism was pointed out as early as 1932 by Quastel and Wheatley, and its involvement in the mechanism of cerebral excitability suggested by Hayashi (1954). Phillis and Ochs (1971), while studying the mechanisms of spreading depression, speculated that excessive glutamate release may provide a substrate for seizure activity. On the other hand, glutamate and glutamine had been used earlier for treatment of corticoreticular epilepsy and partial complex seizure (Price, Waelsch and Putman, 1943).

Whereas there is little doubt that glutamate is an excitatory neurotransmitter, nevertheless detailed characterization of its neurotransmitter function is complicated by the following factors:

(1) Glutamate plays a general role in cerebral metabolism and it is a constituent of all cells. Glucose and acetate are general precursors of glutamate but the administration of those two compounds yield variable amounts of glutamate (Fonnum, 1984). Glutamate metabolism is compartmentalized in a large neuronal pool, but also in a small glial pool where glutamate is derived via glutamine from glutamine synthetase. The overwhelming majority of glutamate is contained in the large neuronal pool (Cremer *et al.*, 1975) which, however, has to be further subdivided to account for the various functions and turnover rates of glutamate. Lesion studies suggest that the transmitter pool represents only 20–40% of the total endogenous glutamate content.
(2) The strict metabolic relationship between glutamate, aspartate, GABA and taurine (TAU) further confuses the issue of an appropriate interpretation of glutamate variations in relation to the state of excitability of the cerebral grey matter. This intertwined relationship renders many speculative hypotheses on the role of these compounds in epileptogenesis possible and plausible (Van Gelder, 1981).
(3) The characterization of the glutamate receptor system is also not as well defined as for the GABA system. Three types of receptors are currently

recognized: N methyl-d-aspartate (NMDA), the quisqualate and the kainate receptors. In general, the agonists show poor correlation between their affinity to the receptor and their pharmacological activity and there is a need for a clearer differentiation between glutamate and aspartate at the receptor level (*see* Fonnum, 1984).

(4) The best available knowledge of glutamate mode of action at the synaptic cleft derives from studies on the spinal cord (Puil, 1981, 1983). Thus, many assumptions on glutamate action must be extrapolated from spinal cord to cerebral neurons.

In conclusion, the poor differentiation between metabolic and transmitter glutamate pool, between aspartate and glutamate as transmitters and between quisqualate, kainate and NMDA receptors, and the intertwined relationships among glutamate, aspartate, GABA and taurine dim the attempt to make solid correlations between changes in glutamate and seizure discharges.

Physiological action of glutamate–aspartate

Iontophoretic application of glutamate to most neurons within the neuraxis elicits crisp, fast onset excitation which terminates briskly upon shutting off the releasing current. The cessation of the excitation is not dependent upon either the length or

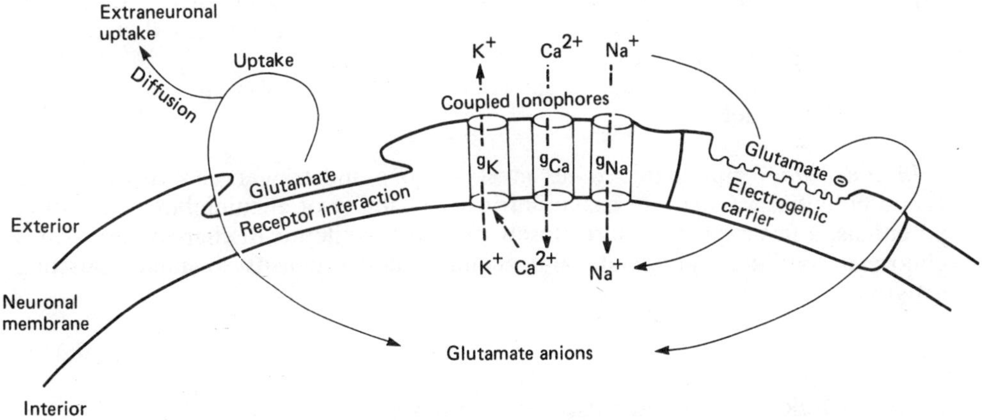

Figure 1.2 Schematic representation of glutamate action at the postsynaptic site. The binding of glutamate to the receptor sites increases membrane conductance to Na^+ and possibly Ca^{2+}. These changes provide the substrate for the excitation resulting in the action potential. Ca^{2+} entry into the cell triggers an increase in membrane K^+ conductance with extrusion of K^+. This cellular loss of positive ions underlies the membrane hyperpolarization that follows the action potential and limits the chances of bursting activity. The action of glutamate is terminated by diffusion (passively) and by extraneural, probably glial, uptake (actively). (From E. Puil, unpublished, with author's permission)

intensity of glutamate release. Repetitive applications of glutamate, but not aspartate, may induce desensitization (Dostrovsky and Pomeranz, 1977). Iontophoretic application of glutamate, though, does not induce bursting activity which instead has been observed after release of aspartate to cortical neurons (Herring, Morris and Salt, 1983). For detailed reviews of all these features see Puil (1981, 1983). The mechanisms whereby glutamate excites neuronal membrane have been elucidated in recent years. The ligation of glutamate to the receptor results in a change of the membrane conductance, particularly for Na^+ and probably Ca^{2+} (*Figure 1.2*). The Na^+-induced depolarization is followed by an afterhyperpolarization (AHP) which is believed to be due to an increase in K^+ conductance triggered by the entrance of Ca^{2+} concomitant to Na^+ channel activation. The cellular extrusion of K^+ is probably the most important physiological mechanism that limits the depolarizing phenomena and prevents repetitive firing which is an important substrate of epileptogenesis. The action of glutamate is terminated by diffusion and/or by an active uptake system, probably glial (*see Figure 1.2*). From the above it appears that in physiological conditions glutamate cannot elicit bursts of action potentials in neurons and consequently does not predispose to seizure discharges. This, however, contrasts with the observation that topical, intraventricular or systemic injection of glutamate and its analogs produce electrographic and behavioral seizures (Hayashi, 1959; Johnston, 1972). It seems therefore that there may exist certain conditions which are favorable to the generation of glutamate-induced burst discharges. These conditions include (Puil, 1984):

(1) reduction of the hyperpolarizing increase in K^+ conductance (gK)
(2) decrease in synaptic inhibition, particularly the GABA-mediated increase in Cl^- conductance;
(3) metabolic derangements such as extracellular accumulation of K^+, decreased activity of the sodium–potassium (Na–K) pump and decreased uptake of excitatory transmitters;
(4) change in membrane properties, increased inward Ca^{2+} currents, and blockade of Na^+ channels.

In conclusion, glutamate excites most neurons and triggers a series of single action potentials. Aspartate has an intrinsic capability of eliciting bursts of action potentials, a firing pattern more closely related to epileptic discharges. In various abnormal conditions glutamate also acquires the propensity to induce bursting activity.

Evidence linking glutamate–aspartate to seizures

Indirect evidence

SYSTEMIC OR TOPICAL APPLICATIONS

Systemic or topical application of glutamate–aspartate produces convulsions in animals (Johnston, 1972). Kainic acid, which is supposed to act through stimulation of the receptors for the excitatory amino acids, is a powerful tool to induce prolonged status epilepticus in various animal species (Ben Ari *et al.*, 1979).

VALPROIC ACID AND RELATED ANTICONVULSANTS
Valproic acid and related anticonvulsant compounds inhibit glutamate–aspartate release. Such inhibition is proportional to their anticonvulsant efficacy (Chapman, Meldrum and Mendes, 1983). A new series of mixed glutamate–aspartate antagonists administered by superfusion are capable of preventing or temporarily suppressing clinical seizures induced by cobalt application to the rat cortex (Coutinho-Netto *et al.*, 1981); some of these glutamate antagonists exert an anticonvulsant effect against a genetic model of murine epilepsy (Croucher, Collins and Meldrum, 1982). On the other hand, glutamate administration does not aggravate clinical epilepsy. Actually, Price, Waelsch and Putman (1943) reported improvement in five out of eight seizure patients, with the best responses observed in cases of possible corticoreticular epilepsy of the petit mal type. Thus, the data on anticonvulsant effects of glutamate antagonist appear to be counterbalanced by some therapeutic effects observed after glutamate administration. Neither set of data is extensive or convincing.

More direct evidence

In the cobalt model of partial seizures, excessive release of glutamate has been observed in parallel to the evolution of clinical partial simplex seizures as judged by behavioral observation (Dodd and Bradford, 1976; Dodd *et al.*, 1980; Koyama, 1972). Craig and Hartman (1973) found marked decrease of glutamate–aspartate and taurine in cobalt-treated rats. No mention was made in this study of the presence or absence of seizures in rats. In the feline model of corticoreticular epilepsy induced by large parenteral injections of penicillin, Van Gelder *et al.* (1983) found a decrease of tissue content of glutamate in the pre-epileptic period when augmented evoked potentials suggested increased neuronal excitability. Such disappearance of glutamate (and to a lesser extent of aspartate) from cerebral tissue was interpreted as indicating excessive release of transmitter. Although this is an acceptable and appealing hypothesis, other explanations are possible. The content of cerebrospinal fluid and/or extracellular glutamate were not assessed and, therefore, the validity of this hypothesis could not be confirmed.

Human studies

Glutamate levels in cerebral tissue from surgically removed human epileptogenic foci were found decreased by Van Gelder, Sherwin and Rasmussen (1972) but not by Perry *et al.* (1975). Sherwin and Van Gelder (1984) found a highly significant 16% increase of glutamic acid dehyrogenase (GDH) activity but no changes in glutamine synthetase (GS) in the spiking cortex of a group of 51 patients undergoing surgery for their epileptic disorder. Glutamine synthetase was elevated in a small subpopulation of patients with severe astrogliosis, thus confirming the value of glutamine synthetase as an enzymatic marker of glial metabolism (Sherwin, Robitaille and Olivier, 1982). On the basis of their data and of the excess of glutamate efflux found in experimental foci, Sherwin and Van Gelder (1984) suggest an imbalance of the various compartments of glutamate metabolism in the epilepsies. They recognize that it is impossible, in the light of the present knowledge, to decide if this is a cause or an effect of the epileptic activity.

Other human studies are even more difficult to interpret since they are concerned with measurements of glutamate in various body fluids. Mutani *et al.* (1974) found severely lowered glutamate in the cerebrospinal fluid of ten epileptic patients in contrast to increased glutamate values found by Logothetis and Bovis (1962) and Plum (1974). Janjua, Metrakos and Van Gelder (1982) suggest that increased plasma glutamate levels are associated with the genetic factors responsible for the expressivity of the corticoreticular epilepsy of petit mal type. Several of these studies suffer from lack of patient population definition, or adequately matched controls, and altogether they are belittled by the poor understanding of the relationship between glutamate concentration in body fluids and its neuro-transmitter function within the CNS. Further studies in this regard should address the issues of type of seizures, presence and type of antiepileptic medications, dietary influences, possible craniocaudal gradient for glutamate and, in particular should elucidate the relevance of the findings to the synaptically available glutamate.

Conclusions

The most appealing speculation on the relationship between glutamate–aspartate and seizures is the one about the possible correlations between an hyperfunctioning glutamate system and corticoreticular epilepsy of petit mal type. This was observed in both experimental models (Van Gelder *et al.*, 1983) and clinical conditions (Janjua, Metrakos and Van Gelder, 1983) but further evidence is needed to consolidate this speculation. A clever explanation for the combined changes in taurine, glutamate, glutamine and aspartate found in studies of epileptic tissues and body fluids has been proposed by Van Gelder (1978, 1981); the epileptic cortex would release excessive glutamate and taurine with extracellular accumulation of the two amino acids due to saturation of the mechanisms for transport and glutamine synthesis. As appealing as it appears the available evidence is too conflicting to offer solid support to this hypothesis, which must await further studies for confirmation. In light of the present knowledge it seems premature to predict if compounds interfering with the glutamate–aspartate system may have any specific utilization in the treatment of epilepsy, except for a general regulation of the cerebral excitability threshold. Also, an improvement of the deranged metabolism of several amino acids in the brain, which is seen in association with several epileptic conditions, may result from glutamate administration. It is presently unknown and unpredictable whether or not this will result in any beneficial effect clinically.

References

ALGERS, B. E. and NICOLL, R. A. (1982) Pharmacological evidence for two kinds of GABA receptors on rat hippocampal pyramidal cell studies *in vitro*. *Journal of Physiology,* **328,** 125–141

ARENSON, M. S. and NISTRI, A. (1983) The inhibitory amino acid GABA hyperpolarizes motor axons: an intracellular study. *Experientia,* **39,** 225–228

AYALA, G. F., DICHTER, M., GUMNIT, R. Y., MATSUMOTO, H. and SPENCER, W. A. (1973) *Brain Research,* **121,** 259–270

BABB, T. L., MITCHELL, A. G. JR and CRANDALL, P. H. (1974) Fastigiobulbar and dentatothalamic influences on hippocampal cobalt epilepsy in the cat. *Electroencephalography and Clinical Neurophysiology,* **36,** 141–154

BAKAY, R. A. E. and HARRIS, A. B. (1981) Neurotransmitters, receptors and biochemical changes in monkey cortical epileptic foci. *Brain Research,* **206,** 387–408

BARKER, J. L. and RANSOM, B. R. (1978) Amino acid pharmacology of mammalian central neurons grown in tissue culture. *Journal of Physiology (London),* **280,** 355–372

BEN ARI, Y., LAGOWSKA, J., TREMBLEY, E. and LE GAL LASALLE, G. (1979a) A new model of focal status epilepticus: intra-amygdaloid application of kainic acid elicits repetitive second generalized convulsive seizures. *Brain Research,* **163,** 176–179

BEN ARI, Y., TREMBLEY, E., OTTERSEN, O. P. and NAQUET, R. (1979b) Evidence suggesting secondary epileptogenic lesions after kainic acid: pretreatment with diazepam reduces distant but not local brain damage. *Brain Research,* **165,** 362–365

BOWERY, N. G. and BROWN, D. A. (1974) Depolarizing action of γ-aminobutyric acid and related compounds on rat superior cervical ganglia *in vitro. British Journal of Pharmacology,* **50,** 205–218

BOWERY, N. G., HILL, D. R., HUDSON, A. L. *et al.* (1980) Baclofen decreases neurotransmitter release in the mammalian CNS by an action at a novel GABA receptor. *Nature (London),* **283,** 92–94

BROWN, D. A. and CONSTANTI, A. (1978) Interaction of pentobarbitone and γ-aminobutyric acid on mammalian sympathetic ganglia cells. *British Journal of Pharmacology,* **63,** 217–224.

BROWN, D. A. and GALVAN, M. (1979) Responses of the guinea pig isolated olfactory cortex slice to γ-aminobutyric acid recorded with extracerebellar electrodes. *British Journal of Pharmacology,* **65,** 247–353

CHAPMAN, A., MELDRUM, B. S. and MENDES, E. (1983) Acute anticonvulsant activity of structural and analogs of valproic acid and changes in brain GABA and aspartate content. *Life Sciences,* **32,** 2023–2031

CHERUBINI, E. and NORTH, R. A. (1984) Inhibtion of calcium spikes and transmitter release by γ-aminobutyric acid in the guinea pig myoenteric plexus. *British Journal of Pharmacology*, **82,** 101–105

COURSIN, D. B. (1954) Convulsive seizure in infants with pyridoxine deficient diet. *Journal of the American Medical Association,* **154,** 406–408

COUTINHO-NETTO, J., ABDUL-GHANI, A. S., COLLINS, J. F. and BRADFORD, H. F. (1981) Is glutamate a trigger factor in epileptic hyperactivity? *Epilepsia,* **22,** 289–297

CRAIG, C. R. and HARTMAN, E. R. (1973) Concentration of amino acids in the brain of cobalt-epileptic rat. *Epilepsia,* **14,** 409–414

CREMER, J. E., HEATH, D. F., PATEL, A. J., BALAZS, R. and CAVANAUGH, J. B. (1975) An experimental model of CNS changes associated with chronic liver disease: portocaval anastomosis in the rat. In *Metabolic Compartmentation and Neurotransmission: Relation to Brain Structure and Function*, edited by S. Berl, D. D. Clarke and D. Schneider, pp. 461–478. New York: Plenum Press

CROUCHER, M. J., COLLINS, J. F. and MELDRUM, B. S. (1982) Anticonvulsant action of excitatory amino acid antagonists. *Science,* **216,** 899–901

DEISZ, R. A. and LUX, H. D. (1977) Diphenylhydantoin prolongs postsynaptic inhibition and iontophoretic GABA action in the crayfish stretch receptor. *Neuroscience Letters,* **5,** 199–203

DODD, P. R. and BRADFORD, H. F. (1976) Release of amino acids from the maturing cobalt-induced epileptic focus. *Brain Research,* **111,** 377–388

DODD, P. R., BRADFORD, H. F., ABDUL-GHANI, A. S., COX, D. W. G. and COUTINHO-NETTO, J. (1980) Release of amino acids from chronic epileptic and subepileptic foci *in vivo. Brain Research,* **193,** 505–517

DOSTROVSKY, J. O. and POMERANZ, B. (1977) Desensitization of glutamate responses – evidence for glutamate receptors in cat spinal cord. *Neuroscience Letters,* **4,** 315–319

EMSON, P. C. and JOSEPH, M. H. (1975) Neurochemical and morphological changes during the development of cobalt-induced epilepsy in the rat. *Brain Research,* **93,** 91–110

ENNA, S. J. and GALLAGHER, J. P. (1983) Biochemical and electrophysiological characteristics of mammalian GABA receptors. *International Review of Neurobiology,* **24,** 181–212

FARIELLO, R. G. (1979) Action of inhibitory amino acids on acute epileptic foci: an electrographic study. *Experimental Neurology,* **66,** 55–63

FARIELLO, R. G. (1984) The role of GABAergic mechanisms in the epilepsies. In *Advances in Epileptology,* Vol. XV. New York: Raven Press, pp. 17–24

FARIELLO, R. G. and GOLDEN, G. T. (1985) The THIP-induced model of bilateral synchronous spike and wave in rats. (In preparation)

FARIELLO, R. G., GOLDEN, G. T., ALEXANDER, G. W., REYES, P. F. and SCHWARTZMAN, R. J. (1984) Metabolic correlates of GABAmimetic-induced EEG abnormalities. In *Neurotransmitters, Seizures and Epilepsy II*, edited by R. G. Fariello, P. L. Morselli, K. G. LLoyd, L. F. Quesney and J. Engle Jr, New York: Raven Press, pp. 245–252

FARIELLO, R. G., GOLDEN, G. T. and BLACK, J. A. (1981) Activating effects of homotaurine and taurine on cortico-reticular epilepsy. *Epilepsia,* **22,** 217–224

FARIELLO, R. G., GOLDEN, G. T. and PISA, M. (1983) Homotaurine (3-aminopropanesulfonic acid, 3APS) protects from the convulsant and cytotoxic effect of systemically administered kainic acid. *Neurology,* **31,** 241–245

FARIELLO, R. G. and HORNYKIEWICZ, O. (1979) Substantia nigra and metrazol convulsions in rats: correlation with striated dopamine metabolism. *Experimental Neurology,* **65,** 202–208

FARIELLO, R. G. and LALLEY, P. M. (1981) Microelectrode studies of the action of 3APS on spontaneous-glutamate-evoked and epileptiform neuronal activity. *Epilepsia,* **22,** 226

FARIELLO, R. G. and TICKU, M. K. (1983) Minireview: the perspective of GABA replenishment treatment in the epilepsies: a critical evaluation of hopes and concerns. *Life Sciences,* **33,** 1629–1640

FARIELLO, R. G., ZEEMAN, B., GOLDEN, G. T., REYES, P. F. and RAMACCI, T. (1984) Transient seizure activity induced by acetylcarnitine. *Neuropharmacology,* **23,** 585–587

FELTZ, P. and RASMINSKY, M. (1974) A model for the mode of action of GABA on primary afferent terminals: depolarizing effects of GABA applied iontophoretically to neurons of mammalian dorsal root ganglia. *Neuropharmacology,* **13,** 553–563.

FONNUM, F. (1984) Short review. Glutamate: a neurotransmitter in mammalian brain. *Journal of Neurochemistry,* **42,** 1–11

GALE, K. (1984) The role of the substantia nigra in the anticonvulsant actions of GABAergic drugs. In *Neurotransmitters, Seizures and Epilepsy II,* edited by R. G. Fariello, P. L. Morselli, K. G. Lloyd, L. F. Quesney and J. Engel Jr. New York: Raven Press, pp. 57–80

GALE, K. and CASU, M. (1981) Dynamic utilization of GABA in substantia nigra: regulation by dopamine and GABA in the striatum and its clinical and behavioral implications. *Molecular and Cellular Biochemistry,* **39,** 369–409

GEDDES, J. W. and WOOD, J. D. (1984) Changes in the amino acid content of nerve endings (synaptosomes) induced by drugs that alter the metabolism of glutamate and γ-aminobutyric acid. *Journal of Neurochemistry,* **42,** 16–24

GELLER, H. M., TAYLOR, D. A. and HOFFER, B. J. (1978) Benzodiazepines and central inhibitory mechanisms. *Naunyn-Schmiedeberg's Archives of Pharmacology,* **304,** 81–88

GLOOR, P., PELLEGRINI, A. and KOSTOPOULOS, G. K. (1979) Effects of changes in cortical excitability upon the epileptic bursts in generalized penicillin epilepsy of the cat. *Electroencephalography and Clinical Neurophysiology,* **46,** 274–289

GOLDEN, G. T. and FARIELLO, R. G. (1984) The epileptogenic action of some direct GABA agonists. Effects of manipulation of the GABA and glutamate systems. In *Neurotransmitters, Seizures and Epilepsy II,* edited by R. G. Fariello, P. L. Morselli, K. G. Lloyd, L. F. Quesney and J. Engel Jr. New York: Raven Press, pp. 237–244

GOWERS, W. R. (1881) *Epilepsy and Other Chronic Convulsive Diseases: Their Causes, Symptoms and Treatment,* p. 309. London: Churchill

HAYASHI, T. (1954) Effects of sodium glutamate on the nervous system. *Keio Journal of Medicine,* **3,** 183–192

HAYASHI, T. (1959) The inhibitory action of β-hydroxy-γ-aminobutyric acid upon the seizure following stimulation of the motor cortex of the dog. *Journal of Physiology (London),* **145,** 570–578

HAYASHI, T. and NEGISHI, K. (1979) Suppression of retinal spike discharge by dipropylacetate (Depakene): a possible involvement of GABA. *Brain Research,* **175,** 271–278

HERRING, P. L., MORRIS, R. and SALT, T. E. (1983) Effects of excitatory amino acids and their antagonists on membrane and action potentials of cat caudate neurons. *Journal of Physiology,* **339,** 207–222

HUNT, A. D., STOKES, J., MCCRORY, W. W. and STROUD, H. H. (1954) Pyridoxine dependency: report of a case of intractable convulsions in an infant controlled by pyridoxine. *Pediatrics,* **13,** 140–145

IADAROLA, M. J. and GALE, K. (1979) Dissociation between drug-induced increases in nerve terminal and non-nerve terminal pools of GABA *in vivo. European Journal of Pharmacology,* **59,** 125–129

IADAROLA, M. J. and GALE, K. (1981) Cellular compartments of GABA in brain and their relationship to anticonvulsant activity. *Molecular and Cellular Biochemistry,* **30,** 305–330

JACKSON, H. H. (1890) Convulsive seizures. *Lancet,* **1,** 685–688

JANJUA, N. A., METRAKOS, J. D. and VAN GELDER, N. M. (1982) Plasma amino acids in epilepsy. In *Genetic Basis of the Epilepsies,* edited by V. E. Anderson, W. A. Hauser, J. R. Penry and C. F. Sing, pp. 181–197. New York: Raven Press

JOHNSTON, G. A. R. (1972) Convulsions induced in 10-day-old rats by intraperitoneal injection of monosodium glutamate and related excitant amino acids. *Biochemical Pharmacology,* **22,** 137

KAMRIN, R. P. and KAMRIN, A. A. (1961) The effects of pyridoxine antagonists and other convulsive agents on amino acid concentrations of the mouse brain. *Journal of Neurochemistry,* **6,** 219–225

KELLY, P. A. T. and MCCULLOCH, J. (1978) Heterogeneous depression of glucose utilization in the caudate nucleus by GABA agonists. *Brain Research,* **209,** 458-463

KELLY, P. A. T. and MCCULLOUCH, J. (1982a) Effects of putative GABAergic agonists, muscimol and THIP, upon local cerebral glucose metabolism. *Journal of Neurochemistry,* **39,** 613–624

KELLY, P. A. T. and MCCULLOUCH, J. (1982b) The effects of the GABAergic agonist muscimol upon the relationship between local cerebral blood flow by glucose utilization. *Brain Research,* **258,** 338–342

KIM, Y. S., BAK, J. J., HASSLER, R. and OKADA, V. (1971) Role of γ-aminobutyric acid (GABA) in the extrapyramidal motor system – some evidence of existence of a type of GABA rich strio-nigral neurons. *Experimental Brain Research,* **14,** 95–104

KING, G. A. (1979) Effects of systemically applied GABA agonists and antagonists on wave spikes ECoG activity in rat. *Neuropharmacology,* **13,** 47–55

KOYAMA, I. (1972) Amino acids in the cobalt-induced epileptogenic and non-epileptogenic cat's cortex. *Canadian Journal of Physiology and Pharmacology,* **50,** 740–752

KRNJEVIČ, K. (1974) Chemical nature of synaptic transmission in vertebrates. *Physiological Review,* **54,** 418–540

KRNJEVIČ, K. (1983) GABA-mediated inhibitory mechanisms in relation to epileptic discharges. In *Basic Mechanisms of Neuronal Hyperexcitability*

KRNJEVIČ, K., REIFFENSTEIN, R. J. and SILVER, A. (1970) Inhibition and paroxysmal activity in long isolated cortical slabs. *Electroencephalography and Clinical Neurophysiology,* **29,** 283–294

LLOYD, K. G., MUNARI, C., BOSSI, L. and MORSELLI, P. L. (1984) The GABA hypothesis of human epilepsy: neurochemical evidence from surgically resected identified foci. In *Neurotransmitters, Seizures and Epilepsy II*, edited by R. G. Fariello, P. L. Morselli, K. G. Lloyd, L. F. Quesney and J. Engel Jr. New York: Raven Press, pp. 285–294

LLOYD, K. G., MUNARI, C., WORMS, P., BOSSI, L. and MORSELLI, P. L. (1983) Indications for the use of γ-aminobutyric acid (GABA) agonists in convulsant disorders. In *Progress in Clinical and Biological Research. Epilepsy: An Update on Research and Therapy*, edited by G. Nistico, R. Di Perri and H. Meinardi, pp. 285–297. New York: Alan R. Liss, Inc.

LOGOTHETIS, J. and BOVIS, M. (1962) Free amino acid changes in the spinal fluid of patients with central nervous system degeneration and chronic epileptic disorders. *World Neurology,* **6,** 474–483

MACON, J. B. and KING, D. W. (1979) Penicillin iontophoresis and the response of somatosensory cortical neurons to amino acids. *Electroencephalography and Clinical Neurophysiology,* **47,** 52–63

MAYNERT, E. W., MARCZYNSKI, T. J. and BROWNING, R. A. (1975) The role of neurotransmitters in the epilepsies. *Advances of Neurology,* **13,** 79–147

MACDONALD, R. L. and BERGEY, G. K. (1979) Valproic acid augments GABA-mediated postsynaptic inhibition in cultured mammalian neurons. *Brain Research,* **170,** 558–562

MACDONALD, R. L. and MCLEAN, M. J. (1984) Barbiturate and hydantoin actions on vertebrate neurons in cell culture. In *Neurotransmitters, Seizures and Epilepsy II,* edited by R. G. Fariello, P. L. Morselli, K. G. Lloyd, L. F. Quesney and J. Engel Jr. New York: Raven Press, pp. 139–152

MCNAMARA, J. O., RIGSBEE, L. C., GALLOWAY, N. J. and SHIN, C. (1984) Evidence that activation of substantia nigra is necessary for limbic seizures. In *Neurotransmitters, Seizures and Epilepsy II,* edited by R. G. Fariello, P. L. Morselli, K. G. Lloyd, L. F. Quesney and J. Engle Jr. New York: Raven Press, pp. 49–56

MELDRUM, B. S. (1975) Epilepsy and γ-aminobutyric acid mediated inhibition. *International Review of Neurobiology,* **17,** 1–36

MELDRUM, B. S. (1978) γ-aminobutyric acid and the search for new anticonvulsant drugs. *Lancet,* **2,** 304–306

METCALF, B. W. (1979) Inhibitors of GABA metabolism. *Biochemical Pharmacology,* **28,** 1705–1712

MÖHLER, H. and OKADA, T. (1977) Benzodiazepine receptors: demonstration in the central nervous system. *Science,* **198,** 849–851

MUTANI, R., BERGAMINI, L. and DORIGUZZI, T. (1969) Experimental evidence for the existence of an extrarhinencephalic control of the activity of the cobalt rhinencephalic epileptogenic focus, Part 2. Effects of paleocerebellar stimulation. *Epilepsia,* **10,** 351–362

MUTANI, R., MONACO, F., DURELLI, L. and DELSEDIME, M. (1974) Free amino acids in the cerebrospinal fluid in epileptic subjects. *Epilepsia,* **15,** 593–597

MUTANI, R., DURELLI, L., MAZZARINO, M. *et al.* (1977) Longitudinal changes of brain amino acid content occurring before, during, and after epileptic activity. *Brain Research,* **122,** 513–521

MYSLOBODSKY, M. S., ACKERMAN, R. F. and ENGEL, J. JR. (1979) Effects of γ-acetylenic GABA γ-vinyl-GABA on metrazol activated and kindle seizures. *Pharmacologic and Biochemical Behavior,* **11,** 265–271

NEWBERRY, N. R. and NICOLL, R. A. (1984) Direct hyperpolarizing action of baclofen on hippocampal pyramidal cells. *Nature,* **308,** 450-452

NICOLL, R. A., ECCLES, J. C., OSHIMA, T. C. and RUBIA, F. (1975) Prolongation of hippocampal inhibitory postsynaptic potentials by barbiturates. *Nature,* **258,** 625–627

PALACIOS, J. M., KUHAR, M. J., RAPOPORT, S. I. and LONDON, E. D. (1982) Effects of γ-aminobutyric acid agonist and antagonist drugs on local cerebral glucose utilization. *Journal of Neuroscience,* **2,** 853–860

PALFREYMAN, M. G., SCHECTER, P. T., BUCKETT, W. R., TELL, G. P. and KOCH-WESTER, T. (1981) The pharmacology of GABA transaminase inhibitors. *Biochemical Pharmacology,* **30,** 817–824

PEDLEY, T. A., HORTON, R. W. and MELDRUM, B. S. (1979) Electroencephalographic and behavioral effects of a GABA agonist (muscimol) on photosensitive epilepsy in the baboon *Papio papio. Epilepsia,* **20,** 409–416

PERRY, T., L., HANSEN, S., KENNEDY, J., WADA, J. A. and THOMPSON, G. B. (1975) Amino acids human epileptogenic foci. *Archives of Neurology,* **32,** 752–754

PHILLIS, J. W. and OCHS, S. (1971) Excitation and depression of cortical neurons during spreading depression. *Experimental Brain Research,* **12,** 132–149

PLUM, C. M. (1974) Free amino acid levels in the cerebrospinal fluid of normal humans and their variations in cases of epilepsy and Spielmeyer–Vogt–Batter disease. *Journal of Neurochemistry,* **23,** 595–600

PRICE, J. C., WAELSH, H. and PUTNAM, T. J. (1943) D-L Glutamic acid hydrochloride in treatment of petit mal and psychomotor seizures. *Journal of the American Medical Association,* **122,** 1153–1156

PRINCE, D. A. and SCHWARTZKROIN, P. A. (1978) Nonsynaptic mechanisms in epileptogenesis. In *Abnormal Neuronal Discharges,* edited by N. Chalazonitis and M. Boisson. New York: Raven Press

PRIOR, P. F., MCLAIN, G. F., SCOTT, D. F. and LAURANCE, M. M. (1972) Tonic status epilepticus precipitated by intravenous diazepam in a child with petit mal status. *Epilepsia,* **13,** 467–472

PUIL, E. A., REIFFENSTEIN, R. J. and TRIGGLE, C. (1974) Epileptiform afterdischarges and chemical responsiveness of cortical neurons. *Electroencephalography and Clinical Neurophysiology,* **36,** 265–273

PUIL, E. A. (1981) S-Glutamate: its interaction with spinal neurons. *Brain Research Reviews,* **3,** 224–322

PUIL, E. A. (1983) Actions and interaction of S-glutamate in the spinal cord. In *Handbook of the Spinal Cord, Vol. I: Pharmacology,* edited by R. A. Davidoff, pp. 105–169. New York: Marcel Dekker, Inc.

PUIL, E. A. (1984) Glutamate excitation of central neurons and their burst discharges. In *Advances in Epileptology, The Thirteenth Epilepsy International Symposium.* New York: Raven Press, pp. 32–37

QUASTEL, T. J. and WHEATLEY, A. H. M. (1932) Oxidations by the brain. *Journal of Biochemistry,* **26,** 725–744

RAMANJANEYULU, R. and TICKU, M. K. (1984) Binding characteristics and interactions of depressant drugs with [35S] *t*-butylbicyclophosphorothionate, a ligand that binds to the picrotoxinin site. *Journal of Neurochemistry,* **42,** 221–229

RIBAK, C. E., HARRIS, C. B., VAUGHN, J. E. and ROBERTS, E. (1979) Inhibitory GABAergic nerve terminals decrease at site of focal epilepsy. *Science,* **205,** 211–214

ROSS, S. M. and CRAIG, C. R. (1981a) Studies on γ-aminobutyric acid transport in cobalt experimental epilepsy in the rat. *Journal of Neurochemistry,* **36,** 1006–1011

ROSS, S. M. and CRAIG, C. R. (1981b) γ-Aminobutyric acid concentration, L-glutamate, L-decarboxylase activity and properties of the γ-aminobutyric acid postsynaptic receptor in cobalt epilepsy in the rat. *Journal of Neuroscience,* **1,** 1388–1396

SCHWARTZKROIN, P. A. and PRINCE, D. A. (1980) Changes in excitatory acid inhibitory synaptic potential leading to epileptogenic activity. *Brain Research,* **183,** 61–76

SCHWARTZKROIN, P. A. and WYLER, A. R. (1980) Mechanisms underlying epileptiform burst discharge. *Annals of Neurology,* **7,** 95–107

SHERWIN, A. L., QUESNEY, L. F., GAUTHIER, S. *et al.*, (1984) Enzymic-changes in activity spiking areas of human epileptic cerebral cortex. *Neurology,* **34,** 927–933

SHERWIN, A. L., ROBITAILLE, Y. and OLIVIER, A. (1982) Comparative study of glutamine synthetase activity in human seizure foci and primary brain tumors. In *Proceedings of the Canadian Association of Neuropathology* (Montreal, 1982)

SHERWIN, A. L. and VAN GELDER, N. M. (1984) Biochemical markers of metabolic abnormalities in human focal epilepsies (in press)

SIMMONDS, M. A. (1981) Distinction between the effects of barbiturates, benzodiazepines and phenytoin on responses to α-aminobutyric acid receptor activation and antagonism by bicuculline and picrotoxinin. *British Journal of Pharmacology,* **73,** 739–747

SNEAD, O. C. III (1983) Sacred disease: neurochemistry of epilepsy. *International Review of Neurobiology,* **24,** 93–180

SNYDER, S. H. (1984) Drug and neurotransmitter receptor in the brain. *Science,* **224,** 22–31

SQUIRES, R. F., CASIDA, J. E., RICHARDSON, M. and SAEDERUP, E. (1983) [35S] t-Butylbicyclophosphorothionate binds with high affinity to brain specific sites couples to γ-aminobutyric acid-A and ion recognition istes. *Molecular Pharmacology,* **23,** 326–336

STONE, W. E., TEWS, J. K. and MITCHELL, E. N. (1960) Chemical concomitants of convulsive activity in the cerebrum. *Neurology,* **10,** 241–248

SYTINSKY, I. A. and THINH, N. T. (1964) The distribution of γ-aminobutyric acid in the monkey brain during picrotoxin in induced seizures. *Journal of Neurochemistry,* **11,** 551–556

TALLMAN, J. F., PAUL, S. J., SKOLNICK, P. and GALLAGER, D. W. (1980) Receptors for the age of anxiety: pharmacology of the benzodiazepines. *Science,* **207,** 274–281

TASSINARI, C. A., DRAVET, C., ROGER, J., CAND, J. P. and GASTAUT, H. (1972) Tonic status epilepticus precipitated by intravenous benzodiazepines in five patients with Lennox–Gastaut syndrome. *Epilepsia,* **13,** 467–472

TIBBLE, J. A. R. and MCGREAL, D. A. (1963) Trial of γ-amino-oxyacetic acid, an anticonvulsant. *Canadian Medical Association Journal* **88,** 881–886

TICKU, M. K. and DAVIS, W. C. (1981) Effect of valproic acid on [^{3}H] diazepam and [^{3}H] dihydropicrotoxinin binding sites at the benzodiazepine-GABA receptor-ionophore complex. *Brain Research* **223,** 218–222

TICKU, M. K., FARIELLO, R. G. and GOLDEN, G. T. (1983) Effects of chronic treatment with some direct GABA agonists on GABA receptor binding. *Society for Neuroscience* (Abstract), **9,** 403

TICKU, M. K. and MAKSAY, G. (1983) Minireview: convulsant/depressant site of action at the allosteric benzodiazepine–GABA receptor–ionophore complex. *Life Sciences,* **33,** 2363–2375

TICKU, M. K. and OLSEN, R. W. (1978) Interaction of barbiturates with dihydropicrotoxinin binding sites relative to the GABA receptor–ionophore system. *Life Sciences,* **22,** 1643–1651

TOWER, D. B. (1976) GABA and seizures: clinical correlates in man. In *Inhibition in the Nervous System and γ-Aminobutyric Acid,* edited by E. Roberts, T. N. Chase and D. B. Tower. New York: Raven Press. pp. 461–478

TOWER, D. B. (1960) The administration of γ-aminobutyric acid to man: suppressive effects and anticonvulsant action. In *Inhibition in the Nervous System and γ-Aminobutyric Acid,* edited by E. Roberts, C. F. Baxter, A. van Harreveld, C. A. G. Wiersma, W. R. Adey and K. F. Killam. New York: Pergamon Press, pp. 562–578

VAN GELDER, N. M. (1978) Taurine, the compartmentalized metabolism of glutamic acid and the epilepsies. *Canadian Journal of Physiology and Pharmacology,* **56,** 362–374

VAN GELDER, N. M. (1981) Glutamic acid in nervous tissue and changes of the taurine content: its implication in the treatment of epilepsy. In *Amino Acids Neurotransmitters*, edited by F. V. Defeudis and P. Mandel, pp. 115–125. New York: Raven Press.

VAN GELDER, N. M., SHERWIN, A. L. and RASMUSSEN, T. (1972) Aminoacid content of epileptogenic human brain: focal versus surrounding regions. *Brain Research,* **40,** 385–393

VAN GELDER, N. M., SIATITAS, I., MENINI, C. and GLOOR, P. (1983) Feline generalized penicillin epilepsy; changes in glutamic acid and taurine parallel the progressive increase in excitability of the cortex. *Epilepsia,* **24,** 200–213

2

Neurophysiological approaches to basic mechanisms of seizures

Eli S. Goldensohn

INTRODUCTION

This chapter deals with two subjects: (1) the generation of EEG epileptogenic activity from the cerebal cortex; and (2) the relevance of kindling and the mirror focus to the clinical management of epilepsy.

The dysfunction underlying a partial seizure disorder is the excessive excitability of a local population of cells in the cerebral cortex (Ward, Schmidt and Thomas, 1959). Abnormally low threshold for excitation in cells distributed throughout the cerebral cortex is the basic condition underlying primary generalized seizures (Gloor, 1979). In primary generalized seizures excessive excitability of the thalamoreticular system plays a secondary role because epileptiform discharges from the cerebral cortex regularly precede those found in deep gray structures (Avoli and Gloor, 1982). Thalamocortical connections are, nevertheless, essential in the production of typical generalized spike and wave paroxysms in the experimental animal (Avoli and Gloor, 1982).

In both partial and generalized seizures the common dysfunction at a cellular level is manifested by excessive discharging of cortical neurons. In normal function a balance of excitatory and inhibitory influences is harmoniously maintained, but in the center of an epileptogenic focus nearly every cell penetrated by microelectrodes shows evidence of excessive excitatory or decreased inhibitory synaptic influences (Goldensohn, 1975) and fires excessively (Matsumato and Ajmone-Marsan, 1964a and b).

Agents capable of causing seizures appear to enhance excitation of neurons either by interfering with inhibitory synaptic mechanisms or by increasing excitatory synaptic activity. Direct action of epileptogenic agents on intrinsic cell properties may also occur. Among the factors affecting the generation of epileptiform activity that results from the topical application of an epileptogenic agent such as penicillin are the action of the drug surrounding the neurons, the intrinsic properties of the neurons themselves, and the location of the neurons within the complex organized neural synaptic networks in the cerebral cortex. Topically applied penicillin is widely used to produce experimental epileptogenic foci for studying the development and spread of epileptiform activity because it can involve a limited aggregate of chemically affected neurons (Goldensohn, Zablow and Salazar, 1977) and because it produces interictal and ictal cortical EEG activity which closely resembles that seen in human focal epilepsy.

The characteristic feature in the EEG which indicates the presence of seizures is the EEG spike. Intracellular recordings with microelectrodes show that the main generators of the EEG spikes are synchronous paroxysmal depolarization shifts (PDSs) across the cell membranes (Goldensohn and Purpura, 1963; Matsumato and Ajmone-Marsan, 1964a and b). Postsynaptic potentials and other transmembranal potentials related to the paroxysmal depolarization shifts contribute to the EEG spike and are responsible for the remainder of the paroxysmal electrical activity found in the EEG. This includes the synchronized participation of organized interconnected populations of cortical neurons whose usual functions are altered to contribute to the production of recurrent synchronous discharges.

The distribution of electrical excitation of neurons participating in focal epileptogenesis progressively increases as the center of the focus is approached. Prolonged inhibitory postsynaptic potentials (IPSPs) are found at the periphery, larval and truncated paroxysmal depolarization shifts in a zone of transition, and highly excited neurons exhibiting sustained paroxysmal depolarization shifts are found near the center of the focus as shown in *Figures 2.1 and 2.2* (Goldensohn, 1969, 1975; Salazar, 1980). Fully developed paroxysmal depolarization shifts have durations similar to their associated EEG spikes and are referred to as sustained shifts. These are usually preceded by a short burst of action potentials and followed successively by rapid repolarization and a long-lasting hyperpolarizing afterpotential. The action potentials in an initial burst progressively decrease in amplitude and complete spike inactivation occurs with maximal depolarization. Paroxysmal depolarization shifts of similiar amplitude, having the same sequence but which begin repolarizing before the EEG spike is over, are called truncated paroxysmal depolarization shifts. The term larval PDS is applied when depolarizations are of lower amplitude and briefer. Although bursts of action potentials decrease in amplitude they do not become inactivated (*see Figure 2.1*). Each of the three types of paroxysmal depolarization shifts has its own separate axially symmetrical distribution within the focus (*see Figure 2.2*). Fully developed shifts are found in a radius of approximately 1.5 mm from the center of the penicillin source. Shorter duration transitional forms, termed truncated and larval paroxysmal depolarization shifts, predominate at radial distances between 1.5 and 2.5 mm (*see Figure 2.2*).

The paroxysmal deplorization shifts which are the principal generators of recurrent negative EEG spikes found at the focus are of much greater amplitude and much longer in duration than usual excitatory postsynaptic potentials (EPSPs). Mechanisms underlying the generation of the paroxysmal depolarization shift are now beginning to be understood. A frequently cited hypothesis holds that the shift at the cell body represents a giant EPSP activated by abnormally large synchronous synaptic excitation (Ayala, Matsumato and Gumnit, 1970; Johnston and Brown, 1982). The input for the giant excitatory postsynaptic potential has been ascribed to a number of synaptic mechanisms, including excessive recurrent excitation, bursting of axon terminals, facilitation of excitatory postsynaptic potentials, and suppression of inhibition. An alternate hypothesis suggests that paroxysmal depolarization shift generation may be the result of changes in intrinsic membrane properties of the neurons and that synaptic events serve only to generate them (Wong and Prince, 1978, 1979). Support for this hypothesis includes the finding that paroxysmal depolarization shift-like bursts may be evoked non-synaptically by brief intracellular current pulses in mouse hippocampal membrane in tissue culture

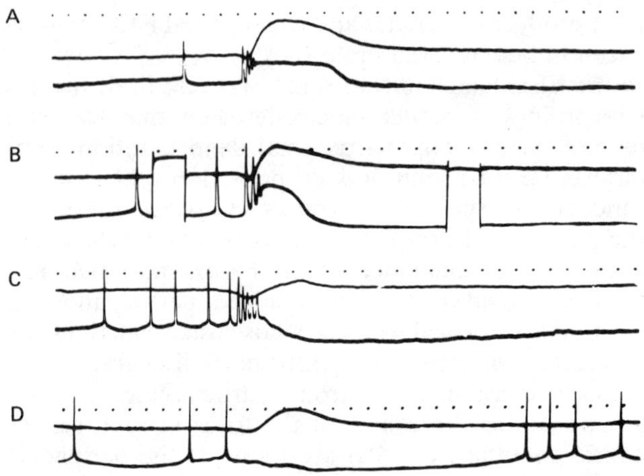

Figure 2.1 Types of intracellular activity seen during interictal EEG spiking at penicillin-induced focus. Upper traces, corticogram. Lower traces, intracellular recordings showing: A, Sustained paroxysmal deplorization shift (PDS); B, truncated paroxysmal depolarization shift; C, larval paroxysmal depolarization shift, D, prolonged inhibitory postsynaptic potential (IPSP). Time marker 10 msec. DC voltage calibration is shown in B, 50 MV (from Goldensohn, 1975)

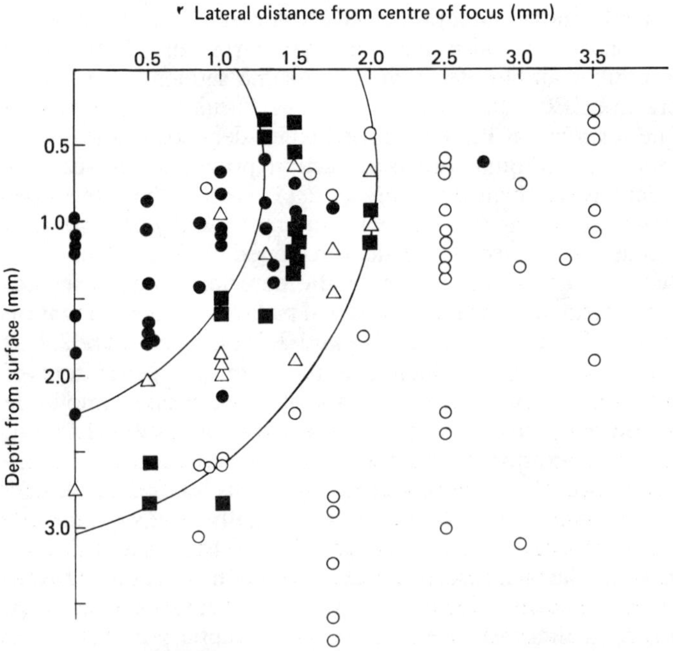

Figure 2.2 Distribution of paroxysmal depolarization shifts and inhibitory postsynaptic potentials during EEG spiking. Nearly all sustained shifts are located within 1–½ mm lateral to the center of the focus. At 2 mm and beyond inhibitory postsynaptic potentials are preponderant. (●) Sustained paroxysmal depolarization shift, (■) truncated paroxysmal depolarization shift, (△) larval paroxysmal depolarization shift, (○) prolonged inhibitory postsynaptic potentials, no involvement (from Goldensohn, 1975; Salazar, 1980)

(Zipser, Crain and Bornstein, 1973) and in molluscan neurons isolated from synaptic influences (Barker and Smith, 1978). Also spontaneous paroxysmal depolarization shift-like bursts occur in CA-3 hippocampal pyramidal cells *in vitro* which are free of unusual synaptic influence. CA-3 paroxysmal depolarization shifts are related to an interplay between inward movements of Ca^{2+} and outward currents generated by K^+ (Johnston, Hablitz and Wilson, 1981). Summations of Ca^{2+} spikes or other voltage-dependent Ca^{2+} potentials, possibly located on dendrites, have been postulated to contribute to the maintenance of the depolarization envelope during the late phase of the paroxysmal depolarization shift (Schwartzkroin and Wyler, 1980; Wong and Prince, 1978).

The controversy over the giant excitatory postsynaptic potential and intrinsic mechanisms hypotheses for being responsible for the paroxysmal depolarization shift is not a valid one as both mechanisms must be involved and each contributes to the shifts. First, cells must be capable of generating the shift, and second, excitatory postsynaptic potentials of great intensity are essential for promoting the degree of excitation needed to initiate the intrinsic mechanisms. Paroxysmal depolarization shifts have been observed to originate in cells in the fourth and fifth layers of the neocortex and it has been suggested that they act as initiators or pacemakers of epileptogenic discharges (Ebersole, 1977; Ebersole and Chatt, 1980). From our data, it seems likely that nearly all large pyramidal cells in the cortex have this capacity, as practically all cells in the center of the penicillin focus that can be penetrated show paroxysmal depolarization shifts (*see Figure 2.2*).

The paroxysmal deplorization shift is followed by an hyperpolarizing after potential (HAP) which lasts several hundred msec (Matsumato and Ajmone-Marsan, 1964a; Salazar, 1980). As shown in *Figure 2.3* the hyperpolarizing afterpotential is associated with suppression of spontaneous unit activity. Both larval and truncated as well as sustained paroxysmal deplorization shifts are followed by hyperpolarizing afterpotentials. Earlier studies indicated that the hyperpolarizing afterpotential was generated by inhibitory postsynaptic potentials (IPSPs) triggered by recurrent inhibition from interneurons which had been activated by axon collaterals of the pyramidal cells exhibiting paroxysmal depolarization shifts. More recently, a non-synaptic mechanism has been proposed for the hyperpolarizing afterpotential which involves a Ca^{2+} or Ca^{2+}–Na^+ activated slow increase in K^+ conductance at pyramidal cell dendrites (Hotson, Schwartzkroin and Prince, 1977; Hotson, Prince and Schwartzkroin, 1979). The hyperpolarizing afterpotential appears to serve as a limiting factor in the frequency of recurrence of epileptiform EEG spikes since the population of neurons which produce the spikes remain hyperpolarized and resistant to generating action potentials for up to more than 500 msec (*Table 2.1*).

Another type of neuronal activity which occurs in association with spontaneous interictal spike discharges is the prominent prolonged inhibitory postsynaptic potential in cells covering a relatively large area at the periphery of the focus (*see Figure 2.2*). The term 'surround inhibition' has been used to describe the activity of this population of neurons (Prince and Wilder, 1967). Surround inhibition may serve to restrict the propagation of epileptiform activity into adjacent cortex by providing an encircling field of strong inhibition coincident with the central focal excitation. Neurons without paroxysmal depolarization shifts which show long-lasting hyperpolarizations coincident with the EEG spike and suppression of spontaneous action potentials are classified as prolonged inhibitory postsynaptic potentials (Salazar, 1980). Some prolonged inhibitory postsynaptic potentials

Table 2.1 Relationshp of duration of hyperpolarization afterpotential (HAP) to type of paroxysmal depolarization shift

Type of paroxysmal depolarization shift	*Paroxysmal depolarization shift duration (msec)*	*Hyperpolarizing afterpotential onset to its maximum hyperpolarization (msec)*	*Onset to first action potential (msec)*	*Maximum amplitude hyperpolarization (mV)*
Sustained paroxysmal depolarization shift	82±22	201±50	1240±438	6±3
Truncated paroxysmal depolarization shift	55±15	141±54	645±360	9±5
Larval paroxysmal depolarization shift	35±10	103±35	475±150	10±3

* Total duration of hyperpolarization afterpotential is a difficult measurement but is estimated as more than twice the figures shown (modified from Salazar, 1980)

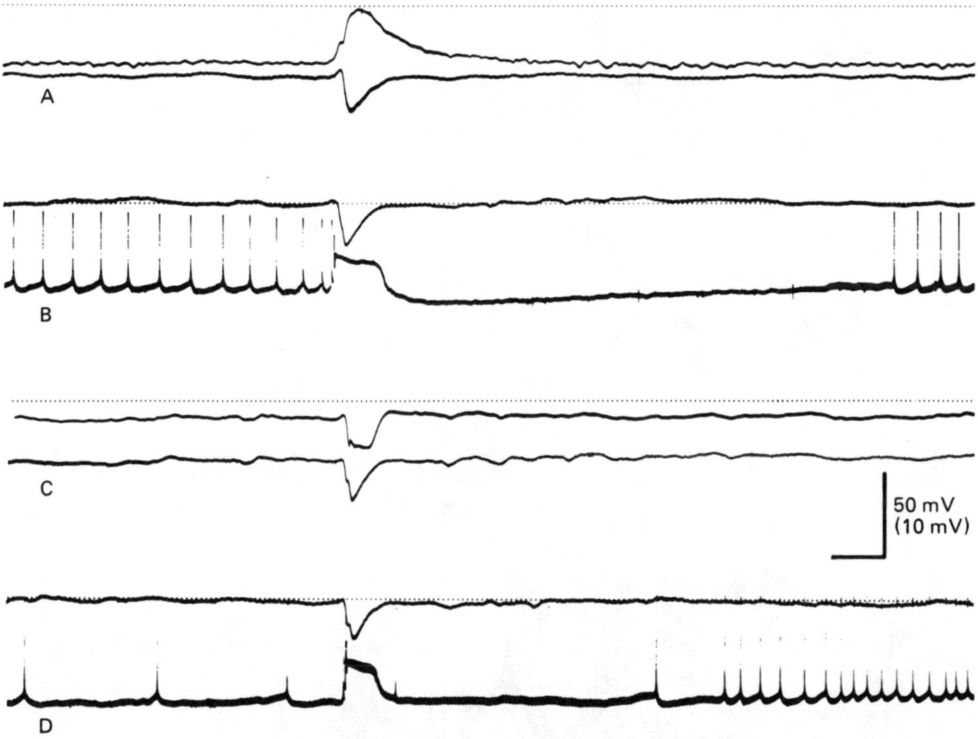

Figure 2.3 Examples of a sustained and a truncated paroxysmal depolarization shift and hyperpolarizing afterpotentials recorded during microelectrode penetrations in two different locations within the same focus. *A and C.* Recorded from the cortical surface. Upper trace of A: focal negative spike from a microelectrode positioned on the pial surface at the center of the focus. Upper trace of C: focal positive spike recorded from the same microelectrode repositioned 1.5 mm laterally. Lower traces: positive spike recorded from a ball electrode located on the pial surface approximately 2 mm lateral to the center of the focus. *B and D.* Surface and intracellular recordings: Lower trace of B; sustained paroxysmal depolarization shift at depth of 1.62 mm. Lower trace of D; truncated paroxysmal depolarization shift at depth of 1.14 mm. Upper traces show positive spikes coincident with intracellular events. Time marker 10 msec. Voltage calibration: intracellular record 50 mV, surface record 10 mV (from Goldensohn and Salazar, 1985)

contain an early brief depolarizing hump. The early depolarizations which sometimes precede the prolonged inhibitory postsynaptic potentials are coincident with a variable brief positive EEG spike component that often immediately precedes the longer more prominent negative EEG spike.

ANATOMICAL ORGANIZATION FOR EPILEPTOGENIC DISCHARGES

The cerebral cortex is the structure from which both focal and generalized seizures begin. Pyramidal cells are vertically oriented with their cell bodies in the deeper layers and their long apical dendrites extending into the superficial layers (*Figure 2.4*). The dendrites receive mainly excitatory contacts, up to several thousand per

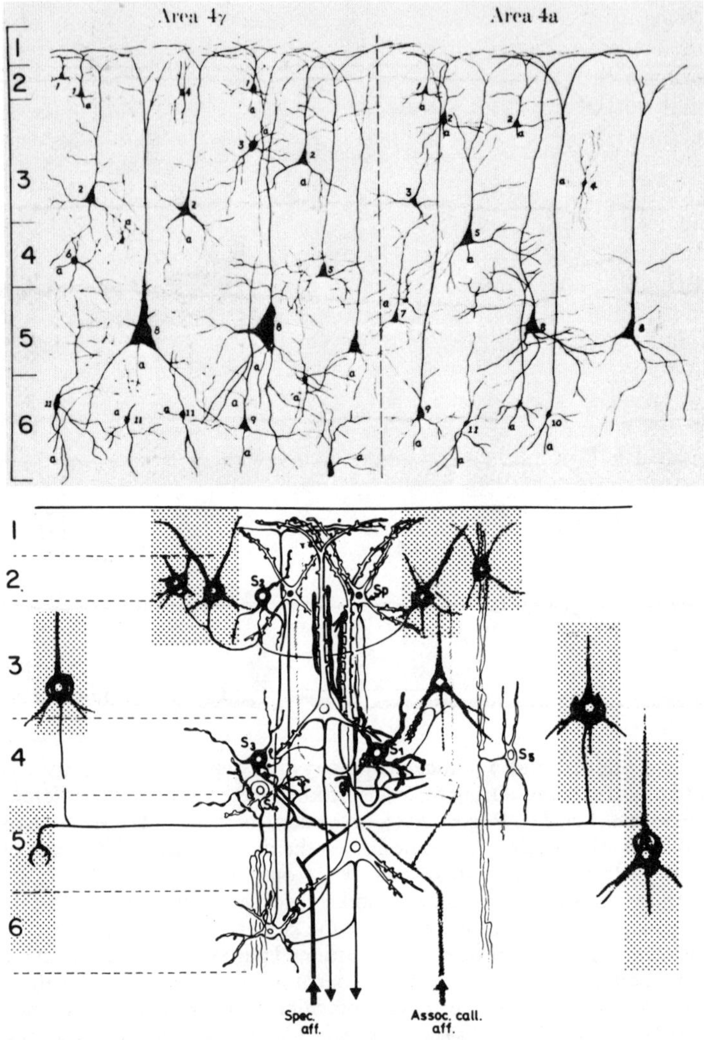

(*a*)

(*b*)

Figure 2.4a Stratification of cells and their processes in the cerebral cortex of man. Note deeply located pyramidal cell bodies in layer 5 and superficially located apical dendrites in layers 1 and 2. Drawn after Golgi preparations (from Von Bonin, 1949). (*b*) Cell types in neocortex and their interconnections. Basket type stellate interneurons (S_2) have short-range pericellular connections in (S_3) distribute processes in wider areas of 500 μ and more in layers 3 and 4 and perhaps in still wider areas in layers 5 and 6. If basket cells are inhibitory this distribution would indicate greater inhibition in the deeper layers. Excitation is greatest in the superficial neurophil of layers 1 and 2 (from Szentagothai, 1969)

dendritic tree. The cell body receives mostly inhibitory contacts that number only between 50 and 100. Athough excitatory synapses greatly outnumber inhibitory ones the latter are more strategically placed on the cell body for preventing the cell from firing. Impulses from any part of the cortex go predominantly to other regions of the cortex and only a small fraction are directed toward subcortical structures such as the specific and associational nuclei of the thalamus. The vertical organization of the excitatory and inhibitory synapses on the pyramidal cells is in keeping with the idea that the structural design of the cortex is based upon interconnections among a large number of small mosaic-like verticular columnar units. Such functional vertical columns have been clearly demonstrated in the occipital lobe (Hubel and Wiesel, 1965). The data of Prince and Wilder (1967) also support the idea of functionally distinct vertically oriented columns in the sensorimotor cortex of the cat. They found that cells along a single electrode track perpendicular to the cortical surface showed either predominantly paroxysmal depolarization shifts or predominantly inhibitory postsynaptic potentials. Our data supports this concept in still another way by demonstrating that cortical areas in animals and man are capable of generating epileptiform EEG spikes from surfaces less than 2 mm in diameter (*Figure 2.5*). This concept is further supported by the fact that the epileptogenic focus has its greatest negativity about 1 mm below the surface, indicating that the surface negative spike is generated in superficial lamina. Slow wave portions of the experimental EEG spike-and-wave complexes are also surface-negative on the EEG but they are generated as positive waves in deeper sites which appear as negativities at the surface (Pollen, 1969; Pollen, Reid and Perot, 1964). The intracellular correlates of the slow wave portion appear to be mainly inhibitory postsynaptic potentials.

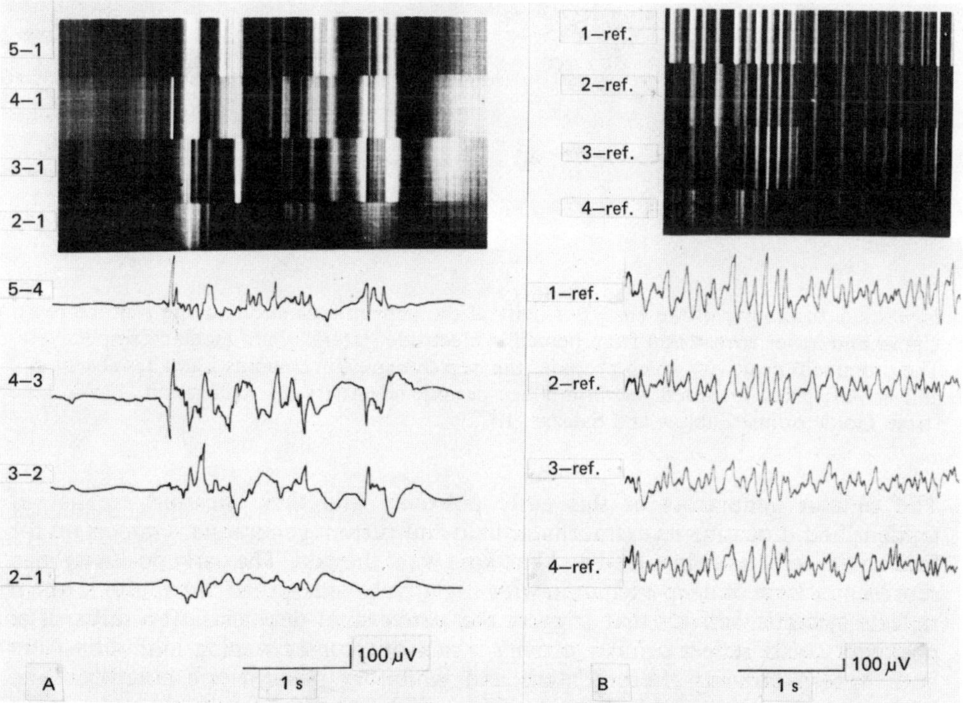

Figure 2.5 Corticograms with computer display of electrical fields. The corticogram and computer display above it record simultaneously from four closely spaced electrodes 2.5 mm apart. A: Non-synchronous high-voltage spikes in corticogram are seen at single electrodes; simultaneous computer display above shows asynchrony of potentials at adjacent electrodes. B: Synchronous spindles in corticogram; synchrony of negative and positive potentials is seen in computer display. Negative, darker areas; positive, lighter areas (from Goldensohn, 1975)

This anatomical–physiological analysis serves as the basis for the idea that the paroxysmal activity from the cortex depends on small, vertically oriented columnar organizations in which excitation occurs at the apical dendrites, predominantly near the surface and in which inhibition occurs predominantly in the deeper layers. Recordings from epileptogenic human cortex revealing minute spike generators are shown in *Figure 2.5*.

ELECTRICAL FIELDS OF EPILEPTOGENIC DISCHARGES

In a strong penicillin focus an early positivity lasting 10–30 msec (*Figure 2.6*) precedes the negative surface element of the EEG spike surface. The negative element is known to be generated mainly by the paroxysmal depolarization shift.

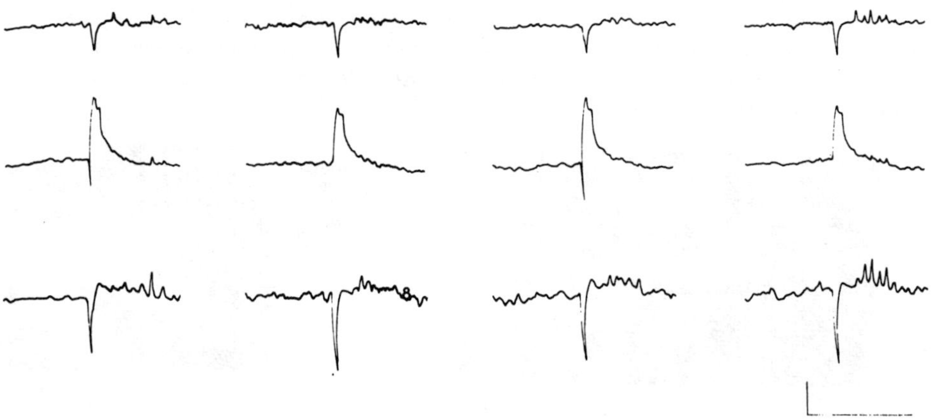

Figure 2.6 Instability of the early positivity at the penicillin electrode alone (middle row). Upper and lower rows 2 mm from penicillin electrode, laterally and medially respectively. The prominent positivity which precedes the negative spike in columns 1 and 3 is absent in 2 and 4. All spikes recorded within a 30 sec period; negativity up, calibration, 1 mV, 1 sec (from Goldensohn, Zablow and Salazar, 1977)

The cellular generators of this early positivity and their location are as yet unidentified. Locating its extracellular field and current generators is important for finding the structures involved and knowing what they do. The early positivity may represent a form of deep excitation with a relatively widespread distribution, which reflects synaptic activity that triggers the paroxysmal depolarization shifts. The positivity could reflect cellular activity which overcomes waning inhibition from both hyperpolarizing afterpotentials and inhibitory postsynaptic potentials and initiates the next interictal discharge. The variability of its amplitude and relative size in relation to the relatively stable negative spike is puzzling (Goldensohn, Zablow and Stein, 1970). The positive spike has a wider field than the negative spike which follows. It is less likely, but also possible considering its wider field, that the early positivity is part of the inhibitory surround. The fact that two adjacent penicillin foci can interact and become synchronous when separated by less than 4 mm but become asynchronous when 6 mm apart (Lüders *et al.*, 1981) suggests that the surround positivity is composed of a number of populations, some of which reflect deep excitation as well as inhibition.

A polarity reversal of negative spindles to positive precedes the appearance of the negative surface spike (*Figure 2.7*) which appears shortly thereafter, as penicillin penetrates further into the cortex. Recent evidence (Kostopoulos *et al.*, 1982) shows that spindles and spike and wave discharges have rather similar fields in the vertical dimension and that the polarity of the individual waves of both reverse between a depth of 200 and 400 mm. In developing foci in which penicillin involves only the superficial layers of the cortex, full-blown paroxysmal depolarization shifts may occur. They occur at 150–200 mm below the surface, and even after 15–20 min of recording prolonged paroxysmal depolarization shifts can continue to be found in the superficial layers (Elgerand Speckman, 1983).

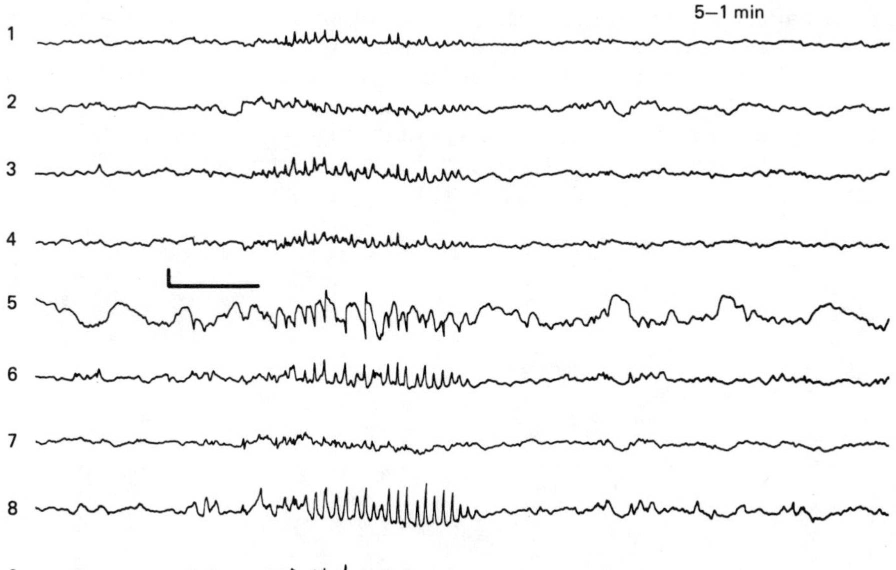

Figure 2.7 Inversion of spindles at the penicillin-containing capillary (channel 5) 1 min after its placement and just before spiking starts. Recording is from 12 electrodes covering a rectangular area of 4 × 6 mm. Recording electrodes for channels 2, 4, 6, and 8 are each separated from the penicillin capillary by 2 mm. Calibration, 500 μV, 1 sec; negative up. Reference is neck muscle (Goldensohn, Zablow and Salazar, 1977)

Nevertheless, it is the pyramidal cells residing in layers IV, V and VI that lie considerably farther below the surface which produce the large numbers of paroxysmal depolarization shifts (Goldensohn, 1975; Salazar, 1970). Also, layer IV in cats (1000 μ deep) is the lamina most sensitive to applied penicillin (Ebersole, 1977; Ebersole and Chatt, 1980). These conflicting data and unresolved questions indicate that definition of the three-dimensional spatial and temporal distributions of extracellular fields and current generators is essential for understanding the generation and spread of epileptiform activity. In a discrete established penicillin focus the cortical EEG shows similar configurations from spike to spike over periods up to several hours (Goldensohn, Zablow and Salazar, 1977). Because of this, information recorded at different depths and horizontal distances from the focus over an extended period of time can describe essentially the same field. The extracellular potential distribution at multiple depths from the cortical surface to a depth of 3.5 mm with plunges at different lateral distances from the center of the focus were made in each experiment. This enabled determination of a composite field potential distribution at multiple locations within the focus. Axial symmetry was found at the surface and assumed to hold for the potential in the third dimension. The three-dimensional extracellular potential field was characterized geometrically by describing the recording sites in terms of two coordinates, depth from the pial surface and radius from the axis of the penicillin electrode. Data from a typical experiment are shown in *Figure 2.8*. The negative spike at the surface near

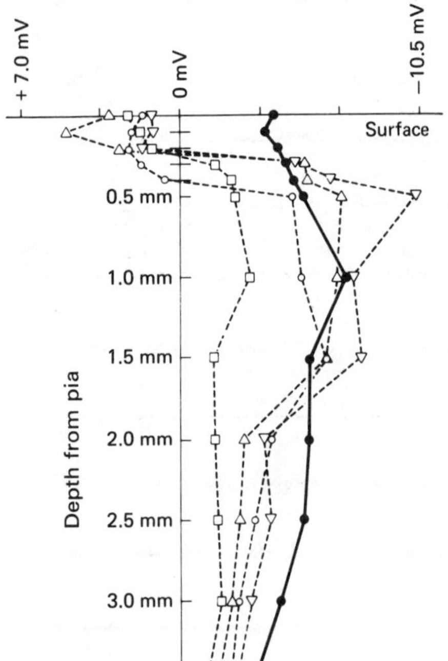

Figure 2.8 Potential distribution in three dimensions at a spike focus (no. 26). Maximal negativities and positivities and found within 1 mm of the surface, indicating superficial cortical generators (from Goldensohn, Zablow and Salazar, 1977)

the center of the focus keeps the same polarity throughout the depth of the cortex with voltage peaks at 0.5–1.0 mm below the surface. The positive spikes in the surround, however, inverted at a depth of about 0.3 mm to become negative and peaked in amplitude at depths similar to the surface negative spikes.

Intensity modulated displays of the field in a plane normal to the surface during the interictal spike are shown in *Figure 2.9*. Initiation of the major negative phase of the surface interictal spike is preceded by the rise of a wave of negativity at a depth of 0.5–1.0 mm below the penicillin source in most foci examined. A lower amplitude negativity occurs almost simultaneously but at the greater depth of 2.0–2.5 mm. Occasionally the earliest potential change from baseline occurs at the periphery of the focus at this same depth. This may be part of the source of the early positivity seen in the EEG spike.

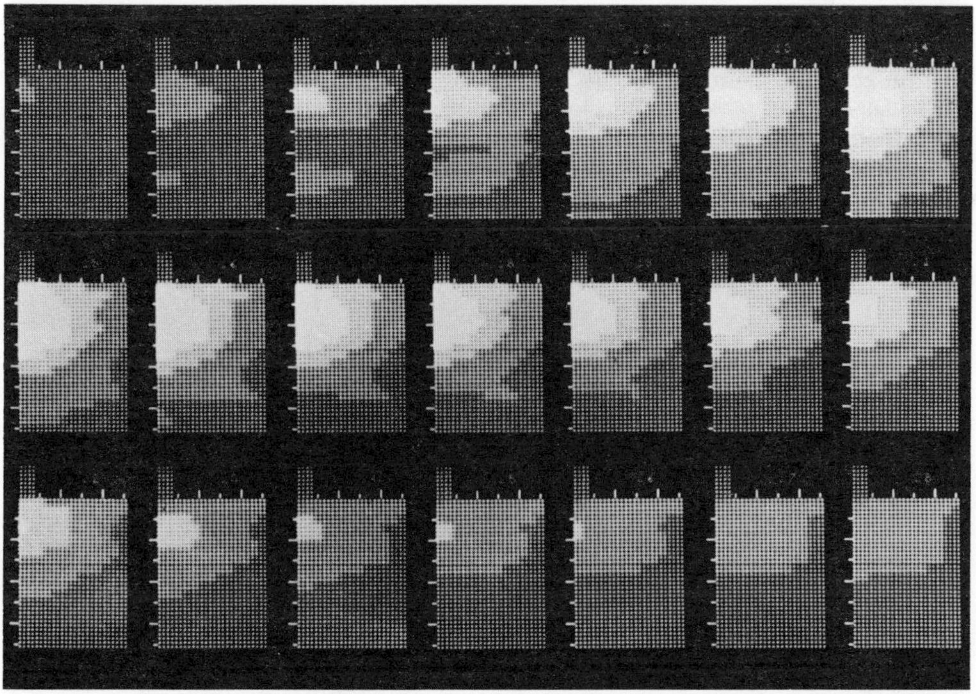

Figure 2.9 Spread of field potential in the cortex during an interictal spike. Successive computed intensity modulated displays represent changes in the distribution of potential in a plane normal to the cortical surface during a single composite spike. Initially and later the most intense negativity occurs at about 0.6 mm and spreads in all directions during the first 36 msec to involve a relatively large cortical volume before receding. Surface positivity in surrounding cortex occurs but is not resolved in these displays because of scaling technique 4 msec epoch. Whiteness indicates negativity. The rectangle at the upper left of each display shows the location of the penicillin source and its shading represents zero potential. The absolute value of the potential at any point is scaled relative to the maximum negativity attained during the spike. Ordinate: axis of the penicillin capillary; depth in 0.5 mm steps from surface; abscissa: lateral distance in 0.5 mm steps from axis of the focus (from Goldensohn and Salazar, 1985)

SPREAD OF POTENTIAL FIELD IN THE FOCUS

In order to estimate the spread of potential field in the focus, the latencies of paroxysmal depolarization shift onsets in individual cells were measured with reference to the interictal spike on the cortical surface after defining the moment of their respective onsets. The dependence of these latencies on the location of the cells in the focus was examined by an analysis of the multiple linear regression of latencies on the distance of the cells from the center of the focus at the surface and on their depths in the cortex. The lateral velocity of propagation paroxysmal depolarization shift initiation from cell to cell is about 0.25 msec, as shown in *Figure 2.10*.

Recognizing the developing negative extracellular potential in the depths is more difficult. An arbitrary chosen fraction of the maximum negativity attained is represented by the edge of the lightest white contour in the sequence of potential distributions. This allows measurement of the velocity of lateral spread of the negative field during the developing spike. From data the rate of development of the negative potential outward from the axis of the focus is also approximately 0.25 msec as shown in *Figure 2.11*. The correspondence with the rate at the surface provides evidence that the development of the negative extracellular potential is due to the sequential onsets of paroxysmal depolarization shifts which occur progressively more distant from the axis of the focus at the rate 0.25 msec.

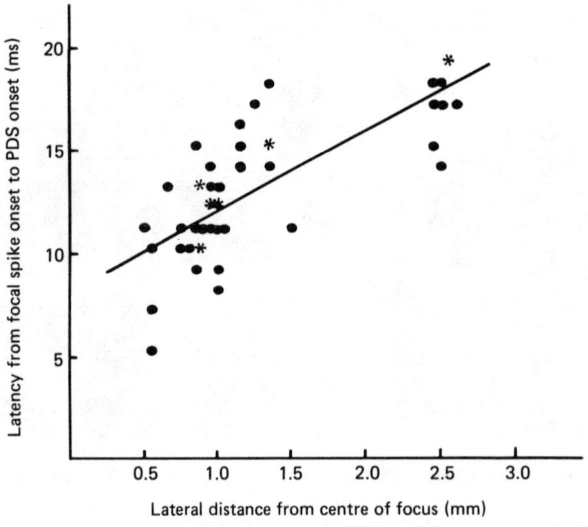

Figure 2.10 Scatter plot of paroxysmal depolarization shift (PDS) onset latencies relative to focal spike onsets as a function of horizontal distance of a cell from the center of a stable focus. Paroxysmal depolarization shift onset latencies are shortest near the center of the focus increasing from about 8 msec at a distance of 0.5 mm to 18 msec at 2.5 mm. The outward velocity of propagation of paroxysmal depolarization shift activity from cell to cell is 0.25 msec^{-1}. The portion of the paroxysmal depolarization shift onset latency contributed by depth dependency has been removed by the multiple linear regression analysis. Each point represents the average shift onset latency of 10 successive interictal spikes (from Goldensohn and Salazar, 1985)

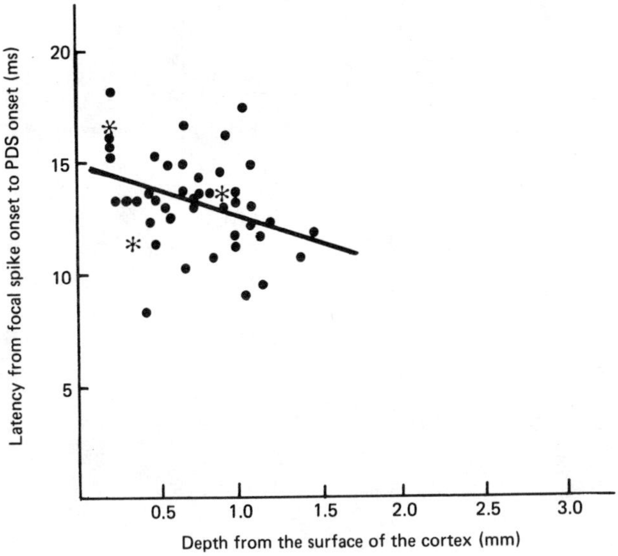

Figure 2.11 Scatter plot similar to *Figure 2.10* demonstrating latencies of propagation of paroxysmal depolarization shifts (PDSs) in the depths. Shift onsets which occur with distance from the axis of the focus show propagation rate similar to that in *Figure 2.10*

RELATIONSHIPS OF POTENTIALS TO CONCENTRATION OF THE EPILEPTOGENIC AGENT

The distribution of electrical activity of neurons participating in focal epileptogenesis exhibits a continuous decrease in excitation as distance increases from the center of the focus, as has been shown. Prolonged inhibitory postsynaptic potentials are found at the periphery, larval and truncated paroxysmal depolarization shifts in the zone of transition, and highly excited neurons evincing sustained paroxysmal depolarization shifts occur near the center of the focus. A mathematical model was developed which estimates the distribution of penicillin in the cortex (Salazar, 1980) and the four categories of intracellular activity are plotted as a function of the radial distances and the various local concentrations of pencillin in *Figure 2.12*. There is a strong relationship with local concentrations (Salazar, 1980). The effects of lamina and columnar organization remain, in spite of the fact that concentration curves fit reasonably well with the distributions of the two markedly different types of activity; the prolonged inhibitory postsynaptic potentials and truncated paroxysmal depolarization shifts. The results imply that the instantaneous local concentration of penicillin determines the synaptic activity of the cells in the columnar organization by the specific action of overcoming gamma-aminobutyric acid (GABA) mediated postsynaptic inhibition at the site of highest concentration of the drug.

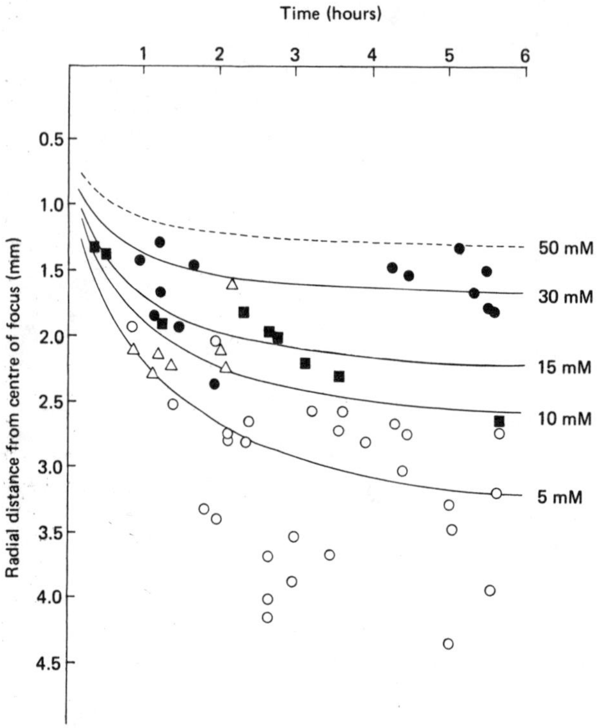

Figure 2.12 Paroxysmal depolarization shift categories and prolonged inhibitory postsynaptic potentials plotted against distance from the focus, time of cell penetration and penicillin concentration. Solid lines: mean concentration for each category of cellular activity; dashed line: concentration boundary above which no cellular activity was recorded. (●) Sustained paroxysmal depolarization shift, (■) truncated paroxysmal depolarization shift, (△) larval paroxysmal depolarization shift, (○) prolonged inhibitory postsynaptic potentials (Salazar, 1980)

KINDLING AND THE MIRROR FOCUS – SECONDARY EPILEPTOGENESIS

Two experimental physiological phenomena – kindling and the mirror focus – bear directly on the management of patients with seizures. Both phenomena have had a remarkable impact on research into the mechanisms of epilepsy (Goldensohn, 1978). Kindling was observed first in rats by Goddard (1976, 1981) and was pursued by him and his Canadian colleagues (Goddard and Douglas, 1975; Goddard, McIntyre and Leech, 1969; Racine, 1978), by Wada (1976, 1981; Wada and Osawa, 1976; Wada, Osawa and Mizoguchi, 1976), and by many others. Kindling as a method for investigating the development of seizures has already added much to our knowledge of the basic mechanisms of epilepsy. Among its remarkable attributes is that the kindling model can produce chronic seizures without evidence of tissue damage.

The mirror focus, a related phenomenon, was first discussed in terms of human epilepsy by Pope *et al.* (1946) and later by Morrell (1959, 1960, 1969) in animals, and in man (Morrell, 1979; Torres and French, 1973). Like kindling, the mirror focus is of physiological importance and is potentially significant in clinical epilepsy. A review of both phenomena, together referred to as secondary epileptogenesis, was recently published (Mayersdorf and Schmidt, 1982).

In addition to presenting the physiological data on kindling and the mirror focus that relate to the development and persistence of seizures in various species, it is necessary to critically evaluate existing evidence that supports or fails to support the idea that kindling and the mirror focus play roles in human epilepsy that should currently influence clinical decisions.

The term mirror focus is used to describe a new, apparently independent epileptogenic focus in an area of the brain contralateral and homotopic to an original focus. It presumes that the secondary focus has been induced by the firing of an original focus, and that over time the secondary focus has become completely independent and capable of producing seizures (Mayersdorf and Schmidt, 1982). Several recent studies in monkeys have failed to produce independent mirror discharges (Harris and Lockard, 1982; Lowrie and Ettlinger, 1980).

The term kindling is used to describe the progressive enhancement of electrical and behavioral responses to short duration, initially subthreshold stimuli that are applied at intervals of days or hours to a discrete area of grey matter of the brain (Goddard, McIntyre and Leech, 1969). Electrical afterdischarges that outlast the stimuli are noted first. The responses increase in intensity over time and repetition of the initial stimulus can lead to complete generalized convulsions. The enhanced responses to ordinarily subthreshold stimuli can persist for many months without reinforcement. A wide variety of stimulus frequencies can result in kindling but a minimum interval between successive trains of stimuli is critical. The enhanced responses can transfer to the homologous areas of the opposite hemisphere. Kindling has resulted in seizures in all species tested, including some primates.

At this time, some 16 years after kindling was first described in the rat, it seems important to examine its possible role in human epilepsy. We do not know whether

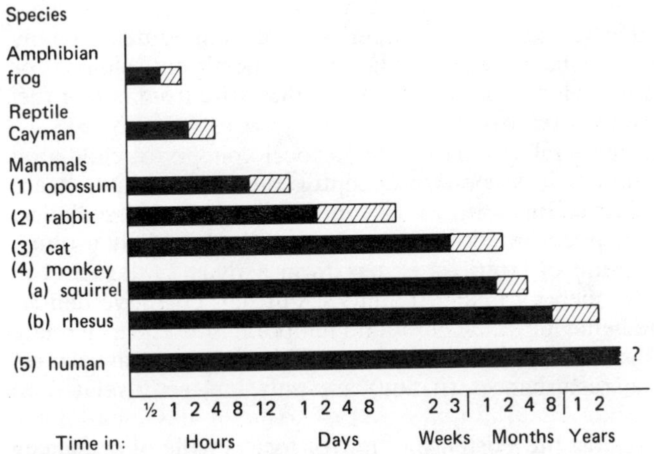

Figure 2.13 Timetable for secondary epileptogenesis; approximate times required for genesis of independent secondary epileptic foci in certain vertebrates (from Wilder, King and Schmidt, 1968)

kindling occurs in the human, and if it should occur, what the effective trigger parameters might be. As with the mirror focus (*Figure 2.13*) we know that evolutionary advancement is associated with progressively greater difficulty in producing kindling (Raine, 1978). Also, spontaneous seizures unrelated to a triggering stimulus are rare even in fully kindled animals and are not observed in primates except in those with genetic convulsive tendencies (Racine, 1978). While it is clear from clinical and experimental experience that interictal discharges indicate seizure susceptibility, their long-term or permanent effects on the process of epileptogenesis are not established. The question of the clinical relevance of kindling and the mirror focus can be explored by examining human cases. Such cases must show electrical activity of repetitive spontaneous electrical discharging at intervals over a long time so that the processes of kindling and the mirror focus might be expected to develop. In each case it may be asked: (1) Do findings suggest that secondary epileptogenesis has occurred? (2) Do they persist? (3) Did kindling occur? (4) Did a mirror focus become established?

Case reports and other clinical data question the occurrence of secondary epileptogenesis in human epilepsy. One study (Wilder, King and Schmidt, 1968) found no evidence of progressive changes in epileptiform activity in human cases of persistent seizures with active foci after 5-year periods of observation. Pope *et al.*, (1948) stated that EEG 'mirror foci' are frequently observed in association with unilateral foci but they regularly disappear after the primary epileptogenic focus is removed. In other studies (Falconer and Cavanaugh, 1959; Falconer and Kennedy, 1961; Falconer, Driver and Serefetinides, 1962; Goldensohn, 1964; Van Buren *et al.*, 1975; Goldring and Gregorie, 1984) contralateral spiking also disappeared promptly after removal of the primary foci and did not reappear during several years of follow-up. Three patients were recently reviewed who had a total of 56 years of uncontrolled seizures. Each showed frequent independent discharges from a contralateral area as well as from the area of a single structural brain lesion. In each case after the unilateral primary focus with the histologically verified lesion was removed, the distant focus disappeared as did the seizures (Goldensohn, 1984). Torres and Jacome (1982) state that they were unable to find in the literature concerned with localized resections for epilepsy any case that would be strongly supportive of the concept that secondary epileptogenesis occurs in humans. To my knowledge, there is no convincing documentation of persistent clinical or electrographic seizures, either in lower primates or man, that arise from mirror foci after the primary focus has been removed.

The very frequent focal interictal spiking in benign focal epilepsy of childhood ('sylvian seizures') never results in secondary epileptogenesis. The children are normal between attacks, their seizures are easily controlled and both the clinical and EEG manifestations disappear in adolescence. There is at best only a rough correlation between the amount of interictal epileptiform activity in the EEG at any point in time and the frequency of clinical attacks. Further, cognitive deficits (Bear and Fedio, 1977) and behavioral changes found temporal lobe epilepsy relate to the duration of illness but not to seizure frequency. This suggests that seizures and interictal psychological disturbances (if any) are only indirectly related to epileptiform discharges.

At present, evidence is against the existence of mirror foci capable of producing chronic seizures in man. Clinical evidence is lacking and contralateral apparently independent EEG changes are not persistent. For these reasons, the concept of the mirror focus should have no place in affecting decisions in the treatment of epilepsy. Kindling remains a useful experimental model for studying epilepsy. Observations in man, however, suggest that as with the mirror focus kindling concept currently should not influence decisions in the diagnosis and management of patients with epilepsy.

References

AVOLI, M. and GLOOR, P. (1982) Interaction of cortex and thalamus in spike and wave discharges of feline generalized penicillin epilepsy. *Experimental Neurology,* **64,** 155–173

AYALA, G. F., MATSUMATO, H. and GUMNIT, R. J. (1970) Excitability changes and inhibitory mechanisms in neocortical neurons during seizures. *Journal of Neurophysiology,* **33,** 73–85

BARKER, J. L. and SMITH, T. G. JR (1978) Electrophysical studies of molluscan neurons generating bursting pacemaker potential activity. In *Abnormal Neuronal Discharges,* edited by N. Chalazonitis and M. Boisson, pp. 359–389. New York: Raven Press

BEAR, D. M. and FEDIO, P. (1977) Quantitative analysis of interictal behavior in temporal lobe epilepsy. *Archives of Neurology,* **34,** 454–467

EBERSOLE, J. S. (1977) Initial abnormalities of neuronal responses during epileptogenesis in visual cortex. *Journal of Neurophysiology,* **40,** 514–526

EBERSOLE, J. S. and CHATT, A. B. (1980) The laminar susceptibility of cat visual cortex to penicillin-induced epileptogenesis. *Neurology,* **30,** 355

ELGER, E. C. and SPECKMAN, E. J. (1983) Penicillin-induced epileptic foci in the motor cortex: vertical inhibition. *Electroencephalography and Clinical Neurophysiology,* **56,** 604–622

FALCONER, M. A. and CAVANAUGH, J. B. (1959) Clinico-pathological considerations of temporal lobe epilepsy due to small focal lesions. *Brain,* **82,** 483–504

FALCONER, M. A. and KENNEDY, W. A. (1961) Epilepsy due to small focal temporal lesions bilateral independent spike-discharging foci. *Journal of Neurology, Neurosurgery and Psychiatry,* **24,** 205–212

FALCONER, M. A., DRIVER, M. V. and SEREFETINIDES, E. A. (1962) Temporal lobe epilepsy due to distant lesions: two cases relieved by operation. *Brain,* **85,** 521–534

GLOOR, P. (1979) Generalized epilepsy with spike-and-wave discharge; a reinterpretation of its electrographic and clinical mainfestations. The 1977 William G. Lenox Lecture, American Epilepsy Society. *Epilepsia,* **20,** 571–588

GODDARD, G. V. and DOUGLAS, R. M. (1975) Does the engram of kindling model the engram of long-term daily memory? *Canadian Journal of Neurological Science,* **2,** 385–394

GODDARD, G. V., MCINTRYE, D. C. and LEECH, C. K. (1969) A permanent change in brain function resulting from daily electrical stimulation. *Experimental Neurology,* **25,** 294–330

GODDARD, G. V. (1967) Development of epileptic seizures through brain stimulation at low intensity. *Nature,* **214,** 1020–1021

GOLDENSOHN, E. S. (1969) Discussion: experimental seizure mechanisms. In *Basic Mechanisms of the Epilepsies*, edited by H. H. Jasper, A. A. Ward. Jr. and A. Pope, pp. 289–298. Boston: Little Brown

GOLDENSOHN, E. S. (1975) Initiation and propagation of epileptogenic foci. In *Complex Partial Seizures and Their Treatment,* edited by J. K. Penry and D. Daly, pp. 141–162. New York: Raven Press

GOLDENSOHN, E. S. (1978) Epileptogenesis: recent neurobiological advances. In *Modern Perspectives in Epilepsy,* edited by J. Wada, pp. 172–184. Montreal: Eden Press

GOLDENSOHN, E. S. (1984) The relevance of secondary epileptogenesis to the treatment of epilepsy: kindling and the mirror focus. *Epilepsia* **25** (Suppl. 2), S156–S168

GOLDENSOHN, E. S. and PURPURA, D. P (1963) Intracellular potentials of cortical neurons during focal epileptogenic discharges. *Science,* **193,** 840–842

GOLDENSOHN, E. S. and SALAZAR, A. M. (1985) Temporal and spatial distribution of intracellular potentials during generation and spread of epileptogenic discharges. In *Basic Mechanisms of the Epilepsies*, edited by A. V. Delgado-Escueta, A. A. Ward, Jr and D. M. Woodbury, New York: Raven Press (in press)

GOLDENSOHN, E. S., ZABLOW, L. and SALAZAR, A. M. JR (1977) The penicillin focus. I. Distribution of potential at the cortical surface. *Electroencephalography and Clinical Neurophysiology,* **42,** 480–492

GOLDENSOHN, E. S., ZABLOW, L. and STEIN, B. (1970) Interrelationships of form and latency of spike discharges from small areas of human cortex. *Electroencephalography and Clinical Neurophysiology,* **29,** 32

GOLDRING, S. and GREGORIE, E. M. (1984) Surgical management of epilepsy using epidural recordings to localize the seizure focus: review of 100 cases. *Journal of Neurosurgery,* **60,** 457–466

HARRIS, A. B. and LOCKARD, J. S. (1981) Absence of seizures or minor foci in experimental epilespy after excision of alumina and astrogliotic scar. *Epilepsia,* **22,** 107–122

HOTSON, J. R., SCHWARTZKRION, P. A. and PRINCE, D. A. (1977) Calcium activated after hyperpolarization in hippocampal slices maintained *in vitro. Social Neuroscience Abstracts,* **3,** 218

HOTSON, J. R., PRINCE, D. A. and SCHWARTZKROIN, P. A. (1979) Anomalous inward rectification in hippocampal neurons. *Journal of Neurophysiology,* **42,** 889–895

HUBEL, D. H. and WIESEL, T. N. (1965) Receptive fields and functional architecture in two nonstriate visual areas (18 and 9) of the cat. *Journal of Neurophysiology,* **28,** 229

JOHNSTON, D., HABLITZ, J. J. and WILSON, W. A. (1981) Voltage clamp discloses slow inward current in hippocampal burst-firing neurones. *Nature,* **286,** 391–393

JOHNSTON, D. AND BROWN, T. H. (1982) Giant synaptic potential hypothesis for epileptiform activity. *Science,* **216,** 745–747

KOSTOPOULOS, G., AVOLI, M., PELLEGRINI, A. and GLOOR, P. (1982) Laminar analysis of spindles and of spikes of the spike and wave discharge of feline generalized penicillin epilepsy. *Electroencephalography and Clinical Neurophysiology,* **53,** 1–13

LÜDERS, H., BUSTAMANTE, L. A., ZABLOW, L. and GOLDENSOHN, E. S. (1981) The independence of closely spaced discrete experimental spike foci. *Neurology,* **31,** 846–851

LOWRIE, M. B. and ETTLINGER, G. (1980) The development of independent secondary ('minor') discharge in the monkey: failure to replicate earlier findings. *Epilepsia,* **22,** 107–122

MATSUMATO, H. and AJMONE-MARSAN, C. (1964a) Cortical cellular phenomena in experimental epilepsy: interictal manifestations. *Experimental Neurology,* **9,** 286–304

MATSUMATO, H. and AJMONE-MARSAN, C. (1964b) Cortical cellular phenomena in experimental epilepsy: ictal manifestations. *Experimental Neurology,* **9,** 305–326

MAYERSDORF, A. and SCHMIDT, R. P. (1982) *Secondary Epileptogenesis.* New York: Raven Press

MORRELL, F. (1959) Experimental epilespy in animals. *Archives of Neurology,* **1,** 141–147

MORRELL, F. (1960) Secondary epileptogenic lesions. *Epilepsia,* **1,** 538–560

MORRELL, F. (1969) Physiology and histochemistry of the mirror focus. In *Basic Mechanisms of the Epilepsies,* edited by H. H. Japser, A. A. Ward Jr. and A. Pope, pp. 357–370. Boston: Little, Brown

MORRELL, F. (1979) Human secondary epileptogenic lesions (abstract). *Neurology,* **29,** 558

POLLEN, D. A., REID, K. H. and PEROT, P. (1964) Microelectrode studies of experimental 3/sec wave and spike in the cat. *Electroencephalography and Clinical Neurophysiology,* **17,** 57–67

POLLEN, D. A. (1969) On the generation of neocortical potentials. In *Basic Mechanisms of the Epilepsies,* edited by H. H. Jasper, A. A. Ward, Jr. and A. Pope. Boston: Little, Brown

POPE, A., MORRIS, A. A., JASPER, H., ELLIOT, K. A. C. and PENFIELD, W. (1946) Histochemical and action potential studies on epileptogenic areas of cerebral cortex in man and the monkey. *Research Publications Association for Research into Nervous and Mental Diseases,* **26,** 218–233

PRINCE, D. A. and WILDER, B. J. (1967) Control mechanisms in cortical epileptogenic foci: 'surround' inhibition. *Archives of Neurology,* **16,** 194–202

RACINE, R. (1978) Kindling: the first decade. *Journal of Neurosurgery,* **3,** 234-252

SALAZAR, A. M. (1980) *Penicillin as an Epileptogenic Agent.* PhD Thesis, State University of New York at Sony Brook, June

SCHWARTZKROIN, P. A. and WYLER, A. R. (1980) Mechanisms underlying epileptiform burst discharge. *Annals of Neurology,* **7,** 95–107

SZENTAGOTHAI, J. (1969) Architecture of the cerebral cortex. In *Basic Mechanisms of the Epilepsies,* edited by H. H. Jasper, A. A. Ward Jr., and A. Pope, pp. 13–28. Boston: Little, Brown

TORRES, F. and FRENCH, L. A. (1973) Acute effect of section of the corpus callosum upon 'independent' epileptiform activity. *Acta Neurologica Scandinavica,* **49,** 47–62

TORRES, F. and JACOME, D. (1982) Secondary epileptogenesis in the human. In *Secondary Epileptogenesis,* edited by A. Mayersdorf and R. P. Schmidt. New York: Raven Press

VAN BUREN, J. M., AJMONE–MARSAN, C., MATSUGA, N. and SADOWSKY, D. (1975) Surgery of temporal lobe epilepsy. *Advances in Neurology,* **8,** 155–196

VON BONIN, G. (1969) *Architecture of the Precentral Motor Cortex,* edited by P. Bucy. Urbana: University of Illinois Press

WADA, J. A. (Editor) (1976) *Kindling.* New York: Raven Press

WADA, J. A. (Editor) (1981) *Kindling 2.* New York: Raven Press

WADA, J. A. and OSAWA, T. (1976) Spontaneous recurrent seizure state induced by daily electric amygdaloid stimulation in Senegalese baboons *Papio papio. Neurology,* **26,** 73–86

WADA, J. A., OSAWA, T. and MIZOGUCHI, T. (1976) Recurrent spontaneous seizure state induced by prefrontal kinding in Senegalese baboons *Papio papio.* In *Kindling,* edited by J. A. Wada. New York: Raven Press

WARD. A. A., JR, SCHMIDT, R. P. and THOMAS, L. B. (1959) The hyperexcitable neurone microelectrode studies of chronic epileptic foci in monkey. *Journal of Neurophysiology,* **22,** 285–296

WILDER, B. J. KING, R. L. and SCHMIDT, R. P. (1968) Comparative study of secondary epileptogenesis. *Epilepsia,* **9,** 275–289

WONG, R. K. S. and PRINCE, D. A. (1978) Participation of calcium spikes during intrinsic burst firing in hippocampal neurons. *Brain Research,* **159,** 385–390

WONG, R. K. S. and PRINCE, D. A. (1979) Dendritic mechanisms underlying penicillin-induced epileptiform activity. *Science,* **204,** 1228–1231

ZIPSER, B., CRAIN, S. M. and BORNSTEIN, M. B. (1973) Directly evoked paroxysmal deplorization of mouse hippocampal neurons in synaptically organized explants in long term culture. *Brain Research (Amsterdam),* **60,** 489–495

3
Mechanism of action of antiepileptic drugs

Paolo L. Morselli and Kenneth G. Lloyd

INTRODUCTION

For many years antiepileptic drugs (AEDs) have been considered as a rather non-homogeneous therapeutic class, their chemical, pharmacological or clinical profiles varying considerably from one drug to another. Furthermore, antiepileptic drugs are used to treat a disorder that also cannot be defined as homogeneous in its clinical expressions, but rather identified as several different syndromes whose aetiopathogenetic mechanisms are still poorly defined.

Within this frame it is understandable that today we really do not have a clear picture of the mechanism(s) of action of the various antiepileptic drugs, and we are confronted with a variety of (sometimes conflicting) hypotheses developed over 20–25 years, implying or describing effects of the various drugs on individual synaptic events.

However, in the last five years, thanks both to the development of more refined techniques permitting the study of drug effects and actions, at molecular level and to the recognition and acceptance of the pharmacokinetic concept of 'therapeutic concentrations', a more consistent picture appears to be emerging, together with an increased knowledge of the biochemical alterations underlying epileptic phenomena.

FUNDAMENTAL FACTORS REGARDING CENTRAL NERVOUS SYSTEM ACTIVITY AND POSSIBLE INTERACTIONS WITH DRUGS

Ionic factors

It is a fundamental tenet of neurophysiology that hyperpolarization and hypopolarization of cell membranes result from alterations in ion conductance via specific, neurotransmitter receptor-mediated ion channels (ionophores).

Chloride ion conductance increases are the result of stimulation of gamma-aminobutyric acid (GABA) and glycine receptors which are the major inhibitory (in terms of neuronal activity) neurotransmitters in the brain and spinal cord (Curtis, 1979; Krnjevic, 1974; Phillis, 1970). Usually, the opening of the chloride ionophore results in hyperpolarization, but this is not universal, especially outside the central nervous system (Gallagher and Shinnick-Gallagher, 1983; Simmonds, 1984). Thus, the chloride ionophore, the opening of which results in decreased neuronal activity, is a potential and desirable site of drug action, especially when disinhibition is the underlying basis of the development of the focal discharge, and especially when it occurs in foci deficient in GABA synthesis (Lloyd *et al.*, 1981a).

Conversely, membrane depolarization and increased neuronal activity is associated with an opening of sodium and potassium ion channels (Krnjevic, 1974; Phillis, 1970). Together with disinhibition, increased excitation is a basis for abnormally increased neuronal activity and is also probably responsible for the spread of seizure activity. These ionophores are also potential sites for antiepileptic drug action in controlling membrane excitability. The calcium channel is also a potential site for antiepileptic drug action, although its role in hyperpolarization or depolarization of central neurones is not completely understood; it may vary between synapses.

Other ion-dependent events are also potential targets for drug action. Neurotransmitter release, for example, is both potassium and calcium dependent; in the hypothetical case of excess excitation due to overabundant release of excitatory neurotransmitter, a mechanism of action involving these ion channels is appealing.

The Na^+–K^+ ATPases are also potential ion-related targets for antiepileptic drug action. These enzymes serve as the 'electrogenic' pumps of the cells, maintaining ionic gradients and membrane stability. Drug action on this pump would be desirable in instances of sodium–potassium imbalance or other causes of membrane hyperexcitability. In addition to its role in maintaining ionic balances, a functional Na^+–K^+ ATPase is necessary for neurotransmitter reuptake, a major means of inactivation of synaptically released transmitter. As all known uptake mechanisms are similar in this regard, it is unlikely that a compound could have a sufficiently high specificity to affect these ATPases and alter neurotransmitter uptake in a selective manner.

Obviously, many other ionic sites are possible for antiepileptic drug action. Such targets include active sites on those synthesizing and metabolizing enzymes for both neurotransmitters and for energy production.

Synapses and membranes

As emphasized above in the section on ionic factors, one of the end results of neurotransmission is an alteration in ionic permeability of neuronal membranes. However, modulation of membrane depolarization can be achieved by mechanisms other than those which have direct action at the ionophores. Such actions can generally be divided into those which alter specific aspects of neurotransmission and those which are associated with a membrane-stabilizing action.

In the latter case the principle involved is the modification of the neuronal plasma membranes to a state of relative insensitivity to depolarization. This action is mediated by inhibition of the large transient increase in the permeability of the membrane to sodium ions (Taylor, 1959) and to calcium ions (Bernard and Bohm, 1965; Ritchie and Cohen, 1975). Such an action of a compound is referred to as a 'local anaesthetic effect', and it is difficult to envisage how a specificity for epileptic tissue could be achieved without resulting in a similar action on other excitable membranes (such as cardiac pacemaker cells). However, this was the original hypothesis for the mechanism of action of several antiepileptic drugs (Bernard and Bohm, 1965).

In contrast to the membrane-stabilizing action, it is possible to obtain a specificity of drug action for individual synaptic events. For presynaptic mechanisms the most accessible targets are processes which regulate the synthesis, release, uptake and metabolism of neurotransmitters (for postsynaptic receptor-mediated events see section on receptors. Such an approach has been shown to be efficacious for the development of antidepressant drugs, for the inhibition of both neurotransmitter uptake (noradrenaline, serotonin, dopamine) and metabolism (monoamine oxidase). Such an approach should also be applicable to the development of antiepileptic drugs. Indeed, specific GABA uptake inhibitors which are capable of entering the brain are anticonvulsant in animal models of epilepsy (Krosgaard-Larsen *et al.*, 1981; Löscher, 1981a and c).

Inhibition of GABA metabolism at the GABA-transaminase step is also an effective means of anticonvulsant action in animal models (Gale, 1984; Gale and Iadarola, 1980; Löscher, 1981a and b; Worms and Lloyd, 1981) and preliminary clinical data with gamma-vinyl-GABA indicate an antiepileptic effect (Rimmer and Richens, 1984). A possible limiting factor in the use of agents enhancing the availability of endogenous GABA is that in some forms of epilepsy the synthesis of GABA may be severely impaired (Lloyd *et al.*, 1981a). In such a case, either postsynaptic action at GABA receptors (see below) or a non-GABAergic mechanism of action is necessary.

Presynaptic actions of antiepileptic drugs at non-GABAergic synapses are also a possibility. In addition to GABA (the major inhibitory neurotransmitter in the brain), other neuronal systems (such as dopamine) also have an inhibitory influence on cell excitability. Experimental evidence indicates an antiepileptic action on noradrenergic neurones by carbamazepine (Morselli *et al.*, 1978). Other appealing potential presynaptic sites of action for antiepileptic drugs include the synthesis and release of excitatory transmitters such as aspartate, glutamate, a host of neuropeptides (Henriksen *et al.*, 1983; Meldrum and Menini, 1981), and arachidonic acid metabolites (leukotrienes, thromboxanes, prostaglandins).

An additional possibility for presynaptic action of antiepileptic drugs could be inhibition of the production and/or release of endogenous epileptogenic agent. Although still in its initial stages, data point to quinolinic acid as a possible endogenous epileptogen; details on its synthesis, release and relation to seizure induction are still preliminary (French *et al.*, 1984; Schwarcz and Foster, 1984).

Receptors

Affinity for a neurotransmitter receptor site is potentially the most specific action of a drug. For a given neurotransmitter there are multiple receptor subtypes (such as for GABA, glutamate, noradrenaline, dopamine, opiates, adenosine), each of which has its own pharmacological profile. This confers a greater specificity on postsynaptic as compared to presynaptic events. In contrast, for ionic mechanisms an ionophore may subserve different neurotransmitter receptors (for example, the chloride ionophore for GABA and glycine); however, each receptor subtype apparently controls only one ionophore, or may plausibly mediate non-ionophore-linked events such as energy production.

For the mechanisms of action of antiepileptic drugs, an agonistic or mimetic effect at inhibitory receptors and an antagonistic action at excitatory receptors are the most appealing prospects. With the inhibitory receptors the major emphasis has been directed towards the GABA A receptor, as the GABA B receptor has been demonstrated only relatively recently (Hill and Bowery, 1981), and baclofen (the prototypic GABA B agonist) has a very limited spectrum of anticonvulsant action (Worms and Lloyd, 1981). Highly specific agonists for GABA A receptors all have an anticonvulsant action in a variety of animal models for epilepsy, and compounds without inherent toxicity are active in all animal models tested [(including kindling, chemical and sensory stimuli in rodents, penicillin focus in the cat, photosensitive *Papio papio* (Cepeda *et al.*, 1982; Joy, Albertson and Stark, 1984; Löscher, 1982; Meldrum, 1981; Worms and Lloyd, 1981; Worms *et al.*, 1982)]. The potent and immediate induction of seizures following blockade of GABA A receptors by bicuculline, or of its subunits by picrotoxin, by convulsant barbiturates, and by convulsant benzodiazepines (Haefely *et al.*, 1981; Lloyd *et al.*, 1983a; Olsen, 1982; Schlosser and Franco, 1979) strongly suggest that GABA A receptors play an essential role in the control of cerebral excitability and are a highly desirable target for antiepileptic drug action.

In addition to the GABA recognition site, the GABA receptor macromolecular complex contains other subunits which are likely targets for antiepileptic drug action. These subunits have in common the facilitation and/or prolongation of GABA-receptor-mediated opening of chloride ionophores. These subunits include recognition sites for drug classes such as the barbiturates and the anxiolytic anticonvulsants (such as benzodiazepines) (Barker, Owen and Segal, 1984; Barker *et al.*, 1984; Braestrup, Nielsen and Honore, 1984; Haefely *et al.*, 1981; Olsen, 1982; Skolnick and Paul, 1981; Squires and Saederup, 1982). The high specificity of these different subunits enables sophisticated and flexible pharmacological manipulation of GABA-receptor-mediated transmission and thus of cerebral excitability and the control of seizures.

Other inhibitory neurotransmitter receptors are less evident as sites of action for antiepileptic drugs. Glycine receptors are mainly distributed in the brainstem and spinal cord although they coexist with GABA receptors in the substantia nigra (Lloyd *et al.*, 1983b), a region involved in the antiepileptic action of certain compounds such as valproic acid (Gale and Iadarola, 1984). However, to date no anticonvulsant compound has been identified which has an agonist action at glycine receptors, although the potent convulsant strychnine is an antagonist at these receptors (Curtis, Duggan and Johnston, 1971).

A potential site of antiepileptic drug action is the dopamine receptor, as apomorphine is reported to have an anticonvulsant effect in generalized photosensitive epilepsy (Quesney, 1981). However, the role of dopamine receptors in different models of epilepsy is complex, as dopamine receptor blockers prevent bicuculline-induced seizures (Worms and Lloyd, 1979). Although not generally recognized as a neurotransmitter, adenosine is a ligand for a high-affinity (A1) binding site in the brain, and purinergic maintenance of inhibitory tone has been proposed (Williams, 1983). It is very possible that this A1 site is important for both the induction of convulsions (for example, by theophylline) and for participating in the action of some antiepileptics. Carbamazepine displaces ligands for the A1 site at concentrations (25–50 μM) well within the therapeutic range (Skerritt, Davies and Johnston, 1983; Skerritt, Johnston and Chow, 1983; Weir *et al.*, 1984). However, it is still not clear whether carbamazepine is an agonist or partial agonist at this A1 site.

Within the overall concept that seizures are due to a loss of inhibition and/or an excess of excitation, a logical mechanism for antiepileptic drug action would be as an antagonist at one of the excitatory receptors such as the aspartate receptor or one of the subclasses of glutamate receptors (NMDA, glutamate, kainate, etc.). Data from both rodent and primate models show an anticonvulsant action of compounds in this class; however, problems of absorption and toxicity must be overcome before the therapeutic potential of this site of action can be realized (Czueczwar and Meldrum, 1982).

It is entirely possible that some antiepileptic drugs are acting at receptors for neurotransmitters as yet unidentified. Thus the benzodiazepines have a highly specific action at a binding site (see below) and 'agonists' (anticonvulsant), 'antagonists' and 'inverse agonists' (convulsant), exist for this site (Meldrum and Braestrup, 1984; Möhler, 1984). It is now well-established that this binding site modulates the GABA-receptor, mediated chloride ionophore (Barker, Owen and Segal, 1984; Barker *et al.*, 1984; Simmonds, 1984), and there is mounting evidence that an endogenous ligand exists for this binding site (Guidotti, 1984). Diphenylhydantoin may also interact with as yet unidentified neurotransmitters, as this antiepileptic binds to a site on brain membranes with a high specificity and affinity which apparently does not correlate with any known receptor (Burnham *et al.*, 1981; Shah, Chambon and Guidotti, 1981).

Drug–brain distribution

It is generally assumed that a drug, in order to exert its effect, must interact with a given component (protein, lipoprotein, etc.) of cellular membranes, a component usually defined as a 'receptor' or 'binding site'. By such an interaction with membrane proteins, drugs may enhance or depress the function which is linked to that given 'binding site'. The specificity or selectivity of a given drug toward a given component of cellular membranes is usually conditioned by its steric tridimensional configuration. However, before reaching its 'site of action', a drug must undergo a long journey through various body compartments and pass several biological membranes. Depending on the characteristics of the drug, the membrane passage may take place by either 'active transport' or by 'passive diffusion'. In the case of antiepileptic drugs, all distribute into various organs and tissues by passive (gradient-dependent) diffusion. In other words, their distribution is regulated by the liposolubility intrinsic to the drug and by regional blood flow.

It is also assumed that all antiepileptic drugs are rather liposoluble compounds, and that the drug–brain concentrations are rather homogeneous and in equilibrium with the drug plasma concentrations during steady state conditions. In general, the brain-to-plasma ratios for various antiepileptic drugs may vary from 0.1 to 0.2 for valproic acid, from 0.4 to 1.5 for phenobarbital, phenytoin and carbamazepine, and from 5 to 10 for benzodiazepines (Houghton *et al.*, 1975; Morselli *et al.*, 1977; Morselli, unpublished observation; Morselli and Franco-Morselli, 1980; Sherwin, Eisen and Sokolowski, 1973; Vajda *et al.*, 1974). It has been shown, however, at experimental and clinical levels, that antiepileptic drugs do not distribute in the brain in a homogeneous manner, and that important differences among various structures may exist which are linked to vascularity and time. During the early phase of distribution into the brain (corresponding to the absorption peak), the liposolubility of the compound, the regional blood flow and the vascularity of various cerebral areas do play a major role. Higher drug concentrations are found in grey matter structures such as cortical grey matter, thalamus, mesencephalon, and olfactory bulb. At a later time, factors such as 'binding to' or 'affinity for' the various tissue components play a more important role. Higher concentrations are observed in cortical white matter and in subcortical areas such as corpus callosum, pons and bulb. This pattern of distribution has been observed in the rat and cat for both acidic compounds such as phenobarbitone and phenytoin and 'neutral' compounds such as diazepam and progabide (Ferrandes *et al.*, 1984; Garrigou *et al.*, 1984; Morselli *et al.*, 1973; Placidi *et al.*, 1976; Roth and Barlow, 1965; Van der Kleijn *et al.*, 1973). These laboratory observations suggesting a blood flow-dependent, non-homogeneous brain distribution of antiepileptic drugs have been confirmed at a clinical level in a series of ongoing studies conducted on discrete human brain specimens, derived from tumoral and non-tumoral epileptic neurosurgery patients (Munari *et al.*, 1980, 1982; Morselli *et al.*, unpublished observation). Brain concentrations and brain: plasma ratios of phenobarbitone, phenytoin, carbamazepine, valproic acid and diazepam not only varied considerably from one patient to another but also varied up to 2–4-fold (100–200%) in neighbouring brain areas from the same patient. In general, brain antiepileptic drug concentrations tended to be higher in normal than in pathological zones. As one would expect (Rapport *et al.*, 1975), tumoral tissues had lower antiepileptic drug levels, but areas defined by stereo EEG as 'epileptogenic' or 'irritative' (*see* Munari and Bancaud, Chapter 14 of this volume) also had antiepileptic drug concentrations lower than 'normal' tissue specimens. The low antiepileptic drug concentrations (even in the presence of 'therapeutic' plasma levels) in 'epileptogenic' areas might partially explain the 'resistance' to pharmacological treatment in these patients. Furthermore, these findings appear to be in agreement with recent positron emission tomography (PET) observations, suggesting that in some epileptic patients, during interictal periods, blood flow and metabolism are lower in focal areas than in surrounding tissues (*see* Engel, Chapter 13 of this volume).

In conclusion, antiepileptic drug–brain distribution depends on each drug's intrinsic liposolubility; it occurs by passive (gradient-dependent) diffusion, and is blood flow-dependent. The differential distribution pattern may partially explain the variability of clinical response for both therapeutic and toxic effects.

AVAILABLE EVIDENCE ON POSSIBLE MODIFICATIONS OF FUNDAMENTAL FACTORS IN SEIZURES AND EPILEPSY

Fundamental biological alterations in animal models for epilepsy

Our knowledge of possible alterations in fundamental biological mechanisms in different models of epilepsy is obviously limited to the number of experiments which have been performed. Furthermore, in *no* model have most of the self-evident experiments related to inhibitory and excitatory neurotransmission been performed.

Several rodent models and one primate model (allylglycine in *Papio papio*) (Cepeda *et al.*, 1982) are based upon specific pharmacologically induced alterations in synaptic function. Examples include the disruption of normal GABAergic tone by inhibition of synthesis (allyglycine and several hydrazide derivatives of pyridoxal phosphate), the direct blockade of receptors (by bicuculline), and the disruption of the chloride ionophore opening either directly (picrotoxin) or by associated allosteric binding sites (convulsant barbiturates and convulsant benzodiazepines); all result in the rapid onset of a seizure state. Similarly, inhibition by strychnine of the glycine receptor mediation of the chloride ionophore results in convulsions (see above, and also Orlowski, Reingold and Stanley, 1977; Tapia, 1974; Wood, Kurylo and Peesker, 1978). A potentially relevant observation is the seizure state induced by opiate peptides when administered intraventricularly (Henriksen *et al.*, 1983; Siggins, 1984). Although interesting, such animal models do not yield any real insight into possible pathogenic factors in human epilepsy.

Of greater interest are genetic animal models of epilepsy and epileptogenic agents which induce convulsions by irritation or cell loss. In those models the most thorough investigations have been performed on the GABA system, with catecholaminergic systems also receiving some attention. At the present time, however, hyperactivity of excitatory neurotransmission in animal models of epilepsy has yet to be demonstrated.

As far as the GABA system is concerned, a marked decrease in L-glutamic acid decarboxylase (the enzyme synthesizing GABA from glutamate) has been noted in such diverse models as the cobalt focus in the rat cortex (Altamura *et al.*, 1978; Emson and Joseph, 1975; Ross and Craig, 1981a), the penicillin focus in the cat cortex (Gottesfeld and Elazar. 1975) and the alumina gel focus in the monkey cortex (Bakay and Harris, 1981; Ribak *et al.*, 1979). These findings strongly suggest a decrease in the ability to synthesize GABA at the site of epileptic activity. This hypothesis is supported by parallel decreases in GABA levels (Bakay and Harris, 1981; Gottesfeld and Elazar, 1972; Ross and Craig, 1981b; Van Gelder and Courtois, 1972) and GABA uptake (Balcar *et al.*, 1978; Ross and Craig, 1981b), indicating that GABA nerve terminals have probably degenerated under these conditions. In the alumina gel model in the monkey cortex a decrease in the number of GABA A receptors has also been noted (Bakay and Harris, 1981). These findings of a decrease in glutamic acid decarboxylase levels and in GABA A binding at the focus have also been found in human foci (Lloyd *et al.*, 1981a).

In the cobalt focus other neurotransmitter systems are also likely to be involved, notably noradrenergic innervation. Thus, decrease in noradrenaline and elevation of its metabolite 3-methoxy-4-hydroxy-phenylethyleneglycol (MHPG) occur (Chauvel, Trottier and Bancaud, 1985; Morselli *et al.*, 1978; Scatton *et al.*, 1981). The observation, however, that alterations in the function of serotonin and acetylcholine neurons also occur in the same foci (Morselli *et al.*, 1978; Scatton *et al.*, 1981) questions the specificity of such changes.

In genetic models of convulsions, decreased GABA synthesis, GABA A binding and potassium-stimulated GABA release have been demonstrated in sound sensitive (DBA/2 strain) mice (Al-Ani *et al.*, 1970; Hertz *et al.*, 1974; Horton, Prestwick and Meldrum, 1982; Ticku, 1979), although no alterations in GABA levels have been documented in epileptic tissue from dogs (Van Gelder *et al.*, 1980) or from photosensitive *Papio papio* (Hansen *et al.*, 1973). In the latter model, however, decreased GABA levels in the cerebrospinal fluid appear to correlate with the photosensitive state of individual animals. Under such conditions metabolites of serotonin (5-HIAA), dopamine (HVA) and noradrenaline (MHPG) are unaltered (Naquet, Lloyd and Scatton, unpublished observation). In genetically epileptic mice, levels of biogenic amines are similar to those in non-epileptic strains (Al-Ani *et al.*, 1970); in epileptic rats, however, noradrenaline may play an important role either in the pathogenesis of the model and/or in the mechanism of action of some anticonvulsant drugs (Jobe and Laird, 1981).

Because of insufficient biochemical data, no definitive statements can as yet be made about the kindling model of epilepsy. However, amygdaloid kindling does not alter GABA levels or GABA A binding sites in several brain regions (Fabisiak and Schwark, 1982; Kalichman, 1982). Benzodiazepine binding in the hippocampus is apparently specifically increased (McNamara, Peper and Patrone, 1980; McNamara *et al.*, 1980). Alterations in monoaminergic neuron activity, especially an increase in hypothalamic noradrenaline levels, have been demonstrated in amygdala-kindled animals (Burnham *et al.*, 1981). However, what is most impressive is the lack of consistent changes after establishment of kindled seizures (Kalichman, 1982). For example, noradrenaline levels and synthesis in most brain regions (including amygdala and hippocampus) and striatal dopamine levels and amygdala dopamine synthesis are unaltered in amygdala-kindled rats (Blackwood, 1981; Burnham *et al.*, 1981). Thus, in the kindling model of epilepsy there is as yet little biochemical support for the behavioural observations suggesting that in various animal models noradrenergic tone is important in determinating the convulsant threshold (Crunelli *et al.*, 1981; Kalichman, 1982). The kindling model in epilepsy therefore stands in contrast to the cobalt model and some genetic models of epilepsy (see above).

'Epileptic' cultured cells

Mouse spinal cord cells exhibit convulsive activity consisting of paroxysmal depolarizing events when grown in tissue culture and exposed in the bath medium to convulsive agents such as picrotoxin (Barker and MacDonald, 1980), bicuculline, penicillin, pentetrazole, strychnine and 4-aminopyrine (Barker *et al.*, 1981, 1984). The convulsive activity evoked by these agents appears to be at least partially due to intense excitatory synaptic activity, the neurotransmitters for which are as yet unidentified. On an ionic level, the convulsant activity is associated with blockade of the transient activations of potassium conductances, resulting in the enhancement of cell excitability. It has been proposed that these transient potassium conductance mechanisms rectify the membrane near spike threshold, thus modulating spike frequency, and are thus a site for opposing actions of convulsant and anticonvulsant compounds (Barker, Owen and Segal, 1984).

Neurotransmitter alterations in epileptic patients

Available evidence of possible modifications of fundamental factors in epileptic patients are mainly derived from measurements of neurotransmitters, the metabolites of these neurotransmitters, and the enzymes which regulate their synthesis and degradation; this data comes from lumbar and ventricular CSF of treated and untreated patients and from brain specimens obtained from epileptic patients undergoing neurosurgery for intractable epilepsy. A series of reports concern observations on brain monoamine metabolites in lumbar and/or ventricular CSF of treated and untreated epileptic patients (Bossi *et al.*, 1981; Chadwick, Jenner and Reynolds, 1977; Garelis and Sourkes, 1974; Papeschi *et al.*, 1972; Shaywitz, Cohen and Bowers, 1975; Young *et al.*, 1980).

On the whole, the results of various studies are not consistent; there is no evidence at all to suggest a primary alteration of monoamine function in patients suffering from either generalized or partial seizures. However, a significant reduction of 5-HIAA (5-hydroxyindoleacetic acid) CSF concentrations, without concomitant modifications of HVA levels, has been observed in infantile spasms, suggesting an abnormal 5-HT (serotonin) function in this syndrome (Silverstein and Johnston, 1984). Within this perspective it is interesting to recall that serotoninergic mechanisms may be important for the regulation of ACTH release from the pituitary. An alteration of 5-HT function is also recognized to be present in myoclonus and progressive myoclonal epilepsy (Airaksinen and Leino, 1982; Van Woert and Hwang, 1981).

An epileptic syndrome which is apparently related to a deficit in cortical dopaminergic transmission is epileptic photosensitivity. Specific dopaminergic agonists, such as apomorphine, block the photosensitive response without modifying the spontaneous spike and wave activity (Quesney, 1981; Quesney and Reader, 1984).

Both an increase (Sherwin and Van Gelder, 1984) and a decrease (Chauvel, Trottier and Bancaud, 1985) in tyrosine hydroxylase activity in epileptic brain specimens have been recently described. A consistent finding in both studies was a decrease in the alpha-1 noradrenergic binding sites in such tissue. A reduction in GABA lumbar CSF levels has been observed in a variety of adult and paediatric epileptic patients (Airaksinen and Leino, 1982; Enna *et al.*, 1977; Manyam *et al.*, 1980; Schmidt and Löscher, 1981; Wood *et al.*, 1979) and the results appear to be rather consistent, suggesting reduced GABA function in most epileptic syndromes. An increased glutamate CSF level has been described by Plum (1974).

A series of studies attempting to define possible alterations of transmitter amino acid content in epileptic tissues has led to inconsistent results (McGeer, McGeer and Wada, 1971; Perry and Hansen, 1981; Perry *et al.*, 1975; Tower, 1960; Van Gelder, Sherwin and Rasmussen, 1972); an exception was the very low GABA levels in cortical material from a vitamin B_6-deficient patient who died in status epilepticus (Lott *et al.*, 1978). Several methodological problems may be the causes of the controversial findings. More recently Lloyd *et al.* (1981a, 1981b, 1983a, 1984a) reported evidence for an alteration of GABA functions in a number of epileptic patients undergoing neurosurgery because of drug-resistant epilepsy.

Brain specimens derived from areas defined by stereoelectroencephalography as normal, epileptogenic, lesional and irritative (see Munari and Bancaud, Chapter 14 of this volume) were analyzed, and a significant reduction of glutamic acid decarboxylase activity was observed in the epileptogenic zones when compared to normal areas of the same patients in about 60% of the cases. Furthermore, a reduction in 3H-GABA binding was also noticed, whereas no modifications were found for GABA-T activity and 3H-kainic acid binding. These results have been confirmed in a subsequent study where, together with a reduction of GABA function, a trend towards an increase in glutamate levels (Rougier *et al.*, 1984) and glutamate dehydrogenase (GDH) activity (Lloyd *et al.*, 1984) was observed. At variance with these findings on glutamic acid decarboxylase are the results of McGeer, McGeer and Wada (1971) and Sherwin and Van Gelder (1985). The latter, analyzing brain specimens from temporal, frontal and occipital cortex, identified by electrocorticography as 'spiking' and 'not spiking' areas, observed a significant increase in glutamic acid dehydrogenase (GDH) but no modification in glutamic acid decarboxylase or GABA-T and glutamine synthetase (GS) activities. Different methodological approaches could explain the different findings. An increase in glutamine synthetase was noticed in patients with focal seizures whose syndromes were characterized by proliferation of astrocytes (Sherwin and Van Gelder, 1985).

LIKELY MECHANISM OF ACTION OF SPECIFIC ANTIEPILEPTIC DRUGS

Phenytoin (PHT)

Among antiepileptic drugs, phenytoin is undoubtedly one of the most studied compounds; a very large body of data is available on its effects on excitable and non-excitable tissues (Woodbury, 1980a, 1982). However, it is still unclear which of the various effects ascribed to phenytoin are relevant or even related to its anticonvulsant action. Very recent data suggest that most of the previously proposed mechanisms are rather non-specific and probably not relevant to its antiepileptic effect.

While a consensus regarding phenytoin's action exists at the neurophysiological level, several hypotheses exist at biochemical or molecular levels. These are an effect on sodium; an effect on membrane transport components; an effect on calcium fluxes; an effect on brain biogenic amines such as 5-HT, norepinephrine and acetylcholine; and an effect on brain amino acids and/or the GABA receptor ionophore complex.

At the neurophysiological level, phenytoin elevates the membrane potential, reduces conduction velocity and spike amplitude, reduces or abolishes repetitive firing, suppresses bursting activity, and inhibits or blocks post-tetanic potentiation (PTP) (Esplin, 1957; Johnston and Ayala, 1975; MacDonald and McLean, 1982; Woodbury, 1980a, 1982).

The 'stabilizing effect' of phenytoin on excitable neuronal membranes is thought to explain its block of post-tetanic potentiation, which has been considered the basis for its suppressive effect on local seizure discharge and for the inhibition of the propagation of sustained seizure activity (Morrel, Bradley and Ptashne, 1959; Wilder, 1969; Wilder and Schmidt, 1965). Phenytoin may have a facilitatory effect on Purkinje cell discharge in the cerebellum (Julien and Halpren, 1972). Phenytoin has been found to alter the threshold for initiation of seizure discharge in the cerebral cortex, hippocampus, amygdala and anterior-dorsal nucleus of the thalamus (ADNT) but not in other areas (Albright, 1983; Aston and Domino, 1961; Delgado and Mihailovic, 1956; Schallek and Kuehn, 1963). Furthermore, the thresholds for electroshock, metrazol, picrotoxin and strychnine-induced convulsions are not elevated by phenytoin – on the contrary they may even be lowered (Woodbury, 1982).

Studies on cultured neurons have shown that at concentrations over 2 μg/ml phenytoin reduces or blocks the spontaneous activity of the cultured cells (MacDonald and McLean, 1982). *In vivo* however, phenytoin does not appear to interfere (at therapeutic concentrations) with the normal function of excitable tissues (Morrell, Bradley and Ptashne, 1959; Wilder and Bruni, 1982; Woodbury, 1982).

At a biochemical level the first hypothesis was that phenytoin interferes with sodium transport (Woodbury, 1955). A number of papers today indicate that phenytoin does significantly decrease the passive sodium influx in excitable tissue by blocking sodium channels in a manner similar to that exerted by local anaesthetics and tetradotoxin (Lewin and Bleck, 1971; Perry, McKinney and De Weer, 1978; Pincus, 1972; Rawson and Pincus, 1968; Woodbury, 1955, 1980a, 1982). The block of passive sodium movements which occurs during depolarization is, according to the same authors, the primary action of phenytoin which, through this mechanism, inhibits the electrical activity of excitable tissues. According to

Courtney and Etter (1983), phenytoin selectively blocks the inactive form of closed sodium channels, thus giving the drug a capacity for selective action in depolarized tissues. On other tissues phenytoin appears to affect the active transport of sodium by increasing the membrane permeability to sodium through a stimulation of Na–K ATPase activity (Lewin and Bleck, 1971; Woodbury, 1955, 1982); although this effect is also observed with the inactive metabolite 5-(4, hydroxyphenyl)-5-phenylhydantoin (HPPH) (Seigel and Goodwin, 1972); it therefore does not appear to be specific.

Recently MacDonald and McLean (1982) observed that the effects of phenytoin on sodium influx in cultured cell neurons are evident only at high drug concentrations – well above the so-called 'therapeutic range'. It appears, as a consequence, that the relevance of the effect of phenytoin on sodium transport (which for many years has been considered the basis of the mechanism of action of the drug) for its anticonvulsant and antiepileptic effect is today questionable.

A second hypothesis concerns the effects of phenytoin on calcium fluxes. Several reports clearly document an effect of phenytoin on calcium (Ca^{2+}) influx across cellular and subcellular presynaptic terminal membranes (Baker and Blaustein, 1968; Blaustein and Wiesmann, 1970; Hasbany, Pincus and Lee, 1974; Lowe *et al.*, 1976; Pincus and Lee, 1973; Sohn and Ferrendelli, 1973, 1976). Apparently phenytoin blocks the initial calcium (Ca^{2+}) entry which occurs through sodium channels; it also reduces the late Ca^{2+} entry into presynaptic axon terminals which is responsible for neurotransmitter release during repetitive stimulation (Hasbany, Pincus and Lee, 1974; Pincus and Lee, 1973). Still under debate is whether such an effect on Ca^{2+} is due to a primary effect of phenytoin on sodium influx, or whether the drug interacts competitively with calcium ions at cell membranes and presynaptic axonal endings, thereby inhibiting Ca^{2+}-dependent processes such as neurotransmitter release and membrane sodium conductance. According to Woodbury (1982) the primary effect is through a reduction in sodium influx, the direct effect being observed only at 'toxic' concentrations.

More recently it has been shown that phenytoin may block calcium-dependent phosphorylation of synaptosomal proteins involved in the synthesis of neurotransmitters, the action antagonizing the activation of a vesicle-associated protein kinase by a calcium–calmodulin complex (DeLorenzo, 1980). These effects of phenytoin on presynaptic calcium fluxes may also explain some of the endocrine effects of the drug (Woodbury, 1982) as well as some of its effects on neurotransmitter release and protein synthesis. Whether they are relevant to the anticonvulsant effect remains to be demonstrated.

As for the effect on sodium transport, moreover, the above-mentioned phenomena are manifest only at concentrations well above those which are 'therapeutic'. At phenytoin concentrations capable of reducing repetitive firing in cultured cell neurons yet not suppressing the spontaneous cell activity, no effect on sodium or calcium fluxes could be observed (MacDonald and McLean, 1982). As a consequence, the mechanism by which phenytoin reduces or blocks repetitive firing is probably not linked to its effects on cation transport. The effect of phenytoin on calcium fluxes and sodium transport is probably the basis of the drug's capability to inhibit the accumulation of cAMP and cGMP which occurs after depolarization of excitable tissue (Ferrendelli, 1980; Ferrendelli and Kinscherf, 1979; Study, 1980).

Phenytoin could exert a direct effect on membrane components; the drug interacts with brain proteins and phospholipids, increasing several-fold the binding of calcium ions to dipalmitoyl and dioleoyl lecithins (Goldberg and Todoroff, 1973,

1976). Such an interaction with membrane proteins and phospholipids could underlie the effect of phenytoin on cation transport as well as on Na–K ATPase (Woodbury, 1982). Furthermore, according to Carnay and Grundfest (1974), phenytoin could bind to hydrophobic complexes of the excitable membrane, thus increasing the hydrophobic forces within it and enhancing the tendency of the membrane to remain in its resting configuration.

The available data on possible effects of phenytoin on biogenic amines are quite fragmentary, and the relevance to its anticonvulsant action is difficult to interpret. The anticonvulsant activity of phenytoin may be reduced significantly by a depletion of brain monoamines (Meyer and Frey, 1973; see also Woodbury, 1980a; Crunelli, Cervo and Samanin, 1981). On this basis it was postulated that part of the anticonvulsant action of phenytoin might be mediated through an effect on either 5-HT, norepinephrine or dopamine systems via 'an enhancement of the inhibitory tone' in the central nervous system.

An increase in brain serotonin (5-HT) following phenytoin administration has been found in brain of experimental animals by Bonnycastle, Giarman and Paasonen (1957) and Chase, Kats and Kopin (1969). The significance of such an observation is still uncertain, as is the rise in CSF 5-hydroxyindoleacetic acid (5-HIAA) described by Chadwick, Jenner and Reynolds (1977) in epileptic patients with toxic phenytoin plasma levels. More recently De Boer, Stoof and Van Duij (1982) observed, at therapeutic concentrations, that phenytoin inhibits the release of 5-HT from rat cortical slices. Phenytoin inhibits the calcium-dependent release of norepinephrine (NE) in brain slices, acts as a non-competitive inhibitor of norepinephrine uptake (De Boer, Stoof and Van Duij, 1982; Hadfield, 1972; Hadfield and Boykin, 1974; Pincus and Lee, 1973; Weinberger, Nichlas and Berl, 1976), has an inhibitory effect on monoamine oxidase activity (Azzaro, Gutrecht and Smith, 1973) and may also increase the turnover rate of norepinephrine (Airaksinen, 1983). Phenytoin is reported to increase dopamine uptake in the hypothalamus and inhibit uptake in the caudate (Hadfield, 1972). Most of the above data have been obtained at high or toxic drug concentrations. Nevertheless, there is very little evidence that the above-mentioned systems play an important direct role in the therapeutic action of phenytoin, although the effects on the dopaminergic system could explain some of the drug's side-effects.

The possible effect of phenytoin on the cholinergic system has received very little attention. According to Bianchi, Beani and Bertelli (1975), phenytoin reduces the abnormally high cortical outflow of acetylcholine induced by seizures in guinea-pigs. Whether this is a direct effect on the presynaptic release of neurotransmitter or a secondary response to reduced paroxysmal neuronal activity was not elucidated.

There is increasing evidence that phenytoin exerts a variety of actions within the GABA synapse and the GABA macromolecular receptor complex at concentrations which are relevant to its therapeutic effect. An increase in GABA brain concentrations in experimental animals subsequent to phenytoin treatment has been reported by several authors (Bhattacharya, Kishor and Saxena, 1964; Saad, El-Masry and Scott, 1972; Vernadakis and Woodbury, 1960) together with a modest inhibitory effect on succinic semialdehyde dehydrogenase (SSAD) (Sawaya, Horton and Meldrum, 1975) and a decrease in glutamic acid brain concentrations (Vernadakis and Woodbury, 1960). Phenytoin may also antagonize the isoniazide-induced depletion of GABA in mouse brain (Saad, Horton and Meldrum, 1972).

These effects of phenytoin are substantiated by neurophysiological observations: a prolongation of the GABA-mediated IPSP and enhancement of both recurrent inhibition and postsynaptic inhibition have been described in invertebrate synapses and in pyramidal cortical cells (Ayala *et al.*, 1977a and b; Ayala and Johnston, 1980; Deisz and Lux, 1977; Raabe and Ayala, 1976). *In vivo* high doses (100 mg/kg i.p.) of phenytoin have no effect *per se* on the firing rate of cells in the dorsal raphe nucleus; such a dose, however, greatly potentiated postsynaptic inhibition in rat cortex (Raabe and Ayala, 1976) and diazepam-induced inhibition of cell firing (Gallager, Mallorga and Tallman, 1980). In mouse spinal cord neurones in culture, Barker *et al.* (1984) demonstrated that phenytoin (100 μM) had no action on basal, GABA-stimulated or benzodiazepine-stimulated chloride conductance. However, much lower doses (10 μM) completely blocked the spontaneous discharges and the rhythmic firing of bicuculline induced by GABA receptor blockade. In the rat cuneate slices (100 μM) phenytoin potentiated muscimol-stimulated depolarization; alone, however, the antiepileptic drug hyperpolarized the cells (Simmonds, 1981). Furthermore, the drug antagonizes excitatory responses induced by glutamate (Sastry and Phillis, 1976) and it selectively depresses the high K^+-evoked release of the excitatory amino acid D-aspartate as well as that of GABA (Skerritt and Johnston, 1983). Such an inhibition of the release of amino acid neurotransmitters requires, according to the authors, a 'modulation' of both calcium and sodium permeabilities.

The electrophysiological data suggest that phenytoin interacts with GABA synaptic components, but not via a direct interaction with the GABA receptor. The latter is substantiated by *in vitro* data showing that phenytoin does not displace 3H-ligand binding at the GABA receptor recognition site (Gallager, Mallorga and Tallman, 1980).

Several potential sites of action exist for the indirect effect of phenytoin on the GABA synapse–macromolecular receptor complex. Within the range of 50–150 μM, phenytoin decreases GABA uptake (100 μM; Essman and Essman, 1980), (although Weinberger, Nichlas and Berl (1976) reported an enhanced uptake of GABA and glutamate), increases total 3H-diazepam binding (50 μM) but diminishes clonazepam-displaceable 3H-benzodiazepine binding (100 μM; Gallager *et al.*, 1981), and displaces dihydropicrotoxinin binding to the chloride ionophore (140 μM; Olsen *et al.*, 1978). The interaction at the anticonvulsant–anxiolytic recognition site may be the most relevant of these. At a low anticonvulsant dose *in vivo* (10 mg/kg i.p.), phenytoin induces an increase in the number of 3H-diazepam binding sites in the rat cortex measured *in vitro*, or after a higher dose (100 mg/kg i.p.) increases 3H-diazepam binding *in vivo* (Gallager, Mallorga and Tallman, 1980). It should be noted that at these concentrations phenytoin has effects on systems other than the GABA synaptic–macromolecular receptor complex. For example, 3H-ligand binding at the voltage-sensitive sodium channel is diminished with an IC_{50} of 40 μM (Willow and Catterall, 1982).

From the data described above it is not easy to present a synthesis of the basic mechanisms underlying the antiepileptic action of phenytoin. Very probably the antiepileptic action is the result of multiple effects at several levels involving both potentiation of GABA-mediated postynaptic inhibition through a direct effect on Cl-ion channels, and a 'modulation' of sodium and calcium movements across cellular and subcellular membranes – movement essential for the uptake and release of neurotransmitters. On the other hand, the blocking effects on either sodium transport or calcium fluxes occurring at higher drug concentrations are probably not related to the antiepileptic action but to its adverse or toxic effects.

Globally these effects of phenytoin, exerted at therapeutic concentrations at both presynaptic and postsynaptic membranes, appear to confirm the hypothesis put forward by Woodbury in 1969 that the drug could act by decreasing excitatory amino acid transmission and increasing the GABA-mediated postsynaptic inhibition.

Phenobarbital (PB) and related anticonvulsant barbiturates

A number of papers available on the possible mechanisms of action of barbiturates imply that all members of this therapeutic class act through very similar mechanisms. Recent data, however (Barker *et al.*, 1984; MacDonald and Barker, 1979b; Simmonds, 1984) point out the potential danger in extrapolating from anticonvulsant barbiturates to sedative or anaesthetic barbiturates, and vice versa. Also important is the dose or concentration at which certain effects of phenobarbital have been observed. Most of the effects noted at high doses are non-specific and are very probably related more to the sedative and/or anaesthetic effect than to the anticonvulsant action. The data reported in this chapter are limited to phenobarbital. However they may be applied to (a) mephobarbital, which in the body is transformed into phenobarbital, and (b) probably also to primidone (see below). Phenobarbital has little or no effect on post-tetanic potentiation (Raines and Standaert, 1969) and preferentially depresses polysynaptic responses (Esplin, 1963). It elevates seizure thresholds more at the cortical than at the reticular level by both inhibiting the spread and suppressing the firing from the foci (Aston and Domino, 1961; Gangloff and Monnier, 1957; Morrell, Bradley and Prashne, 1959; Prichard, 1980; Straw and Mitchell, 1966). The latter effect is not shared by phenytoin, suggesting that phenobarbital could act on abnormal neurones, while phenytoin acts on normal neurones (Prichard, 1982). Among the various antiepileptic drugs, phenobarbital is probably the most active in the kindling model (Albright and Burnham, 1980; Bruni and Albright, 1984; Straw and Mitchell, 1966).

The drug appears to enhance presynaptic inhibition (Eccles, 1964; Nicoll, 1978) but it also greatly prolongs postsynaptic inhibitory potentials (Nicoll *et al.*, 1975). Phenobarbital is effective against repetitive stimulation, but with single stimuli there is a trend towards an enhanced response. According to Wilder and Bruni (1982) this could partially explain the apparently paradoxical effect of phenobarbital in absence seizures. Several possible modes of action have been postulated or described from a biochemical or molecular point of view. At high concentrations, as for phenytoin, phenobarbital decreases sodium and potassium transcellular transport, reducing membrane sodium and potassium conductances (Blaustein, 1968; Heyer and MacDonald, 1982; Schwartz, 1979), and has also been shown to reduce Ca^{2+} influx in presynaptic endings in both synaptosomal preparations and sympathetic ganglia (Blaustein, 1976; Ondrusek, Belknap and Leslie, 1979; Sohn and Ferrendelli, 1976).

These effects on membrane conductances and calcium influx could result in decreased neurotransmitter release as well as reduction in the generation of those excitatory and inhibitory postsynaptic potentials which depend on increased sodium conductance (Wilder and Bruni, 1982). A reduction in the release of several neurotransmitters, such as GABA, glutamate, acetylcholine and aspartate has been described (Cutler and Young, 1979; MacDonald and McLean, 1982; Proctor and Weakly, 1976; Skerritt and Johnston, 1984). However, as all these effects occur only at high concentrations of phenobarbital, they are most likely more important for sedation than for anticonvulsant action. Another effect observed at high doses or concentrations is the depression of the cytochrome–oxidase system, which is responsible for the synthesis of high-energy phosphate compounds necessary for the maintenance of membrane potentials (Prichard, 1980, 1982; Wilder and Bruni, 1982). More recently, it has been shown that phenobarbital at high doses binds to dihydropicrotoxinin receptors and that it may directly activate GABA-related chloride channels thereby enhancing postsynaptic chloride conductance (Olsen, 1981).

At 'therapeutic' concentrations, however, phenobarbital produces few changes in membrane conductances when applied directly to single neurones (MacDonald and Barker, 1979a; MacDonald and McLean, 1982). Postsynaptic inhibitory responses to GABA are enhanced, and excitatory responses to glutamic acid are antagonized while responses to glycine and beta-alanine remain unaffected (Ransom and Barker, 1976).

The magnitude of these effects is remarkably different. The antagonism of the glutamate-response amplitude reached a maximum at 40–50%, whereas the enhancement of the GABA-response amplitude attained 250–500%. According to MacDonald and Barker (1979a), the phenobarbital effect on GABAergic synaptic transmission is more significant than its action on glutamatergic excitation. Such an enhancement of GABAergic transmission is probably due either to an increase in the affinity of the active site for GABA (at the receptor ionophore complex) or to an increase in the duration of the unitary conductance changes.

In a subsequent paper, the same authors (MacDonald and Barker, 1979b) compared the effect of phenobarbital, pentobarbital and chlordiazepoxide and observed that in contrast to phenobarbital, pentobarbital completely abolished the spontaneous activity of cultured spinal cord neurones. Furthermore, the postsynaptic direct membrane effect of pentobarbital was about a hundred times more potent than that of phenobarbital, while the threshold for GABA response modulation was of the same magnitude. While phenobarbital appears to increase IPSC (inhibiting postsynaptic current) amplitude, pentobarbital prolongs IPSC decay without changing IPSC amplitude (MacDonald and Barker, 1979b; Barker, Owen and Segal, 1984). In contrast, diazepam in the same system appears to enhance amplitude and prolong decay (Barker, Owen and Segal, 1984). Unlike pentobarbital, the 'modulating' effect of phenobarbital on GABAergic transmission appears to have a much lower threshold than its direct membrane effect. This difference could explain the different profiles of the two drugs. Another dissimilarity between the two barbiturates is evident from recent papers: repeated treatment with phenobarbital reduces diazepam binding and increases receptor affinity (Sonowane, Yaffe and Shapiro, 1980) whereas pentobarbital treatment leads to an increased apparent affinity of the benzodiazepine binding site without changing the number of binding sites (Skolnick, Paul and Barker, 1980).

Recently it has been reported that phenobarbital may selectively inhibit the K^+-evoked release of the excitatory amino acid D-aspartate (Skerritt and Johnston, 1983). On the whole it appears that at 'therapeutic' concentrations, phenobarbital exerts its anticonvulsant action by specifically increasing postsynaptic GABAergic inhibition and simultaneously reducing glutamatergic excitation. At higher concentrations, less specific effects on ion transport and high energy phosphate synthesis may alter membrane potentials, leading to a global reduction in central nervous system function with intense sedation and depression of consciousness.

Primidone (PRI)

The antiepileptic effect of primidone is due both to the activity of the compound itself and to that of its two active metabolites: phenobarbital and phenylethymalonamide (PEMA) (Woodbury and Pippenger, 1982). However, no data are available at the biochemical level on the possible mechanism of action of the drug; only hypotheses based on the similarity of its effects with phenytoin and carbamazepine can be put forward. According to Woodbury and Pippenger (1982), primidone could act through an alteration of ionic fluxes, but no proof of this exists to date.

Trimethadione (TMO) and related oxalidinediones

Most of the data relating to the possible mechanism of action of this series of compounds are derived from neurophysiological studies. Very few data exist at the biochemical level. It is known that trimethadione, unlike phenytoin, does not affect post-tetanic potentiation and does not modify the synaptic transmission of single impulses (Esplin and Curto, 1957). Trimethadione, however, markedly depresses the response to repetitive electrical stimulation (as shown by Esplin and Curto, (1957) in spinal cord preparations), prolongs postictal depression (Esplin and Freston, 1960) and raises seizure thresholds, probably through an enhancement of presynaptic inhibition (Kreisman, Murphy and King, 1978; Schallek and Kuehn, 1963). Furthermore, trimethadione may significantly depress afterdischarge activity evoked by visual stimuli (Shearer, Fleming and Bigler, 1976; Turkanis *et al.*, 1977). From a neurophysiological point of view the drug appears to be more active on subcortical structures, and may exert an antifacilitatory action by affecting inhibitory and excitatory thalamic circuits (Wilder and Bruni, 1982).

From a biochemical or molecular point of view trimethadione is considered to have little or no effect on major neurotransmitter systems (McMillen and Isaac, 1978; Withrow, 1980) and does not interfere with cAMP and cGMP functions (Ferrendelli and Kinscherf, 1979). Trimethadione reduces or blocks several biochemical alterations induced by a convulsant dose of pentylenetetrazole, such as: (a) increased cortical release of ACh (Gardner and Webster, 1977); (b) increased monoamine metabolites (McMillen and Isaac, 1978); and (c) K^+ hyperpermeability (Gross and Woodbury, 1972). It is, however, difficult to say whether such effects are the results of the protective action of trimethadione against pentylenetetrazole-induced convulsions or a specific action on these biochemical systems. The reduction of potassium hyperpermeability subsequent to pentylenetetrazole could not be confirmed by Tannhauser and Izquierdo (1974); there is, however, the possibility that *in vivo* an action on potassium balance is exerted by the metabolite dimethadione, which may induce intracellular acidosis with consequent changes in potassium balance (Withrow, 1982).

Regarding the possible role of neurotransmitters in the action of trimethadione, Diaz in 1974 described a 28–44% increase in the rate of 5-HT synthesis, and more recently Löscher and Frey (1977) reported that trimethadione may antagonize the inhibition of glutamic acid dehydrogenase activity (and the consequent fall in GABA concentrations) induced by isoniazide. According to these authors, GABA could play a role in the action of trimethadione. This hypothesis is plausible considering that the neurophysiological profile of the drug bears similarities to those agents known to act by enhancing GABA-mediated inhibition. Recently Skerritt and Johnston (1983) observed that trimethadione may inhibit K^+-evoked release of D-aspartate, an excitatory amino acid in rat cerebral cortex slices.

Ethosuximide (ETS) and related succinimides

Ethosuximide and related succinimides reduce synaptic transmission during repetitive stimulation but do not depress transmission of single impulses (Radan and Esplin, 1977). Ethosuximide is thought to exert its effects either on ascending reticular activation or directly on inhibitory cells in the thalamic relay nuclei (Englander *et al.*, 1977; Nowack *et al.*, 1979; Wenzel, Krueger and Mueller, 1971). According to Fromm and Kohli (1972), ethosuximide acts preferentially on corticofugal inhibition of afferent activation in the spinal trigeminal nucleus with an effect opposite to that observed for phenytoin and carbamazepine.

At the biochemical and molecular levels several effects of ethosuximide have been described; however, their relevance to therapeutic activity in absence seizures is still not clarified. At concentrations of 2.5–25 mM, ethosuximide inhibits Na^+–K^+ ATPase but not Mg^{2+} ATPase (Gilbert and Wyllie, 1974; Leznicki and Dymecki, 1974), and it depresses the brain metabolic rate, reducing brain oxygen consumption (Nahorski, 1972). At elevated concentrations, ethosuximide may inhibit GABA-T and succinic semialdehyde dehydrogenase (Sawaya, Horton and Meldrum, 1975), but such activity is not seen at therapeutic concentrations (Leznicki and Dymecki, 1974). Ethosuximide non-competitively inhibits NADPH-linked aldehyde reductase, the enzyme responsible for the conversion of succinic semialdehyde to gamma-hydroxybutyrate, and when used chronically it decreases brain levels of gamma-hydroxybutyrate (Erwin and Dietrich, 1973; Snead, Bearden and Pegram, 1980; Tabakoff and Von Wartburg, 1975). In this perspective, it may be worthwhile to recall that gamma-hydroxybutyrate induces EEG and clinical features similar to absence seizures in animal models (Snead, 1978a and b). At the ionic level, Sohn and Ferrendelli (1976) reported that ethosuximide has no effect on Ca^{2+} movements and that there is no evidence for an effect on other ion conductances. Like other antiepileptic drugs, ethosuximide reduces basal levels of cerebellar cGMP in rodents (Lust *et al.*, 1978) and may increase dopaminergic transmission (Klunk and Ferrendelli, 1980). Barnes and Dichter (1984) recently reported that in cultured cortical neurones ethosuximide decreased GABA responses, which suggests that the action of ethosuximide is not due to an enhancement of GABA-mediated inhibition on cortical neurones. Furthermore, ethosuximide appeared to enhance the picrotoxin antagonism of the GABA response and to reduce the glycine-mediated increase in membrane conductance. These authors agree with the hypothesis of Ferrendelli and Klunk (1982) that the action of ethosuximide may be related to a non-identified neurotransmitter system as suggested by the data of Capek and Esplin (1977). In conclusion, none of the biochemical or molecular effects described or observed for ethosuximide may be taken as a basis for its antiepileptic activity; the mechanism of action of this class of drug is completely unknown.

Carbamazepine (CBZ)

While at the clinical level the therapeutic profile of carbamazepine (CBZ) is quite similar to that of phenytoin (Porter, 1982), the drug appears to exert its effects through a mechanism of action quite dissimilar from that of phenytoin. In fact, at therapeutic doses, carbamazepine does not alter post-tetanic potentiation (Krupp, 1969), and it affects ionic membrane conductances only at very high doses (Schauf, Davis and Marder, 1974). Unlike phenytoin, carbamazepine does not increase the discharge rate of cerebellar Purkinje cells (Julien and Hollister, 1975). However, like phenytoin, carbamazepine depresses synaptic transmission in the spinal trigeminal nucleus and elevates the threshold for electrically induced afterdischarges in cortex and amygdala (Albright, 1983; Fromm and Killian, 1967; Julien and Hollister, 1975). According to the data of Holm *et al.* (1970) the drug could exert a selective effect on the ventral anterior thalamus since it depresses transmission in the nucleus ventralis anterior thalami (NVAT) at doses which do not modify transmission in other brain areas, such as reticular formation, hippocampus and amygdala. Such an effect on the nucleus ventralis anterior thalami may be of importance since this brain area has been implicated in the generalization and spread of seizure discharges (Holm *et al.*, 1970; Kusske, Ojemann and Ward, 1972; Verzeano, 1972).

On the biochemical side, various reports suggest a possible effect of carbamazepine on several brain neurotransmitters and cyclic nucleotides; however, currently available data do not provide a clear definition of the mechanism of action of the antiepileptic activity of carbamazepine. A selective increase in striatal acetylcholine concentrations has been described by Consolo, Bianchi and Landinsky (1976), while according to Purdy *et al.* (1977) the drug may interfere with noradrenaline uptake by brain synaptosomes.

In a series of experiments on control and cobalt-treated rats, Morselli *et al.* (1978) found that in control animals carbamazepine (after both acute and repeated administration) induced a significant rise in brain 3-methoxy-4-hydroxyphenylethyleneglycol sulphate (MOPEG-SO_4) and 5-HIAA levels with concomitant decreases in noradrenaline concentrations. Furthermore. carbamazepine in cobalt-treated rats restored the reduced brain levels of MOPEG-SO_4 and 5-HIAA. These observations agree with the data reported by Quattrone and Samanin (1977) who noticed that a depletion of brain catecholamines (by 6-OH-dopamine) may significantly decrease the anticonvulsant activity of the drug in rats, and who suggested a possible involvement of the noradrenergic and serotoninergic systems in the mechanism of action of carbamazepine. As further indirect support of this hypothesis, Post *et al.* (1983) suggest a therapeutic effect of carbamazepine in mood disorders which are supposedly due to an alteration of noradrenergic and serotoninergic brain systems. Unlike phenytoin, carbamazepine fails to alter the potassium-evoked release of brain amino acids, such as GABA, glutamate and aspartate (Skerritt and Johnston, 1983; Lewin and Bleck, 1971), but according to Bernasconi and Martin (1979) it may reduce or inhibit GABA turnover.

Another series of reports concerns the effects of carbamazepine on cyclic nucleotides and adenosine receptors. At high concentrations (0.1–1.0 mM) carbamazepine may block the ouabain-induced rise in cAMP in cerebral cortical slices (Lewin and Bleck, 1977), and administered chronically to rabbits the drug reduces basal cAMP in the CSF and prevents the cAMP rise following convulsions (Myllyla, 1976). More recently, Skerritt, Davies and Johnston (1982) reported that carbamazepine selectively inhibits purine receptor binding and suggested that a purinergic component exists in the anticonvulsant action of the drug. In subsequent papers (Skerritt, Davies and Johnston, 1983; Skerritt, Johnston and Chow, 1983), the same authors suggest that carbamazepine may exert part of its anticonvulsant effect by acting as a 'partial agonist' of adenosine receptors. Such an effect appears to be specific and is not shared by other antiepileptic drugs. On the basis of the different effects of various purines on adenosine-linked adenylcyclases, subclasses fo adenosine receptors have been proposed (Daly, Bruns, and Snyder, 1981; Daly, Butts-Lamb and Padgett, 1983; Londos, Cooper and Wolff, 1980; Van Calder, Muller and Haprecht, 1979). According to Weir *et al.* (1984) carbamazepine could act as an agonist of adenosine A1 receptors (inhibitory to adenylate cyclase) and as an antagonist of adenosine A2 receptors (stimulatory to adenylate cyclase).

All these data suggesting a pharmacologically relevant action of carbamazepine on the receptors of neuromodulator adenosine in the central nervous system are very interesting because A1 adenosine receptor agonists have been shown to possess anticonvulsant activity (Dunwiddie and Worth, 1982) and they could help to interpret some of the above-mentioned effects of carbamazepine on brain catecholamines.

Benzodiazepines (BZP)

Almost every putative neurotransmitter has been associated with the many actions of the benzodiazepines since their development 30 years ago (Haefely *et al.*, 1981; Skolnick and Paul, 1981). However, over the past five years convincing evidence has accumulated which indicates that benzodiazepines exert the majority of their central activities via an action at highly specific recognition sites which form an integral part of the GABA receptor macromolecule (Barker, Owen and Segal, 1984; Braestrup, Nielsen and Honore, 1984; Costa and Guidotti, 1979; Haefely *et al.*, 1981; Möhler, 1984; Olsen, 1982; Skolnick and Paul, 1981; Squires and Saederup, 1982). Depending on the localization of this macromolecule, there will be secondary effects on noradrenergic, cholinergic, serotoninergic, etc. pathways.

The evidence that a specific membrane site exists to which many anxiolytic/anticonvulsant compounds bind with a high affinity cannot be denied. Squires and Braestrup (1977) and Möhler and Okada (1977) simultaneously demonstrated the high-affinity (nM) binding of 3H-diazepam to rat brain membranes. Following these observations an enormous literature has gathered, supporting and extending these findings. Other benzodiazepines and different chemical series of anxiolytic/anticonvulsant drugs (such as triazolopyridazenes, cyclopyrolones, beta-carbolines, pyrazoloquinolines and purines) displace 3H-diazepam (or similar ligands) from this high affinity site. This activity is highly correlated with the compounds' anticonvulsant (pentelenetetrazole convulsions) activity (Meldrum and Braestrup, 1984). Other series of compounds which have anxiolytic but not anticonvulsant activity are not active at this site (Lloyd *et al.*, 1984b; Taylor *et al.*, 1984) suggesting that the anticonvulsant action is specific for activity at this site. This recognition site (which is heterogeneous, at least between hippocampal and cerebellar sites) has a complex interaction with GABA receptors. Indeed, sophisticated solubilization, immunological and autoradiographic techniques demonstrate that this recognition site is a subunit which integrates with other components to form the GABA-chloride ionophore macromolecular complex (Braestrup, Nielsen and Honore, 1984; Costa and Guidotti, 1979; Möhler *et al.*, 1984; Olsen, 1982; Squires and Seaderup, 1982; Tallman, 1983). The most elegant demonstration of the physical association of GABA and benzodiazepine recognition sites uses monoclonal antibodies to show coexistence of the GABA and benzodiazepine binding sites in the same macromolecular complex (Möhler *et al.*, 1984) and combined autoradiography-immunofluorescence to show coexistence of the benzodiazepine recognition site in the same synapse as GAD activity (Möhler, Richards and Wu, 1981). GABA receptor activation alters the displacement of 3H-flunitrazepam (or similar ligands) binding by different compounds in a manner highly consistent with the compounds' pharmacological activity within the different chemical series active at this recognition site (Briley and Langer, 1978; Meldrum and Braestrup, 1984; Tallman, 1983). The displacement by anticonvulsant compounds is enhanced by the presence of GABA whereas the displacement by convulsant members of the group is diminished (the 'GABA shift') (Möhler, 1984; Tallman, 1983). This implies that GABA receptor activation modulates, and underlies, the biological signal resulting from interactions with this recognition site.

Of potentially greater interest for the anticonvulsant activity of benzodiazepines is the effect of these compounds on GABA receptor function. The *in vitro* incubation of benzodiazepines – or other anxiolytic/anticonvulsants acting at the same recognition site – increases 3H-GABA binding by enhancing the affinity of the GABA receptor site (Guidotti *et al.*, 1979). This effect is also observed *in vivo* (Guidotti and Ferrero, 1984), that is the efficacy of GABAergic transmission is enhanced. This enhanced binding is believed to be modulated by a polypeptide such as GABA modulin (Guidotti, 1984) or GABArins (Johnston and Skerritt, 1984). Antagonists of the anxiolytic/anticonvulsant recognition site block the increase in GABA binding as well as the anticonvulsant activity (Hunkeler *et al.*, 1981; Lloyd *et al.*, 1981b; Meldrum and Braestrup, 1984; Möhler, 1984).

These binding studies are confirmed by experiments with fetal mouse spinal cord neurones in tissue culture, neurones which exhibit binding characteristics identical to the cortex/hippocampal recognition site for anticonvulsant/anxiolytic drugs (Barker *et al.*, 1981, 1984). In these studies, benzodiazepines enhanced the increase in GABA-mediated chloride conductance by augmenting the frequency with which GABA activates the chloride ion-channels with little or no effect on the average conductance or duration of a single channel (Study and Barker, 1981). In some cases benzodiazepines (diazepam, lorazepam) had a intrinsic effect on chloride ion conductance (Barker, Owen and Segal, 1984). Using a different approach Baraldi *et al.* (1979) demonstrated a similar action; diazepam enhanced the increase in chloride ion flux elicited by threshold concentrations of GABA and muscimol in NB 2a neuroblastoma cells. Further *in vitro* examples of the mediation by GABA of the action of benzodiazepines can be found in recent review monographs devoted to this topic (Haefely *et al.*, 1981; Skolnick and Paul, 1982; Tallman, 1983).

The experimental evidence available indicates that the action of the benzodiazepines *in vivo* is mediated by the same mechanisms which can be shown *in vitro*. Thus, 3H-benzodiazepines are ligands for the same recognition sites *in vivo* as they are *in vitro*, as determined by the kinetics, the distribution and the specificity of the *in vivo* binding (Haefely *et al.*, 1981). The data suggest that the mediation of benzodiazepine activity *in vivo* by GABA receptors is similar to the *in vitro* situation. Thus GABA A agonists enhance, and GABA A antagonists diminish, the *ex vivo* binding of 3H-benzodiazepines to their binding sites (Gallager, Thomas and Tallman, 1978). These *ex vivo* studies are confirmed by PET scanning, which shows the actual *in vivo* binding (Maziere *et al.*, 1984). That these sites are related to the anticonvulsant action of the benzodiazepines is suggested by the observation that compounds which are antagonists *in vitro* (that is, displace 3H-benzodiazepines binding without intrinsic pharmacological activity and do not exhibit the 'GABA shift') block the anticonvulsant action of the benzodiazepines (such as diazepam) (Hunkeler *et al.*, 1981; Lloyd *et al.*, 1981a; Meldrum and Braestrup, 1984; Möhler, 1984).

The neurophysiological data is consistent with the binding data; at several different sites in the central nervous system (for example, amygdala, cortex, spinal cord, cerebellar Purkinje cell), different benzodiazepines (chlordiazepoxide, diazepam, flurazepam) at low doses enhance GABA-mediated inhibition – but not other neurotransmitter-mediated responses (Geller, Taylor and Huffer, 1978; Nestoros and Nistri, 1979; Nistri and Constant, 1978; for further reference see Haefely *et al.*, 1981). Furthermore, the benzodiazepines exhibit a mutually antagonist action with GABA antagonists such as bicuculline or picrotoxin (Bowery and Dray, 1978; Dray and Straughan, 1976; Haefely *et al.*, 1981; Polc, Möhler and Haefely, 1974). At spontaneously active synapses where GABA has been identified as the neurotransmitter (such as cerebral and cerebellar cortex, dorsal Deiters nucleus, presynaptic inhibition in the spinal cord), benzodiazepines enhance the action of the physiological transmitter (Lloyd *et al.*, 1979; Polc, Möhler and Haefely, 1974; Raabe and Gumnit, 1977; Wolf and Haas, 1977; Lloyd *et al.*, 1979). It is important to note that after inhibition of GABA synthesis the benzodiazepines are no longer active in enhancing physiological inhibition (Polc, Möhler and Haefely, 1974). Finally, a convulsant benzodiazepine reduces GABA-mediated neurotransmission in the spinal cord (Schlosser and Franco, 1979).

Thus, benzodiazepines appear to act both *in vitro* and *in vivo* via a specific recognition-binding site whose function is to modulate GABA receptor function. Other effects of benzodiazepines either occur at concentrations much higher than those relevant for clinical actions (for instance, the 150 μM IC_{50} at sodium channels; Willow and Catterall, 1982) or may be mediated via recognition sites linked to GABA receptors, (for example, on monoaminergic neurones – Gallager, 1978; Scatton *et al.*, 1982). However, a major question unanswered is whether or not all of the actions (such as anxiolytic, myorelaxant, hypnotic in addition to anticonvulsant) of benzodiazepines are mediated via GABA receptor modulation. If so, then it must still be determined which GABAergic neurones are responsible for which actions of the benzodiazepines.

Another important aspect not directly addressed in this review is the nature of a possible ligand for the recognition site of anxiolytic/anticonvulsant compounds such as the benzodiazepines. It is presumed that the action of benzodiazepines (and related compounds) actually mimics or antagonizes the action of an endogenous substance. Recently a 105 amino acid polypeptide was identified (Guidotti *et al.*, 1984) which displaces 3H-benzodiazepine binding and diminishes GABA-mediated chloride conductance. This compound is thought to be related to the anxiolytic action of benzodiazepines (Guidotti *et al.*, 1984) and its role in the anticonvulsant effect of these compounds is yet to be studied.

Valproic acid (VPA)

Valproic acid is the oldest chemical compound among the currently available antiepileptic drugs. Although its anticonvulsant properties were not discovered until the early 1960s (Meunier *et al.*, 1963), its synthesis was accomplished more than a century ago (Burton, 1882). For several years the basic mechanism of valproic acid was attributed to an increase in brain GABA levels due to a reduction of the metabolism of this amino acid; valproic acid's anticonvulsant action was based on an enhanced presence of GABA at the synaptic level. More recently several other hypotheses have been put forward to explain the mechanism of action of valproic acid. Two appear to be based on more consistent experimental evidence. The first suggests that valproic acid may have a direct membrane effect on neurones (Slater and Johnston, 1978), the second proposes that valproic acid enhances GABA-mediated postsynaptic inhibition (MacDonald and Bergey, 1979). Possible actions of valproic acid on other brain amino acids, cyclic nucleotides and brain monoamines have recently been reviewed by Chapman *et al.* (1982) and will be described here only very briefly.

An increase in GABA concentration following administration of valproic acid has been observed and described by several authors both in animal brain (Cisielski *et el.*, 1975; Godin *et al.*, 1969; Horton *et al.*, 1977; Löscher, 1979, 1980, 1981a and b; Simler *et al.*, 1973) and in the CSF of epileptic patients (Löscher, 1979; Schmidt and Löscher, 1981). Although there is general agreement that valproate increases brain GABA concentrations, there is considerable controversy regarding the mechanism by which GABA brain levels are increased, and the possible relevance of this phenomenon for the anticonvulsant activity of the compound. According to Godin *et al.* (1969), Simler *et al.*, (1973), Maitre, Csielski and Mandel (1974), Horton *et al.* (1977) and Cisielski *et al.* (1975), the increase in brain GABA concentrations is due to the inhibition of GABA-T, while according to Fowler, Beckford and John (1975) the doses necessary to elicit such an effect are much higher than those required for the anticonvulsant effect. On the other hand, Harvey, Bradford and Davison (1975), Anzelark *et al.* (1976) and Sawaya, Horton and Meldrum (1975) reported that valproic acid is a potent inhibitor of succinic semialdehyde dehydrogenase (SSAD) and that the effect on GABA-T is probably secondary to an effect on SSAD. *In vivo* data, however, failed to demonstrate a positive relationship between anticonvulsant effects and inhibition of SSAD, while such a correlation was observed for the inhibition of GABA-T (Schechter, Tranier and Grove, 1978; Simler *et al.*, 1973; Wood, Kurylo and Tsui, 1981). According to Löscher and Frey (1977) valproic acid probably acts by activating the glutamic acid decarboxylase system. Lust *et al.* (1976) described a lowering of cGMP in the cerebellum which according to the authors, could lead to an increase in cerebellar Purkinje cell output; however, no modifications of cortical cGMP and cAMP were observed by McCandless *et al.* (1979).

To complicate matters further, Löscher (1980), working at therapeutic concentrations, was unable to demonstrate any effect of valproic acid on GABA metabolism, and Kerwin, Olpe and Schmutz (1980) and Kerwin and Taberner (1981) observed that the anticonvulsant action precedes any increase in brain GABA levels. However, at the clinical level, a significant increase in CSF GABA concentrations has been observed following chronic valproic acid treatment, and such an increase appears to correlate with the therapeutic effect of the drug (*see* Schmidt and Löscher, 1981). Although there is presently a consensus of opinion that appropriate doses of valproic acid increase GABA levels in the biological fluids and brains of several animal species and man, the link between the GABA elevations and the anticonvulsant or antiepileptic effect of valproate is not yet clarified and is questioned by several authors. Slater and Johnston first demonstrated in 1978 that valproic acid applied to aplysia neurones *in vitro* at doses of 5–20 mM induces a concentration-dependent increase in potassium conductance accompanied by a hyperpolarization of the membrane and a decrease in input resistance. In the aplysia abdominal ganglion, valproic acid decreases the repetitive firing of pacemaker cells as well as the duration of excitatory postsynaptic potentials. These interesting data could offer an alternative explanation to some of the controversial points described above; however, before this hypothesis can be considered, a confirmation of the effect in a mammalian preparation is needed. Such data are still missing six years after the publication of the original hypothesis. In fact, Blume *et al.* (1979) reported that iontophoretic application of valproic acid to cortical neurones may lead to an increased firing rate which, according to the authors, may be due to an effect on glutamic and aspartic acids.

MacDonald and Bergey (1979) reported that in cultured spinal cord neurones valproic acid applied by iontophoresis enhanced the responses of iontophoretically applied GABA, but not those of glutamate and glycine. Such a selective increase in GABA-mediated postsynaptic inhibition was confirmed by other authors on cortical and brainstem neurones both *in vitro* and *in vivo* (Baldino and Geller, 1981a and b; Gent and Phillips, 1980; Kerwin, Olpe and Schmutz, 1980). This attractive and apparently well-documented hypothesis suffers, however, from the fact that some of the observed effects could be due to the high pH of the solutions used for iontophoresis. More recent studies using neutral pH solutions confirm this finding but only at very high drug concentrations. No potentiation could be observed at concentrations close to those considered therapeutic in man (Harrison and Simmonds, 1982; MacDonald, 1984, personal communication). Thus, further *in vivo* data are necessary to confirm the validity of this hypothesis, which in our opinion can best explain the drug's immediate onset of action in animals, where the peak concentrations achieved in biological fluids and brain are probably several-fold the steady state 'through' concentrations considered therapeutic in man.

A decrease in brain aspartate levels has been observed after acute valproic acid administration. There is apparently a positive correlation between this decrease and the drug's anticonvulsant activity against audiogenic seizures in DBA/2 mice (Godin *et al.*, 1969; Perry and Hansen, 1978; Schechter,1978). However, a marked increase in brain aspartate, glutamate, taurine and glutamine levels following chronic valproate administration has been described (Patsalos and Lascelles, 1981; Williams *et al.*, 1980) while only minimal modifications (or none at all) were observed after acute dosing (Chapman *et al.*, 1982). Valproic acid does not appear to have any consistent effect on brain monoamine metabolism. The minor modifications reported are not directly related to the anticonvulsant activity of valproic acid since manipulation of brain monoamine synthesis or turnover does not alter the anticonvulsant effects of the drug (Horton *et al.*, 1977; McMillen and Isaac, 1978). Finally, valproic acid does not bind to GABA A receptors, to GABA B receptors (Löscher, 1980; Lloyd, unpublished observation) or to the benzodiazepine recognition site (Burnham, King and Lloyd, 1981; Ticku and Davis, 1981), but it may inhibit the binding of 3H-dihydropicrotoxin to the picrotoxin receptor (Ticku and Davis, 1981). Whether this action is related to the anticonvulsant and antiepileptic activity of valproate is still unknown.

None of the three major hypotheses presently proposed for the possible mechanism of action of valproic acid are fully convincing. Further experimental data obtained in conditions closer to those observed in experimental models of epilepsy are needed. Moreover, two of these hypotheses could very well coexist, since the potentiation of GABA-mediated postsynaptic inhibition could be responsible for the immediate (peak-related) action of the drug, while the increase in brain GABA concentrations could explain the persistence of the effect even when valproic acid concentrations in biological fluids are well below those considered 'therapeutic' (Rowan *et al.*, 1979). The action of valproate by a direct effect on membranes is more difficult to accept, especially in view of the data of Blume et al. (1979) and Kerwin, Olpe and Schmutz (1980) which show that *in vivo* valproic acid directly applied to cortical and hippocampal neurones does not have a direct depressant action on the excitability of these neurones. Finally the possibility that valproic acid exerts its anticonvulsant effects through one or more metabolites cannot be excluded on the basis of our present knowledge.

Progabide (PGB)

Progabide is a new antiepileptic drug with a broad spectrum of activity both in animal models and in man. In animal models progabide is active against convulsions and/or mortality induced by allylglycine, bicuculline, picrotoxin, pentetrazole, penicillin, strychnine, kainic acid and electroshock. It is also effective in spontaneously photosensitive *Papio papio*, in sound-sensitive DBA/2 mice and in kindling in rats (Cepeda *et al.*, 1982; Joy, Albertson and Stark, 1984; Worms *et al.*, 1981, 1982). As well as being metabolized to another active anticonvulsant, SL 75.102, progabide possesses inherent activity. That each compound has inherent activity is demonstrated by (a) the different rank orders in convulsant models; (b) the fact that the absolute potency of progabide is greater than SL 75.102 in the penicillin focus although SL 75.102 is more potent than progabide in some other models; (c) the ability of progabide to displace GABA receptor binding (see below); and (d) the rapid onset of progabide's anticonvulsant action (less than 2 min) which occurs before the appearance of substantial levels of SL 75.102 (Lloyd *et al.*, 1982; Worms *et al.*, 1982).

From the available data it appears that progabide and SL 75.102 are highly specific agonists for both GABA A and GABA B receptors (Bowery *et al.*, 1985; Lloyd *et al.*, 1982). It is generally assumed that GABA A receptor agonist activity is responsible for the anticonvulsant profile since baclofen (the prototypic GABA B agonist) has only a limited anticonvulsant spectrum in animal models (Worms and Lloyd, 1981); and furthermore compounds which are agonists (such as THIP, muscimol) or enhancers (such as benzodiazepine, barbiturates) specifically for GABA A receptors have a much wider range of anticonvulsant activity than does baclofen (Worms and Lloyd, 1981).

Binding techniques have shown that progabide and SL 75.102 displace various 3H-ligands (GABA, muscimol, isoguvacine) from GABA A receptors in both rat and human membrane preparations. The IC_{50} for 3H-GABA in the human brain preparation for SL 75.102 is about 0.8 μM, whereas under these conditions (no triton X-100) that of the neurotransmitter itself is 0.2 μM. In rat brain membranes, progabide is less active than SL 75.102 by a factor of 5–15-fold. The results of these membrane-binding techniques are confirmed by autoradiography on cerebellar slices which shows that SL 75.102 prevents the specific grain pattern of 3H-GABA labelling (Bowery *et al.*, 1985). The GABA receptor–agonist activity of progabide and SL 75.102 are confirmed by inhibition of GABA release from tissue slices and by the enhancement of 3H-diazepam binding *in vitro* (Bowery, Hill and Hudson, 1982; Koe, 1983; Lloyd *et al.*, 1982). Within the GABA synapse, progabide appears specific for GABA receptors, as neither GABA synthesis (glutamic acid decarboxylase activity) nor GABA metabolism (GABA-T activity) are altered by concentrations of progabide or SL 75.102 much greater than that needed to displace 3H-GABA from its receptor (Lloyd *et al.*, 1982). The specificity of these compounds for the GABA receptor is demonstrated *in vitro* by the lack of activity (at 100 μM) at recognition sites for alpha and beta-adrenoreceptors, histamine receptors, muscarine receptors, and binding sites for antidepressants and kainic acid. At 100 μM 3H-strychnine binding (for glycine receptors) is displaced (Lloyd *et al.*, 1982). In neurophysiological experiments (dorsal root ganglia and superior cervical ganglia), SL 75.102 (used because of its much greater solubility than progabide) mimics the action of GABA in all aspects. The depolarization caused by GABA or SL 75.102 has the same off-rate, shows cross-desensitization, is blocked by bicuculline and picrotoxin, and, most importantly, has the same reversal potential, indicating that both compounds act at the same recognition site controlling the chloride ionophore (Bowery *et al.*, 1985; Desarmenien *et al.*, 1981; Gallagher, Nakamura and Shinnick-Gallagher, 1983).

The specificity of progabide and SL 75.102 for GABA receptors demonstrated *in vitro* is reflected by their activity *in vivo*. Thus progabide displaces specific 3H-muscimol binding to GABA A receptors in the mouse brain in addition to its anticonvulsant action (Guidotti and Ferrero, 1985), and after administration of progabide *in vivo* 3H-diazepam binding to brain membrane preparations is increased (Koe, 1983). Both of these actions are specific for GABA receptor agonists and mimetics. Similarly, *in vivo* administration of progabide has no effect on cardiovascular noradrenergic, serotoninergic or cholinergic receptors, or on the muscarinic responses (central or peripheral) induced by oxytremorine (Cavero and Lloyd, unpublished data). This confirms the specificity of progabide and SL 75.102 for GABA receptor activation. Furthermore, within the GABA-receptor macromolecular complex, progabide functions independently of the subunit recognition site for anxiolytic/anticonvulsant compounds (the so-called benzodiazepine recognition site). A specific antagonist for this site, RO 15–1788, does not in any way influence the anticonvulsant activity of progabide (Lloyd *et al.*, 1981b). Consistent with the hypothesis that progabide and SL 75.102 exert their anticonvulsant action via GABA receptor activation is the observation that anticonvulsant action of progabide is accompanied by brain levels of progabide and SL 75.102 which are sufficient for GABA receptor activation (Worms *et al.*, 1982). Thus, both the *in vitro* and *in vivo* data provide evidence indicating that the anticonvulsant action of progabide can only be explained by the stimulation of GABA receptors, either by progabide itself or together with its acidic metabolite SL 75.102.

Acetazolamide (ACZ)

Most of the available evidence on the possible mechanism of action of acetazolamide is derived from rather old studies, since the compound is now uncommonly used at the clinical level. There is a consensus on the only well-documented biochemical effect of the drug: its inhibition of cerebral carbonic anhydrase with subsequent accumulation of intracellular CO_2 and H_2CO_3 (Gray *et al.*, 1957; Millichap, Thatcher and Williams, 1955). Interestingly, carbonic anhydrase is located mainly in glial cells and myelin, and glial cells regulate the acid–base balance in the brain as well as the potassium homeostasis (Woodbury, 1980a and b; Woodbury and Kemp, 1982). The result of the inhibition of carbonic anhydrase is a reduction in intracellular sodium (Woodbury, 1980b) with a concomitant increase in intracellular potassium and consequent neuronal hyperpolarization and reduction of cellular excitability.

According to Woodbury and Kemp (1982), acetazolamide may induce two opposite effects: (a) at low doses, it induces a decrease or a block in the spread of seizures by increasing CO_2 in neurones; (b) at high doses, it may exert an excitatory effect due or related to blockade of the glial anion transport system (Cl^-, HCO_3).

In light of the present hypotheses on the role of GABA in central nervous system transmission, it is interesting to recall that an increase in brain GABA concentrations following acetazolamide was described in 1959 by Woodbury and Esplin. An increase in both glutamic and aspartic acid was also observed. One cannot ignore the possibility that the compound's effects on the acid–base balance and potassium homeostasis may induce a modification of the transmitter amino acid release.

CONCLUDING REMARKS

It is evident from the data reviewed above and summarized in *Table 3.1* that the mechanism of action of most of the currently used antiepileptic drugs is still poorly understood. According to the available data and hypotheses, each drug may exert several different actions depending on the doses or concentrations employed and/or on the experimental model tested. Furthermore, since the basic mechanisms underlying the epilepsies are not yet understood, it is not easy to identify which of the proposed mechanisms of action is really relevant to antiepileptic activity in patients, and it is very likely that several actions concur in the final antiepileptic effect in man.

However, despite the variety of hypotheses put forward, data acquired in the last three or four years all suggest a common site of action for phenytoin, phenobarbital, primidone, trimethadione, benzodiazepine, valproic acid and progabide. At therapeutic concentrations all these drugs interact (even if at different sites or subunits) with the GABA receptor–ionophore macromolecular complex altering Cl^- conductance. The result of such an interaction is a potentiation and/or a prolongation of the GABA-mediated postsynaptic inhibition. Depending on both the drug and the dose, such an interaction with the GABA-receptor–Cl–ionophore complex may or may not be accompanied by a reduction of excitatory amino acid release and/or by a 'modulatory' effect on cation (N^+, K^+, Ca^{2+}) movements which may further modify the response of excitable tissues.

Ethosuximide, on the contrary, appears to antagonize GABA-mediated responses, increase the dopaminergic transmission, and act by reducing the brain levels of gamma-hydroxybutyrate.

Apart from acetazolamide, which has not been studied in recent years, an exception is shown by carbamazepine for which there are no data suggesting an interaction with the GABA receptor–ionophore complex; an interaction with the noradrenergic system and adenosine receptors appears to be relevant for its antiepileptic action.

Table 3.1 Proposed mechanism(s) of action of antiepileptic drugs

Proposed effects	*Phenytoin*	*Phenobarbital*	*Trimethadione*	*Ethosuximide*	*Carbamazepine*	*Benzodiazepine*	*Valproic acid*	*Progabide*	*Acetazolamide*
Effects on movements of cations *	↓ Passive Na^+ influx ↑ Na/K-ATPase activity ↑ Active Na^+ transport ↓ Ca^{2+} influx *	↓ Na^+ and K^+ transcellular transport ↓ Ca^{2+} influx *	↓ K^+ permeability *	↓ Na/K-ATPase activity No effect on Ca^{2+} *	↓ Na^+ conductance *	↓ Na^+ influx ↓ K^+ permeability *	↑ K^+ conductance ↓ Ca^{2+} fluxes		↓ Intracellular Na^+ ↑ Intracellular K^+
Effects on cyclic nucleotides	↓ cAMP and cGMP accumulation }	↓ cAMP and cGMP accumulation }		↓ Basal levels cGMP }	↓ cAMP Inhibits purine receptor binding partial agonist adenosine receptor		↓ cGMP	↓ cGMP	
Effects on cerebral energy metabolism		↓ Cytochrome oxydase system *							
Effects on brain monoamines	Variable effects on 5-HT system ↑ Dopamine 'tonus' ↑ Norepinephrine turnover rate ↓ Monoamine oxidase activity ↓ Acetylcholine release *	Minor variable effects ↑ Turnover norepinephrine and 5-HT *	Antagonizes: pentylenetetra-zole induced ↑ in monodamine metabolism ↑ Acetylcholine release ↑ 5-HT synthesis *	↑ Dopamine transmission	↑ Norepinephrine and 5-HT systems ↑ Striatal acetylcholine		Minor effects	↑ Norepinephrine turnover ↓ 5-HT and dopamine turnover	

Table 3.1 continued

Proposed effects	*Phenytoin*	*Phenobarbital*	*Trimethadione*	*Ethosuximide*	*Carbamazepine*	*Benzodiazepine*	*Valproic acid*	*Progabide*	*Acetazolamide*
Effects on neurotransmitter amino acids (a) Inhibitory	↑ Brain GABA levels ↓ SSAD activity antagonizes isoniazide-induced GABA depletion	↓ GABA release ↑ Postsynaptic responses to GABA	Antagonizes isoniazide induced glutamic acid decarboxylase inhibition Antagonizes isoniazide induced GABA depletion	↓ Glycine-mediated increased in membrane conduction ↓ Postsynaptic responses to GABA	↓ GABA turnover	↑ GABAergic transmission	↑ GABA brain level (GABA-T ↓; ↓ SSAD/ ↑ GAD ↑ Postsynaptic responses to GABA	↓ GABA release No effect on GAD, GABA-T, SSAD	↑ GABA brain levels
(b) Excitatory	↓ Glutamate-release ↓ K^+-evoked aspartase release	↓ Glutamate release ↓ Postsynaptic responses to glutamate ↓ K^+-evoked aspartate release	↓ K^+-evoked aspartate release				↓ Aspartate brain levels		
Effects on (at) GABA-receptor–ionophore complex	Displaces dihydropicrotoxin binding to Cl-ionophore	↑ Affinity of active site for GABA on receptor–ionophore complex ↑ Inhibiting postsynaptic current amplitude	↑ Cl^- conductance	↑ Picrotoxin antagonist to GABA responses		↑ GABA-mediated Cl^- conductance ↑ Affinity for GABA receptor site	↓ Binding of dihydropicrotoxin; does not bind to GABA A nor GABA B receptors	Specific agonist of GABA A and GABA B receptors ↑ DZ binding	
Other effects	↓ Ca^{2+} dependent phosphorylation of synaptosomal proteins *		↑ Intracellular CO_2 }	↓ Brain gamma-hydroxybutyrate					↓ Cerebral carbonic anhydrase activity ↑ Intracellular CO_2 and H_2CO_3

5HHT = serotonin; GABA-T = GABA-transaminase; SSAD = succinic semialdehyde dehydrogenase; GAD = glutamic acid decarboxylase; DZ = diazepam; ↓ = decrease or block; ↑ = increase;
* = high doses only

The more marked effects observed for most drugs at high doses and/or concentrations on the movement of cations and the release of transmitters are surely less specific and probably more related to the toxic or adverse effects of the drugs than to their therapeutic action.

In conclusion, most of the available data support the hypothesis that an action at the GABA-receptor–ionophore macromolecular complex (observed for most antiepileptic drugs at therapeutic concentrations) is a common mechanism of action for several antiepileptic drugs accounting for their therapeutic efficacy in tonic, tonic-clonic and partial seizures. Furthermore, these data agree with the biochemical findings in animals and in man which suggest that a deficit of GABA function may play an important role in either the genesis or the maintenance of several epileptic syndromes.

Acknowledgements

The authors wish to thank Miss Béatrice Chapelier, Miss Béatrice Panteste and Miss Sophie Squazzaventre for the careful typing and editing of the manuscript.

References

AIRAKSINEN, M. M. (1983) The role of receptors in the action of antiepileptic drugs. *Acta Neurologica Scandinavica,* **67,** 31–46

AIRAKSINEN, M. M. and LEINO, E. (1982) Decrease of GABA in the cerebrospinal fluid of patients with progressive myoclonus epilepsy and its correlation with the decrease of 5HIAA and HVA. *Acta Neurologica Scandinavica,* **66,** 666–672

AL-ANI, A. T., TUNNICLIFF, G., RICK, J. T. and KERKUT, G. A. (1970) GABA production, acetylcholinesterase activity and biogenic amine levels in brains from mouse strains differing in spontaneous activity and reactivity. *Life Sciences,* **91,** 21–27

ALBRIGHT, P. S. (1983) Effects of carbamazepine, clonazepam and phenytoin on seizure threshold in amygdala and cortex. *Experimental Neurology,* **79,** 11–17

ALBRIGHT, P. S. and BURNHAM, W. M. (1980) Development of a new pharmacological seizure model: effects of anticonvulsants on cortical and amygdala-kindled seizures in the rat. *Epilepsia,* **21,** 681–689

ALTAMURA, A. C., BONATI, M., GIORDANO, P. L. and ALGERI, S. (1978) The activity of some neurotransmitter-synthesizing enzymes in experimental cobalt epilepsy. *Neuroscience Letters,* **7,** 83–87

ANZELARK, G., HORTON, R. W., MELDRUM, B. S. and SAWAYA, M. C. B. (1976) Anticonvulsant action of ethanolamine-o-sulfate and di-n-propylacetate and the metabolism of gamma aminobutyric acid (GABA) in mice with audiogenic seizures. *Biochemical Pharmacology,* **25,** 413–417

ASTON, R. and DOMINO, E. F. (1961) Differential effects of phenobarbital, pentobarbital, and diphenylhydantoin on motor cortical and reticular thresholds in the rhesus monkey. *Psychopharmacologia,* **2,** 304–317

AYALA, G. F. and JOHNSTON, D. (1980) Phenytoin: electrophysiological studies in simple neuronal systems. *Advances in Neurology,* **27,** 339–351

AYALA, G. F., LIN, S. and JOHNSTON, D. (1977a) The mechanism of action of diphenylhydantoin on invertebrate neurons. I. Effects on basic membrane properties. *Brain Research,* **121,** 245–258

AYALA, G. F., JOHNSTON, D., LIN, S. and DICHTER, H. N. (1977b). The mechanism of action of diphenylhydantoin on invertebrate neurons. II. Effects on synaptic mechanisms. *Brain Research,* **121,** 259–270

AZZARO, A. J., GUTRECHT, J. A. and SMITH, D. J. (1973) Effect of diphenylhydantoin on the uptake and catabolism of L-3H norepinephrine *in vitro* in rat cerebral cortex issue. *Biochemical Pharmacology,* **22,** 2719–2729

BAKAY, R. A. E. and HARRIS, A. B. (1981) Neurotransmitter, receptor and biochemical changes in monkey cortical epileptic foci, *Brian Research,* **206,** 387–404

BAKER, P. F. and BLAUSTEIN, M. P. (1968) Sodium-dependent uptake of calcium by crab nerve. *Biochemica Biophysica Acta,* **150**, 167–170

BALCAR, V. J., PUMAIN, R., MARK, J., BORG, J. and MANDEL, P. (1978) GABA-mediated inhibition in the epileptogenic focus, a process which may be involved in the mechanism of the cobalt-induced epilepsy. *Brain Research*, **154,** 182–185

BALDINO, F. and GELLER, H. M. (1981a) Sodium valproate enhancement of gamma-aminobutyric acid (GABA) inhibition: electrophysiological evidence for anticonvulsant activity. *Journal of Pharmacology and Experimental Therapeutics*, **217**, 445–450

BALDINO, F. and GELLER, H. M. (1981b) Effect of sodium valproate on hypothalamic neurones *in vivo* and *in vitro*. Brian Research, **219,** 231–237

BARALDI, M., GUIDOTTI, A., SCHWARTZ, J. P. and COSTA, E. (1979) GABA receptors in clonal cell lines: a model for the study of benzodiazepines at molecular level. *Science,* **205,** 821–823

BARKER, J. L. and MACDONALD, J. F. (1980) Picrotoxin convulsions involve synaptic and nonsynaptic mechanisms on cultured mouse spinal neurons. *Science,* **208,** 1054–1056

BARKER, J. L., MACDONALD, J. F., MATHERS, D. A., MCBURNEY, R. N. and STUDY, R. E. (1981) Convulsant and anticonvulsant pharmacology of cultured mouse spinal neurons. In *Neurotransmitters, Seizures and Epilepsy,* edited by P. L. Morselli, K. G. Lloyd, W. Loscher, B. Meldrum and E. H. Reynolds, pp. 49–62. New York: Raven Press

BARKER, J. L., OWEN, D. G. and SEGAL, M. (1984) Clinically important drugs modulate GABA-activated Cl-conductance. *Clinical Neuropharmacology,* **7** (Suppl. 1), 564–565

BARKER, J. L., GRATZ, E., OWEN, D. E. and STUDY, R. E. (1984) Pharmacological effects of clinically important drugs on the excitability of cultured mouse spinal neurons. In *Actions and Interactions of GABA and Benzodiazepines*, edited by N. G. Bowery, pp. 203–216. New York: Raven Press

BARNES, D. M. and DICHTER, M. A. (1984) Effects of ethosuximide and tetramethyl succinimide on cultured cortical neurons. *Neurology,* **34,** 620–625

BERNARD, G. G. and BOHM, E. (1965) *Local Anesthetics as Anticonvulsants: A Study on Experimental and Clinical Epilepsy.* Stockholm: Almqvist and Wiksell

BERNASCONI, R. and MARTIN, P (1979) Effects of antiepileptic drugs on the GABA turnover rate. *Naunyn Schmiedeberg's Archives of Pharmacology,* **307** (Suppl.), 271

BHATTACHARYA, S., KISHOR, K. and SAXENA, P. (1964) A neuropharmacological study of gamma-aminobutyric acid (GABA). *Archives Internationales de Pharmacodynamie et Therapie,* **150,** 295–305

BIANCHI, C., BEANI, L. and BERTELLI, A. (1975) Effects of some anti-epileptic drugs on brain acetylcholine. *Neuropharmacology.* **14,** 327–332

BLACKWOOD, D. (1981) The role of noradrenaline and dopamine in amygdaloid kindling. In *Neurotransmitters, Seizures and Epilepsy,* edited by P. L. Morselli, K. G. Lloyd, W. Loscher, B. Meldrum and E. H. Reynolds, pp. 203–214. New York: Raven Press

BLAUSTEIN, M. P. (1968) Barbiturates block sodium and potassium conductance increases in voltage-clamped lobster axons. *Journal of General Physiology,* **51,** 293–307

BLAUSTEIN, M. P. (1976) Barbiturates block calcium uptake by stimulated and potassium-depolarized rat sympathetic ganglia. *Journal of Pharmacology and Experimental Therapeutics,* **196,** 80–86

BLAUSTEIN, M. P. and WIESMANN, W. P. (1970) The effect of sodium ions on calcium movements in isolated synaptic terminals. *Proceedings of the National Academy of Sciences of the USA,* **66,** 664–671

BLUME, H. W., LUMOUR, Y., ARNAULD, E., LAYTON, B. S. and RENAULD, L. P. (1979) Sodium di-n-propylacetate (valproate) action on single neurons in rat cerebral cortex and hippocampus. *Brain Research,* **171,** 182–185

BONNYCASTLE, D. D., GIARMAN, N. J. and PAASONEN, M. K. (1957) Anticonvulsant compounds and 5-hydroxytryptamine in rat brain. *British Journal of Pharmacology,* **12,** 228–231

BOSSI, L., ZIVKOVIC, B., SCATTON, B. *et al.* (1981) Ventricular CSF concentrations of NA, DA, HVA and 5HIAA in epileptic patients. In *Neurotransmitters, Seizures and Epilepsy,* edited by P. L. Morselli, K. G. Lloyd, W. Loscher, B. Meldrum and E. H. Reynolds, pp. 307–314. New York: Raven Press

BOWERY, N. G. and DRAY, A. (1978) Reversal of the action of amino acid antagonists by barbiturates and other hypnotic drugs. *British Journal of Pharmacology,* **63,** 197–215

BOWERY, N. G., HILL, D. R. and HUDSON, A. L. (1982) Evidence that SL 75102 is an agonist at GABA B as well as GABA A receptors. *Neuropharmacology,* **21,** 391–395

BOWERY, N. G., HILL, D. R., HUDSON, A. L. and PRICE, G. W. (1985) GABA-mimetic action of SL 75102 at neuronal receptors. In *Epilepsy and GABA Receptor Agonists: Basic and Therapeutic Research*, edited by G. Bartholini, L. Bossi, K. G. Lloyd and P. L. Morselli, pp. 63–80. New York: Raven Press

BRAESTRUP, C., NIELSEN, M. and HONORE, T. (1984) Molecular interactions in the GABA/benzodiazepine receptor, chloride ion channel complex. High energy radiation inactivation studies. *Clinical Neuropharmacology,* **7** (Suppl. 1), 562–563

BRILEY, M. S. and LANGER, S. Z. (1978) Influence of GABA receptor agonists and antagonists on the binding of 3H-diazepam to the benzodiazepine receptor. *European Journal of Pharmacology,* **52,** 129–132

BRUNI, J. and ALBRIGHT, P. S. (1984) The clinical pharmacology of antiepileptic drugs. *Clinical Neuropharmacology,* **7,** 1–34

BURNHAM, W. M., KING, G. A. and LLOYD, K. G. (1981) Extra-focal catecholamine levels in 'kindled' rat forebrains. *Progress in Neuropsychopharmacology,* **5,** 537–541

BURNHAM, P. M., SPERO, L., OKAZAKI, M. M. and MADRAS, B. K. (1981) Saturable binding of (3H) phenytoin to rat membrane fraction. *Canadian Journal of Physiology and Pharmacology,* **59,** 402–407

BURTON, B. S. (1982) On the propyl derivatives and decomposition products of ethylacetoacetate. *American Chemical Journal,* **3,** 385–395

CAPEK, R. and ESPLIN, B. (1977) Effects of ethosuximide on transmission of repetitive impulses and apparent rates of transmitter turnover in the spinal monosynaptic pathway. *Journal of Pharmacology and Experimental Therapeutics,* **201,** 320–325

CARNAY, L. and GRUNDFEST, S. (1974) Excitable membrane stabilization by diphenylhydantoin and calcium. *Neuropharmacology,* **13,** 1097–1108

CEPEDA, C., WORMS, P., LLOYD, K. G. and NAQUET, R. (1982) Action of progabide in the photosensitive baboon, *Papio papio. Epilepsia,* **24,** 463–470

CHADWICK, D., JENNER, P. and REYNOLDS, E. H. (1977) Serotonin metabolism in human epilepsy: the influence of anticonvulsant drugs. *Annals of Neurology,* **1,** 218–224

CHAPMAN, A., KEANE, P. E., MELDRUM, B. S., SIMIAND, J. and VERNIERES, J. C. (1982) Mechanism of anticonvulsant action of valproate. *Progress in Neurobiology,* **19,** 315–359

CHASE, T. N., KATZ, R. I. and KOPIN, I. J. (1969) Effect of anticonvulsants on brain serotonin. *Transactions of the American Neurological Association,* **94,** 236–238

CHAUVEL, P., TROTTIER, S. and BANCAUD, J. (1985) Catecholamines in experimental and human epilepsy. In *Basic Mechanisms of the Epilepsies,* edited by A. V. Delgado-Escueta, A. A. Ward, Jr and D. Woodbury. New York: Raven Press

CISIELSKI, L., MAITRE, J., CASH, C. and MANDEL P. (1975) Regional distribution and effects of cerebral mitochondrial respiration of the anticonvulsive drug n-dipropylacetate. *Biochemical Pharmacology,* **24,** 1055–1058

CONSOLO, S., BIANCHI, S. and LADINSKY, H. (1976) Effect of carbamazepine on cholinergic parameters in rat brain areas. *Neuropharmacology,* **35,** 653–657

COSTA, E. and GUIDOTTI, A. (1979) Molecular mechanisms in the receptor action of benzodiazepines. *Annual Reviews of Pharmacology and Toxicology,* **19,** 531–545

COURTNEY, K. R. and ETTER, E. F. (1983) Modulated anticonvulsant block of sodium channels in nerve and muscle. *European Journal of Pharmacology,* **88,** 1–9

CRUNELLI, V., CERVO, L. and SAMANIN, R. (1981) Evidence for a preferential role of central noradrenergic neurons in electrically induced convulsions and activity of various anticonvulsants in the rat. In *Neurotransmitters, Seizures and Epilepsy,* edited by P. L. Morselli, K. G. Lloyd, W. Löscher, B. Meldrum and E. H. Reynolds, pp. 195–202. New York: Raven Press

CURTIS, D. (1979) GABAergic transmission in the mammalian central nervous system. In *GABA – Neurotransmitters,* edited by P. Krogsgaard-Larsen. J. Scheel-Kruger and H. Kofod, pp. 17–27. Copenhagen: Munksgaard

CURTIS, D. R., DUGGAN, A. W. and JOHNSTON, G. A. R. (1971) The specificity of strychnine as a glycine antagonist in the mammalian spinal cord. *Experimental Brain Research,* **12,** 547–565

CUTLER, R. W. P. and YOUNG, J. (1979) Effect of barbiturates on release of endogenous amino acids from rat cortex slices. *Neurochemical Research,* **4,** 319–329

CZUECZWAR, S. J. and MELDRUM, B. (1982) Protection against chemically induced seizures by 2-amino-7-phosphono-heptanoic acid. *European Journal of Pharmacology,* **83,** 335–338

DALY, J. W., BRUNS, R. F., and SNYDER, S. H. (1981) Adenosine receptors in the central nervous system: relationship to the central action of methylxanthines. *Life Sciences,* **28,** 2083–2097

DALY, J. W., BUTTS-LAMB, P., and PADGETT, W. (1983) Subclasses of adenosine receptors in the central nervous system: interactions with caffeine and related methylxanthines. *Cellular and Molecular Neurobiology,* **3,** 69–80

DE BOER, T., STOOF, J. C., and VAN DUIJ, N. H. (1982) The effects of convulsant and anticonvulsant drugs on the release of radiolabelled GABA, glutamate, noradrenaline, serotonin and acethylcholine from rat cortical slices. *Brain Research,* **253,** 153–160

DEISZ, R. A. and LUX, H. D. (1977) Diphenylhydantoin prolongs post-synaptic inhibition and iontophoretic GABA action in the crayfish stretch receptor. *Neuroscience Letters,* **5,** 199–203

DELGADO, J. M. R. and MIHAILOVIC, L. (1956) Use of intracerebral electrodes to evaluate drugs that act on the central nervous system. *Annals of the New York Academy of Sciences,* **64,** 644–666

DELORENZO, R. J. (1980) Phenytoin:calcium – and calmodulin-dependent protein phosphorylation and neurotransmitter release. *Advances in Neurology,* **27,** 399–414

DESARMENIEN, M., FELTZ, P., HEADLEY, P. M. and SANTANGELO, F. (1981) SL 75102 as a gamma-aminobutyric acid agonist: experiments on dorsal root ganglion neurons *in vitro. British Journal of Pharmacology,* **72,** 355–364

DIAZ, P. M. (1974) Interaction of pentylenetetrazol and trimethadione on the metabolism of serotonin in brain and its relation to the anticonvulsivant action of trimethadione. *Neuropharmacology,* **13,** 615–621

DRAY, A. and STRAUGHAN, D. W. (1976) Benzodiazepines: GABA and glycine receptors on single neurons in the rat medulla. *Journal of Pharmacy and Pharmacology,* **28,** 314–315

DUNWIDDIE, T. V. and WORTH, T. (1982) Sedative and anticonvulsant effects of adenosine analogs in mouse and rat. *Journal of Pharmacology and Experimental Therapeutics,* **220,** 70–76

ECCLES, J. C. (1964) *Physiology of Synapses.* New York: Academic Press

EMSON, P. C. and JOSEPH, M. H. (1975) Neurochemical and morphological changes during the development of cobalt-induced epilepsy in the rat. *Brain Research,* **93,** 91–110

ENGLANDER, R. M., JOHNSON, R. N., BRICKLEY, J. J. and HANNA, G. R. (1977) Effects of anticonvulsant drugs on thalamocortical excitability. *Neurology (Minneapolis),* **27,** 1134–1139

ENNA, S. J., STERN, L. Z., WASTEK, G. J. and YAMAMURA, H. (1977) Cerebrospinal fluid aminobutyric acid variations in neurological disorders. *Archives of Neurology,* **34,** 683–685

ERWIN, V. G. and DIETRICH, R. A. (1973) Inhibition of bovine brain aldehyde reductase by anticonvulsant compounds. *Biochemical Pharmacology,* **2,** 2615–2624

ESPLIN, D. (1957) Effect of diphenylhydantoin on synaptic transmission in the cat spinal cord and stellate ganglion. *Journal of Pharmacology and Experimental Therapeutics,* **120,** 301–323

ESPLIN, D. W. (1963) Criteria for assessing effects of depressant drugs on spinal cord synaptic transmission, with examples of drug selectivity. *Archives Internationales de Pharmacodynamie et de Therapie,* **143,** 479–497

ESPLIN, D. W. and CURTO, E. M. (1957) Effects of trimethadione on synaptic transmission in the spinal cord: antagonism of trimethadione and pentylenetetrazol. *Journal of Pharmacology and Experimental Therapeutics,* **121,** 457–467

ESPLIN, D. W. and FRESTON, J. W. (1960) Physiological and pharmacological analysis of spinal cord convulsions. *Journal of Pharmacology and Experimental Therapeutics,* **130,** 68–80

ESSMAN, W. B. and ESSMAN, E. (1980) Anticonvulsant effects upon regional synaptosomal GABA uptake: differences in convulsed rats. *Brain Research Bulletin,* 5 Suppl. 2, 821–824

FABISIAK, J. P. and SCHWARZ, W. S. (1982) Cerebral free amino acids in the amygdaloid kindling model of epilepsy. *Neuropharmacology,* **21,** 179–182

FERRANDES, B., DURAND, A., PADOVANI, P. *et al.* (1984) Metabolism of progabide in four animal species and in man. In *Epilepsy and GABA Receptor Agonists: Basic and Therapeutic research*, edited by G. Bartholini, L. Bossi, K. G. Lloyd and P. L. Morselli. New York: Raven Press

FERRENDELLI, J. A. (1980) Phenytoin: cyclic nucleotide regulation in the brain. *Advances in Neurology,* **27,** 429–433

FERRENDELLI, J. A. and KINSCHERF, D. A. (1979) Inhibitory effects of anticonvulsant drugs on cyclic nucleotide accumulation in brain. *Annals of Neurology,* **5,** 533–538

FERRENDELLI, J. A. and KLUNK, W. E. (1982) Ethosuximide: mechanism of action. In *Antiepileptic Drugs,* edited by D. M. Woodbury, J. K. Penry and C. E. Pippenger, pp. 655–661. New York: Raven Press

FOWLER, L. J., BECKFORD, J. and JOHN, R. A. (1975) An analysis of the kinetics of the inhibition of rabbit brain gamma-aminobutyrate aminotransferase by sodium n-dipropylacetate and some other simple carboxylic acids. *Biochemical Pharmacology,* **24,** 1267–1270

FRENCH, E. D., FOSTER, A. C., VEZZANI, A. and SCHWARCZ, R. (1984) Quinolinate and kynurenate, two endogenous tryptophan metabolites with potential links to epileptic disorders. *Clinical Neuropharmacology,* **7** (Suppl. 1), 456–457

FROMM, G. H. and KILLIAN, J. M. (1967) Effect of some anticonvulsant drugs on the spinal trigeminal nucleus. *Neurology* (*Minneapolis*), **17,** 275–280

FROMM, G. H. and KOHLI, C. M. (1972) The role of inhibitory pathways in petit mal epilepsy. *Neurology (Minneapolis),* **22,** 1012–1020

GALE, K. (1984) Role of the substantia nigra in the anticonvulsant action of GABAergic drugs. In *Neurotransmitters, Seizures and Epilepsy*, edited by R. G. Fariello, J. Engel, K. G. Lloyd, P. L. Morselli and L. F. Quesney, pp. 57–80. New York: Raven Press

GALE, K. and IADAROLA, M. (1980) Seizure protection and increased nerve terminal GABA: delayed effects of GABA transaminase inhibition. *Science,* **208,** 288–291

GALLAGER, D. W. (1978) Benzodiazepines: potentiation of a GABA inhibitory response in the dorsal raphe nucleus. *European Journal of Pharmacology,* **49,** 133–143

GALLAGER, D. W., THOMAS, J. W. and TALLMAN, J. F. (1978) Effect of GABAergic drugs on benzodiazepine site sensitivity in rat cerebral cortex. *Biochemical Pharmacology,* **27,** 2745–2749

GALLAGER, D. W., MALLORGA, P. and TALLMAN, J. F. (1980) Interaction of diphenylhydantoin and benzodiazepines in the CNS. *Brain Research,* **189,** 209–220

GALLAGER, D. W., MALLORGA, P., SWAIMAN, K., NEALE, E. A. and NELSON, P. G. (1981) Effects of phenytoin on 3H-diazepam binding in dissociated primary cell culture. *Brain Research,* **218,** 319–330

GALLAGHER, J. P. and SHINNICK-GALLAGHER, P. (1983) Electrophysiological characteristics of GABA-receptor complexes. In *The GABA Receptors,* edited by S. J. Enna, pp. 25–62. Clifton: Humana Press

GALLAGHER, J. P., NAKAMURA, J. and SHINNICK-GALLAGHER, P. (1983) Effects of glial uptake and desensitization on the activity of gamma-aminobutyric acid (GABA) and its analogs at the cat dorsal root ganglion. *Journal of Pharmacology and Experimental Therapeutics,* **226,** 876–884

GANGLOFF, H. and MONNIER, M. (1957) The action of anticonvulsant drugs tested by electrical stimulation of the rabbit cortex, diencephalon and rhinencephalon in the unanesthetized rabbit. *Electroencephalography and Clinical Neurophysiology,* **9,** 43–58

GARDNER, C. R. and WEBSTER, R. A. (1977) Convulsant–anticonvulsant interactions on seizure activity and cortical acetylcholine release. *European Journal of Pharmacology,* **42,** 247–256

GARELIS, E. and SOURKES, T. L. (1974) Use of cerebrospinal fluid drawn during pneumoencephalography in the study of monoamine metabolism in man. *Journal of Neurology, Neurosurgery and Psychiatry,* **37,** 704–710

GARRIGOU, D., DURAND, A., FERRANDES, B. and MORSELLI, P. L. (1984) Kinetics of the distribution of progabide and related metabolites in various areas of the rat brain. *14th CINP, Florence, June 19–23 1984.* Abstract, 723

GELLER, H. M., TAYLOR, D. A. and HOFFER, B. J. (1978) Benzodiazepines and central inhibitory mechanisms. *Naunyn-Schmiedeberg's Archives of Pharmacology,* **304,** 81–88

GENT, J. P. and PHILLIPS, N. I. (1980) Sodium di-n-propylacetate (valproate) potentiates responses to GABA and muscimol on single central neurones. *Brain Research,* **197,** 275–278

GILBERT, J. C. and WYLLIE, M. G. (1974) The effects of anticonvulsant ethosuximide on adenosine triphosphatase activities of synaptosomes prepared from rat cerebral cortex. *British Journal of Pharmacology,* **52,** 139P–140P

GODIN, Y., HEINER, L., MARK, J. and MANDEL, P. (1969) Effects of di-n-propylacetate, an anticonvulsive compound, on GABA metabolism. *Journal of Neurochemistry,* **16,** 869–873

GOLDBERG, M. A. and TODOROFF, T. (1973) Binding of diphenylhydantoin to brain protein. *Biochemical Pharmacology,* **22,** 2973–2980

GOLDBERG, M. A. and TODOROFF, T. (1976) Diphenylhydantoin binding to brain lipids and phospholipids. *Biochemical Pharmacology,* **25,** 2079–2083

GOTTESFELD, Z. and ELAZAR, Z. (1972) GABA and glutamate in different EEG stages of the penicillin focus. *Nature,* **240,** 478–479

GOTTESFELD, Z. and ELAZAR, Z. (1975) GABA synthesis and uptake in penicillin focus. *Brain Research,* **84,** 346–350

GRAY, W. D., MAREN, T. H., SISSON, G. M. and SMITH, F. H. (1957) Carbonic anhydrase inhibition. VII. Carbonic anhydrase inhibition and anticonvulsant effect. *Journal of Pharmacology and Experimental Therapy,* **121,** 160–170

GROSS, G. J. and WOODBURY, D. M. (1972) Effects of pentylenetetrazole on ion transport in the isolated toad bladder. *Journal of Pharmacology and Experimental Therapeutics,* **181,** 257–272

GUIDOTTI, A. (1985) Role of benzodiazepines/GABA receptors in the neurobiological mechanisms of anxiety. *Clinical Neuropharmacology,* **7** (Suppl. 1), 568–569

GUIDOTTI, A. and FERRERO, P. (1985) *Ex vivo* binding of 3H muscimol to GABA A recognition sites: a tool to characterize GABA receptor agonists. In *Epilepsy and GABA Receptor Agonists: Basic and Therapeutic Research,* edited by G. Bartholini, L. Bossi, K. G. Lloyd and P. L. Morselli, pp. 31–41. New York: Raven Press

GUIDOTTI, A., CORDA, M. G., VACCARINO, F. and WISE, B. C. (1984) Role of GABA-modulin and of an endogenous effector of beta-carboline binding sites in the GABA-benzodiazepine receptor interaction. In *Actions and Interactions of GABA and Benzodiazepines,* edited by N. G. Bowery, pp. 191–202. New York: Raven Press

GUIDOTTI, A., TOFFANO, G., BARLAKI, M., SCHWARTZ, J. P. and COSTA, E. (1979) A molecular mechanism for the facilitation of GABA receptor function by benzodiazepines. In *GABA-Neurotransmitters,* edited by P. Krogsgaard-Larsen, J. Scheel-Kruger and H. Kofod, pp. 406–415. Copenhagen: Munskgaard

HADFIELD, M. G. (1972) Uptake and binding of catecholamines: effect of diphenylhydantoin and a new mechanism of action. *Archives of Neurology,* **26,** 78–84

HADFIELD, M. G. and BOYKIN, M. E. (1974) Effect of diphenylhydantoin administered *in vivo* on 3H-1-norepinephrine uptake in rat synaptosomes. *Research Communications in Chemical Pathology and Pharmacology,* **7,** 209–212

HAEFELY, W., PIERI, L., POLC, P. and SCHAFFNER, T. (1981) General pharmacology and neuropharmacology of benzodiazepine derivatives. In *Handbook of Experimental Pharmacology,* Volume 55/II, edited by F. Hoffmeister and G. Stille, pp. 13–262. Berlin: Springer Verlag

HANSEN, S., PERRY, T. L., WADA, J. A. and SOKOL, M. (1973) Brain amino acids in baboons with light induced epilepsy. *Brain Research,* **50,** 480–483

HARRISON, N. L. and SIMMONDS, M. A. (1982) Sodium valproate enhances responses to GABA receptor activation only at high concentrations. *Brain Research,* **250,** 201–204

HARVEY, P. K. P., BRADFORD, H. F. and DAVISON, A. N. (1975) The inhibitory effect of sodium n-dipropylacetate on the degradative enzymes of the GABA shunt. *FEBS Letters,* **52,** 251–254

HASBANY, M., PINCUS, J. H. and LEE, S. H. (1974) Diphenylhydantoin and calcium movement in lobster nerves. *Archives of Neurology,* **31,** 250–254

HENRIKSEN, S. J., CHOUVET, G., MCGINTY, J. and BLOOM, F. E. (1983) Neuropeptides and the epilepsies: current perspectives. In *Epilepsy: an Update of Research and Therapy*, edited by G. Nistico, R. DiPerri and H. Meinardi, pp. 105–120. New York: Alan Liss

HERTZ, L., SCHOUSBOE, A., FORNBY, B. and LENNOX-BUCHTHAL, M. (1974). Some age-dependent biochemical changes in mice susceptible to seizures. *Epilepsia,* **15,** 619–631.

HEYER, E. J. and MACDONALD, R. L. (1982) Barbiturate reduction of calcium dependent action potentials. *Brain Research,* **236,** 157–171

HILL, N. and BOWERY, N. G. (1981) 3H-Baclofen and 3H-GABA bind to bicuculline insensitive GABA B sites in rat brain. *Nature,* **290,** 149–152

HOLM, E., KELLETER, R., HEINEMANN, H. and HAMANN, K. F. (1970). Elektrophysiologische analyse der wirkungen von carbamazepin anf das behirn der katze. *Pharmakopsychiatrie Neuro-Psychopharmakologie,* **3,** 187–200

HORTON, R. W., ANLEZARK, G. M., SAWAYA, M. C. B. and MELDRUM, B. S. (1977) Monoamine and GABA metabolism and the anticonvulsant action of di-n-propylacetate and ethanolamine-O-sulphate. *European Journal of Pharmacology,* **41,** 387–397

HORTON, R. W., PRESTWICK, S. A. and MELDRUM, B. S. (1982) Gamma aminobutyric acid and benzodiazepine binding sites in audiogenic seizure-susceptible mice. *Journal of Neurochemistry,* **39,** 864–870

HOUGHTON, G. W., RICHENS, A., TOSELAND, P. A., DAVIDSON, S. and FALCONER, M. A. (1975) Brain concentrations of phenytoin, phenobarbitone and primidone in epileptic patients. *European Journal of Clinical Pharmacology,* **9,** 73–78

HUNKELER, W., MÖHLER, H., PIERI, L. *et al.* (1981) Selective antagonists of benzodiazepine receptors. *Nature,* **290,** 514–516

JOBE, P. C. and LAIRD, H. E. (1981) Neurotransmitter abnormalities as determinants of seizure susceptibility and intensity in the genetic models of epilepsy. *Biochemical Pharmacology,* **30,** 3137–3144

JOHNSTON, D. and AYALA, G. F. (1975) The action of a common anticonvulsant on bursting pacemaker cells in aplysia. *Science,* **189,** 1009–1011

JOHNSTON, G. A. R. and SKERRITT, J. H. (1984) Gabarins and the nexus between GABA and benzodiazepine receptors. In *Actions and Interactions of GABA and Benzodiazepines,* edited by N. G. Bowery, pp. 179–190. New York: Raven Press

JOY, R. M., ALBERTSON, T. F. and STARK, L. G. (1984) Analysis of the actions of progabide, a specific GABA receptor agonist, on kindling and kindling seizures. *Experimental Neurology,* **83,** 144–154

JULIEN, R. M. and HALPREN, L. M. (1972) Effects of diphenylhydantoin and other acid on epileptiform activity and Purkinje cells discharge rate. *Epilepsia,* **13,** 387–400

JULIEN, R. M. and HOLLISTER, R. P. (1975) Carbamazepine: mechanism of action. In *Advances in Neurology,* Vol. 11, edited by J. K. Penry and D. D. Daly, pp. 263–276. New York: Raven Press

KALICHMAN, M. W. (1982) Neurochemical correlates of the kindling model of epilepsy. *Neuroscience and Biobehavioral Reviews,* **6,** 165–181

KERWIN, R. W. and TABERNER, P. V. (1981) The mechanism of action of sodium valproate. *General Pharmacology,* **12,** 71–75

KERWIN, R. W., OLPE, H. R. and SCHMUTZ, M. (1980) The effect of sodium-n-dipropylacetate on gamma-aminobutyric acid dependent inhibition in the rat cortex and substantia nigra in relation to its anticonvulsant activity. *British Journal of Pharmacology,* **71,** 545–551

KLUNK, W. E. and FERRENDELLI, J. A. (1980) Reversal of the anticonvulsant action of ethosuximide by drugs that diminish CNS dopaminergic neurotransmission. *Neurology (Minneapolis),* **30,** 421

KOE, B. K. (1983) Enhancement of benzodiazepine binding by progabide (SL 76002) and SL 75102. *Drug Development Research,* **3,** 421–432

KREISMAN, N. R., MURPHY, M. F. and KING, W. M. (1978) Effects of the anticonvulsant, trimethadione, on bursting pacemaker activity and recruitment of inhibition in the abdominal ganglion of *Aplysia californica. Computer Biochemistry,* **60C,** 145–154

KRNJEVIC, K. (1974) Chemical nature of synaptic transmission in vertebrates. *Physiological Reviews,* **54,** 418–432

KROGSGAARD-LARSEN, P., LABOUTA, J. M., MELDRUM, B., CROUCHER, M. and SCHOUSBOE, A. (1981) GABA uptake inhibitors as experimental tools and potential drugs in epilepsy research. In *Neurotransmitters, Seizures and Epilepsy,* edited by P. L. Morselli, K. G. Lloyd, W. Loscher, B. Meldrum and E. H. Reynolds, pp. 23–33. New York: Raven Press

KRUPP, P. (1969) The effect of Tegretol on some elementary neuronal mechanisms. *Headache,* **9,** 42–46

KUSSKE, J. A., OJEMANN, G. A. and WARD, A. A. JR (1972) Effects of lesions in ventral anterior thalamus on experimental focal epilepsy. *Experimental Neurology,* **34,** 279–290

LEWIN, E. and BLECK, V. (1971) The effect of diphenylhydantoin administration on sodium potassium activated ATPase in cortex. *Neurology,* **21,** 647–651

LEWIN, E. and BLECK, V. (1977) Cyclic AMP accumulation in cerebral cortical slices effect of carbamazepine, phenobarbital and phenytoin. *Epilepsia,* **18,** 237–242

LEZNICKI, A. and DYMECKI, J. (1974) The effect of certain anticonvulsants *in vitro* and *in vivo* on enzyme activities in rat brain. *Neurologia Neurochirurgia Polska,* **24,** 413–419

LLOYD, K. G., WORMS, P. P., DEPOORTERE, H. and BARTHOLINI, G. (1979) Pharmacological profile of SL 76002, a new GABA-mimetic drug. In *GABA-Neurotransmitters* edited by P. Krogsgaard-Larsen, J. Scheel-Kruger and H. Kofod, pp. 308–324. Copenhagen: Munksgaard

LLOYD, K. G., BOVIER, P., BROEKKAMP, C. L. and WORMS, P. (1981a) Reversal of the antiaversive and anticonvulsant actions of diazepam, but not progabide, by a selective antagonist of benzodiazepine receptors. *European Journal of Pharmacology,* **75,** 77–78

LLOYD, K. G., MUNARI, C., BOSSI, L., STOEFFELS, C. TALAIRACH, J. and MORSELLI, P. L. (1981b) Biochemical evidence for the alterations of GABA-mediated synaptic transmission in pathological brain tissue (stereo EEG or morphological definition) from epileptic patients. In *Neurotransmitters, Seizures and Epilepsy*, edited by P. L. Morselli, K. G. Lloyd, W. Loscher, B. Meldrum and E. G. Reynolds, pp. 325–338. New York: Raven Press

LLOYD, K. G., ARBILLA, S., BEAUMONT, K. *et al.* (1982) Gamma-aminobutyric acid (GABA) receptor stimulation. II. Specificity of progabide (SL 76002) and SL 75102 for the GABA receptor. *Journal of Pharmacology and Experimental Therapeutics,* **220,** 672–677

LLOYD, K. G., MUNARI, C., WORMS, P., BOSSI, L. and MORSELLI, P. L. (1983a) Indications for the use of gamma-aminobutyric acid (GABA) – agonists in convulsant disorders. In *Epilepsy: An Update on Research and Therapy,* edited by G. Nistico, R. Di Perri and H. Meinardi, pp. 285–297. New York: Alan Liss

LLOYD, K. G., DEMONTIS, G., BROEKKAMP, C. L., THURET, F. and WORMS, P. (1983b) Neurochemical and neuropharmacological indications for the involvement of GABA and glycine receptors in neuropsychiatric disorders. In *CNS Receptors – From Molecular Pharmacology to Behavior*, edited by P. Meudel and F. V. DeFeudis, pp. 137–148. New York: Raven Press

LLOYD, K. G., MUNARI, C., BOSSI, L. and MORSELLI, P. L. (1984a) The GABA hypothesis of human epilepsy: neurochemical evidence from surgically resected identified foci. In: *Neurotransmitters, Seizures and Epilepsy II,* edited by R. G. Fariello, P. L. Morselli, K. G. Lloyd and J. Engel, L. F. Quesney, pp. 285–294. New York: Raven Press

LLOYD, K. G., DEPOORTERE, H., MANOURY, P., SCATTON, B., ZIVKOVIC, B., LANGER, S. Z., MORSELLI, P. L. and BARTHOLINI, G. (1984b) Non-benzodiazepine anxiolytics: potential activity of phenylpiperazines without 3H-diazepam displacing action. *Clinical Neuropharmacology,* **7** (Suppl. 1), 896–897

LONDOS, C., COOPER, D. M. F. and WOLFF, J. (1980) Subclasses of external adenosine receptors. *Proceedings of the National Academy of Sciences of the USA,* **74,** 2551–2554

LÖSCHER, W. (1979) GABA in plasma and cerebrospinal fluid of different species. Effects of gamma-acetylenic GABA, gamma-vinyl GABA and sodium valproate. *Journal of Neurochemistry,* **32,** 1587–1591

LÖSCHER, W. (1980) Effect of inhibitors of GABA transmission on the synthesis, binding, uptake and metabolism of GABA. *Journal of Neurochemistry,* **34,** 1603–1608

LÖSCHER, W. (1981a) Anticonvulsant activity of metabolites of valproic acid. *Archives Internationales de Pharmacodynamie et de Therapie,* **249,** 158–163

LÖSCHER, W. (1981b) Valproate induced changes in GABA metabolism at the subcellular level. *Biochemical Pharmacology,* **30,** 1364–1366

LÖSCHER, W. (1981c) Biochemical pharmacology of inhibitors of GABA metabolism and valproic acid. In *Neurotransmitters, Seizures and Epilepsy,* edited by P. L. Morselli, K. G. Lloyd, W. Löscher, B. Meldrum and E. H. Reynolds, pp. 93–102. New York: Raven Press

LÖSCHER, W. (1982) Comparative assay of anticonvulsant and toxic potencies of sixteen GABA mimetic drugs. *Neuropharmacology,* **21,** 803–810

LÖSCHER, W. and FREY, H. H. (1977) Effect of convulsant and anti-convulsant agents on levels and metabolism of gamma aminobutyric acid in mouse brain. *Naunyn Schmiedeberg's Archives of Pharmacology,* **296,** 263–269

LOTT, I. T., COULOMBE, T., DIPAOLO, R. V., RICHARDSON, E. P. and LEVY, H. L. (1978) Vitamin B-6 dependent seizures: pathology and chemical findings in brain. *Neurology,* **28,** 47–54

LOWE, D. A., RICHARDSON, B. P., TAYLOR, P. and DONATSCH, P. (1976) Increasing intracellular sodium triggers calcium release from bound pools. *Nature,* **260,** 337–338

LUST, W. D., KUPFERBERG, H. J., PASSONNEAU, J. V. and PENRY, J. K. (1976) Metabolite levels in brain following experimental seizures: the effects of isoniazid and sodium valproate in cerebellar and cerebral cortical layers. *Journal of Neurochemistry,* **32,** 755–760

LUST, W. D., KUPFERBERG, H. J., JONEKAWA, W. D., PENRY, J. K., PASSONEAU, J. V. and WHEATON, A. B. (1978) Changes in brain metabolites induced by convulsants or electroshock: effects of anticonvulsant agents. *Molecular Pharmacology,* **14,** 347–350

MACDONALD, R. L. and BARKER, J. L. (1979a) Enhancement of GABA-mediated postsynaptic inhibition in cultured mammalian spinal cord neurons: a common mode of anticonvulsant action. *Brain Research,* **167,** 323–336

MACDONALD, R. L. and BARKER, J. L. (1979b). Anticonvulsant and anesthetic barbiturates: different postsynaptic actions in cultured mammalian neurons. *Neurology,* **29,** 432–447

MACDONALD, R. L. and BERGEY, G. K. (1979) Valproic acid augments GABA mediated postsynaptic inhibition in cultured mammalian neurons. *Brian Research,* **170,** 558–562

MACDONALD, R. L. and MCLEAN, M. J. (1982) Cellular bases of barbiturate and phenytoin anticonvulsant drug action. *Epilepsia,* **23** (Suppl. 1), S7–18

MAITRE, M., CISIELSKI, L. and MANDEL, P. (1974) Effect of 2-methyl 2-ethyl caproic acid and 2-2-dimethyl valeric acid on audiogenic seizures and brain gamma-aminobutyric acid. *Biochemical Pharmacology,* **23,** 2363–2368

MANYAM, N. V. B., KATZ, L., HARE, T. A., GERBER, J. C. and GROSSMAN, M. N. (1980) Levels of gamma-aminobutyric acid in cerebrospinal fluid in various neurologic disorders. *Archives of Neurology,* **37,** 352–355

MAZIERE, M., HANTRAYE, P., GUIBERT, B. *et al.* (1984) RO15-1788-C: a specific radioligand for an *in vivo* study of central benzodiazepine receptors by positron emission tomography. *Clinical Neuropharmacology,* **7** (Suppl. 1), 662–663

MCCANDLESS, D. W., FEUSSNER, G. K., LUST, W. D. and PASSONNEAU, J. V. (1979) Metabolite levels in brain following experimental seizures: the effects of isoniazid and sodium valproate in cerebellar and cerebral cortical layers. *Journal of Neurochemistry,* **32,** 755–760

MCGEER, P. L., MCGEER, E. G. and WADA, J. A. (1971) Glutamic acid decarboxylase in Parkinson's disease and epilepsy. *Neurology,* **21,** 1000–1007

MCMILLEN, B. A. and ISAAC, L. (1978) Effects of pentylenetetrazol and trimethadione on feline brain monoamine metabolism. *Biochemical Pharmacology,* **27,** 1815–1820

MCNAMARA, J. O., PEPER, A. M. and PATRONE, V. (1980) Repeated seizures induce long-term increase in hippocampal benzodiazepine receptors. *Proceedings of the National Academy of Sciences of the USA,* **77,** 3029–3032

MCNAMARA, J. O., BYRNE, M. C., DASHIEFF, R. M. and FITZ, J. G. (1980) The kindling model of epilepsy: a review. *Progress in Neurobiology,* **15,** 139–159

MELDRUM, B. (1981) GABA agonists as anti-epileptic agents. In *GABA and Benzodiazepine Receptors,* edited by E. Costa, G. Di Chiarra and G. L. Gessa, pp. 207–218. New York: Raven Press

MELDRUM, B. and BRAESTRUP, C. (1984) GABA and the anticonvulsant action of benzodiazepines and related drugs. In *Actions and Interactions of GABA and Benzodiazepines,* edited by N. G. Bowery, pp. 133–154. New York: Raven Press

MELDRUM, B. and MENINI, C. (1981) Effects of morphine, enkephalins, beta-endorphin and related compounds on seizure thresholds. In *Neurotransmitters, Seizures and Epilepsy,* edited by P. L. Morselli, K. G. Lloyd, W. Loscher, B. Meldrum and E. H. Reynolds, pp. 185–194. New York: Raven Press

MEUNIER, H., CARRAY, G., MEUNIER, Y., EYMARD, P. and AIMARD, M. (1963) Pharmacology of 2 propylvaleric acid. *Therapie,* **18,** 435–483

MEYER, H. and FREY, H. H. (1973) Dependence of anticonvulsant drug action on central monoamines. *Neuropharmacology,* **12,** 939–947

MILLICHAP, J. G., THATCHER, L. D. and WILLIAMS, P. (1955) Anticonvulsant action of acetazolamide alone and in combination with ammonium chloride. *Federation Proceedings,* **14,** 370

MÖHLER, H. (1984) Benzodiazepine receptors and their ligands. In *Actions and Interactions of GABA and Benzodiazepines,* edited by N. G. Bowery, pp. 155–166. New York: Raven Press

MÖHLER, H. and OKADA, T. (1977) Benzodiazepine receptor: demonstration in the central nervous system. *Science,* **198,** 849–851

MÖHLER, H., SCHOCH, P., HARING, P., TAKACS, B. and STAHLI, C. H. (1984) A purified GABA/benzodiazepine receptor: biochemical, pharmacological and immunological characterization. *Clinical Neuropharmacology,* **7** (Suppl. 1), 560–561

MÖHLER, H., RICHARDS, J. G. and WU, J. Y. (1981) Autoradiographic localization of benzodiazepine receptors in immunocytochemically identified gamma-aminobutyrergic synapses. *Proceedings of the National Academy of Sciences of the USA,* **78,** 1935–1938

MORRELL, F., BRADLEY, W. and PTASHNE, M. (1959) Effects of drugs on discharge characteristics of chronic epileptogenic lesions. *Neurology (Minneapolis),* **9,** 492–498

MORSELLI, P. L., CASSANO, G. B., PLACIDI, G. F., MUSCETTOLA, G. B. and RIZZO, M. (1973) Kinetics of the distribution of 14C-diazepam and its metabolites in various areas of cat brain. In *The Benzodiazepines,* edited by S. Garattimi, E. Mussini and L. O. Randall, pp. 129–143. New York: Raven Press

MORSELLI, P. L., BARUZZI, A., GERNA, M., BOSSI, L. and PORTA, M. (1977) Carbamazepine and carbamazepine-10,11-epoxide concentrations in human brain. *British Journal of Clinical Pharmacology,* **4,** 535–540

MORSELLI, P. L., CALDERINI, G., CONSOLAZIONE, A., RIVA, E. and ALTAMURA, C. (1978) Effect of carbamazepine on brain mediators in control and cobalt-treated rats. In *Advances in Epileptology,* edited by H. Meinardi and A. J. Rowan, pp. 176–182. Amsterdam, Lisse: Swets and Zeitlinger BV

MORSELLI, P. L. and FRANCO-MORSELLI, R. (1980) Clinical pharmacokinetics of antiepileptic drugs in adults. *Pharmacology and Therapeutics,* **10,** 65–101

MUNARI, C., ROVEI, V., TALAIRACH, J., SANJUAN, E., BANCAUD, J. and MORSELLI, P. L. (1980) AED concentrations in discrete brain areas of epileptic patients undergoing surgical intervention. In *Advances in Epileptology, IX Symposium,* edited by J. Wada and J. K. Penry, pp. 129. New York: Raven Press

MUNARI, C., BOSSI, L., STOFFELS, C., BRUNET, P., BANCAUD, J., TALAIRACH, J. and MORSELLI, P. L. (1982) Concentrations cérébrales des médicaments anti-comitiaux chez les malades ayant une epilepsie tumorale. *Revue d'E.E.G. et de Neurophysiologie,* **12,** 38–43

MYLLYLA, V. V. (1976) Effect of convulsions and anticonvulsive drugs on cerebrospinal fluid acid cyclic AMP in rabbits. *European Neurology,* **14,** 97–107.

NAHORSKI, S. R. (1972) Biochemical effects of the anticonvulsants trimethadione, ethosuximide and chlordiazepoxide in rat brain. *Journal of Neurochemistry,* **19,** 1937–1946

NESTROS, J. N. and NISTRI, A. (1979) Effects of iontophoretically applied flurazepam on responses of cerebral cortical neurons to putative neurotransmitters. *Canadian Journal of Physiology and Pharmacology,* **57,** 1324–1329

NICOLL, R. A. (1978) Pentobarbital: differential postsynaptic actions on sympathetic ganglion cells. *Science,* **199,** 451–452

NICOLL, R. A., ECCLES, J. C., OSHIWA, T. amd RUBIA, F. (1975) Prolongation of hippocampal inhibitory postsynaptic potentials by barbiturates. *Nature,* **258,** 265–267

NISTRI, A. and CONSTANTI, A. (1978) Effects of flurazepam on amino acid evoked responses recorded from the lobster muscle and the frog spinal cord. *Neuropharmacology,* **17,** 127–135

NOWACK, W. J., JOHNSON, R. N., ENGLANDER, R. M. and HANNA, G. R. (1979) Effects of valproate and ethosuximide on thalamocortical excitability. *Neurology (Minneapolis),* **29,** 96–99

OLSEN, R. W. (1981) GABA–benzodiazepine–barbiturate receptor interaction. *Journal of Neurochemistry,* **37,** 1–13

OLSEN, R. W. (1982) Drug interactions at the GABA receptor ionophore complex. *Annual Reviews of Pharmacology and Toxicology,* **22,** 245–277

OLSEN, R. W., TICKU, M. K., VAN NESS, P. C. and GREENLEE, D. (1978) Effects of drugs on gamma-aminobutyric acid receptors, uptake, release and synthesis *in vitro. Brain Research,* **139,** 277–294

ONDRUSEK, M. G., BELKNAP, J. K. and LESLIE, S. W. (1979) Effects of acute and chronic barbiturate administration on synaptosomal calcium accumulation. *Molecular Pharmacology,* **15,** 386–395

ORLOWSKI, M., REINGOLD, D. F. and STANLEY, M. E. (1977) D-and L-isomers of allylglycine: convulsive action and inhibition of brain L-glutamate decarboxylase. *Journal of Neurochemistry,* **28,** 349–353

PAPESCHI, R., MOLINANEGRO, P., SOURKES, T. L. and ERBA, G. (1927) The concentration of homovanillic and 5-hydroxyindolacetic acids in ventricular and lumbar GSF. *Neurology,* **22,** 1151–1159

PATSALOS, P. N. and LASCELLES, P. T. (1981) Changes in regional brain levels of amino acid putative neurotransmitters after prolonged treatment with the anticonvulsant drugs diphenylhydantoin, phenobarbitone, sodium valproate, ethosuximide, and sulthiame in the rat. *Journal of Neurochemistry,* **36,** 688–695

PERRY, T. L. and HANSEN, S. (1978) Biochemical effects in man and rat of three drugs which can increase brain GABA content. *Journal of Neurochemistry,* **30,** 679–684

PERRY, J. G., MCKINNEY, L. and DE WEER, P. (1978) The cellular mode of action of the antiepileptic drug 5,5-diphenylhydantoin. *Nature,* **272,** 272–273

PERRY, T. L., HANSEN, S., KENNEDY, J., WADA, J. A. and THOMPSON, G. B. (1975) Amino acids in human epileptogenic foci. *Archives of Neurology,* **32,** 752–754

PHILLIS, J. W. (1970) *The Pharmacology of Synapses.* New York: Pergamon Press

PINCUS, J. H. (1972) Diphenylhydantoin and ion flux in lobster nerve. *Archives of Neurology,* **26,** 4–10

PINCUS, J. H. and LEE, S. H. (1973) Diphenylhydantoin and calcium. Relation to norepinephrine release from brain slices. *Archives of Neurology,* **29,** 239–244

PLACIDI, G. F., TOGNONI, G., PACIFICI, G. M., CASSANO, G. B. and MORSELLI, P. L. (1976) Regional distribution of diazepam and its metabolites in the brain of cat after chronic treatment. *Psychopharmacology,* **48,** 133–137

PLUM, C. M. (1974) Free amino acid levels in the cerebrospinal fluid of normal humans and their variations in cases of epilepsy and Spielmeyer-Vogt-Batter disease. *Journal of Neurochemistry,* **23,** 595–600

POLC, P., MÖHLER, H. and HAEFELY, W. (1974) The effect of diazepam on spinal cord activities: possible sites and mechanisms of actions. *Naunyn Schmiedeberg's Archives of Pharmacology,* **284,** 319–333

PORTER, R. (1982) Clinical efficacy and use of antiepileptic drugs. In *Antiepileptic Drugs,* 2nd edition, edited by D. M. Woodbury, J. K. Penry and C. E. Pippenger, pp. 167–175. New York: Raven Press

POST, R. M., UNDE, T. W., VALLENGER, J. C., CHATTERJE, D. C., GREENE, R. F. and BUNNEY, W. E. (1983) Carbamazepine and its 10-11-epoxide metabolite in plasma and CSF: relationship to antidepressant response. *Archives of General Psychiatry,* **40,** 673–676

PRICHARD, J. W. (1980) Antiepileptic drugs – phenobarbital: proposed mechanisms of antiepileptic action. In *Antiepileptic Drugs: Mechanisms of Action,* edited by G. H. Glaser, J. K. Penry and D. M. Woodbury, pp. 553–562. New York: Raven Press

PRICHARD, J. W. (1982) Phenobarbital – mechanisms of action. In *Antiepileptic Drugs,* edited by D. M. Woodbury, J. K. Penry and C. E. Pippenger, pp. 365–376. New York: Raven Press

PROCTOR, W. R. and WEAKLY, J. N. (1976) A comparison of the presynaptic and postsynaptic actions of pentobarbitone and phenobarbitone in the neuromuscular junction of the frog. *Journal of Physiology (London),* **258,** 257–268

PURDY, R. E., JULIEN, R. M., FAIRHURST, A. S. and TERRY, M. D. (1977) Effect of carbamazepine on the *in vitro* uptake and release of norepinephrine in adrenergic nerves of rabbit aorta and in whole brain synaptosomes. *Epilepsia,* **18,** 251–257

QUATTRONE, A. and SAMANIN, R. (1977) Decreased anticonvulsant activity of carbamazepine in 6-hydroxydopamine-treated rats. *European Journal of Pharmacology,* **41,** 333–336

QUESNEY, L. F. (1981) Dopamine and generalized photosensitive epilepsy. In *Neurotransmitters, Seizures and Epilepsy,* edited by P. L. Morselli, K. G. Lloyd, W. Löscher, B. Meldrum and E. H. Reynolds, pp. 263–274. New York: Raven Press

QUESNEY, L. F. and READER, T. (1984) Role of cortical catecholamine depletion in the genesis of epileptic photosensitivity. In *Neurotransmitters, Seizures and Epilepsy,* Volume II, edited by R. Fariello, P. L. Morselli, K. G. Lloyd, L. F. Quesney and J. Engel, pp. 11–22. New York: Raven Press

RAABE, W. and AYALA, G. F. (1976) Diphenylhydantoin increases cortical post-synaptic inhibition. *Brain Research,* **105,** 597–601

RAABE, W. and GUMNIT, R. J. (1977) Anticonvulsant action of diazepam; increase of cortical postsynaptic inhibition. *Epilepsia,* **18,** 117–120

RADAN, C. and ESPLIN, B. (1977) Effects of ethosuximide on transmission of repetitive impulses and apparent rate of transmitter turnover in the spinal monosynaptic pathway. *Journal of Pharmacology and Experimental Therapeutics,* **201,** 320–325

RAINES, A. and STANDAERT, F. G. (1969) Effects of anticonvulsant drugs on nerve terminals. *Epilepsia,* **10,** 211–227

RANSOM, B. R. and BARKER, J. L. (1976) Pentobarbital selectively enhances GABA-mediated postsynaptic inhibition in tissue cultured mouse spinal neurons. *Brain Research,* **114,** 530–535

RAPPORT, R. L., HARRIS, A. B., FRIEL, P. N. and DJEMANN, G. A. (1975) Human epileptic brain Na, K, Atpase activity and phenytoin concentrations. *Archives of Neurology,* **32,** 549–554

RAWSON, M. D. and PINCUS, J. H. (1968) The effect of diphenylhydantoin on sodium, potassium, magnesium, activated adenosine triphosphatase in microsomal fractions of rat and guinea pig brain and on whole homogenates of human brain. *Biochemical Pharmacology,* **17,** 573–579

RIBAK, C. E., HARRIS, A. B., VAUGHAN, J. E. and ROBERTS, E. (1979) Inhibitory GABAergic nerve terminals decrease at sites of focal epilepsy. *Science,* **205,** 211–214

RIMMER, E. M. and RITCHIE, A. (1984) Double-blind study of gamma-vinyl-GABA in patients with refractory epilepsy. *Lancet,* **1,** 189–190

RITCHIE, J. M. and COHEN, P. J. (1975) Cocaine: procaine and other synthetic local anesthetics. In *The Pharmacological Basis of Therapeutics,* edited by L. S. Goodman and A. Gilman, pp. 379–403. New York: Macmillan

ROSS, S. M. and CRAIG, C. R. (1981a) Gamma-aminobutyric acid concentrations, L-glutamic acid decarboxylase activity and properties of the gamma-aminobutyric acid postsynaptic receptor in cobalt epilepsy in the rat. *Journal for Neuroscience,* **1,** 1388–1396

ROSS, S. M. and CRAIG, C. R. (1981b) Studies on gamma-aminobutyric acid transport in cobalt experimental epilepsy in the rat. *Journal of Neurochemistry,* **36,** 1006–1011

ROTH, L. T. and BARLOW, C. F. (1965) Autoradiography of drugs in the brain. In *Isotopes in Experimental Pharmacology,* edited by L. J. Roth, pp. 49–62. Chicago and London: University of Chicago Press

ROUGIER, A., LOISEAU, G., COHADON, F., LLOYD, K. G. and MORSELLI, P. L. (1984) GABA and other amino acids in cortical and hippocampal foci removed neurosurgically from epileptic patients. In *Advances in Epileptology,* XVth Epilepsy International Symposium, edited by R. J. Porter, R. H. Mattson, A. A. Ward and M. Dam, pp. 43–48. New York: Raven Press

ROWAN, A. J., BINNIE, C. D., DE BEER-PAWLIKOWSKI, N. K. B., GOEDHART, D. M., GUTTER, T., VAN DER GEEST, P., MEINARDI, H. and MEIJER, J. W. A. (1979) Sodium valproate: serial monitoring of EEG and serum levels. *Neurology (Minneapolis),* **29,** 1450–1459

SAAD, S. F., EL-MASRY, A. M. and SCOTT, P. M. (1972) Influence of certain anticonvulsants on the concentration of gamma-aminobutyric acid in the cerebral hemisphere of mice. *European Journal of Pharmacology,* **17,** 386–392

SASTRY, S. R. and PHILLIS, J. W. (1976) Antagonism of glutamate and acetylcholine excitation of rat cerebral cortical neurons by diphenylhydantoin. *General Pharmacology,* **7,** 411–413

SAWAYA, M. C. B., HORTON, R. W. and MELDRUM, B. S. (1975) Effects of anticonvulsant drugs on the cerebral enzymes metabolizing GABA. *Epilepsia,* **16,** 649–655

SCATTON, B., DEBEK, J., ZIVKOVIC, B., LIEGOIS, C., TROTTIER, S., CHAVEL, P. and BANCAUD, J. (1981) Alterations in catecholamine, serotonin, acetylcholine and cyclic nucleotides in brain regions after cobalt induced epilepsy in the rat: influence of anticonvulsant treatment. In *Neurotransmitters, Seizures and Epilepsy,* edited by P. L. Morselli, K. G. Lloyd, W. Löscher, B. Meldrum and E. H. Reynolds, pp. 215–226. New York: Raven Press

SCATTON, B., ZIVKOVIC, B., DEBEK, J., LLOYD, K. G., CONSTANTONIDIS, J., TISSOT, R. and BARTHOLINI, G. (1982) Gamma-aminobutyric acid (GABA) receptor stimulation. III. Effect of progabide (SL 76002) on norepinephrine, dopamine and 5-hydroxytryptamine turnover in rat brain areas. *Journal of Pharmacology and Experimental Therapeutics,* **220,** 678–687

SCHALLEK, W. and KUEHN, A. (1963) Effects of trimethadione, diphenylhydantoin and chlordiazepoxide on afterdischarges in the brain of the cat. *Proceedings of the Society for Experimental Biology and Medicine,* **112,** 813–817

SCHAUF, C. L., DAVIS, F. A. and MARDER, J. (1974) Effects of carbamazepine on the ionic conductances of myxicola giant axons. *Journal of Pharmacology and Experimental Therapeutics,* **189,** 538–543

SCHECHTER, P. J., TRANIER, Y. and GROVE, J. (1978) Effect of n-dipropylacetate on amino acid concentrations in mouse brain: correlation with anti-convulsant activity. *Journal of Neurochemistry,* **31,** 1325–1327

SCHECHTER, P. J., HANKE, N. F. J., GROVE, J., HUEBERT, N. and SJOERDSMA, A. (1984) Biochemical and clinical effects of gamma vinyl GABA in patients with epilepsy. *Neurology,* **34,** 182–186

SCHLOSSER, W. and FRANCO, S. (1979) Reduction of gamma-aminobutyric acid (GABA)-mediated transmission by a convulsant benzodiazepine. *Journal of Pharmacology and Experimental Therapeutics,* **211,** 290–295

SCHMIDT, D. and LÖSCHER, W. (1981) GABA concentrations in cerebrospinal fluid acid plasma of patients with epileptic seizures. In *Neurotransmitters, Seizures and Epilepsy,* edited by P. L. Morselli, K. G. Lloyd, W. Löscher, B. Meldrum and E. H. Reynolds, pp. 315–324. New York: Raven Press

SCHWARCZ, R. and FOSTER, A. C. (1984) Studies of quinolinic acid metabolism in rat brain. *Clinical Neuropharmacology,* **7** (Suppl. 1), 450–451

SCHWARTZ, J. R. (1979) The mode of action of phenobarbital on the excitable membrane of the node of Ranvier. *European Journal of Pharmacology,* **56,** 51–60

SEIGEL, G. J. and GOODWIN, B. B. (1972) Sodium–potassium activated adenosine triphosphatase of brain microsomes: modification of sodium inhibition by diphenylhydantoin. *Journal of Clinical Investigation,* **51,** 1164–1169

SHAH, D. S., CHAMBON, P. and GUIDOTTI, A. (1981) Binding of (3H)-5,5-diphenylhydantoin to rat brain membranes. *Neuropharmacology,* **20,** 1115–1119

SHAYWITZ, B. A., COHEN, D. J. and BOWERS, M. B. (1975) Reduced cerebrospinal fluid-5-hydroxyindoleacetic acid and homovanillic acid in children with epilepsy. *Neurology,* **25,** 72–79

SHEARER, D. E., FLEMING, D. E. and BIGLER, E. D. (1976) The photically evoked afterdischarge; a model for the study of drugs useful in the treatment of petit mal epilepsy. *Epilepsia,* **17,** 429–433

SHERWIN, A. L. and VAN GELDER, N. M. (1985) Biochemical markers of metabolic abnormalities in human focal epilepsy. In *Basic Mechanisms of the Epilepsies,* edited by A. V. Delgado-Escueta, A. A. Ward and D. Woodbury. New York: Raven Press

SHERWIN, A. L., EISEN, A. A. and SOKOLOWSKI, C. D. (1973) Anticonvulsant drugs in human epileptogenic brain – correlation of phenobarbital and diphenylhydantoin levels with plasma. *Archives of Neurology,* **29,** 73–77

SHERWIN, A. L., QUESNEY, L. F., GAUTHIER, S., OLIVER, A., ROBITAILLE, Y., MCQUAID, P., HARVEY, C. and VAN GELDER, N. M. (1984) Enzymatic changes in activity spiking areas of human epileptic cerebral cortex. *Neurology,* **34,** 927–933.

SIGGINS, G. R. (1984) Epileptogenic mechanisms of opioid peptide actions in the limbic system. In *Basic Mechanisms of the Epilepsies,* edited by A. V. Delgado-Escueta, A. A. Ward, Jr and D. Woodbury. New York: Raven Press

SILVERSTEIN, F. and JOHNSTON, M. V. (1984) Cerebrospinal fluid monoamine metabolites in patients with infantile spasms. *Neurology,* **34,** 102–105

SIMLER, S., CIESIELSKI, L., MAITRE, M., RANDRIANARIOSA, H. and MANDEL, P. (1973) Effect of sodium n-dipropylacetate on audiogenic seizures and brain gamma aminobutyric acid level. *Biochemical Pharmacology,* **22,** 1701–1708

SIMMONDS, M. A. (1981) Distinctions between the effects of barbiturates, benzodiazepines and phenytoin on responses to gamma-aminobutyric acid receptor activation and antagonisms by bicuculline and picrotoxin. *British Journal of Pharmacology,* **73,** 739–747

SIMMONDS, M. A. (1984) Physiological and pharmacological characteristics of the actions of GABA. In *Actions and Interactions of GABA and Benzodiazepines,* edited by N. G. Bowery, pp. 27–41. New York: Raven Press

SKERRITT, J. H. and JOHNSTON, G. A. R. (1983) Inhibition of amino acid transmitter release from rat brain slices by phenytoin and related anticonvulsants. *Clinical and Experimental Pharmacology and Physiology,* **10,** 527–533

SKERRITT, J. H. and JOHNSTON, G. A. R. (1984) Modulation of excitatory amino acid release by convulsant and anticonvulsant drugs. In *Neurotransmitters, Seizures and Epilepsy,* Volume II, edited by R. Fariello, P. Morselli, K. G. Lloyd, L. F. Quesney and J. Engel, pp. 215–226. New York: Raven Press

SKERRITT, J. H., DAVIES, L. P. and JOHNSTON, G. A. R. (1982) A purinergic component in the anticonvulsant action of carbamazepine. *European Journal of Pharmacology,* **82,** 195–197

SKERRITT, J. H., DAVIES, L. P. and JOHNSTON, G. A. R. (1983) Interaction of the anticonvulsant carbamazepine with adenosine receptors. 1: Neurochemical studies. *Epilepsia,* **24,** 634–642

SKERRITT, J. H., JOHNSTON, G. A. R. and CHOW, S. C. (1983) Interaction of the anticonvulsant carbamazepine with adenosine receptors. 2: Pharmacological studies. *Epilepsia,* **24,** 643–650

SKOLNICK, P., PAUL, S. M. and BARKER, J. L. (1980) Pentobarbital potentiates GABA enhanced 3H-diazepam binding to benzodiazepine receptors. *European Journal of Pharmacology,* **65,** 125–127

SKOLNICK, P. and PAUL, S. M. (1981) The mechanism(s) of action of the benzodiazepines. *Medicinal Research Reviews,* **1,** 3–22

SLATER, G. E. and JOHNSTON, D. (1978) Sodium valproate increases potassium conductance in *Aplysia* neurons. *Epilepsia,* **19,** 379–384

SNEAD, O. C. (1978a) Gamma-hydroxybutyrate in the monkey: II – Effect of chronic oral anticonvulsant drugs. *Neurology (Minneapolis),* **28,** 643–648

SNEAD, O. C. (1978b) Gamma-hydroxybutyrate in the monkey: III – Effect of intravenous anticonvulsant drugs. *Neurology (Minneapolis),* **28,** 1173–1178

SNEAD, O. C., BEARDEN, L. J. and PEGRAM, V. (1980) Effect of acute and chronic anticonvulsant administration on endogenous gamma-hydroxybutyrate in rat brain. *Neuropharmacology,* **19,** 47–52

SOHN, R. S. and FERRENDELLI, J. A. (1973) Inhibition of Ca^{2+} transport into rat brain synaptosomes by diphenylhydantoin (DPH). *Journal of Pharmacology and Experimental Therapeutics,* **185,** 272–275

SOHN, R. S. and FERRENDELLI, J. A. (1976) Anticonvulsant drug mechanisms phenytoin, phenobarbital, and ethosuximide and Ca^{2+} flux in isolated presynaptic endings. *Archives of Neurology,* **33,** 626–629

SONAWANE, B. R., YAFFE, S. J. and SHAPIRO, B. H. (1980) Changes in mouse brain diazepam receptor binding after phenobarbital administration. *Life Sciences,* **27,** 1335–1338

SQUIRES, R. F. and BRAESTRUP, C. (1977) Benzodiazepine receptors in rat brain. *Nature,* **266,** 732–734

SQUIRES, R. and SAEDERUP, E. (1982) Gamma-aminobutyric acid receptors modulate cation binding sites coupled to independent benzodiazepine, picrotoxin and anion binding sites. *Molecular Pharmacology,* **22,** 327–334

STRAW, R. N. and MITCHELL, C. L. (1966) Effect of phenobarbital on cortical afterdischarge and overseizure patterns in the rat. *International Journal of Neuropharmacology,* **5,** 323–330

STUDY, R. E. (1980) Phenytoin inhibition of cyclic guanosine 3′, 5′-monophosphate (cGMP) accumulation in neuroblastoma cells by calcium channel blockade. *Journal of Pharmacology Experimental and Therapeutics,* **215,** 575–581

STUDY, R. E. and BARKER, J. L. (1981) Diazepam and (-) pentobarbital: fluctuation analyses reveal different mechanisms for potentiation of GABA responses in cultured neurons. *Proceedings of the National Academy of Sciences of the USA,* **78,** 7180–7184

TABAKOFF, B. and VON WARTBURG, J. P. (1975) Separation of aldehyde reductases and alcohol dehydrogenase from brain by affinity chromatography: metabolism of succinic semialdehyde and ethanol. *Biochemical and Biophysical Research Communications,* **63,** 957–966

TALLMAN, J. F. (1983) GABA and benzodiazepine receptors. In *The GABA Receptors,* edited by S. J. Enna, pp. 93–107. Clifton: Humana Press

TANNHAUSER, M. and IZQUIERDO, I. (1974) Effect of seizures and anticonvulsant agents on hippocampal RNA concentration. *Pharmacology,* **11,** 139–145

TAPIA, R. (1974) The role of gamma-aminobutyric acid metabolism in the regulation of cerebral excitability. In *Neurohumoral Coding of Brain Function,* edited by R. D. Meyers and R. R. Drucker-Collin, pp. 3–26. New York: Plenum Press

TAYLOR, D. P., EISON, A. S., EISON, M. S., RIBLET, L. A., TEMPLE, O. L. and VAN DER MAELEN, C. P. (1984) Biochemistry and pharmacology of the anxioselective drug buspirone. *Clinical Neuropharmacology,* **7** (Suppl. 1), 886–887

TAYLOR, R. E. (1959) Effect of procaine on electrical properties of squid axon membrane. *American Journal of Physiology,* **196,** 1071–1078

TICKU, M. (1979) Differences in gamma-amino acid receptor sensitivity in inbred strains of mice. *Journal of Neurochemistry,* **33,** 1135–1138

TICKU, M. K. and DAVIS, W. C. (1981) Effect of valproic acid on 3H-diazepam and 3H-dihydropicrotoxinin binding sites at the benzodiazepine–GABA receptor–ionophore complex. *Brain Research,* **223,** 218–222

TOWER, D. B. (1960) *Neurochemistry of Epilepsy.* Springfield, Ill.: Charles C. Thomas

TURKANIS, S. A., CHIU, P., BORYS, H. K. and KARLER, R. (1977) Influence of delta-9-tetrahydrocannabinol and cannabidiol on photically evoked after-discharge potentials. *Psychopharmacology,* **52,** 207–212

VAJDA, F., WILLIAMS, F. M., DAVIDSON, S., FALCONER, M. A. and BRECKENRIDGE, A. (1974) Human brain, cerebrospinal fluid and plasma concentrations of diphenylhydantoin and phenobarbital. *Clinical Pharmacology and Therapeutics,* **15,** 597–603

VAN CALDER, D., MULLER, M. and HAMPRECHT, B. (1979) Adenosine regulates, via two different types of receptors, the accumulation of cyclic AMP in cultured brain cells. *Journal of Neurochemistry,* **33,** 999–1005

VAN DER KLEIJN, E., GUELEN, P. J. M., BEELEN, T. C. M., RIJNJES, N. V. M. and ZUIDGEEST, T. L. B. (1973) Kinetics of general and regional brain distribution of closely related 7-chloro-1, 4-benzodiazepines. In *The Benzodiazepines,* edited by S. Garattini, E. Mussini and L. O. Randall, pp. 145–164. New York: Raven Press

VAN GELDER, N. M. and COURTOIS, A. (1972) Close correlation between changing content of specific amino acids in epileptogenic cortex of cats, and severity of epilepsy. *Brain Research,* **43,** 477–484

VAN GELDER, N. M., EDMONDS, H. C. HEGERBERG, G. A., CHATBURN, C. C., CLEMMONS, M. R. and SYLVESTER, D. M. (1980) Amino-acid changes in a genetic strain of epileptic beagle dogs. *Journal of Neurochemistry,* **35,** 1087–1091

VAN GELDER, N. M., SHERWIN, A. L. and RASMUSSEN, T. (1972) Amino acid content of epileptogenic human brain: focal versus surrounding regions. *Brain Research,* **40,** 385–393

VAN WOERT, M. H. and HWANG, E. C. (1981) Role of brain serotonin in myoclonus. In *Neurotransmitters, Seizures and Epilepsy,* edited by P. L. Morselli, K. G. Lloyd, W. Löscher, B. Meldrum and E. H. Reynolds, pp. 239–247. New York: Raven Press

VERNADAKIS, A. and WOODBURY, D. M. (1960) Effects of diphenylhydantoin and adrenocortical steroids on free glutamic acid, glutamine, and gamma aminobutyric acid concentrations of rat cerebral cortex. In *Inhibition in the Nervous System and Gamma-aminobutyric Acid*, edited by E. Roberts, pp. 47–63. New York: Macmillan (Pergamon)

VERZEANO, M. (1972) Pacemakers, synchronization and epilepsy. In *Synchronization of EEG Activities in Epilepsies,* edited by H. Petsche and M. A. B. Brazier, pp. 154–188. New York: Springer-Verlag

WEINBERGER, J., NICHLAS, W. J. and BERL, S. (1976) Mechanism of action of anticonvulsants. *Neurology (Minneapolis),* **26,** 162–166

WEIR, R. L., PADGETT, W., DALY, J. W. and ANDERSON, J. (1984) Interaction of anticonvulsant drugs with adenosine receptors in the central nervous system. *Epilepsia,* **25(4),** 492–498

WENZEL, J., KRUEGER, E. and MUELLER, M. (1971) Hemmung Pentetrazol-induzierter hypersynchroner Aktivität im thalamokortikalen System durch Ethosuximid. *Acta Biologica et Medica Germanica,* **26,** 567–572

WILDER, B. J. (1969) Laboratory evaluation of antiepileptic drugs. *Epilepsia,* **10,** 237, 260–261, 380

WILDER, B. J. and BRUNI, J. (1982) Mechanisms of action of AED. *Clinical Neuropharmacology,* **5,** 23–43

WILDER, B. J. and SCHMIDT, R. P. (1965) Propagation of epileptic discharge from chronic neocortical foci in monkey. *Epilepsia,* **6,** 297–309

WILLIAMS, M. (1983) Adenosine receptors in the mammalian central nervous system. *Progress in Neuro-Psychopharmacology and Biological Psychiatry,* **7,** 443–450

WILLIAMS, R. J. H., PATSALOS, P. N., LOWE, R. and LASCELLES, P. T. (1980) Changes in brain amino acid neurotransmitters induced by sodium valproate and their relevance to epilepsy and interactions with other anticonvulsants. In *The Place of Sodium Valproate in the Treatment of Epilepsy.* Royal Society of Medicine, International Congress and Symposium No. 30, pp. 95–102. London: Academic Press and Royal Society of Medicine

WILLOW, M. and CATTERALL, W. A. (1982) Inhibition of binding of 3H-batrachotoxinin 20-gamma-benzoate to sodium channels by the anticonvulsant drugs diphenylhydantoin and carbamazepine. *Molecular Pharmacology,* **22,** 627–635

WITHROW, C. D. (1980) Oxazolidinediones. In *Antiepileptic Drugs: Mechanisms of Action,* edited by G. H. Glaser, J. K. Penry and D. M. Woodbury, pp. 577–586. New York: Raven Press

WITHROW, C. D. (1982) Trimethadione – mechanisms of actions. In *Antiepileptic Drugs,* edited by D. M. Woodbury, J. K. Penry and C. E. Pippenger, pp. 705–709. New York: Raven Press

WOLF, P. and HAAS, H. L. (1977 Effects of diazepines and barbiturates on hippocampal recurrent inhibition. *Naunyn Schmiedeberg's Archives of Pharmacology,* **299,** 211–218

WOOD, J. D., KURYLO, E. and PEESKER, J. (1978) The possible involvement of GABA and its compartmentation in the mechanism of some convulsant and anticonvulsant agents. In *Amino Acids as Chemical Transmitters,* edited by F. Fonnum, pp. 439–444. New York: Plenum Press

WOOD, J. D., KURYLO, E. and TSUI, S. K. (1981) Interactions of di-n-propylacetate, GABAculine and aminooxyacetic acid: anticonvulsant activity and the gamma-aminobutyrate system. *Journal of Neurochemistry,* **37,** 1440–1447

WOOD, J. H., HARE, J. A., GLAESER, B. S., BALLENGER, J. C. and POST, R. M. (1979) Low cerebrospinal fluid aminobutyric acid content in seizure patients. *Neurology,* **29,** 1203–1208

WOODBURY, D. M. (1955) Effect of diphenylhydantoin on electrolytes and radiosodium turnover in brain and other tissues of normal hyponatremic and postictal rats. *Journal of Pharmacology and Experimental Therapeutics,* **115,** 74–95

WOODBURY, D. M. (1969) Mechanisms of action of anticonvulsants. In *Basic Mechanisms of the Epilepsies,* edited by H. H. Jasper, A. A. Ward and A. Pope, pp. 647–681. Boston: Little, Brown

WOODBURY, D. M. (1980a) Phenytoin: proposed mechanisms of anticonvulsant action. *Advances in Neurology,* **27,** 447–471

WOODBURY, D. M. (1980b) Carbonic anhydrase inhibitors. *Advances in Neurology,* **27,** 617–633

WOODBURY, D. M. and ESPLIN, D. W. (1959) Neuropharmacology and neurochemistry of anticonvulsant drugs. *Research Publications for the Association for Research into Nervous and Mental Diseases,* **37,** 24–56

WOODBURY, D. M. (1982) Phenytoin – mechanisms of actions. In *Antiepileptic Drugs,* edited by D. M. Woodbury, J. K. Penry and C. E. Pippenger, pp. 269–281. New York: Raven Press

WOODBURY, D. M. and KEMP, J. W. (1982) Sulfonamides and derivatives: acetazolamide. In *Antiepileptic Drugs,* edited by D. M. Woodbury, J. K. Penry and C. E. Pippenger, pp. 771–789. New York: Raven Press

WOODBURY, D. M. and PIPPENGER, C. E. (1982) Primidone mechanism of action. In *Antiepileptic Drugs,* edited by D. M. Woodbury, J. K. Penry and C. E. Pippenger. New York: Raven Press

WORMS, P. and LLOYD, K. G. (1979) Differential blockade of bicuculline convulsions by neuroleptics. *European Journal of Pharmacology,* **51,** 85–88

WORMS, P. and LLOYD, K. G. (1981) Functional alterations of GABA synapses in relation to seizures. In *Neurotransmitters, Seizures and Epilepsy,* edited by P. L. Morselli, K. G. Lloyd, W. Löscher, B. Meldrum and E. H. Reynolds, pp. 37–44. New York: Raven Press

WORMS, P., DEPOORTERE, H., DURAND, H., MORSELLI, P. L., LLOYD, K. G. and BARTHOLINI, G. (1982) Gamma-aminobutyric acid (GABA) receptor stimulation. I: Neuropharmacological profiles of progabide (SL 76002) and SL 75102 with emphasis on their anticonvulsant spectra. *Journal of Pharmacology and Experimental Therapeutics,* **220,** 660–671

YOUNG, S. M., GAUTHIER, S., ANDERSON, G. M. and PURDY, W. C. (1980) Trytophan, 5 hydroxyindolacetic acid in human cerebrospinal fluid: inter-relationships and the influence of age, sex, epilepsy, and anticonvulsant drugs. *Journal of Neurology, Neurosurgery and Psychiatry,* **43,** 438–445

4
The empirical use of models in the development of antiepileptic drugs

Roger J. Porter

INTRODUCTION

Although therapies other than antiepileptic drugs will continue to be important in the effort to control epilepsy, most patients are dependent on their medications, either wholly or in part, for their seizure control. Furthermore, the likelihood of continued dependence on such medications in the next several decades seems quite high – certainly higher than the likelihood of a dramatic breakthrough in our understanding of the basic mechanisms of the epilepsies which would lead to a drastic alteration in current therapeutic approaches.

Unfortunately, many patients continue to have seizures in spite of optimal utilization of available medications. In the United States, for example, the total number of patients with uncontrolled partial seizures is estimated to be 350 000 (Ward, 1983), and approximately 200 000 people have seizures more than once per month (Commission for the Control of Epilepsy and its Consequences, 1978). For many patients with epilepsy the development of a new antiepileptic drug offers the only hope of achieving control of their seizures. For those patients whose seizures are controlled by currently available therapy, a new drug may reduce the toxic effects they often tolerate to gain seizure control (Krall *et al.*, 1978). This chapter reviews (1) the history of antiepileptic drug development, (2) the various models used in the search for new drugs, (3) the drug approval process, and (4) clinical trial strategies. Portions of this chapter have been published previously (Porter *et al.*, 1984).

EARLY HISTORY OF ANTIEPILEPTIC DRUG DISCOVERY

In 1857 potassium bromide was introduced for the treatment of epilepsy when Sir Charles Locock used it to treat catamenial seizures (Locock, 1857). Its ability to reduce seizure frequency in many patients who were not helped by other therapies led to the establishment of its efficacy and its subsequent widespread replacement of more primitive, ineffective therapies. During the next 50 years bromide was used regularly to treat epilepsy, in spite of toxicity such as severe skin eruptions and psychosis.

Table 4.1 Antiepileptic drugs marketed in the United States (from Porter *et al.*, 1984)

Year introduced	*International non-proprietary name*	*US trade name*	*Company*
1912	Phenobarbital	Luminal	Winthrop
1935	Mephobarbital	Mebaral	Winthrop
1938	Phenytoin	Dilantin	Parke-Davis
1946	Trimethadione	Tridione	Abbott
1947	Mephenytoin	Mesantoin	Sandoz
1949	Paramethadione	Paradione	Abbott
1950	Phethenylate[a]	Thiantoin	Lilly
1951	Phenacemide	Phenurone	Abbott
1952	Metharbital	Gemonil	Abbott
1952	Benzchlorpropamide[b]	Hibicon	Lederle
1953	Phensuximide	Milontin	Parke-Davis
1954	Primidone	Mysoline	Ayerst
1957	Methsuximide	Celontin	Parke-Davis
1957	Ethotoin	Peganone	Abbott
1960	Aminoglutethimide[c]	Elipten	Ciba
1960	Ethosuximide	Zarontin	Parke-Davis
1968	Diazepam[d]	Valium	Roche
1974	Carbamazepine	Tegretol	Geigy
1975	Clonazepam	Clonopin	Roche
1978	Valproic acid	Depakene	Abbott
1981	Clorazepate dipotassium[d]	Tranxene	Abbott

[a] Withdrawn, 1952
[b] Withdrawn, 1955
[c] Withdrawn, 1966
[d] Approved by FDA as adjunct

Table 4.2 Antiepileptic barbiturates used in the United States (from Porter 1984)

Drug	*Active metabolite*
Phenobarbital	none known
Primidone	phenobarbital, phenylethylmalonamide
Mephobarbital	phenobarbital
Metharbital	barbital
Barbital	none known
Eterobarb (experimental in United States)	phenobarbital

The modern history of drugs marketed in the United States for the treatment of epilepsy (*Table 4.1*) begins with the introduction of phenobarbital in 1912. A new synthetic sedative-hypnotic drug, phenobarbital was shown by Hauptmann (1912) to possess the ability to reduce seizure frequency. Proving to be more effective and less toxic than bromide, phenobarbital soon became the antiepileptic drug of choice. Since the barbituric acid molecule was easily modified, many analogs of phenobarbital were synthesized, approximately 50 of which were marketed in the first 35 years of this century. A few of these, such as metharbital and mephobarbital, demonstrated antiepileptic activity and continue as marketed antiepileptic drugs; many of these analogs are metabolized to phenobarbital (*Table 4.2*), which may exert the major antiepileptic effect (Porter, 1984). The discovery of the antiepileptic action of both bromide and phenobarbital was clearly serendipitous. Later, with the development of seizure models in animals, the search for new antiepileptic drugs was based on a more scientific approach (Porter, 1984).

THE DEVELOPMENT OF MODELS IN THE SEARCH FOR NEW ANTIEPILEPTIC DRUGS

In 1882 an early model of epilepsy was developed in which seizures were elicited in dogs by direct faradic stimulation of the motor cortex; chemicals were thereby tested for anticonvulsant activity (Albertoni, 1882). Later, other seizure models were developed from convulsant chemicals such as picrotoxin, bicuculline, strychnine, and pentylenetetrazol.

In 1937 Merritt and Putnam (1938) and Merritt, Putnam and Schwab (1938) used a seizure model based on a new electroshock technique for producing convulsions in cats and screened a group of compounds supplied to them by Parke-Davis; they discovered the anticonvulsant properties of phenytoin, then called diphenylhydantoin. Because phenytoin was well tolerated by laboratory animals it was subjected to clinical trials in 1938 and marketed that same year. The absence of a sedative effect and the dramatic seizure improvement when phenytoin was added to barbiturate therapy were the key factors in the rapid marketing of this new drug. In addition, its entry into the market was not delayed by regulatory requirements. At that time, the introduction of new drugs in the United States was still regulated by the Federal Food and Drugs Act of 1906 which required only that the drugs be accurately labeled (FFD Act of 1906); no proof of safety or efficacy was required.

The discovery of phenytoin by Merritt and Putnam had implications beyond the drug itself. As both bromides and barbiturates were sedative, it had previously been thought that antiepileptic drugs must sedate to stop seizures; phenytoin is non-sedative and anticonvulsant. The discovery of phenytoin established the meaningfulness of the laboratory search for antiepileptic drugs – more than serendipity could play a role. The discovery was also a first, major step toward laboratory and clinical differentiation of antiepileptic drugs – a differentiation used today. Finally, the discovery led to increased studies of structure–activity relationships, and of both neurophysiological and neurochemical bases of seizures (Swinyard, 1982). The discovery demonstrated that industry could collaborate with academic investigators, a relationship which has flourished in succeeding years.

Following the introduction of phenytoin, several pharmaceutical firms began molecular modification projects dealing with phenytoin and its analogs. Numerous hydantoins were synthesized and tested during this period. In addition, investigators from the pharmaceutical industry as well as from academia began to explore new and improved methods of seizure provocation.

In 1944 Richards and Everett reported that trimethadione, an analgesic compound that was to become the first antiabsence drug, prevented the threshold seizures induced by pentylenetetrazol in rodents. They also showed that these seizures were prevented by phenobarbital but not by phenytoin. At the same time,

Goodman *et al.* (1953) confirmed Richards and Everett's results and further showed that phenytoin and phenobarbital, but not trimethadione, modified the pattern of maximal electroshock seizures. These findings demonstrated the different anticonvulsant actions of these drugs and the qualitative difference between threshold and maximal seizures.

Between 1945 and 1950 several investigators tested clinically active anticonvulsant drugs in a variety of experimental models but failed to find a single model in which all drugs were active. A battery of tests, however, did uncover profiles of anticonvulsant activity which, with few exceptions, correlated well with clinical efficacy and specificity (Swinyard, 1949). In 1951 Chen and colleagues investigated the anticonvulsant activity of approximately 65 phenylsuccinimides, utilizing an abbreviated version of these tests. Among the most potent antipentylenetetrazol compounds were phensuximide and methsuximide, both of which were later approved for the treatment of absence seizures (1953 and 1957 respectively). A third succinimide, ethosuximide, was introduced for the treatment for absence seizures in 1960.

During the same period (1938–60) two analogs of phenytoin (mephenytoin and ethotoin), two analogs of phenobarbital (metharbital and primidone), and an analog of trimethadione (paramethadione) were marketed in the United States. Each of these analogs has a spectrum of activity similar to that of its parent drug and was marketed for similar use.

Three other drugs, phethenylate, benzchlorpropamide, and aminoglutethimide, were also marketed for use in epilepsy during this period. Both phethenylate and benzchlorpropamide, however, were withdrawn from the market by 1960. Phethenylate was found to cause a high incidence of hepatic necrosis, and benzchlorpropamide showed toxic effects with long-term use in animals. Aminoglutethimide was withdrawn in 1966 after it was found to cause a high incidence of goiters.

Interestingly, all antiepileptic drugs developed from 1912 to 1960 were based on a simple, heterocyclic ring structure (*Figure 4.1*). During this period, genuinely

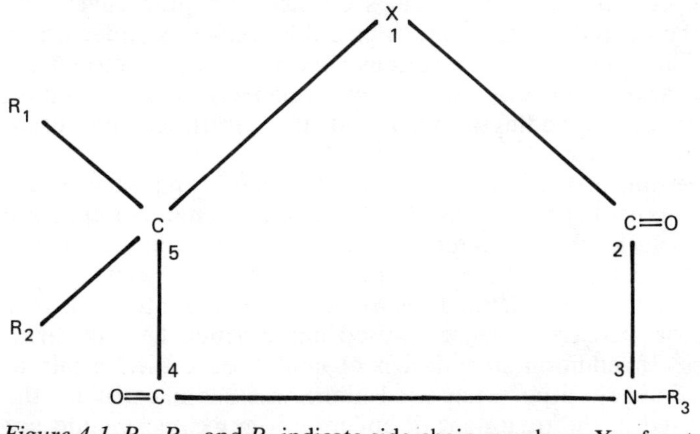

Figure 4.1 R_1, R_2, and R_3 indicate side-chain members. X refers to components of different drug groupings: hydantoinates —NH—, barbiturates —CO—NH—, oxazolidinediones —O—, succinimides —CH_2—, and acetylureas —NH_2— (from Coatsworth and Penry, 1972)

novel structures were ignored in the development of antiepileptic drugs; instead, attention centered on the hydantoins, the barbiturates, the oxazolidinediones, the succinimides, and the acetylureas.

The marketing of all drugs in the United States after 1938 was regulated by the Federal Food, Drug, and Cosmetic Act of 1938, which required proof of safety in addition to the 1906 labeling provisions. Definitive questions about efficacy were usually not resolved until after a new drug was marketed.

DECLINE IN ANTIEPILEPTIC DRUG DEVELOPMENT

The highly productive period of antiepileptic drug development in the 1940s and 1950s was followed by more than a decade of dormancy in the United States. During the 12-year period from 1961 to 1973 there was only one newly marketed drug that had any use in epilepsy; this was diazepam, an adjunctive drug used mostly in status epilepticus (*see Table 4.1*).

There were many reasons for the decline in the development of new drugs for epilepsy. Some clinicians believed that improvements in therapy depended mainly on better utilization of existing drugs. This belief helped to strengthen the impression that there was not a substantial need for new drugs, even though many patients with common seizure types and most patients with rare seizure types failed to respond to the available drugs, and many suffered medication side-effects. Furthermore, the attention of the pharmaceutical industry had shifted to other areas of central nervous system (CNS) therapy. The discovery of tranquilizers and sedative-hypnotics, which achieved remarkable financial success, resulted in the expansion of research into other areas of CNS pharmacology. In addition, the relatively large number of effective, marketed antiepileptic drugs made it questionable, in the view of the pharmaceutical industry, whether a new drug could capture a market large enough to justify the cost of its development. The cost of drug development was increasing, and this increase was made formal in the United States with the passage of the Drug Amendments Act of 1962 to the Federal Food, Drug, and Cosmetic Act of 1938. Known as the Kefauver–Harris amendments, this legislation required the establishment of a drug's efficacy as a prerequisite for marketing approval in the United States and restricted the conditions under which drugs could be tested. This legislation had a serious impact on drug development, not only for epilepsy but also for any disease affecting a relatively small population where the market was correspondingly small and the return on corporate investment was doubtful.

Problems of clinical testing also contributed to the reluctance of pharmaceutical firms to pursue the development of new drugs. Proof of efficacy of new antiepileptic drugs, for example, was seriously hampered by the lack of appropriate patient populations for controlled clinical trials. Patient populations whose seizure types and seizure frequency were well defined were almost non-existent. Either dramatically decreased or increased seizures caused many patients to withdraw from controlled studies. In addition, the design of controlled clinical trials to establish the efficacy of a new drug when used alone was complicated by the multiple drug therapy used in the treatment of epilepsy. Many clinicians did not believe in the need for controlled clinical trials. The resulting lack of controlled trial data was a major impediment to developing new antiepileptic drugs by the newer, more rigorous standards of the 1960s.

A survey of pharmaceutical firms in 1967 (Public Health Service Advisory Committee on the Epilepsies, 1967) revealed that most firms had no new antiepileptic drugs under development and that several drugs that were tested had not gained the approval of the US Food and Drug Administration (FDA) because of inadequate proof of efficacy. The most frequent reason cited for the lack of interest in antiepileptic drug development was financial; the cost of development was prohibitive compared with the expected return from marketing. Furthermore, an informal survey of academic medicinal chemists revealed that those who were synthesizing potential anticonvulsant agents had no access to appropriate pharmacological testing.

RENEWED INTEREST IN DRUGS FOR EPILEPSY

To help reverse the decline in antiepileptic drug development, the Epilepsy Branch of the National Institute of Neurological and Communicative Disorders and Stroke, US, beginning in 1968, in collaboration with other investigators, conducted controlled clinical trials of seven drugs (albutoin, carbamazepine, clonazepam, chlorazepate dipotassium, mexiletine, sulthiame, and valproic acid) that needed definitive proof of efficacy before they could be marketed as antiepileptic drugs in the United States. Support of these trials not only decreased the cost of development for the pharmaceutical sponsors of these drugs but also provided an opportunity for the Epilepsy Branch to develop methodology and standards for the conduct of controlled trials of antiepileptic drugs. Data collected in these trials eventually supported the new drug application (NDA) for carbamazepine, clonazepam, and valproic acid, which were marketed in this country as primary antiepileptic drugs in 1974, 1975, and 1978, respectively, and for chlorazepate dipotassium, which was approved in 1981 as an adjunctive drug for the treatment of epilepsy. Trials of albutoin, mexiletine, and sulthiame failed to support their efficacy in the populations studied, and these drugs have not been marketed in the United States.

In addition to the support of clinical trials of available drugs, the need for involvement in the drug development process at the preclinical stage soon became apparent, and a federally sponsored antiepileptic drug development program was formally established with the introduction of the Anticonvulsant Screening Project in 1975 (Porter *et al.*, 1984).

ANTIEPILEPTIC DRUG DEVELOPMENT PROGRAM

Several other government-sponsored drug development programs set the precedent for federal government assistance in antiepileptic drug development. These programs vary but are concerned primarily with drugs that for various reasons would not be developed independently by drug companies. Among their many functions, these programs usually embrace two fundamental elements. First, in preclinical development, screening for activity is a common element. Programs seek potential drugs, often in an effort to entice drug companies to become interested in a compound. Second, these drug development programs are often involved in controlled clinical trials of new drugs.

The Antiepileptic Drug Development (ADD) Program, sponsored by the Epilepsy Branch, encompasses both the preclinical and clinical elements of drug development (*Figure 4.2*). The preclinical portion contributed by the Epilepsy Branch comprises the Anticonvulsant Screening Project and the Toxicology Project; the clinical portion involves controlled clinical trials (Porter, 1983).

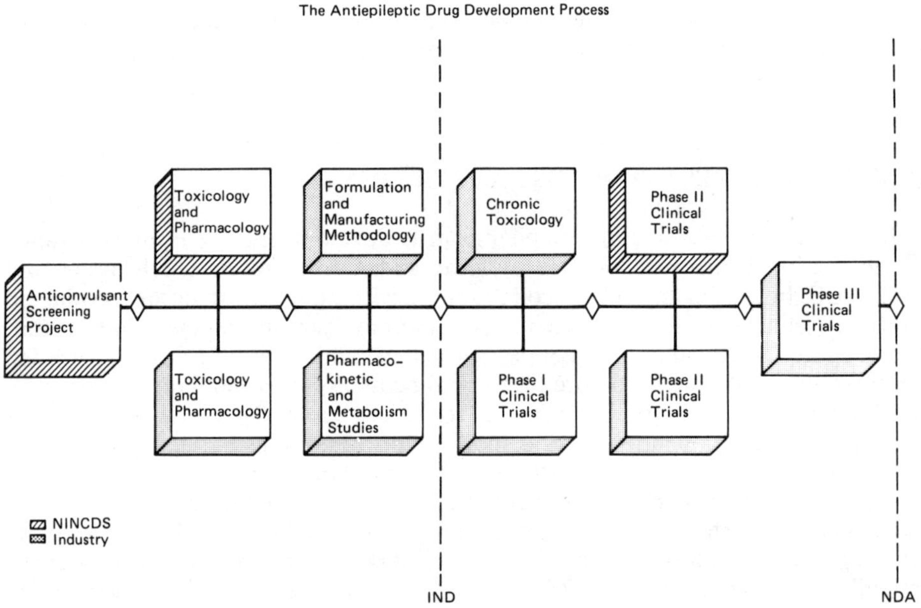

Figure 4.2 The antiepileptic drug development process (IND, Investigational New Drug Application; NDA, New Drug Application) (from Porter, 1983)

In the preclinical process the ADD Program receives compounds from academic medicinal chemists and the pharmaceutical industry for screening in seven phases. When a compound shows exceptional anticonvulsant activity in the later phases of the screening project, toxicology studies in animals are required to support initial human use of the drug; one is conducted in rodents and the other in non-rodents, usually dogs. Generally, the ADD Program supports one of the studies and the sponsor supports the other.

The clinical segment of the program begins after the sponsor is granted an investigational exemption for a new drug (IND). Studies in healthy volunteers (phase I) are supported by the sponsor or infrequently by the ADD Program. The initial controlled clinical trials in epileptic patients (phase II) are supported by the ADD Program. Finally, broader clinical trials (phase III) are conducted by the sponsor. Successful completion of the clinical phases of evaluation is generally followed by marketing of the new drug.

Because the seven steps in the Anticonvulsant Screening Project and the three stages of clinical evaluation are all referred to as phases, the former are designated by arabic numerals (phases 1–7) and the latter by Roman numerals (phases I–III) to help avoid confusion (Porter *et al.*, 1984).

Anticonvulsant screening project

Medicinal chemists from academia and the pharmaceutical industry submit chemical compounds to the Anticonvulsant Screening Project for evaluation of anticonvulsant activity and antiepileptic potential. The testing is done at no cost to them, and they retain their patent rights to all compounds offered for testing. As of October 1983, more than 8000 compounds had been tested. By testing the compounds in a standardized, consistent manner, the project has developed a database by which the structure–activity relationships of anticonvulsants can be predicted.

The Anticonvulsant Screening Project includes seven distinct testing phases to evaluate anticonvulsant activity, describe neurotoxic effects, and delineate possible mechanisms of action. The most commonly used antiepileptic drugs marketed in the United States were tested in phases 2–6; the results have been previously reported (Porter *et al.*, 1984).

The profiles of experimental anticonvulsant activity of all clinically useful antiepileptic drugs are characterized by their ability to prevent seizure spread and/or to increase minimal seizure threshold. Drugs useful in generalized tonic/clonic seizures and partial seizures (such as phenytoin) prevent seizure spread and may or may not increase minimal seizure threshold. Drugs useful in absence seizures (such as ethosuximide) elevate seizure threshold and have only limited, if any, value to prevent seizure spread.

The screening project, therefore, initially utilizes two tests for the detection of anticonvulsant activity in candidate compounds: the maximal electroshock seizure (MES) test to detect agents that prevent seizure spread, and the subcutaneous pentylenetetrazol (Metrazol) (scMet) seizure threshold test to detect agents that elevate minimal seizure threshold. Neurological toxicity is evaluated initially by the rotorod ataxia test. If a compound shows significant anticonvulsant activity and minimal neurotoxicity, it is advanced to further screening.

The screening project is divided into seven phases. The number of compounds is decreased at each phase, such that only the most promising compounds are advanced to toxicology evaluation. Phase 1 estimates the potency and protective index of active compounds using MES and scMet and eliminates inactive compounds from further testing. Neurotoxic compounds are also eliminated, using the rotorod test. Phase 2 testing quantitates the anticonvulsant activity and neurotoxicity estimated in phase 1 testing. Phase 3 testing reveals the dose–time relations in the profile of overt toxic manifestations, as well as the median hypnotic dose (HD_{50}) and the 24-hour median lethal dose (LD_{50}). Phase 4 testing provides the same kind of information as phase 2, except that the test compound is given orally. Phase 5 further delineates the antiepileptic potential of the candidate compounds. A part of this phase utilizes four chemical convulsants: pentylenetetrazol, bicuculline, picrotoxin, and strychnine. Because each of these convulsants acts through a somewhat different neurotransmitter system, the ED_{50}s obtained by these procedures help reflect the profile of antiepileptic activity of the test compound. This profile can be compared with the profiles of clinically effective antiepileptic drugs, helping to differentiate the activity of the test compound and giving some insight into its possible mechanism of action. Phase 6 verifies the anticonvulsant activity and neurotoxicity in another rodent species. The ED_{50}s in the MES and scMet tests and the TD_{50} are determined after oral administration of the compound to rats. Phase 7 provides the dosage information essential for subsequent toxicity studies by estimating the minimal lethal dose and effect of prolonged administration on anticonvulsant activity in rats who receive the drug orally. Further discussion of these phases is described in detail elsewhere (Porter *et al.*, 1984).

Toxicology project

If the results from all phases of the Anticonvulsant Screening Project are favorable, compounds may be scheduled for further testing in the Toxicology Project. This project provides the toxicity evaluation required by the FDA before humans are exposed to the drugs; it consists of 91-day evaluations of the compound after oral administration to rats and beagle dogs. The selection of compounds for toxicity studies is based on the following criteria:

(1) adequate absorption after oral administration of the compound to mice and rats;
(2) adequate protective indices after oral and intraperitoneal administration of the compound to mice and rats;
(3) novel chemical structure of the compound; and
(4) absence of tolerance to the anticonvulsant effects of the compound.

Emphasis is given to potent compounds of novel structure, that is, compounds with activity equal to or greater than that of known antiepileptic drugs but of a different chemical family.

Controlled clinical trials

Once a compound has progressed through the aforementioned projects, it is potentially ready for one of the most important steps in drug development: introduction to humans. Because of important species differences in drug metabolism and drug action, the ultimate value of any new drug must obviously be proven clinically.

Human studies do not usually begin in patients, but in healthy volunteers. The studies are designed primarily to test the clinical safety of the drugs. Such studies often last less than a month and determine the range of tolerated doses. These investigations are sometimes referred to as phase I studies (Porter, 1984).

Following the volunteer studies, patient studies begin. Pilot studies are usually followed by controlled clinical trials, which are commonly double-blind; that is, neither the patient nor the doctor knows whether the drug or a placebo is being taken. In the United States two well-controlled clinical trials are necessary; both must demonstrate antiepileptic effectiveness. Long-term evaluation of the compound in a large number of patients follows the definitive efficacy testing. Such studies often include patients tested in earlier clinical investigations. Exposing the drug to a large number of patients helps uncover unusual reactions and provides further evidence of its effectiveness. The clinical studies in patients are often termed phase II and phase III studies (Porter, 1984).

Phase II studies evaluate the safety and efficacy of the drug in epileptic patients and determine the therapeutic dose range and its variability in individual patients. The ADD Program has concentrated on the support of phase II clinical trials, first with the sponsorship of clinical trials leading to the marketing of four drugs from 1974 to 1981, and more recently with the evaluation of promising compounds emerging from the screening and toxicity projects.

The design and execution of controlled clinical trials of antiepileptic drugs is not a trivial task. The subtleties of seizures and clinical observations require close interaction between clinical neurologists experienced in conducting controlled clinical trials and biostatisticians with experience in the design of clinical trials and knowledge of neurological disease. The patient population must be carefully defined. Practical limitations imposed on the study design by the problems of patient availability must also be considered. A small patient sample is typical. Highly efficient statistical designs and accompanying analyses are imperative in testing new antiepileptic therapies if the trials are to yield the maximum amount of clinically useful information.

Accurate classification of the seizure type is crucial to the success of the trial. Because multiple terminologies are used to describe seizures, the clinical trial must clearly define the seizure type in order to make the trial comprehensible to others. Classification of seizures is usually based on the description given by the patient or an observer, but this description is often inadequate. For drug trials, the seizure type should be diagnosed by video monitoring whenever possible, and the seizures should be classified according to the International Classification of Epileptic Seizures (Commission on Classification and Terminology of the International League against Epilepsy, 1981).

Wide disparity in seizure frequency is common among epileptic patients. Because some patients experience more seizures than others, antiepileptic drug testing requires maximal statistical efficiency with minimal danger to the patient. The use of the classic two-period crossover design has become a standard technique to alleviate this problem.

Clinical trials are further complicated by the fact that many potential participants have multiple seizure types. A new drug effective for one type of seizure may have no effect on another type. Other antiepileptic drugs may be required when multiple seizure types coexist, but most of them are enzyme inducers and may affect the metabolism of the test drug.

Several difficulties may be encountered in selecting a seizure type for study. It would be desirable to have the drug marketed for all types of seizures for which it is effective, but the cost of mounting controlled studies for several seizure types is considerable. In practice, a new drug application (NDA) is usually sought for a specific seizure type, and additional indications are requested later.

The parameters used to measure drug efficacy must be sensitive and meaningful indicators of a true treatment effect. Sophisticated statistical analyses of poorly defined clinical parameters could lead to studies which in themselves are appropriately analyzable, but which have very little inferential credence.

Finally, moral and ethical considerations limit the testing of new drugs for some seizure types to individuals who are continuing to have seizures despite optimal therapy with existing drugs or to those who are experiencing severe adverse reactions to these drugs. Comparison of a test drug with a placebo is usually the best way of revealing drug effects. The use of a placebo alone, however, is only rarely permissible because of medical and ethical objections to not treating seizures. Thus, in clinical trials of antiepileptic drugs, there is an increased emphasis on the need for clinically relevant endpoints and effective statistical design (Porter *et al.*, 1984).

The ADD Program has played a major role in advancing clinical trial methodology to help solve the aforementioned problems. With the use of new and better methods of evaluation, the convincing power and sensitivity of antiepileptic drug trials has increased significantly. Controlled trials and double-blind studies of new antiepileptic drugs are now general practice; they were used, for example, in a cooperative study at eleven Veterans Administration Medical Centers (Mattson, 1983). Guidelines for antiepileptic drug testing have been developed by the Epilepsy Branch and adopted by the International League Against Epilepsy and the FDA (US Food and Drug Administration, 1981).

Phase III studies evaluate the long-term efficacy of the new drug, usually in patients who have been treated successfully with the drug during the phase II trials. Generally, in an open protocol, about 150 of these patients are allowed to continue on the new drug for at least one year.

Clearly, although the clinical study of epilepsy is fraught with a multitude of difficult scientific and ethical problems, antiepileptic drug development is in a stage of expansion that allows greater and greater specificity of medication tailored to the specific seizure type. As new drugs are developed, old ones will be replaced. No regimen should be considered infinitely useful. There is always the distinct possibility of change in the light of new drugs and technological advances.

References

ALBERTONI, P. (1882) Untersuchungen uber die Wirkung einiger Arzneimittel auf die Erregbarkeit des Grosshirns nebst Beitragen zur Therapie der Epilepsie. *Archiv für Experimentelle Pathologie und Pharmakologie,* **15,** 248–288

COATSWORTH, J. J. and PENRY, J. K. (1972) Clinical efficacy and use. In *Antiepileptic Drugs*, edited by D. M. Woodbury, J. K. Penry and R. P. Schmidt, pp. 87–96. New York: Raven Press

CHEN, P. G., PORTMAN, R., ENSOR, C. R. and BRATTON, A. C. JR (1951) The anticonvulsant activity of a-phenylsuccinimides. *Journal of Pharmacology and Experimental Therapy,* **103,** 54–61

COMMISSION FOR THE CONTROL OF EPILEPSY AND ITS CONSEQUENCES (1978) *Plan for Nationwide Action on Epilepsy,* Vol. 1. DHEW Publication No. (NIH) 78–276. Washington, DC: US Department of Health Education and Welfare

COMMISSION ON CLASSIFICATION AND TERMINOLOGY OF THE INTERNATIONAL LEAGUE AGAINST EPILEPSY (1981) Proposal for revised clinical and electroencephalographic classification of epileptic seizures. *Epilepsia,* **22,** 489–501

Drug Amendments Act of 1962. Public Law 87–781, 21 USC 355.

Federal Food, Drug, and Cosmetic Act of 1938. Public Law 717, 75th Congress

Federal Food and Drugs Act of 1906. Public Law 384, 59th Congress

GOODMAN, L. S., GREWAL, M. S., BROWN, W. C., and SWINYARD, E. A. (1953) Comparison of maximal seizures evoked by pentylenetetrazol (Metrazol) and electroshock in mice, and their modification by anticonvulsants. *Journal of Pharmacology and Experimental Therapy,* **108,** 168–176

HAUPTMANN, A. (1912) Luminal bei Epilepsie. *Muncher Medizinische Wochenschrift,* **59,** 1907–1909

KRALL, R. L., PENRY, J. K., KUPFERBERG, H. J. and SWINYARD, E. A. (1978) Antiepileptic drug development. I. History and a program for progress. *Epilepsia,* **19,** 393–408

LOCOCK, C. (1857) Discussion of a paper by E. H. Sieveking. Analysis of 52 cases of epilepsy observed by the author. *Lancet,* **1,** 527

MATTSON, R. H. (1983) The design of clinical studies to assess the efficacy and toxicity of antiepileptic drugs. *Neurology,* **33** (Suppl. 1), 1–37

MERRITT, H. H., PUTNAM, T. J. and SCHWAB, D. M. (1938) A new series of anticonvulsant drugs tested by experiments on animals. *Archives of Neurology and Psychiatry,* **39,** 1003–1015

MERRITT, H. H. and PUTNAM T. J. (1938) Sodium diphenylhydantoinate in the treatment of convulsive disorders. *Journal of the American Medical Association,* **111,** 1068–1073

PORTER, R. J. (1984) *Epilepsy: 100 Elementary Principles*. London: Saunders.

PORTER, R. J. (1983) Antiepileptic Drug Development Program. In *Orphan Drugs and Orphan Diseases: Clinical Realities and Public Policy*, edited by G. J. Brewer, pp. 53–66. New York: Alan R. Liss, Inc.

PORTER, R. J., CEREGHINO, J. J., GLADDING, G. D. *et al.* (1984) Antiepileptic Drug Development Program. *Cleveland Clinic Quarterly,* **51,** 293–305

PUBLIC HEALTH SERVICE ADVISORY COMMITTEE ON THE EPILEPSIES (1967) *Minutes of Meeting, 9 February 1967.* National Institutes of Health, Bethesda.

RICHARDS, R. K. and EVERETT, G. M. (1944) Analgesic and anticonvulsive properties of 3,5,5-trimethyloxazolidine-2,4-dione (Tridione). *Federation Proceedings 1944*, **3,** 39

SWINYARD, E. A. (1949) Laboratory assay of clinically effective antiepileptic drugs. *Journal of the American Pharmacological Association,* **38,** 201–204

SWINYARD, E. A. (1982) Introduction. In *Antiepileptic Drugs,* edited by D. M. Woodbury, J. K. Penry and C. E. Pippenger, pp. 1–9. New York: Raven Press

US FOOD AND DRUG ADMINISTRATION (1981) *Guidelines for the Clinical Evaluation of Antiepileptic Drugs (Adults and Children)*. FDA, Rockville, Md.

WARD, A. A. JR (1983) Perspectives for surgical therapy of epilepsy. In *Epilepsy*, edited by A. A. Ward, Jr, J. K. Penry and D. Purpura, pp. 371–375. New York: Raven Press

5
Epidemiology of epilepsy

Bruce S. Schoenberg

EPIDEMIOLOGICAL APPROACH TO THE STUDY OF EPILEPSY

Neuroepidemiology is concerned with the distribution and determinants of neurological disease in human populations (Schoenberg, 1982a). Studies of the distribution of disease address questions related to which particular segments of the population are most affected by the disorder. For example, is the disease more common among children? Does it occur more frequently in a specific region of the world? Answers to such questions provide important clues with regard to factors which may be associated with either the occurrence of the disease or its natural history – in other words, the determinants of the disease.

Unlike the laboratory investigator who is able to manipulate experimental conditions within the limits of technical sophistication, the epidemiologist examines disease occurrence in human populations who cannot be subjected to a milieu controlled by the researcher. Instead, the epidemiologist must employ carefully designed strategies to analyze 'experiments of nature'. During the course of our lives we are exposed to a large number of factors, some of which may play an important role in the etiology of disease. Epidemiological procedures allow us to identify these factors and thereby provide information useful in the design of rational strategies for disease control and prevention. All investigators of disease as it occurs in humans, be they biochemists, clinicians, or epidemiologists, should use these techniques. It is therefore appropriate that a consideration of epidemiological methods appears in this volume, since these same principles apply to all research involving human subjects.

DISEASE DEFINITION AND CLASSIFICATION

> When I use a word . . . it means just what I choose it to mean – neither more nor less.
>
> Lewis Carroll, *Alice Through the Looking Glass*

Perhaps the most frequently neglected element in planning an epidemiological investigation is the design of adequate diagnostic criteria. Without precise definitions of disease it is impossible for other investigators to replicate a study.

Similarly, without such detail, one cannot be certain whether two reports are describing the same disease entity. This is especially important for disorders of the nervous system which generally do not have pathognomonic signs, symptoms, or laboratory findings. Although the need for carefully defined diagnostic criteria may be recognized, it is often overlooked or posed in terms of vague generalities. In many instances, descriptions of disease are substituted for definitions of disease. One must translate descriptions into operational rules which must be adhered to in arriving at a diagnosis.

The situation with regard to epilepsy is further complicated by the fact that we are dealing with a symptom complex which may be a manifestation of a large number of diverse disease entities, each with a different cause(s) (some known and some unknown). For example, individuals with a brain tumor, those with a completed stroke, those who have sustained a head injury, or those with a wide variety of metabolic disorders may each present with recurrent afebrile seizures. There is some disagreement in published reports as to what evidence is required to document a seizure or even the definition of a seizure (for example, some authors include certain abnormal electroencephalographic findings in the absence of overt clinical manifestations). Authors categorize seizures using different systems of classification, some based on presumed etiology, others based on clinical manifestations, responses to therapy, etc. In practice, the situation is even more complex in that a given patient may exhibit multiple types of seizures.

There are similar controversies with regard to the definition of epilepsy. Some investigators include even single, isolated seizures, while others include febrile convulsions. Parallel problems exist in attempting to categorize specific subtypes of epilepsy. Finally, there is no consistency as to what evidence is necessary and sufficient to assign a specific etiology to a given seizure disorder. Results of past and current efforts at classifying seizure types and forms of epilepsy are well-summarized in Chapter 6. It should be emphasized, however, that a given set of rules for diagnosis or classification cannot satisfy all potential applications equally well. For example, the individual physician may use elaborate and extensive laboratory investigations to supplement clinical findings in a given patient in order to establish a rather precise diagnosis. This strategy cannot be implemented in a field study of a large population group in regions far removed from major medical centers, however.

CASE ASCERTAINMENT

The level of case ascertainment varies widely among the large number of published articles. This is a function of (a) the methods used to identify individuals with seizures; and (b) the social customs of the population being investigated. Studies have been based on reviews of medical records, cases reported to a centralized registry, and community-wide case-finding surveys. If a substantial proportion of the population does not have ready access to expert neurological care, then studies based only on cases known to the medical community (investigations which identify those with epilepsy by using medical records or data in a registry) will seriously underestimate the magnitude of seizure disorders in the population. Furthermore, data derived from diagnoses made by medical personnel with little experience with seizure disorders yield results which must be treated with considerable caution.

This problem is nicely summarized in a quotation from a British statistician, who wrote (Stamp, 1929):

> The government are very keen on amassing statistics – they collect them, add them, raise them to the *n*th power, take the cube root and prepare wonderful diagrams. But what you must never forget is that every one of those figures comes in the first instance from the . . . village watchman, who puts down what he damn pleases.

Thus the quality of a study rests with the quality of the diagnostic abilities of the 'village watchman', who is responsible for correctly identifying those with epilepsy in the community.

Social customs and living habits may also have a profound influence on the ease of case ascertainment. If epilepsy is associated with a negative social stigma, patients may be deliberately hidden from the medical investigator, and the presence of seizures may be actively denied. Communities with much social contact and interaction are more likely to notice the presence of seizures in a given individual. If all members of a family sleep together in the same room or in close proximity, nocturnal convulsions are more likely to come to the attention of others. In cultures where individuals gather around a fire, looking at the flames may precipitate a seizure and result in serious burns (Goudsmit, van der Waals and Gajdusek, 1983). Similarly, in communities in which people sleep around a fire, a convulsion is likely to result in moderate or severe burns. The presence of such burns can be utilized to identify epilepsy suspects. The ease of case ascertainment is also related to the seizure type and the seizure frequency. Thus, absence seizures are less likely to come to the attention of others than are generalized tonic-clonic convulsions. Spells of inattention which occur only once or twice each day are less frequently noticed than if such episodes occur multiple times each hour.

In addition, there may be a considerable delay between the onset of seizures and the correct diagnosis of epilepsy. Investigations which are based on medical records must consequently continue to search for diagnoses of epilepsy made several years after the time period of interest to avoid missing any cases. In spite of this rather lengthy list of methodological problems confronting the epidemiological study of epilepsy, many successful investigations have been carried out around the world. However, since researchers applied different solutions to these problems, one must exercise great care in comparing one study with another.

THE INTERNATIONAL MAGNITUDE AND DISTRIBUTION OF EPILEPSY

To obtain an unbiased picture of the spectrum of disease in the community, the epidemiologist attempts to identify all cases in the defined population. In general, referral patterns and patient behavior are such that certain physicians or medical institutions may see an unrepresentative sample of all those with the disorder. One neurologist may see no cases of a certain disorder, while another clinician, working in the same community, may restrict his entire practice to patients with that particular disorder.

By identifying all cases of the disorder in a well-defined population, the epidemiologist attempts to avoid this problem. Through such studies it is possible to estimate the magnitude of the disease burden in the community and the distribution of important factors in the portion of the population affected by the disorder. To state how many people have a given disease or died from that particular disease has little meaning unless one also provides data concerning how many people were at risk of having that same disease or dying from it. To adjust for this, the epidemiologist usually reports the magnitude of the disease burden as a rate or ratio, in which the number of cases of the disease in the community (in the numerator) is related to the population at risk of having the disease (in the denominator). The most commonly used epidemiological indices of disease magnitude are defined in *Table 5.1*.

Table 5.1 Common epidemiologic indices (from Schoenberg, 1981, with permission of Thieme-Stratton, publishers of *Seminars in Neurology*)

Mortality measures the frequency of deaths within a specific population and is calculated for a given time interval and given place. It is often expressed as a death rate: deaths from a given disease per 100 000 persons at risk of dying of the disease per year.

Incidence measures the rapidity with which a disease occurs or the frequency of addition of new cases of a disease within a specific population. It is calculated for a given time interval and given place, and is often expressed as an incidence rate: the number of new cases of a given disease during a specified period (usually 1 year) per 100 000 persons at risk of having the disease for the first time per year.*

Prevalence measures the frequency of all current cases of a disease within a specific population and is calculated for a given time and given place. It is usually expressed as a prevalence ratio: the number of persons with a given disease at a specified time per 100 000 persons capable of having the disease at the same specified time.*

* Prevalence and incidence are related to each other as follows: prevalence approximately equals incidence multiplied by the average duration of the disease.

Mortality estimates

The most readily available data concerning the magnitude of disease on a worldwide basis are derived from mortality tabulations. This makes it possible to examine trends from country to country and to evaluate changes over time. Unfortunately, such data have a number of substantial disadvantages. Mortality statistics are not a good indication of disease frequency since only a small proportion of those with epilepsy die as a result of their seizures (in other words, the case–fatality ratio is low). This results in an under-reporting of the frequency of epilepsy as measured by mortality data. Two studies provide an estimate of the degree of under-reporting. In Rochester, Minnesota (USA), only 11% of all deaths among those with epilepsy had convulsions or epilepsy mentioned on the death certificate (Hauser, 1978). In Warsaw, Poland, epilepsy was listed on the death certificate as an underlying or associated cause of death in only 29% of known cases who died (Zielinski, 1974a).

In addition, most mortality statistics are based on a single, underlying cause of death appearing on the death certificate. In reality, it is often a combination of factors which leads to the person's demise. The extent of this problem has recently been investigated. Newly available data in the United States for the years 1971 and 1973–78 included tabulations for all causes of death listed on the death certificate. During this period of time, for the 29 065 death certificates on which epilepsy was listed (as an underlying, immediate, associated, or contributory cause of death), it was specified as the underlying cause of death in 41% (Chandra, Bharucha and Schoenberg, 1984).

Finally, in dealing with mortality statistics, one must be concerned with the accuracy of death certificate diagnoses, particularly from country to country and over long periods of time. Despite these problems, mortality data have been analyzed in an attempt to determine international patterns. The first such comprehensive review of mortality statistics for epilepsy was carried out by Goldberg and Kurland (1962) for the years 1951–58. Age-adjusted mortality rates for epilepsy varied from 1.0–4.5 deaths/1000 000/year. Chile, Colombia, Portugal and Mexico were found to have the highest rates, while Denmark, Poland, Sweden and the US white population had the lowest figures. More recently these data were updated for the years 1967–73 (Massey and Schoenberg, 1985). With few exceptions, mortality rates for epilepsy have declined. However, countries in Latin America continue to report the highest mortality figures. As more prevalence surveys are carried out around the world, in the future it will no longer be necessary to rely on mortality tabulations to estimate patterns of disease frequency internationally.

A detailed analysis of mortality data in the United States for epilepsy as the underlying cause of death for the years 1959–61 was carried out by Kurtzke *et al.* (1973). Males have higher rates than females, while non-whites have higher rates than whites. Age-specific mortality rates increase only slightly with age, with the exception of data for non-white males. Although the tabulations are based on a relatively small number of deaths, non-white males have a maximal mortality rate between 35–44 years of age and a second smaller peak in the elderly.

As noted previously, US mortality data were recently analyzed for all deaths due to epilepsy (that is, with epilepsy as the underlying cause of death) and all deaths *related to* epilepsy (that is, with epilepsy as the underlying, immediate, associated, or contributory cause of death) for the years 1971 and 1973–78. The average annual age-adjusted rates for all deaths related to epilepsy are more than double the corresponding rates for deaths due to epilepsy. Rates for those whose deaths are due to epilepsy remain relatively unchanged with age. However, for all deaths related to epilepsy, rates increase with advancing age. For deaths due to and all deaths related to epilepsy, rates for either sex are higher for non-whites; and for either race, are higher for males (Chandra, Bharucha and Schoenberg, 1983).

Incidence estimates

Epilepsy incidence rates are much more difficult to obtain since they require special investigations. The range of reported average annual incidence rates is quite broad, varying from a low of 17.3 new cases/100 000/year for Niigata City, Japan (Sato, 1964) to a high of 100 new cases/100 000/year for an Australian study (Crombie *et al.*, 1960). The authors reporting this very high rate included both isolated seizures and febrile seizures in their estimate of the epilepsy incidence rate. However, most of the reported rates for recurrent afebrile seizures are not very different from each other (30–50 new cases/100 000/year) (Hauser, 1978). As suggested by mortality data, incidence rates are generally higher among males. With one exception, reports document that infants and children have the highest age-specific incidence rates (Leviton and Cowan, 1982). The exception is from studies in Rochester, Minnesota, where age-specific incidence rates reveal two peaks: below 1 year of age and in the elderly (Hauser and Kurland, 1975). There has been considerable debate as to the significance of this pattern in the Rochester data. Some have suggested that the peak in the elderly may reflect seizures secondary to brain tumors and stroke, both of which have very high incidence rates in the oldest members of the population (Matsumoto *et al.*, 1973; Schoenberg, Christine and Whisnant, 1978). The occurrence of recurrent afebrile seizures in elderly members of the Rochester population is easily documented through the unique facilities of the records-linkage system available for members of this community (Kurland, Molgaard and Schoenberg, 1982). However, 70% of the incidence cases of epilepsy were classified as having idiopathic seizures. The high rate documented for elderly Rochester residents may simply reflect more complete case ascertainment in this age group compared to the elderly in other populations. A similar phenomenon was reported for brain tumor incidence rates in this same community (Schoenberg, Christine and Whisnant, 1978).

At present there are no uniform standards for categorizing epilepsy as being the result of a specific etiology (that is, symptomatic epilepsy) or being of unknown etiology (that is, idiopathic). In most reports the decision is a clinical judgement on the part of the investigator or the attending physician. In the Rochester, Minnesota, study approximately 5% of the identified epileptics were thought to have seizures secondary to head trauma; in 5% cerebrovascular disease was the presumed etiology; 4% were thought to be due to brain tumor; 4% to congenital or genetic abnormalities; and 3% as a result of infectious diseases (Hauser, 1978). In most morbidity surveys, 65–75% of identified cases of epilepsy are reported to be of unknown etiology (Hauser, 1978).

Although most reports indicate that the majority of patients with epilepsy have seizures which are generalized from onset (Gastaut, 1970), in the Rochester, Minnesota, study 60% of the cases had partial seizures (Hauser and Kurland, 1975). This again may reflect better case ascertainment in the Rochester population (that is, better identification of seizures and of other primary diseases presenting with seizures, particularly among the elderly).

Only Rochester, Minnesota, has sufficient data over an extended period of time to allow measurement of the long-term trends in incidence rates. When data were analyzed for 1935–74, there was an initial rise in rates during the first decade (thought to represent better case identification), but over the subsequent 30 years there was a consistent decline in the number of new cases/unit population/year (Hauser, Annegers and Kurland, 1977).

Based on published age-specific incidence rates, Hauser (1978) estimated the cumulative or lifetime incidence of epilepsy. His estimate of the risk of recurrent afebrile seizures during the course of one's lifetime of 2–4.3% establish that epilepsy is one of the commonest neurological disorders.

Prevalence estimates

Studies of prevalence pose an additional problem because investigators disagree as to the definition of a prevalent case of epilepsy. Some include all individuals residing in the community who have ever had epilepsy and are still alive at the time of the study. Others include only 'active' cases (that is, those with recurrent afebrile seizures who (a) remain on anticonvulsant medication, or (b) have experienced their last afebrile seizure within a specified time interval before the date of the survey). Thus, medical practice can influence whether a given patient is included or excluded in a prevalence survey. Some clinicians may decide to maintain a patient on anticonvulsant medication for as long as possible while another clinician may attempt to withdraw the medication as soon as this appears to be feasible.

Most figures for prevalence ratios based on cases continuing on anticonvulsant medication fall within the narrow range of three to six cases/1000. These figures are largely for Caucasian populations residing in developed countries. The lowest prevalence ratio has been reported for Japan (1.5 cases/1000) (Sato, 1964). The highest prevalence figures have been documented in Africa and in South America (Aall-Jilek, 1965; Gomez, Arciniegas and Torres, 1978; Osuntokun *et al.*, 1982; van der Waals, Goudsmit and Gajdusek, 1983), with figures as high as 15–30 cases/1000. To verify whether these patterns reflect actual excesses and are not the result of methodological differences, the World Health Organization launched a series of neuroepidemiological prevalence surveys, using uniform techniques and standard definitions of a prevalent case of epilepsy (Schoenberg, 1982b). Such investigations are currently under way in Chile, Colombia, Ecuador, India, Italy, Mexico, Nigeria, the People's Republic of China, Peru and Venezuela. Results of initial pilot studies appear to confirm these high prevalence ratios in Africa and Latin America (Cruz *et al.*, unpublished observations).

Of special interest in interpreting prevalence figures is a study by Zielinski (1974b) for residents of Warsaw, Poland. He supplemented his review of medical records by a 10% sample of households to identify those with epilepsy. Data derived from the medical records as the only source of information yielded a prevalence ratio of 5.1/1000. When additional information obtained from the household survey was included, the prevalence ratio increased to 10.4/1000.

Prevalence ratios are generally higher for males, a finding consistent with mortality and incidence data (Hauser, 1978). In order to measure differences by race in the prevalence ratio of epilepsy in a well-defined US community, a door-to-door survey was carried out for the population of a rural, biracial county in south-central Mississippi. Uniform methods were used throughout, and all diagnoses were made by senior, board-certified neurologists. The investigation reported the following prevalence figures: 1.1/100 for white males; 0.7/100 for white females; 1.4/100 for black males; and 1.0/100 for black females. About 7% of identified cases had never been evaluated medically for epilepsy before the survey. In contrast to this, 49% of the black population with epilepsy and 35% of the white population with epilepsy had not previously been evaluated by a neurologist or a neurosurgeon for their seizure disorder (Haerer, Anderson and Schoenberg, 1984).

Studies of the variation in prevalence ratios with age generally show lower figures for the oldest members of the population (de Graaf, 1974; Sato, 1964). Again, the exception is provided by tabulations for the population of Rochester, Minnesota, which reveal an increasing prevalence ratio with increasing age. This pattern is thought to be due at least in part to the very high level of continuing follow-up of previously identified cases, and reflects the curve for age-specific incidence rates in this same population (Hauser and Kurland, 1975).

NATURAL HISTORY OF EPILEPSY AND FACTORS AFFECTING PROGNOSIS

Investigations of the prognosis of individuals with epilepsy have concentrated on two important issues: remission of symptoms and survival. Although the data were not derived from a well-defined population, Hauser *et al.* (1982) studied seizure recurrence after a first unprovoked seizure among patients presenting at four major hospitals serving the population of Minneapolis–St. Paul in the United States. The cumulative risk of a subsequent seizure was 27% at three years following the initial episode. The risk of recurrence was greatest in patients who were known to have suffered a prior neurological insult. Among factors investigated which did not affect the risk of recurrence were age at first seizure, sex, type of seizure, an abnormality on the neurological examination, or status epilepticus at onset. Based on data such as this, most investigators do not include single isolated seizures in the definition of epilepsy.

Even a proportion of those who go on to have recurrent afebrile seizures may experience some resolution of their epilepsy. Using available prevalence and incidence data, Hauser (1978) estimated that the average duration of symptoms among epileptics is approximately 12 years. Hauser and Kurland (1975) were able to provide more detailed information on the resolution of symptoms by investigating the experience of all incidence cases of epilepsy in the Rochester, Minnesota, population. Among all newly diagnosed epileptics in Rochester, 40% of those followed for ten or more years were seizure-free for at least two years as of the date of last follow-up. For those under observation for 15 years, 49% were seizure-free for at least 2 years; the figure rose to 55% for those followed for 20 years. The leading causes of death among newly diagnosed cases of epilepsy in the Rochester population between 1935 and 1974 were neoplasms (21.4%), heart disease (19.8%), cerebrovascular disease (17.1%) and accidents (6.4%) (Hauser, Annegers and Elveback, 1980).

Survival data among epileptics are also available from the Rochester studies. The observed survival of all identified epileptics in the Rochester population was compared to expected survival, based on the experience of an age- and sex-matched comparison group from the same area of the United States. Relative survival (observed/expected) was 91% at five years after diagnosis, and 85% at both 10 and 15 years following the diagnosis. Those whose seizures were due to recognized primary disease (such as brain tumor) and those with seizure onset before age 5 had the poorest prognosis with regard to survival. Other data available from insurance statistics show that insured individuals with epilepsy have two to three times the risk of dying compared to demographically similar individuals free of serious illness at the time of issuance of the insurance policy (Henriksen, Juul-Jensen and Lund, 1967; Schiottz-Christensen and Bruhn, 1973). It should be emphasized that individuals either with or without seizures who elect to take out an insurance policy may not be representative of either the epileptics or those free of epilepsy in the population.

FEBRILE SEIZURES

The relationship between febrile seizures and the subsequent occurrence of recurrent afebrile seizures in the same individual has been the subject of several investigations. The problem of seizures associated with fever presents a dilemma both for the researcher and the attending physician who must distinguish among three alternatives: (a) those with a seizure diathesis who later have recurrent afebrile seizures and in whom fever increases the risk of seizures; (b) those in whom the seizure is a manifestation of some underlying disease (for example meningitis);

and (c) those who tend to have seizures only in the presence of fever and not beyond the age of 4 (Leviton and Cowan, 1982).

Febrile seizures appear to be relatively common events. Data from England (Miller *et al.*, 1960; Ross, 1973), Israel (Costeff, 1965), Mexico (Garcia-Pedroza *et al.*, 1983), and selected areas in the continental United States (Hauser and Kurland, 1975; Meighan, Queener and Weitman, 1976; Schuman and Miller, 1966; Rose *et al.*, 1973; van den Berg, 1974) estimate the cumulative risk of febrile seizures among children to be 2–5%. Two reports derived from studies in the Mariana Islands in the western Pacific yield much higher estimates of between 11 and 14% (Mathai *et al.*, 1968; Stanhope, Brody and Brink, 1972). Between 2.0 and 4.4% of children with febrile seizures are reported to later develop epilepsy (that is, recurrent afebrile seizures) (Leviton and Cowan, 1982).

Attempts have been made to identify factors which are useful in distinguishing those febrile-seizure patients at high risk for the occurrence of recurrent afebrile seizures (Annegers *et al.*, 1979; Nelson and Ellenberg, 1976, 1978). Recognized characteristics of importance include: (a) features of the patient (low Apgar score at birth, neurological abnormalities before the first febrile seizure, or febrile seizures occurring after age 4); (b) features of the febrile seizure itself (focal, predominantly unilateral, recurrent, lasting more than 10–15 minutes, or accompanied by postictal paralysis); or (c) features of the family history (positive for epilepsy). There is as yet no uniform agreement as to the efficacy of treating febrile seizure patients with anticonvulsants in an attempt to reduce the incidence of subsequent epilepsy (Nelson and Ellenberg, 1981).

GENETIC ASPECTS

There are a multitude of inherited disorders involving the nervous system which have recurrent afebrile seizures as part of the clinical manifestations. However, compared to the rather frequent occurrence of epilepsy, these individual genetic conditions are relatively rare and account for only a small proportion of all those with recurrent afebrile seizures (Hauser, Annegers and Anderson, 1983).

A number of studies have tried to measure the relative importance of genetic factors in the more common forms of epilepsy. Such investigations must confront the same problems of diagnostic accuracy and case ascertainment faced by those attempting to measure the frequency of epilepsy in a defined population. There is evidence suggesting that a spike-wave electroencephalographic (EEG) pattern is inherited (Metrakos and Metrakos, 1961, 1969). However, this EEG pattern cannot be equated with clinical seizures. Investigations of the genetic aspects of clinical epilepsy include twin studies, case-control analyses, and cohort investigations (Annegers *et al.*, 1982; Newmark and Penry, 1979). In general, when considering idiopathic epilepsy monozygotic twins have a higher concordance (85–88%) than dizygotic twins (4–16%) (Conrad, 1935; Inouye, 1960; Lennox and Lennox, 1960). It should be pointed out that many of these twin studies are based on case series of twins. Twin pairs with two affected members are more likely to come to medical attention than twin pairs with only one affected member; hence, such case series tend to overestimate the concordance among twins. To avoid this problem, a study of medical records for all twins born in Denmark over a 40-year period was carried out by Harvald and Hauge (1965). The results of this investigation confirmed the higher concordance for epilepsy among monozygotic as compared to dizygotic twin pairs. A possible source of bias remains even in this study, however, since monozygotic twins are reported to have higher frequencies of prematurity and low birth weights than their dizygotic counterparts (Yerushalmy and Sheerar, 1940). Despite these problems, twin studies suggest that genetic factors play an important role in determining the risk of epilepsy.

Several investigators have addressed the question of whether relatives of epileptics have a greater seizure risk than what might be expected from either the experience of a comparison group or from the general population-based morbidity rates for epilepsy (Conrad, 1937; Eisner, Pauli and Livingston, 1959; Harvald, 1954; Lennox and Lennox, 1960; Metrakos and Metrakos, 1960). All were consistent in reporting that relatives of epileptics have a higher risk of seizures.

Annegers *et al.* (1976) investigated the same problem by analyzing the frequency of seizure disorders among the offspring of identified cases of epilepsy in the population of Rochester, Minnesota. The risk of seizures in the offspring of female epileptics was significantly increased; this finding was not duplicated among the children of male epileptics, however. Annegers *et al.* (1982) also studied the risk of seizure disorders among the relatives of epileptics whose seizures began before the age of 15. As before, his index cases were derived from the Rochester, Minnesota, population. The risk of epilepsy through age 20 was higher than expected among the siblings and children of the probands.

In all of these studies demonstrating an increased risk of seizures among family members of identified epileptics, it should be pointed out that families share *both* genetic and environmental factors. Therefore, clusters of multiple cases of disease within members of a family cannot be equated with a genetic etiology. For example, seizures resulting from birth injury secondary to cephalopelvic disproportion may affect multiple children of the same mother.

FUTURE PROSPECTS

Attempts to study the epidemiological features of epilepsy must address the methodological problems of defining, classifying and identifying cases. The lack of uniform procedures in implementing such investigations necessitates using great caution in comparing the results of different studies. Despite these problems, epidemiological studies have consistently demonstrated that epilepsy represents a major health problem wherever it has been investigated throughout the world. This is particularly true in Africa and Latin America. The techniques of experimental epidemiology (controlled clinical trials) are being used to evaluate both the efficacy and safety of new therapeutic modalities introduced to control the clinical manifestations of epilepsy. Finally, analytical epidemiological investigations are just beginning to identify risk factors for the occurrence of recurrent afebrile convulsions. Such studies are urgently needed to design and implement rational programs for the control and prevention of epilepsy on a broad scale.

References

AALL-JILEK, L. M. (1965) Epilepsy in the Wapagoro tribe in Tanganyika. *Acta Psychiatrica et Neurologica Scandinavica,* **41,** 57–86

ANNEGERS, J. F., HAUSER, W. A., ELVEBACK, L. R., ANDERSON, V. E. and KURLAND, L. T. (1976) Seizure disorders in offspring of parents with a history of seizures: a maternal–paternal difference? *Epilepsia,* **17,** 1–9

ANNEGERS, J. F., HAUSER, W. A., ANDERSON, V. E. and KURLAND, L. T. (1982) The risks of seizure disorders among relatives of patients with childhood onset epilepsy. *Neurology (New York)*, **32**, 174–179

ANNEGERS, J. F., HAUSER, W. A., ELVEBACK, L. R. and KURLAND, L. T. (1979) The risk of epilepsy following febrile convulsions. *Neurology (Minneapolis)*, **29**, 297–303

CHANDRA, V., BHARUCHA, N. E. and SCHOENBERG, B. S. (1983) Deaths related to epilepsy in the United States. *Neuroepidemiology*, **2**, 148–155

CONRAD, K. (1935) Erbanlage und epilepsie. Untersuchungen an einer Serie von 253 Zwillingspaaren. *Zentralblatt für die gesamte Neurologie und Psychiatrie*, **153**, 271–326

CONRAD, K. (1937) Erbanlage und epilepsie. Ergebnisse einer Nachkommenschaftsuntersuchung an Epileptikern. *Zentralblatt für die Gesamte Neurologie und Psychiatrie*, **159**, 521–581

COSTEFF, H. (1965) Convulsions in childhood: their natural history and indications for treatment. *New England Journal of Medicine*, **273**, 1410–1413

CROMBIE, D. L., CROSS, K. W., FRY, J., PINSENT, R. J. F. H. and WATTS, C. A. H. (1960) A survey of the epilepsies in general practice: a report by the Research Committee of the College of General Practitioners. *British Medical Journal*, **2**, 416–422

DE GRAAF, A. S. (1974) Epidemiological aspects of epilepsy in Northern Norway. *Epilepsia*, **15**, 291–299

EISNER, V., PAULI, L. L. and LIVINGSTON, S. (1959) Hereditary aspects of epilepsy. *Bulletin of the Johns Hopkins Hospital*, **105**, 245–271

GARCIA-PEDROZA, F., RUBIO-DONNADIEU, F., GARCIA-RAMOS, G., ESCOBEDO-RIOS, F. and GONZALEZ-CORTES, A. (1983) Prevalence of epilepsy in children: Tlalpan, Mexico City, Mexico. *Neuroepidemiology*, **2**, 16–23

GASTAUT, H. (1970) Clinical and electroencephalographic classification of the epilepsies. *Epilepsia*, **11**, 102–113

GOLDBERG, I. D. and KURLAND, L. T. (1962) Mortality in 33 countries from diseases of the nervous system. *World Neurology*, **3**, 444–465

GOMEZ, J. G., ARCINIEGAS, E. and TORRES, J. (1978) Prevalence of epilepsy in Bogota, Colombia. *Neurology (Minneapolis)*, **28**, 90–94

GOUDSMIT, J., VAN DER WAALS, F. W. and GAJDUSEK, D. C. (1983) Epilepsy in the Gbawein and Wroughbarh Clan of Grand Bassa County, Liberia: the endemic occurrence of 'See-ee' in the native population. *Neuroepidemiology*, **2**, 24–34

HAERER, A. F., ANDERSON, D. W. and SCHOENBERG, B. S. (1984) Racial differences in the prevalence and clinical features of epilepsy: population survey of Copiah County, Mississippi. *Annals of Neurology*, **16**, 120 (abstract)

HARVALD, B. (1954) *Heredity in Epilepsy: An Electroencephalographic Study of Relatives of Epileptics*. Copenhagen: University Institute for Human Genetics

HARVALD, B. and HAUGE, M. (1965) Hereditary factors elucidated by twin studies. In *Genetics and the Epidemiology of Chronic Disease*, edited by J. V. Neel, M. W. Shaw, and W. J. Schull. *US Public Health Service Publication 1163*, pp. 61–76. Washington, DC: US Government Printing Office

HAUSER, W. A. (1978) Epidemiology of epilepsy. In *Neurological Epidemiology: Principles and Clinical Applications*, edited by B. S. Schoenberg. *Advances in Neurology*, **19**, 313–338. New York: Raven Press

HAUSER, W. A., ANNEGERS, J. F. and ANDERSON, V. E. (1983) Epidemiology and genetics of epilepsy. In *Epilepsy*, edited by A. A. Ward, Jr, J. K. Penry and D. Purpura. *Research Publications of the Association for Research in Nervous and Mental Disease*, **61**, 267–294

HAUSER, W. A., ANDERSON, V. E., LOEWENSON, R. B. and MCROBERTS, S. M. (1982) Seizure recurrence after a first unprovoked seizure. *New England Journal of Medicine*, **307**, 522–528

HAUSER, W. A., ANNEGERS, J. F. and ELVEBACK, L. R. (1980) Mortality in patients with epilepsy. *Epilepsia*, **21**, 399–412

HAUSER, W. A., ANNEGERS, J. F. and KURLAND, L. T. (1977) Is the incidence of epilepsy declining? *American Journal of Epidemiology*, **106**, 246 (abstract)

HAUSER, W. A. and KURLAND, L. T. (1975) The epidemiology of epilepsy in Rochester, Minnesota, 1935 through 1967. *Epilepsia*, **16**, 1–66

HENRIKSEN, P. B., JUUL-JENSEN, P. and LUND, M. (1967) The mortality of epileptics; a preliminary report. In *Social Studies in Epilepsy, No. 5*, pp. 5–12. London: International Bureau for Epilepsy

INOUYE, E. (1960) Observations on forty twin index cases with chronic epilepsy and their co-twins. *Journal of Nervous and Mental Disease*, **130**, 401–416

KURLAND, L. T., MOLGAARD, C. A. and SCHOENBERG, B. S. (1982) Mayo Clinic records-linkage: contributions to neuroepidemiology. *Neuroepidemiology*, **1**, 102–114

KURTZKE, J. F., KURLAND, L. T., GOLDBERG, I. D., CHOI, N. W. and REEDER, F. A. (1973) Convulsive disorders. In *Epidemiology of Neurologic and Sense Organ Disorders*, edited by L. T. Kurland, J. F. Kurtzke and I. D. Goldberg, pp. 15–40. Cambridge: Harvard University Press

LENNOX, W. G. and LENNOX, M. A. (1960) *Epilepsy and Related Disorders,* Vol. 1. Boston: Little, Brown

LEVITON, A. and COWAN, L. D. (1982) Epidemiology of seizure disorders in children. *Neuroepidemiology,* **1,** 40–83

MASSEY, E. W. and SCHOENBERG, B. S. (1985) Mortality from epilepsy: international patterns and changes over time. *Neuroepidemiology* (in press)

MATHAI, K. V., DUNN, D. P., KURLAND, L. T. and REEDER, F. A. (1968) Convulsive disorders in the Mariana Islands. *Epilepsia,* **9,** 77–85

MATSUMOTO, N., WHISNANT, J. P., KURLAND, L. T. and OKAZAKI, H. (1973) Natural history of stroke in Rochester, Minnesota, 1955 through 1969: an extension of a previous study, 1945 through 1954. *Stroke,* **4,** 20–29

MEIGHAN, S., QUEENER, L. and WEITMAN, M. (1976) Prevalence of epilepsy in children of Multnomah County, Oregon. *Epilepsia,* **17,** 245–256

METRAKOS, J. D. and METRAKOS, K. (1960) Genetics of convulsive disorders. I. Introduction, problems, methods and baselines. *Neurology (Minneapolis),* **10,** 228–240

METRAKOS, K. and METRAKOS, J. D. (1961) Genetics of convulsive disorders. II. Genetic and electroencephalographic studies in centrencephalic epilepsy. *Neurology (Minneapolis),* **11,** 474–483

METRAKOS, J. D. and METRAKOS, K. (1969) Discussion: genetic studies in clinical epilepsy. In *Basic Mechanisms of the Epilepsies,* edited by H. H. Jasper, A. A. Ward, Jr and A. Pope, pp. 700–708. Boston: Little, Brown

MILLER, F. J. W., COURT, S. D. M., WALTON, W. S. and KNOX, E. G. (1960) *Growing up in Newcastle-upon-Tyne. A Continuing Study of Health and Illness in Young Children Within Their Families*, pp. 164–173. London: Oxford University Press

NELSON, K. B. and ELLENBERG, J. H. (1976) Predictors of epilepsy in children who have experienced febrile seizures. *New England Journal of Medicine,* **295,** 1029–1033

NELSON, K. B. and ELLENBERG, J. H. (1978) Prognosis in children with febrile seizures. *Pediatrics,* **61,** 720–727

NELSON, K. B. and ELLENBERG, J. H. (1981) *Febrile Seizures.* New York: Raven Press

NEWMARK, M. E. and PENRY, J. K. (1979) *Genetics of Epilepsy: A Review.* New York: Raven Press

OSUNTOKUN, B. O., SCHOENBERG, B. S., NOTTIDGE, V. A. *et al.* (1982) Research protocol for measuring the prevalence of neurological disorders in developing countries. Results of a pilot study in Nigeria. *Neuroepidemiology,* **1,** 143–153

ROSE, S. W., PENRY, J. K., MARKUSH, R. E., RADLOFF, L. A. and PUTNAM, P. L. (1973) Prevalence of epilepsy in children. *Epilepsia,* **14,** 133–152

ROSS, E. M. (1973) Convulsive disorders in British children. *Proceedings of the Royal Society of Medicine,* **66,** 702–703

SATO, S. (1964) The epidemiological and clinico-statistical study of epilepsy in Niigata City. Part 2. The epidemiological study of epilepsy in Niigata City. *Clinical Neurology (Tokyo),* **4,** 413–424

SCHIOTTZ-CHRISTENSEN, E. and BRUHN, P. (1973) Intelligence, behaviour and scholastic achievement subsequent to febrile convulsions: an analysis of discordant twin pairs. *Developmental Medicine and Child Neurology,* **15,** 565–575

SCHOENBERG, B. S. (1981) Neurologic disease in the elderly: epidemiologic aspects. *Seminars in Neurology,* **1,** 5–12

SCHOENBERG, B. S. (1982a) The scope of neuroepidemiology. *Neuroepidemiology,* **1,** 1–16

SCHOENBERG, B. S. (1982b) Clinical neuroepidemiology in developing countries; neurology with few neurologists. *Neuroepidemiology,* **1,** 137–142

SCHOENBERG, B. S., CHRISTINE, B. W. and WHISNANT, J. P. (1978) The resolution of discrepancies in the reported incidence of primary brain tumors. *Neurology (Minneapolis),* **28,** 817–823

SCHUMAN, S. H. and MILLER, L. J. (1966) Febrile convulsions in families: findings in an epidemiologic survey. *Clinical Pediatrics,* **5,** 604–608

STAMP, J. (1929) *Some Economic Factors in Modern Life,* pp. 258–259. London: P. S. King and Son

STANHOPE, J. M., BRODY, J. A. and BRINK, E. (1972) Convulsions among the Chamorro people of Guam, Mariana Islands. I. Seizure disorders. *American Journal of Epidemiology,* **95,** 292–304

VAN DEN BERG, B. J. (1974) Studies on convulsive disorders in young children. IV. Incidence of convulsions among children. *Developmental Medicine and Child Neurology,* **16,** 457–464

VAN DER WAALS, F. W., GOUDSMIT, J. and GAJDUSEK, D. C. (1983) See-ee: clinical characteristics of highly prevalent seizure disorders in the Gbawein and Wroughbarh Clan Region of Grand Bassa County, Liberia. *Neuroepidemiology,* **2,** 35–44

YERUSHALMY, J. and SHEERAR, S. E. (1940) Studies on twins: II. On the early mortality of like-sexed and unlike-sexed twins. *Human Biology,* **12,** 247–263

ZIELINSKI, J. J. (1974a) Epilepsy and mortality rate and cause of death. *Epilepsia,* **15,** 191–201

ZIELINSKI, J. J. (1974b) Epileptics not in treatment. *Epilepsia,* **15,** 203–210

6
The classification of seizures and the epilepsies

Peter Wolf

> To some extent, the phenomena themselves seem to suggest names; at other times, names imply theories
>
> Temkin (1971)

DISTINCTION BETWEEN SEIZURES AND EPILEPSIES

One of the most common and most confusing inexactitudes in clinical language, but also in written reports, is the indiscriminate use of terminology applicable for epileptic seizures and that of epileptic syndromes. The probable reason for this difficulty is that seizures are the most obvious, the only indispensable and in many respects the characteristic symptoms of the epilepsies.

If a confusion of seizure and epilepsy terminology is thus explicable, it is not excusable for obvious reasons. Many epileptic illnesses are characterized by more than one seizure type; seizures of one type (such as generalized tonic-clonic) may be symptoms of various kinds of epilepsy; an occasional seizure (such as a febrile convulsion) is an epileptic seizure but generally not considered as sufficient for a diagnosis of epilepsy. Clarity of terminology is, therefore, indispensable.

Definitions

Epileptic seizure

The term needs no explanation. Often, epileptic seizures are referred to as just 'seizures'. This must be avoided as there are other kinds of seizures such as tetanic or hysterical.

Epileptic event

A seizure is an epileptic event, but the term epileptic event covers more. On the one hand, it may include subclinical epileptic discharge found with neurophysiological examinations, and on the other, such as in status epilepticus, several seizures in a limited time and a relationship close enough to justify their being looked upon as one event. Finally, the various signs and symptoms composing one seizure are sometimes spoken of as 'seizure events'.

Epileptic syndrome

This is an epileptic disorder that is characterized by a cluster of signs and symptoms customarily occurring together but not necessarily having a common aetiology and prognosis. The signs and symptoms may be clinical (case history, seizure types, modes of recurrence, neurological and psychological findings) or findings detected by ancillary studies (X-ray, EEG, CT scan, etc.).

Epilepsies

There is no uniform use of the term. Some use it synonymously with epileptic syndromes, but others feel it should be reserved for epileptic diseases alone. This, however, would restrict the term to very few and rare cases. At our present state of knowledge we seem to be aware of a substantial number of epileptic syndromes, and guess that some of them might turn out to be diseases in the strict sense when more becomes known about their aetiology and pathogenesis. It seems reasonable, therefore, to apply the term to all chronic disorders characterized by recurring epileptic seizures regardless of whether they are to be considered as syndromes or diseases. Thus it covers more than 'epileptic syndromes' but also less; for instance, febrile convulsions are certainly an epileptic syndrome but *not* an epilepsy.

HISTORY OF CLASSIFICATION IN THE FIELD OF EPILEPSY

Attempts at classification are as old as the literature on epilepsy, indicating that medical men have very early become aware that there is no one and single disease epilepsy. Hippocrates ridicules contemporary belief that attributes the various forms of the disease – identified by details of their symptomatology – to the action of different gods. He himself distinguished chronic epilepsies from occasional seizures, and was aware of age-dependent differences of the latter.

Hellenistic physicians, then, differentiated between seizures of cerebral and extracerebral origin. The latter was assumed to be in that part of the body where the initial seizure symptoms were localized: the stomach in the case of epigastric auras, the limbs in focal motor seizures.

As in many other fields of medicine, the hellenistic ideas remained the prevailing doctrine throughout the middle ages and even longer. Thus, the triple differentiation of epilepsy used by Esquirol in the early 19th century was still very close to the ancient concepts: idiopathic if the origin (whether identified or not) was in the brain; sympathetic if the brain was drawn into a seizure by irritation from other parts of the body (what was later called reflex epilepsy); symptomatic if the seizures were symptoms of an extracerebral disorder such as an exanthematous disease, or retarded dentition.

This classification dealt with grand mal seizures only, but Esquirol and his contemporaries were also aware of other seizures. Such an awareness can be traced throughout the medieval literature (Temkin, 1971), and in 1770, Tissot seems to have been the first to clearly differentiate between major and minor seizures (*grands et petits accès*). His description of the latter includes one of absence seizures as well as many individual forms whose variability seemed infinite to him (Tissot, 1770). The term 'petit mal' was first mentioned by Esquirol (1815) as a term that was in use in common hospital language. It is not quite clear if he himself used it for all minor seizures, and whether he considered his own term '*vertige épileptique*' (epileptic vertigo) as a synonym for petit mal or as something different. His disciple Calmeil (1824) distinguished grand mal, absence and petit mal (for minor seizures other than absences). Prichard (1822) wrote on 'local convulsion, or partial epilepsy'.

Ushered in by Tissot's description of absence, the 19th century became the age of the discovery of the various seizure types: the seizure type that later was baptized Jacksonian, by Bravais (1827); salaam seizures by West (1841); uncinate fits by Jackson (1899); and the jerks of juvenile myoclonic epilepsy by Herpin (1867). Some authors seem to have considered all seizure types that were not grand mal as one category of incomplete (Herpin) or partial seizures whereas others considered several seizure types separately*.

It was at a rather late stage only that the idea presented itself to treat seizures as one subject and epilepsy as another. The main reason seems to have been the discovery that unilateral convulsions, especially of the Jacksonian type, were often a sign of gross organic brain disease and belonged, thus, to a different category of disorders than epilepsy proper (idiopathic, essential, genuine, cryptogenic epilepsy). The distinction between idiopathic and symptomatic epilepsy (the latter, also called epileptiform seizures, closely linked to the concept of the epileptic focus or 'discharging lesion' of Jackson) became for a long period one of the fundamentals of classification of epilepsy. There were, however, always other viewpoints. The syndromatic aspect that was to become especially important seems to have supervened from two channels:

(1) Speculations on the hereditary causes of idiopathic epilepsy where conditions such as consumption (Gowers) and alcoholism were often considered as indicators of a genetic disposition.
(2) The discussion of whether all absences are epileptic or if there exists a separate disease 'pyknolepsy' with frequent absences but which is more closely related to narcolepsy than to epilepsy (Friedmann, 1906–15, quoted by Janz, 1969).

Recent developments

More recently, the EEG became an important instrument of classification as it could discover epileptic foci of various localizations as well as generalized discharge of various appearance.

Towards the middle of this century, the multiplicity of taxonomic aspects increased so much that Merlis (1972) counted some 150 current and frequently overlapping syndromatic terms. Eleven systems of classification would have been necessary to cover them all (*Table 6.1*).

It is no surprise that as a consequence of this development classification and nomenclature became a topic of discussion among epileptologists as it was felt that the confusion of terminology was on the brink of becoming babylonian. The reader with an interest in details of this discussion is referred to the writings of McNaughton (1952), Masland (1959–60, 1974), Symonds (1955), Gastaut (1969), Merlis (1970, 1972) and Wolf (1979), and to the publications of the Commission on

* Those references not included at the end of this chapter are quoted after Janz (1969), Masland (1974) and Temkin (1971).

Table 6.1 Possible criteria of classification of epileptic syndromes (after Merlis, 1972)

Seizure type and EEG
Aetiology
Anatomy and physiology
Precipitating factors
Manifestation age
Severity of seizures (major versus minor)
Severity of the disease and its chronicity
Localization of seizures
Relation to the sleep–wake cycle
Relation to the menstrual cycle
Special syndromes

Classification and Terminology of the International League Against Epilepsy – ILAE (1964, 1969).

This discussion was often fervent and sometimes bitter, as many terms convey theories, and acceptance of such terms by any official scientific body could be considered a benediction, upholding certain theories to the disadvantage of others.

A classification of epileptic seizures was recognized by the ILAE in 1969, revised in 1981, and is still being disputed. A dictionary of epilepsy (Gastaut, 1973) was published under the auspices of the World Health Organization. It has not become the important source of reference that it was intended to be, perhaps because it reflects too exclusively the opinions of one particular school, condemning the divergent terms used in other schools as 'obsolete' or 'incorrect'. A classification of epilepsies was proposed to the ILAE in 1970, but was never accepted. The Commission on Classification and Terminology of the ILAE is working on this classification, which aims to be a comprehensive one acceptable to a broad scientific public.

THE INTERNATIONAL CLASSIFICATION OF EPILEPTIC SEIZURES (ICES)

The now valid ICES was accepted by the General Assembly of the International League against Epilepsy, in Kyoto, on 19 September 1981; it had been published shortly before this meeting (Commission on Classification and Terminology of the ILAE, 1981; *see* Appendix. It is the result of a novel approach. Two ILAE Commissions on Classification and Terminology had for subsequent four-year periods worked on it, basing themselves entirely on the evaluation of video-recorded seizures which were presented and discussed at several workshops of the Commissions. The resulting suggestions were discussed with the national branches of the ILAE; the classification in its accepted form is the result of this process and bears its marks in the form of some compromises. Not everybody approved of everything in it, and it seems possible that further revisions will follow. This would be in line with the feeling of the commission responsible for the 1981 classification, whose preface reads:

> The classification is not sacrosanct. The terminology represents that which can be seen and agreed upon by representative observers. With increasing

knowledge, the categories may change, the skeleton will be 'fleshed out' and the nuances elaborated. It is hoped that the classification in itself will aid in mobilizing those concepts which will lead to its modification in time.

Fundamental aspects

The 1981 classification differs from the previous one in some details of minor importance but also in some fundamental aspects. These are discussed below.

Restriction to individual seizures

The 1969 classification of seizures had included several syndromatic aspects: clinical seizure type, ictal and interictal EEG, anatomical substrate, aetiology and age. Reasons were not given but one can assume that the authors of that classification wished to classify seizures which were 'typical' for individual patients. This requires some abstraction from the variations that may occur from one seizure to the next in one patient, and resembles how a doctor tries to make a differential seizure diagnosis from the descriptions he gets from the patient and from eye witnesses of his seizures.

The 1969 classification even included one syndromatic entity that comprises a group of seizures of quite different appearance: that is, 'infantile spasms'.

Video recording of seizures provides the doctor with a means of evaluating their signs with a hitherto unknown exactitude; repetitive inspection by several experts is also possible. Obviously, full use of this new technique allowed the Commission to reach a high standard of exactitude. Such an approach inevitably resulted in an attempt to classify the *individual* seizures as exactly as possible, notwithstanding their variability in a given patient. The 1981 ICES allows each seizure to be classified very exactly; on the other hand, the individual signs and symptoms are sufficiently grouped to allow the variable but fundamentally similar seizures of one patient to be assigned to one major category.

The variability of the seizures of a single patient, hitherto regarded as 'noise' that blurred the essential seizure typology of this patient, can, based on this system, become the object of study and research; an example is Stefan's investigation of absence seizures (1982).

As a consequence, syndromatic entities were removed from the 1981 seizure classification, as well as most additional findings that would contribute to syndromatic aspects. The logic was not entirely complete, however, as EEG findings are included in the 1981 ICES. With regard to ictal findings, this can be defended, although some hold that a purely clinical classification would be better; the inclusion of interictal EEG findings, however, is in clear disagreement with the principle of classification of individual seizures and apparently reflects one of the compromises mentioned above.

The great importance that video evaluations have had for this classification may have resulted in an over-emphasis on the observable signs at the expense of the subjective symptoms that form part of seizure symptomatology. It is mainly in the practical use of video-monitoring for classifying purposes that this should be borne in mind.

Seizures as sequential events

Traditional terms like 'grand mal', 'psychomotor seizure', and 'aura' are retrospective terms: they look at the seizure after its termination and form a comprehensive statement of all that has happened. This approach has been completely abandoned by the 1981 ICES which looks at every seizure as a sequence of events that develop in time, and where, at the onset, it is not known how these events will progress.

Again, the evaluation of video-recorded seizures by the Commission seems to have had an influence on this because video evaluations are in fact done in this way. It must be noted, however, that the 1969 ICES already had a tendency to look at seizures in this evolutive way, and the idea is fundamentally Jacksonian to study the sequential development of a seizure, as this may teach us much about the source of the epileptic discharge and its propagation through the central nervous system.

Thus, the 1969 ICES had already abandoned the term 'aura', treating auras as the first (and potentially independent) part of a composite seizure. The sequential analysis approach is fully applied in that part of the 1981 ICES that deals with focal or partial seizures, but only in rudimentary form in the section of generalized seizures. This reflects very well the present state of our knowledge but it is noteworthy that the method of video analysis seems to be on the brink of expanding this approach into the realm of generalized seizures. Thus, the above-mentioned study of Stefan (1982) on absences indicates that regular forms of a march of ictal events can also be discovered there.

There is one point where this approach has not been given full credit: the heading of the first part of the ICES (1981) where the terms partial, focal and local are given as synonyms, with 'partial' as the preferred term. These terms, of course, can be considered, to a certain extent, as synonyms because at present they are used for the same seizure types. It must not be forgotten, however, that their meanings are indeed different: focal seizure is a seizure that has a (recognizable) focal onset from which it can develop in different possible ways; the term local seizure is being very little used but would apply to those focal seizures that remain confined to a restricted area; a partial seizure is a seizure that involves not the whole brain (originally: the whole body) but only parts of it; more precisely, only parts that are not bilateral and symmetric.

It is true that the preface of this part of the ICES as well as the dictionary of epilepsy explain 'partial' in a way that makes it a true synonym of 'focal'. It is, however, difficult to see the necessity of substituting for 'focal' a synonym that has precisely the same meaning, to understand why such a synonym should be created by redefinition of a time-honoured term, and to expect that a broad public will follow such a suggestion. In teaching it is always a hard task to explain why a fully developed complex focal seizure with loss of consciousness and a long period of confusion and automatisms should be considered as a 'partial' seizure although involving the whole person in such a profound and distressing way. It is no problem to explain that it is a seizure with focal onset, and thus a focal seizure. Of the three terms, 'focal' is obviously the one of which the meaning is closest to the approach of sequential seizure analysis of the new ICES, and should therefore have been chosen as the preferred term. It will, indeed, be used as such by the present author throughout this chapter.

Classes of focal seizures and their definitions

Principal classes

The 1969 ICES had three classes of focal seizures: elementary, complex, and those with secondary generalization. Whereas it was clear enough that the last category was the same as what was previously called grand mal of focal onset, the distinction of the first two categories was much less precise. Complex, so a footnote said, 'implies an organized, high-level cerebral activity'. 'Elementary' focal seizures seemed to be those with crude sensations or with undifferentiated convulsive movements.

In practice, however, it was less easy than expected to know whether a seizure implied organized, high-level cerebral activity. Further, one subclass of focal seizures of the 1969 ICES, the 'compound forms', created a still greater problem as it implied 'a joining together of elementary or (and/or) complex symptoms'. Video evaluations proved that the majority of focal seizures had to be placed here which depreciated the distinction of elementary and complex.

An attempt was made, therefore, to determine a group of symptoms common to all seizures that were accepted as complex focal but the only such symptom was impairment of consciousness.

The subsequent suggestion by the Commission – that in due course has been accepted – to define as 'complex' focal seizures those where consciousness was impaired, and 'simple' those where this did not happen, was met by vehement criticism and gave rise to much discussion. The criticisms belonged mainly to two groups: one held that 'complex' should not be redefined but kept in its old meaning; this advice was difficult to follow because of the lack of a sufficiently precise definition of 'complex'. The other was ready to accept a dichotomy of seizures into those with impaired and those with preserved consciousness, but did not find 'simple' and 'complex' very appropriate labels for this dichotomy. Some therefore suggested dropping these terms. This suggestion did not have sufficient support by the 1981 vote but has been brought up again as a motion by a group of epileptologists. Whatever the result of the motion may be, whoever makes a distinction between seizures with either retained or with impaired consciousness but prefers not to use the terms 'simple' and 'complex' will still find himself in agreement with the essence of the 1981 ICES.

A more fundamental criticism questioned the feasibility of this consciousness dichotomy, finding it a difficult and, perhaps, often impossible task to tell whether or not consciousness had been impaired. Similarly, it has been pointed out that, philosophically, consciousness is still an open and controversial issue. It is difficult to find a generally acceptable definition of consciousness; did it not enhance rather than diminish taxonomic ambiguities to make consciousness a watershed of classification?

Theoretical refinement, however, was not the major aim of the Commission, and it is, of course, true that any doctor who takes a seizure history will raise the important point of the question of whether consciousness is retained throughout the seizure or not, not least to get an idea of the degree of disability the seizure disorder inflicts on the patient. For this, everyone seems content with an operational definition of consciousness that implies the patient's responsiveness and awareness. This has also been used in the ICES where it is explained that:

operationally, in the context of this classification, consciousness refers to the degree of awareness and/or responsiveness of the patient to externally applied stimuli. Responsiveness refers to the ability of the patient to carry out simple commands or willed movement and awareness refers to a patient's contact with events during the period in question and its recall. A person aware and unresponsive will be able to recount the events that occurred during an attack and his inability to respond by movement or speech. In this context, unresponsiveness is other than the result of paralysis, aphasia or apraxia.

Subclasses

The 1981 ICES recognizes 18 subclasses of simple focal seizures belonging to four groups, four modalities of complex focal seizures, and three types of secondarily generalized seizures (*see* Appendix. It gives many examples of the kind of seizure signs and symptoms that may be encountered. The ICES as it was published comprises a section called 'Definition of Terms' in which further details are given.

SIMPLE FOCAL SEIZURES

The definitions given for groups A.1–3 are short and point mainly to the localizing significance of the first seizure symptom. For group A.4 (simple focal seizures with psychic symptoms) they are more elaborate although still exemplary rather than comprehensive. They will be abstracted here together with a few additional comments.

Dysphasic seizures

These must be carefully distinguished from phonatory seizures with speech arrest (A.1e), because only dysphasic seizures point to a focus in the speech-dominant hemisphere. The most helpful items of distinction are the impairment of not only production but also reception of speech, and the use of dysphasic language (semantic paraphasias, jargon aphasia).

Dysmnesic seizures

These comprise déjà and jamais vécu (vu, entendu) experiences, paramnesias (false recollections) and rare phenomena such as rapid recollections of episodes of one's past life, sometimes in the form of 'panoramic vision' or as one variety of forced thinking.

Cognitive seizures

Most instances of forced thinking belong here, together with other compulsive symptoms, distortions of the time sense and dreamy states. The latter often include dysmnesic experiences.

Affective seizures

Most often, ictal emotions are unpleasant (fear, terror, depression, anger), but sometimes feelings of well being are experienced whereas ictal ecstasy seems extremely rare. Experiences of sexual excitation are also rare, and not necessarily pleasant. It is pointed out that ictal anger or rage unlike temper tantrums appears unprovoked, and abates rapidly. It is often accompanied by the appropriate automatic signs, and may lead to running away. More often, however, running is an automatism or, occasionally, a compulsive symptom (Wolf, 1984). Ictal laughter is most often not accompanied by mirth, and not remembered by the patients, and thus usually an automatism.

Ictal illusions

These may concern the external world in the sense of deformed visual or, less commonly, auditory perception, but also in the form of derealization. They may also concern the patient's person, including disturbances of the body image or experiences of depersonalization.

Illusions may also be understood as cognitive disturbances, and in the ICES definition of terms depersonalization appears under both these headings, but its classification as illusions is probably more specific.

Structured ictal hallucinations

These must be differentiated from simple hallucinations or crude sensations that belong to the special sensory symptoms (A.3). To distinguish them from illusions is sometimes difficult, and they are often combined with dysmnesic experiences.

COMPLEX FOCAL SEIZURES

The subclasses (*see* Appendix) are self-explanatory. The differentiation of B.1a and B.1b is often not immediately understood. B.1b should perhaps better read 'like B.1a but additionally comprising automatisms'. The 'definition of terms' is very specific about automatisms, pointing out that these may occur both in complex focal seizures and in some kinds of generalized seizures. It conveys the Jacksonian concept that ictal automatisms usually represent the release of behaviour belonging to a lower level of central nervous system organization under the influence of the ictal clouding of consciousness, or dissolution of the highest coordinating centres.

Oral automatisms of complex focal seizures as well as other primitive automatisms, including well-coordinated patterns such as laughing, running or verbigeration (speech automatisms) most often belong to the nuclear ictal symptomatology unlike more elaborate and complex automatisms that are commonly seen in the postictal twilight stage. In absence seizures, oral automatisms mark the second step in the march of ictal events and begin, as an average, 5–6 seconds after absence onset (Stefan, 1982), whereas non-oral automatisms occur later.

It is pointed out that most automatisms do not lend themselves to simple anatomic interpretation although they seem to have in common a discharge involving various areas of the limbic system.

Classes of generalized seizures and their definition

There is less systematization in the classification of generalized than that of focal seizures. A differentiation between convulsive and non-convulsive seizures is found in the introduction but not in the classification proper. Instead, the seizures are arranged in six parallel classes: absences; myoclonic seizures; clonic seizures; tonic seizures; tonic-clonic seizures; atonic seizures.

Absences

The ICES differentiates between absence seizures and atypical absences. The section on absence seizures is the most elaborate part of the classification of generalized seizures. It is explained that:

> the hallmark of the absence attack is sudden onset, interruption of ongoing activities, a blank stare, possibly a brief upward rotation of the eyes. If the patient is speaking, speech is slowed or interrupted; if walking, he stands transfixed; if eating, the food will stop on his way to the mouth. Usually the patient will be unresponsive when spoken to. In some, attacks are aborted when the patient is spoken to. The attack lasts from a few seconds to half a minute and evaporates as rapidly as it commenced.

Six kinds of absence seizures are recognized.

WITH IMPAIRMENT OF CONSCIOUSNESS ONLY

This applies to an absence of the above description without any other activities during the attack.

WITH MILD CLONIC COMPONENTS

'Here the onset of the attack is indistinguishable from the above, but clonic movements may occur in the eyelids, at the corner of the mouth, or in other muscle groups which may vary in severity from almost imperceptible movements to generalized myoclonic jerks. Objects held in the hand may be dropped.' This term covers more than seems to be indicated by the terminology 'mild' which probably has been chosen because such movements usually are mild. But there is no separate class of more intensive cloni, and no distinction is made between myoclonic and clonic phenomena.

WITH ATONIC COMPONENTS

'Here there may be a diminution in tone of muscles subserving posture as well as in the limbs leading to drooping of the head, occasionally slumping of the trunk, dropping of the arms, and relaxing of the grip. Rarely, tone is sufficiently diminished to cause this person to fall.'

WITH TONIC COMPONENTS

'Here during the attack tonic muscle contraction may occur, leading to increase in muscle tone which may affect the extensor muscles or the flexor muscles symmetrically or asymmetrically. If the patient is standing the head may be drawn backward and the trunk may arch. This may lead to retropulsion. The head may tonically draw to one or another side.' The comment tries to connect this classification to the different approach of classifying generalized minor seizures according to their motor pattern (Janz, 1969).

WITH AUTOMATISMS

> Purposeful or quasipurposeful movements occurring in the absence of awareness during an absence attack are frequent and may range from lip licking and swallowing to clothes fumbling or aimless walking. If spoken to the patient may grunt or turn to the spoken voice and when touched or tickled may rub the site.

> Automatisms are quite elaborate and may consist of combinations of the above-described movements or may be so simple as to be missed by casual observation.

Automatisms of complex focal seizuresare compared elsewhere in this volume. Not everybody would agree that automatisms in absences are usually elaborate.

WITH AUTONOMIC COMPONENTS

No explanations are given in the ICES but autonomic signs such as changes of respiration and heart rate may be observed in absences or, more rarely, pallor and flushes or enuresis.

The classification notes that all the above, with the exception of impairment of consciousness only, may also be used in combination, and in the 'definition of terms' it is stated that 'mixed forms of absence frequently occur'.

The situation is somewhat similar to the 'compound forms' of focal seizures in the 1969 ICES that became one of the principal reasons for the early revision of that classification (see above). Now the ICES recognizes several possible modes of composition of complex focal seizures that represent the subclasses of this group. For absences, a similar stage has not been reached. Stefan (1982) in his exhaustive analysis of 528 video-recorded absences of 59 patients proposes to differentiate between absences:

with impairment of consciousness only;
with oculomotor manifestations; and
without oculomotor manifestations but with oral or other automatisms, tonic symptoms or sporadic myoclonia.

Not all of his cases, however, belonged to these three categories, and this is presumably only the first step in a new approach to systematize absences, and remains still to be verified and discussed.

Atypical absences

'Atypical absence' is the least well-defined and perhaps most dubious of all the terms in the 1981 ICES; it is definitely a result of compromise. This is not a clinical group at all, but only defined by the EEG (*see* Appendix). It is explained that patients who have a 'more heterogeneous' EEG than described in absence seizures (allowing for spike-wave frequencies between 2/s and 4/s) may have changes in tone that are more pronounced than in absence seizures; the onset or cessation of the seizure may not be abrupt. This is one of the points demonstrating that the inclusion of even the ictal EEG in the ICES introduces a syndromatic feature, and should, perhaps, better have been avoided.

Should the 1981 ICES be followed to the letter a patient with absences of any of the types described above who has, for example, asymmetrical spike-waves or abnormal background activity, would have to be classed as having 'atypical absences'. There are people, however, who do not agree with this, and the author finds himself short of arguments against them.

The very idea of 'typical' and 'atypical' seizures is in discord with the purely descriptive principle of the 1981 ICES as it compares the individual seizure with an abstraction that is supposed to be the ideal of one particular seizure type.

Myoclonic seizures

Of these, only one form is recognized: 'Myoclonic jerks (single or multiple)'. The 'definition of terms' explains that indeed all varieties of myoclonus are supposed to be included in this category. It only draws attention to the existence of non-epileptic forms of myoclonus that do not belong in this category. The EEG, too, recognizes several possibilities (*see* Appendix, p. 378).

The ICES does not say expressly that for a seizure to be included here consciousness should be retained, but the above definition of absence with mild clonic components makes it clear that myoclonic seizures with impaired consciousness are supposed to be classed as absences.

Clonic seizures

The ICES does not attempt to define the difference between clonic and myoclonic. At an earlier stage of discussion a definition of clonic was suggested as multiple jerks of rhythmic or quasi-rhythmic repetition, and as myoclonic, single jerks and those with arrhythmic repetition. It appears that such a major definition was no longer considered necessary because the only type of clonic seizure recognized in the ICES is described as a variant of 'generalized convulsive seizures' (that is, what was before, and in clinical language still is, called grand mal; the feasibility of deleting this term appears somewhat doubtful as it does not seem to be covered entirely by 'generalized tonic-clonic seizure'). The comment seems to indicate that consciousness is lost in clonic seizures, and anyone seeking very precise definitions may perhaps miss a phrase about the differentiation from absence with mild clonic components. Distinction would mainly have to be based on the duration of both seizures, the extent of disturbance of consciousness, the preservation or loss of postural tone, and the immediate or delayed recovery from the seizure.

The clonic seizure as it is described here is certainly an extremely rare type of epileptic seizure. It is not quite clear on what observations are based the very specific statements on ictal and interictal EEG (*see* Appendix).

Tonic seizures

Two varieties of tonic seizures are mentioned in the 'definition of terms'. The first seems, again, to represent a variety of grand mal or generalized convulsive seizures, and is described by a quotation from Gowers defining a tonic seizure as:

> a rigid, violent muscular contraction, fixing the limbs in some strained position. There is usually deviation of the eyes and of the head towards one side, and this may amount to rotation involving the whole body, sometimes actually causing the patient to turn around, even two or three times. The features are distorted; the color of the face, unchanged at first, rapidly becomes pale and then flushed and ultimately livid as the fixation of the chest by the spasms stops the movements of respiration. The eyes are open or closed; the conjunctiva is insensitive; the pupils dilate widely as cyanosis comes on. As the spasm continues, it commonly changes in its relative intensity in different parts, causing slight alterations in the position of the limbs.

It must be pointed out that the classification of such a seizure depends entirely on the question whether the patient is or is not aware of the initial deviation of eyes and head to one side. If he is, the seizure must be classed as focal.

The second variety is that of 'tonic-axial seizures with extension of head, neck and trunk' that have been described in detail by Gastaut *et al.* (1963). According to this paper as well as to the present author's experiences, however, these seizures often comprise a short phase of bilateral symmetric cloni. Thus, in a descriptive rather than abstracting classification like the 1981 ICES, many of them would have to be classed as generalized tonic-clonic.

Tonic-clonic seizures

This term is meant to replace grand mal but only those grand mal seizures that do not have a focal onset. It is supposed to be self-explanatory, and is not further described in the 'definition of terms'. However, as has been pointed out above, in a rigidly descriptive classification there are seizures that would not be considered as grand mal because of their brevity, abrupt cessation and the fact that consciousness is not necessarily lost, but are indeed composed of a sequence of tonic and clonic generalized or at least bilateral convulsions.

Atonic (astatic) seizures

The following definition is given:

> A sudden diminution in muscle tone occurs which may be fragmentary, leading to a head drop with slackening of the jaw, the dropping of a limb or a loss of all muscle tone leading to a slumping to the ground. When these attacks are extremely brief they are known as 'drop attacks'. If consciousness is lost, this loss is extremely brief. The sudden loss of postural tone in the head and trunk may lead to injury by projecting objects. The face is particularly subject to injury. In the case of more prolonged atonic attacks, the slumping may be progressive in a rhythmic, successive relaxation manner. (So-called drop attacks may be seen in conditions other than epilepsy, such as brainstem ischemia and narcolepsy cataplexy syndrome.)

Unclassified seizures

The category includes seizures that cannot be classified because of inadequate or incomplete data, as well as seizures that defy classification in the ICES categories. Here, again, is a field for further research with the help of seizure monitoring.

TOWARDS A SYNDROME CLASSIFICATION

The development of a classification of epileptic seizures – difficult, controversial and time-consuming as it was – is not more than the fundament on which a classification of the epilepsies or epileptic syndromes remains to be constructed.

A first attempt at this was the 'Proposal for an International Classification of Epilepsies (ICE)', published in 1970 (*Table 6.2*). It has never been accepted by any international body nor has there been much discussion about it. Some of its terms became widely used, but not always in the meaning that they were attributed. The

Table 6.2 Proposal for an international classification of the epilepsies (abstracted from Merlis, 1970)

I Generalized epilepsies
  (1) Primary generalized epilepsies (defined by seizure types, normal neurological status, onset in childhood and adolescence, lack of any clear aetiology and various types of bilateral synchronous epileptic discharge in the EEG)
  (2) Secondary generalized epilepsies (defined by seizure types, usually in the presence of abnormal neurological or psychological findings, with onset most frequent in childhood, usually with diffuse or mutlifocal brain lesions, and with slow EEG background activity and epileptic discharges different from I. (1)
  (3) Undetermined generalized epilepsies

II Partial (focal, local) epilepsies (defined by focal seizures, possible neurological deficit – sometimes postictal – onset at any age, usually associated with brain damage and focal EEG signs)

III Unclassifiable epilepsy (either because not belonging to the above types or because of insufficient data)

most widespread misuse is that of 'primary generalized epilepsy' and 'secondary generalized epilepsy'. The former is generally used for all epilepsies with non-focal seizures, whereas the latter is mostly misunderstood to mean epilepsy with grand mal of focal onset. The definitions that Gastaut (1973) has given unfortunately give various parallel explanations for the terms primary and secondary:

> The term 'primary generalized epilepsy' (from primus, first) is certainly imperfect but has the advantage (a) of stressing the historical background of this type of epilepsy, which was the first to be recognized as a distinct morbid entity in the form of 'grand mal' (comitial disease, sacred disease, falling sickness, etc.), since the original meaning of primary is 'first' or 'oldest'; (b) of indicating the lack of any clear aetiology in this form of epilepsy, and perhaps even of suggesting the centrencephalic transmission mechanism of its seizures, since another meaning of primary is 'first to occur'.
>
> The proposed term 'secondary' generalized epilepsy (from secundarius, second in order), although imperfect, has the advantage of indicating the relatively recent nosological identification of these forms of epilepsy, the fact that their aetiology is secondary to chronic encephalopathy, and the fact that they are characterized by a secondary bisynchronous discharge mechanism.*

This explanation may have enhanced the existing confusion.

* The idea that the classical authors understood, by 'grand mal', only generalized tonic-clonic seizures of 'primary generalized epilepsy' would be difficult to defend, and the historical explanations of the terms seem confusing rather than helpful. The views expressed on mechanisms of discharge and transmission appear still too hypothetical to be used in matters of terminology and classification.

It seems clear enough, though, that 'primary' in the proposal means that the epilepsy is the primary disturbance, and 'secondary' that it is the consequence of some underlying disorder. For the sake of clarity, these terms will presumably be dropped in favour of idiopathic (or cryptogenic) and symptomatic. Whereas these two classes seem clear enough, the 'undetermined generalized epilepsies' are a most problematic group as was discussed by Masland (1974) and Wolf (1979). This will not be further discussed as the term seems never to have been in use.

As in the ICES, the ICE proposal juxtaposes 'generalized' and 'partial (focal, local) epilepsies'. No attempt was made to subdivide the focal epilepsies nor was much comment made of the possibility of such a subdivision in the proposal. Some authors have tried to transfer the subdivision of the seizure classification (simple or elementary versus complex) to the syndrome classification but this appears impossible as too many patients have both simple and complex focal seizures.

The term 'partial' which is, in the ICES, one of three acknowledged synonyms, is not applicable for the ICE because it would exclude from classification the many patients whose only seizure type is simple focal evolving to generalized tonic-clonic (or grand mal of focal onset to use the term with which many readers will be more familiar); it would be nonsensical to maintain that such a patient, who perhaps experiences only a short and almost imperceptible aura before his tonic-clonic seizures, suffers from partial (or local) epilepsy. But neither can the term 'focal', that would be appropriate for these cases, be used without reservation because in a case classed as focal *epilepsy* one would expect a well-defined constant epileptic focus. This, however, is not true for the many children suffering from benign epilepsies with focal *seizures* with shifting site and even side of onset. Perhaps the most appropriate term would be 'localization-related epilepsies'.

A small but by no means negligible group of patients belong neither clearly to the generalized nor to the localization-related epilepsies because they present characteristics of both groups (for example, absences with bilateral spike-wave discharge but also with focal seizures and a spike focus in the EEG, or both a family predisposition of generalized epilepsy and a history of brain damage). They have no appropriate place in the ICE proposal.

These and other matters are currently being dealt with by the Commission on Classification and Terminology, so their detailed discussion here would be premature. The reader who is especially interested in the discussion on syndrome classification is referred to the papers of Gastaut (1969), Masland (1959–60, 1969, 1974), McNaughton (1952), Merlis (1970, 1972), Symonds (1955) and Wolf (1979).

References

COMMISSION ON CLASSIFICATION AND TERMINOLOGY OF THE ILAE (1964) A proposed international classification of epileptic seizures. *Epilepsia,* **5,** 297–306

COMMISSION ON CLASSIFICATION AND TERMINOLOGY OF THE ILAE (1981) Proposal for revised clinical and electroencephalographic classification of epileptic seizures. *Epilepsia,* **22,** 489–501

GASTAUT, H. (1969) Classification of the epilepsies. Proposal for an international classification. *Epilepsia,* **10,** S14–S21

GASTAUT, H. (1969 and 1970) Clinical and electroencephalographical classification of epileptic seizures. *Epilepsia,* **10,** S2–S13, and **11,** 102–113

GASTAUT, H. (1973) *Dictionary of Epilepsy.* Geneva: WHO

GASTAUT, H., ROGER, J., OUAHCHI, S., TIMSIT, M. and BROUGHTON, R. (1963) An electro-clinical study of generalized epileptic seizures of tonic expression. *Epilepsia,* **4,** 15–44

HIPPOCRATES *On the Sacred Disease* (Many editions, quoted here after the German translation by W. Capelle (1955) Zürich: Artemis)

JACKSON, J. H. and STEWART, P. (1899) Epileptic attacks with a warning of a crude sensation of smell and with the intellectual aura (dreamy state) in a patient who had symptoms pointing to gross organic disease of the right temporo-sphenoidal lobe. *Brain*, **22**, 534–549

JANZ, D. (1969) *Die Epilepsien.* Stuttgart: Thieme

MASLAND, R. L. (1959–60) Classification of the epilepsies. *Epilepsia,* **1,** 512–520

MASLAND, R. L. (1969) Comments on the classification of epilepsy. *Epilepsia,* **10,** S22–S28

MASLAND, R. L. (1974) The classification of the epilepsies. A historical review. In *Handbook of Clinical Neurology,* edited by P. J. Vinken and G. W. Bruyn, Vol. XV, pp. 1–29. Amsterdam: North Holland

McNAUGHTON, F. L. (1952) The classification of the epilepsies. *Epilepsia 3rd series,* **1,** 7–16

MERLIS, J. K. (1970) Proposal for an international classification of the epilepsies. *Epilepsia,* **11,** 114–119

MERLIS, J. K. (1972) Treatment in relation to classification of the epilepsies. *Acta Neurologica Latin America,* **18,** 42–51

STEFAN, H. (1982) *Epileptische Absencen.* Stuttgart, New York: Thieme

SYMONDS, C. (1955) Classification of the epilepsies. *British Medical Journal*, 1235–1238

TEMKIN, O. (1971) *The Falling Sickness*, 2nd edn., pp. 323, 250. Baltimore and London: Johns Hopkins Press

TISSOT, S. A. (1770) *Traité de l'Épilepsie*. Lausanne: Chapuis, and Paris: Didot. Reprinted (1984) Lausanne: Fondation Eben-Hezer

WOLF, P. (1979) Nomenklatur und Klassifikation epileptischer Anfälle und Syndrome. *Nervenarzt,* **50,** 547–554

WOLF, P. (1984) Lokomotorischer Zwang im epileptischen Anfall (ictal compulsive locomotion). *Nervenarzt,* **55,** 197–201

APPENDIX: THE INTERNATIONAL CLASSIFICATION OF EPILEPTIC SEIZURES (ICES) (1981 revision)

The ICES (Commission on Classification and Terminology of the ILAE, 1981) has in its first part 'partial' as the preferred term. Substitution of 'focal' is possible throughout, and in the first sentence of the introduction avoids the somewhat clumsy explanation that, in partial seizures, the first signs 'indicate initial activation of a system of neurons limited to part of one cerebral hemisphere'. The meaning is the same as 'focal' but differs from the traditional signification of 'partial'. At an intermediate stage of the redefinition of 'partial' (Gastaut, 1969) this read: 'The neuronal discharge results from a lesion more or less localized to part of a hemisphere and nearly always involves directly or indirectly only one part of the cerebral cortex'. The anatomical statement (certainly a correct one) which is part of the definition is an example for the inclusion of syndromatic aspects of the classification of seizures which was still common at that stage of the discussion. It is now being reserved for the syndrome classification. Then, it seems doubtful if the second part of this definition can be applied to focal or partial seizures with impairment of consciousness.

I Focal (partial, local) seizures

Focal seizures are those in which, in general, the first clinical and electroencephalographic changes indicate initial activation of a limited system of neurons. A focal seizure is classified primarily on the basis of whether or not consciousness is impaired during the attack. When consciousness is not impaired, the seizure is classified as a simple focal seizure. When consciousness is impaired, the seizure is classified as a complex focal seizure. Impairment of consciousness may be the first clinical sign, or simple focal seizures may evolve into complex focal seizures. In patients with impaired consciousness, aberrations of behaviour (automatisms) may occur. A focal seizure may not terminate, but instead progress to a generalized motor seizure. Impaired consciousness is defined as the inability to respond normally to exogenous stimuli by virtue of altered awareness and/or responsiveness.

There is considerable evidence that simple focal seizures usually have unilateral hemispheric involvement and only rarely have bilateral hemispheric involvement; complex focal seizures, however, frequently have bilateral hemispheric involvement.

Focal seizures can be classified into one of the following three fundamental groups:

A. Simple focal seizures
B. Complex focal seizures
   1. With impairment of consciousness at onset
   2. Simple focal onset followed by impairment of consciousness
C. Focal seizures evolving to generalized tonic-clonic convulsions (GTC)
   1. Simple evolving to GTC
   2. Complex evolving to GTC (including those with simple focal onset)

Clinical seizure type	*EEG seizure type*	*EEG interictal expression*
A. *Simple focal seizures* (consciousness not impaired) 1. With motor signs (a) Focal motor without march (b) Focal motor with march (Jacksonian) (c) Versive (d) Postural (e) Phonatory (vocalization or arrest of speech)	Local contralateral discharge starting over the corresponding area of cortical representation (not always recorded on the scalp)	Local contralateral discharge
2. With somatosensory or special sensory symptoms (simple hallucinations, e.g., tingling, light flashes, buzzing) (a) Somatosensory (b) Visual (c) Auditory (d) Olfactory (e) Gustatory (f) Vertiginous		
3. With autonomic symptoms or signs (including epigastric sensation, pallor, sweating, flushing, pilo-erection and pupillary dilatation)		
4. With psychic symptoms (disturbance of higher cerebral function). These symptoms rarely occur without impairment of consciousness and are much more commonly experienced as complex focal seizures (a) Dysphasic (b) Dysmnesic (e.g., déjà vu) (c) Cognitive (e.g., dreamy states, distortions of time sense) (d) Affective (fear, anger, etc.) (e) Illusions (e.g., macropsia) (f) Structured hallucinations (e.g., music, scenes)		
B. *Complex focal seizures* (with impairment of consciousness; may sometimes begin with simple symptomatology)	Unilateral or, frequently, bilateral discharge, diffuse or focal in temporal or frontotemporal regions	Unilteral or bilateral generally asynchronous focus; usually in the temporal or frontal regions
1. Simple focal onset followed by impairment of consciousness (a) With simple focal features (A.1–A.4) followed by impaired consciousness (b) With automatisms		
2. With impairment of consciousness at onset (a) With impairment of consciousness only (b) With automatisms		

Clinical seizure type	*EEG seizure type*	*EEG interictal expression*
C. *Focal seizures evolving to secondarily generalized seizures*		
(These may be generalized tonic-clonic, tonic, or clonic)	Above discharges become secondarily and rapidly generalized	
1. Simple focal seizures (A) evolving to generalized seizures		
2. Complex focal seizures (B) evolving to generalized seizures		
3. Simple focal seizures evolving to complex focal seizures evolving to generalized seizures		

II Generalized seizures (convulsive or non-convulsive)

Generalized seizures are those in which the first clinical changes indicate initial involvement of both hemispheres. Consciousness may be impaired and this impairment may be the initial manifestation. Motor manifestations are bilateral. The ictal electroencephalographic patterns initially are bilateral, and presumably reflect neuronal discharge which is widespread in both hemispheres.

Clinical seizure type	*EEG seizure type*	*EEG interictal expression*
A. 1. *Absence seizures*		
(a) Impairment of consciousness only (b) With mild clonic components (c) With atonic components (d) With tonic components (e) With automatisms (f) With autonomic components (b) to (f) may be used alone or in combination)	Usually regular and symmetrical 3 Hz but may be 2–4 Hz spike-and-slow-wave complexes and may have multiple spike-and-slow-wave complexes. Abnormalities are bilateral	Background activity usually normal although paroxysmal activity (such as spikes or spike-and-slow-wave complexes) may occur. This activity is usually regular and symmetrical
2. *Atypical absence*		
May have: (a) Changes in tone that are more pronounced than in A.1 (b) Onset and/or cessation that is not abrupt	EEG more heterogeneous; may include irregular spike-and-slow-wave complexes, fast activity or other paroxysmal activity. Abnormalities are bilateral but often irregular and asymmetrical	Background usually abnormal; paroxysmal activity (such as spikes or spike-and-slow-wave complexes) frequently irregular and asymmetrical
B. *Myoclonic seizures*		
Myoclonic jerks (single or multiple)	Polyspike and wave, or sometimes spike and wave or sharp and slow waves	Same as ictal

Clinical seizure type	*EEG seizure type*	*EEG interictal expression*
C. *Clonic seizures*	Fast activity (10 c/s or more) and slow waves; occasional spike-and-wave patterns	Spike-and-wave or polyspike-and-wave discharges
D. *Tonic seizures*	Low voltage, fast activity or a fast rhythm of 9–10 c/s or more decreasing in frequency and increasing in amplitude	More or less rhythmic discharges of sharp and slow waves, sometimes asymmetrical. Background is often abnormal for age
E. *Tonic-clonic seizures*	Rhythm at 10 or more c/s decreasing in frequency and increasing in amplitude during tonic phase, interrupted by slow waves during clonic phase	Polyspike and waves or spike and wave, or, sometimes, sharp and slow wave discharges
F. *Atonic seizures* (Astatic) (combinations of the above may occur, e.g. B and F, B and D)	Polyspikes and wave or flattening or low-voltage fast activity	Polyspikes and slow wave

III Unclassified epileptic seizures

Includes all seizures that cannot be classified because of inadequate or incomplete data and some that defy classification in hitherto described categories. This includes some neonatal seizures, e.g. rhythmic eye movements, chewing, and swimming movements.

IV Addendum

Repeated epileptic seizures occur under a variety of circumstances: (1) as fortuitous attacks, coming unexpectedly and without any apparent provocation; (2) as cyclic attacks, at more or less regular intervals (e.g. in relation to the menstrual cycle, or the sleep-walking cycle); (3) as attacks provoked by: (a) non-sensory factors (fatigue, alcohol, emotion, etc.), or (b) sensory factors, sometimes referred to as 'reflex seizures'.

Prolonged or repetitive seizures (status epilepticus). The term 'status epilepticus' is used whenever a seizure persists for a sufficient length of time or is repeated frequently enough that recovery between attacks does not occur. Status epilepticus may be divided into focal (e.g. Jacksonian), or generalized (e.g. absence status or tonic-clonic status). When very localized motor status occurs, it is referred to as epilepsia partialis continua.

Reproduced by courtesy of the Editor and Publisher, *Epilepsia*

7
Intensive monitoring: epileptic and non-epileptic seizures

Roger J. Porter

Essential to the appropriate diagnosis and treatment of any disease is an appreciation of the natural history of the disorder – the dynamic changes in the patient that provide clues to whether the suspected diagnosis is correct or whether the therapy is appropriate and effective. In acute disorders, such as appendicitis, the evolution of the disorder is usually rapid, and the collection of data regarding diagnosis and therapy may be complete in a few days or less. In chronic disorders the course is much more difficult to discern, as the patient may not change from week to week or even from year to year. Epilepsy, a chronic disorder, is further complicated by its paroxysmal nature – the physician often makes the diagnosis on the basis of a few events, each lasting at most only a few minutes; the observers of these events, furthermore, are variably reliable in their ability to adequately describe the behavioral manifestations of the seizures. Efforts to improve the physician's ability to gather the needed diagnostic and therapeutic information have concentrated on qualitative and quantitative seizure information and on plasma levels of antiepileptic drugs. The combined use of these techniques, especially useful in the evaluation and treatment of epilepsy, has been termed 'intensive monitoring', and consists primarily of long-term electroencephalographic and video recordings and frequent blood level determinations of the various antiepileptic drugs. This chapter will review the techniques of intensive monitoring and the specific usefulness of these techniques in the diagnosis and therapy of epilepsy; special emphasis will be placed on the differential diagnosis of non-epileptic seizures. The importance of intensive monitoring in the proper conduct of clinical trials will also be briefly discussed.

TECHNIQUES OF INTENSIVE MONITORING

Long-term electroencephalographic (EEG) recording

Prolonged monitoring of the EEG is not new. Many clinicians and investigators have advocated a departure from the routine 20-minute recording, and good laboratories are as flexible with the amount of recording time as they are with modification of montages. Prolongation of a routine recording, however, has such limitations and disadvantages that special techniques of obtaining the long-term EEG have been developed. These disadvantages include (a) artificial environment; (b) confined observation space; (c) the patient's limited ability to move about without risking prominent artifact; (d) electrode problems; and (e) excessive accumulation of paper records. In order to collect long-term EEG data for quantitation, classification, and localization, two acceptable alternatives have been devised to alleviate these problems (Porter, 1980).

The simplest alternative is merely a modification of the 'front end' of the recording system that allows the patient to move about while attached to a 7–10 m cable. Low-voltage scalp potentials cannot be measured over these distances, however, and modification at the source is essential. Successful systems of this type are in use at the Montreal Neurological Institute (Ives, Thompson and Gloor, 1976) and at the Institute voor Epilepsiebestrijding in The Netherlands. Both of these systems utilize preamplification at the head to increase the signal strength for transmission in relatively low-impedance cables. This decreases the likelihood of interference from extraneous sources and presents a reasonable voltage to the recording system. One system (Ives, Thompson and Gloor, 1976) multiplexes the signal at the head so that only one channel of information need be carried to a decoder. The other system uses a multichannel cable with appropriate connections directly to the recording system. Multiplexing at the head and reducing the data to a single channel has the advantage of allowing a hospital unit to be wired with relatively inexpensive cable, using multiple inputs throughout the unit occupied by the patient. The unmultiplexed system, however, has the advantage of relative simplicity and the circumvention of difficulties inherent in encoding and decoding. Both systems are effective (Porter, 1980).

The alternative to direct, 'hard-wired' EEG recording is the radio-telemetered EEG. The patient is allowed much greater freedom of movement because the 'umbilical cord' is absent. Preamplification at the head is an integral part of the system, and the major problems are related to the actual transmitter–receiver characteristics. The systems have been reviewed (Porter, Wolf and Penry, 1971; Porter, Penry and Wolf, 1976), and only the critical features are outlined here. First, the preamplifiers must be sensitive enough to recognize the low-voltage scalp potentials. Second, for multichannel recording, multiplexing is virtually mandatory because it requires only one transmitter and receiver. Third, crystal control is highly desirable to avoid drift in both the transmitter and receiver. Fourth, the transmitted signal should be frequency modulated. Finally, some system of dual antenna-receivers is recommended (Porter, Wolf and Penry, 1971). All of the above features will greatly enhance the quality of the recording and decrease the likelihood of outside interference (Porter, 1980).

Scalp recordings require good technique of electrode application, with impedances below 5000 ohms (Ω) per pair. We use 10 mm silver cup electrodes with a 2 mm hole, which can be refilled with a blunt needle as required. Collodion is used to apply the electrodes, sometimes with double layers of gauze for recordings longer than six hours. Electrode wires should be trimmed short to decrease artifact from movement and extraneous electrical sources (Porter, 1980).

Aside from computer analysis, the final step is the recording of the EEG itself. Both the 'hard-wired' and the telemetered systems are capable of sending the EEG data to a tape recorder or to a standard EEG machine. The advantages of a tape recorder are simplicity of operation and compactness of data storage. Disadvantages are the need for expensive multichannel FM recorders if the signal is not already multiplexed, inability to see the EEG as it is being recorded (an oscilloscope or video reformatter may be added for this purpose), and the need for a time-code generator so that recording time can be multiplexed onto the tape; such a generator is very useful when a certain moment in time is sought for playback onto paper (Porter, 1980).

The use of intensive, long-term electroencephalographic recordings, even in the absence of the other techniques, has specific applications in diagnosis and therapy of certain epilepsies, as well as applications in clinical trials of antiepileptic drugs. These applications are reviewed later in this chapter. A special variant of long-term EEG monitoring is the wearable cassette recorder which allows 24-hour continuous recording. Although such devices are rarely coupled to video recordings, rapid review playback units allow scanning of a prolonged recording in a relatively short time. These recording and playback systems have gradually improved in miniaturization, in technical quality, and in the number of channels simultaneously recorded and displayed. Interpretation of the data may be difficult, and the services of an experienced electroencephalographer are mandatory in the proper use of the system.

Videotape recording

Intensive monitoring with video recording is a more recent advance than EEG monitoring, and it has added a significant dimension to our understanding of seizures. There are three basic elements of any video system: cameras, tape recorders, and video monitors. A number of integrated systems are available for monochromatic (black and white) recordings, and many are relatively inexpensive. Unfortunately, the less expensive systems usually have the least resolution and the least flexibility. The best systems are of modular construction, utilizing the best model and manufacturer for each piece of equipment. Cameras should be reasonably sensitive, and the following features are desirable, although not mandatory: (a) zoom lens, either hand or remote controlled; (b) remote focus; (c) automatic iris and other automatic black and white level controls (highly desirable when light may change as when, for example, a nurse in a white uniform walks in front of the camera); and (d) remote pan-tilt for aiming the camera (Porter, 1980).

Videotape recorders are an important link and, to a large extent, determine the quality of the resulting recording. As a rule, there is a general relationship between the width of the tape and the resultant quality. The most inexpensive machines use 1¼ cm (½ in) tape. The standard U-matic cassettes use 2 cm (¾ in) tape. The better, industrial and the newer broadcast quality open-reel machines use 2½ cm (1 in) tape. In general, therefore, the more expensive machines use the widest tape and obtain the best resolution. Several factors determine what type of machine is required. Expense is a major consideration. The need for transfer and editing is discussed below. Ease of operation and the possibility of remote operation should be considered, as should the value of a second audio track. One of the most difficult decisions concerns the use of open-reel versus cassette video systems. The better open-reel systems offer superior recording characteristics, but the cassettes are relatively convenient, easily stored, and if the U-matic format is chosen, have the advantage of being played on multiple machines with little difficulty. The disadvantages of cassettes are related to the complex mechanisms in the recorder. For example, they may be difficult to 'cue' properly; reviewing a seizure multiple times can be time-consuming and frustrating because the simple 'rewind' procedure does not always return to the beginning of the attack (Porter, 1980).

Two little-publicized facts about video recording are worth emphasizing. The first relates to information transfer. Many investigators record seizures on video tape and then later wish to show them at a different location on a different machine; disappointment is often the result. First, except for the very best, well-aligned machines, the original tape will almost always play best on the machine used for recording. Even an identical machine can have subtle (or severe) differences in mechanical alignment that will affect the reproduction. Even differences in line voltage, temperature, or humidity can cause a decrement in reproduction quality. This whole problem becomes especially noticeable when one tape is transferred to another, or 'edited'. Since the splicing of video tape is complicated and obsolete, the transfer is electronic; 20–30% degradation of quality in the electronic copy is the rule, and more severe degradation occurs with less expensive machines, different types of machines, poorly aligned machines, or original recordings of poor quality. It is no surprise to the experienced technician to see a tape play perfectly on the original machine but very poorly (or not at all) on a similar machine; electronic transfer of the information on such tape is difficult or impossible. The way to avoid this problem is to use high quality, well-aligned machines for both recording and playback. The newest videotape machines, using the so-called 'C' format, claim no degradation of picture quality after editing multiple times, in other words, even after multiple successive copies.

The second fact about video recording that is not widely appreciated is the need for a highly qualified technician, on at least a part-time basis, to keep the various components in good order. Video systems are not merely 'on' or 'off', but are capable of functioning at many levels of efficiency; only the optimal level will give good recordings. Cameras and tape recorders require periodic, expert maintenance to achieve this level of performance, and electronic technicians who have only a passing familiarity with video technology (an electronic world of its own) will likely not provide the expertise needed (Porter, 1980).

The only other mandatory piece of equipment for video recording is the monitor, which resembles a television set without a receiver. The simplest monitor will give only a view of the video information. More sophisticated monitors can help analyze the recorded signal and are extremely useful to the experienced technician. Other equipment can be very useful in video recordings. As previously mentioned, a time-coder generator that projects the year, month, day, hour, minute, and second on the screen is valuable in data retrieval. Similarly, the EEG montages can be placed beside the tracing so that each channel can be readily identified. If more than one camera image is to be combined in a 'split-screen' view, a 'special effects' generator is needed. Equipment that can be valuable in maintaining peak performance includes waveform monitors, oscilloscopes, processing amplifiers, and time-base correctors, but these are primarily useful to the sophisticated technician. Video systems and their uses have been reviewed (Porter, Penry and Wolf, 1976; Penry and Porter, 1977).

The simultaneous use of EEG and video recording

The intensive monitoring unit is most effective if the patient's prolonged EEG recording is teamed with a long-term video recording, thereby providing simultaneous documentation of the clinical and EEG manifestations of the epileptic seizures. The major problem involved in accomplishing this coupling has been in the display of the EEG on the same video screen. Three methods have been previously described (Porter, Penry and Wolf, 1976), but only one of the three will be reviewed here; it involves the use of the analog-TV reformatter developed in the Biomedical Engineering and Instrumentation Branch of the National Institutes of Health and now commercially available. Using this technique, the EEGs may be recorded exclusively on magnetic tape; the EEG machine is used only for playback of a specific recording. Independent of the tape recording, the analog EEG signal is displayed on the video screen by the reformatter. The signal simulates EEG and does not have the oscilloscopic appearance that is unfamiliar to many electroencephalographers. The video display, using a special-effects generator, two cameras, a time-code generator, and a reformatter, is shown in *Figure 7.1*. Videotapes can be routinely erased if no seizures are recorded, allowing reuse of videotapes which contain no useful data.

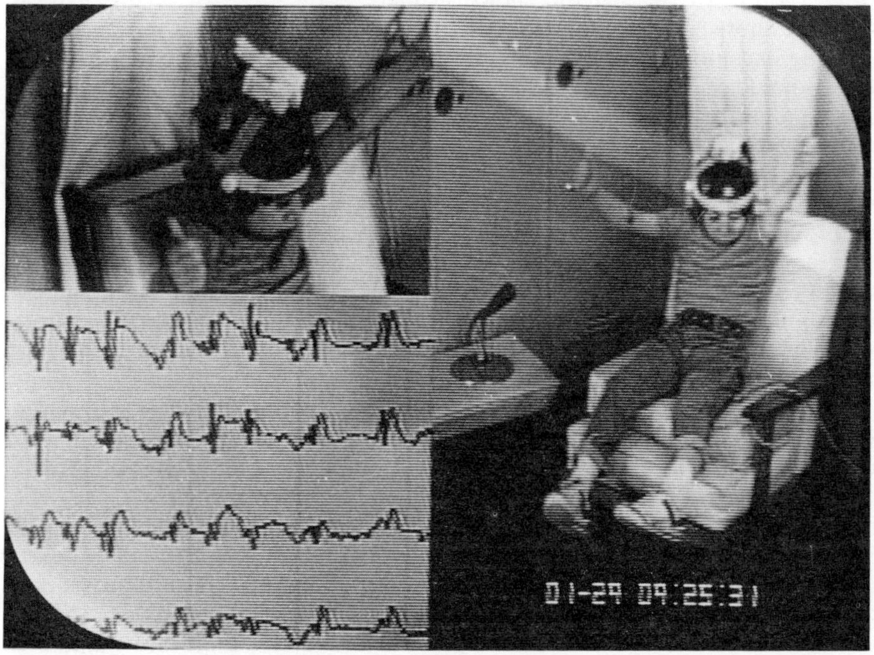

Figure 7.1 Two cameras and reformatted EEG combined into a video display in an intensive monitoring unit (see text for details)

Some mention must be made of the location of the equipment and the type of room used for intensive monitoring. The modified hospital room, with its beds, tables, closets, curtains, and so forth, is often used because of planning and space deficiencies. The disadvantages of such a room are several. The room is more than likely designated for patient care, and control of its use may not be possible or may be limited by the enthusiasm of the nursing staff. If non-epileptic patients share the room, the periods of intensive monitoring may seem to be nothing but an inconvenience, and strife may arise. Furthermore, equipment must be located so that the primary function of the room remains unchanged – in other words, the nursing function remains largely undisturbed. This requirement may limit, for example, the placement of the cameras to a rather high position on the wall that restricts the view of the patient but does not impede the nursing staff. More practical, but less generally available, is the clinical neurophysiology laboratory solely devoted to intensive monitoring. Such a room has much greater flexibility and is obviously under more direct control of the investigative team. The single disadvantage of such a laboratory is its location with respect to a nursing unit. Nurses are available for immediate help when the unit is part of the ward; assistance may be hard to get in a remote laboratory (Porter, 1980).

Plasma antiepileptic drug monitoring

The monitoring of antiepileptic drug levels in plasma is an integral part of intensive monitoring. Although the specific choice of medication for each seizure type is reviewed elsewhere in this volume (Chapters 9 to 11), certain principles of administering and monitoring antiepileptic drugs are reviewed here.

Epilepsy should virtually always be a positive diagnosis; when the diagnosis is uncertain, a therapeutic trial of antiepileptic drugs is rarely successful. When psychogenic seizures are incorrectly diagnosed as epilepsy, for example, administration of antiepileptic drugs may result in a temporary placebo effect, temporary worsening of the condition, or intolerance to the medication. Eventually, confusion reigns as more drugs at higher doses are tried. The chief pitfalls in the diagnosis of epilepsy include not only psychogenic seizures but also acute anxiety attacks, dissociative states, and syncope (Porter, 1984). The diagnosis of epilepsy, therefore, should be firmly established before antiepileptic drug therapy is undertaken.

Numerous studies have shown that a single drug controls seizures in many patients and that 'polytherapy' is often unnecessary. Patients always deserve at least one trial of monotherapy; a different drug can be tried if the first is unsuccessful. Refractory epilepsy, however, will usually be better controlled with more than one drug (Porter, Schulman and Penry, 1980; Porter, 1984).

Many tables of optimal therapeutic plasma drug levels for various antiepileptic drugs have been published, including those in this volume. The usual therapeutic range of phenytoin plasma levels, for example, is 10–20 μg/ml, which suggests that most patients will experience optimal seizure control with minimal toxicity if their plasma phenytoin level is within this range. Unfortunately, there are numerous exceptions to this guideline, and many patients are well controlled at higher or lower levels. Some patients, for example, tolerate phenytoin levels exceeding 20 μg/ml and require these high levels for seizure control. On the other hand the 'usual' neurological dose of 300 mg, which half the time gives a plasma phenytoin level of less than 10 μg/ml (Porter and Layzer, 1975), appears to give adequate seizure control in some patients. The plasma drug level, therefore, is only a guide to optimal use of antiepileptic drugs (Porter, 1984). A summary of the major considerations of the use of plasma drug levels is as follows:

(1) Antiepileptic drug monitoring is used only as a guide to changes in therapy; it is not a substitute for clinical judgement.

(2) Expected therapeutic plasma drug levels are average values; each patient will have an individual optimal value.
(3) The determinations help achieve maximal effects of each medication. The use of gradually increasing doses to establish the maximally tolerated dose is a valid concept in patients with refractory seizures.
(4) The determinations are invaluable in the presence of toxic side-effects, especially in patients taking multiple drugs.
(5) Non-compliance, malabsorption, and altered metabolism can be identified, but only non-compliance is a common problem.
(6) A reliable laboratory is critical to proper interpretation of the results. If the blood samples for determination of plasma drug levels are drawn at various times during the day, such levels may be misleading (Porter, 1983, 1984).

One of the more confusing aspects of monitoring plasma levels of antiepileptic drugs arises because determinations are made on blood samples obtained randomly at various times during the day. Especially with short half-life drugs, it is important to establish a fixed relationship between drug intake and blood sampling. Since it is virtually impossible to obtain blood samples during the day under controlled conditions, the only rational time to take routine samples is in the morning, before the first dose of medication is administered. Such samples reflect the baseline (trough) level and are directly comparable. Changes in doses can thereby be confidently followed by monitoring plasma drug levels without fear of artifactual effects from numerous variables (such as influence of food on rate of absorption,

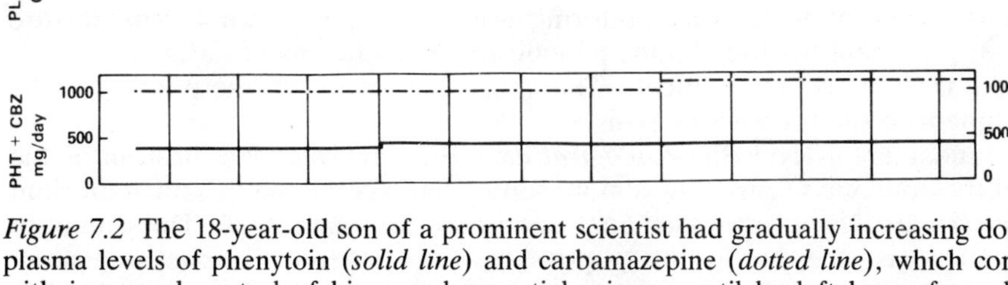

Figure 7.2 The 18-year-old son of a prominent scientist had gradually increasing doses and plasma levels of phenytoin (*solid line*) and carbamazepine (*dotted line*), which correlated with improved control of his complex partial seizures until he left home for college in September 1980. On 19 and 20 September, he had several secondarily generalized tonic-clonic seizures in the college dormitory. He was taken home on 21 September, and blood drug levels were determined three days later on 24 September. The phenytoin (PHT) level had fallen dramatically from the level in May 1980, but the carbamazepine (CBZ) was apparently unchanged. This puzzling observation was explained by the parents' careful monitoring of drug intake during the patient's three days at home. Carbamazepine, with a short half-life, returned quickly to a steady state, and by 24 September the level was again therapeutic. Phenytoin, however, with a relatively long half-life, took much longer to return to the steady state, and the 24 September level was therefore low. Seizure control returned after drug intake was resumed

time of venepuncture). Inconvenience to the patient is often considerable, but the data are well worth the effort, especially in difficult cases. If the epilepsy clinic is held in the morning, rather than in the afternoon, patients can delay taking their morning dose until after the blood sample is obtained (Porter, 1984).

To detect the toxic offender in a multidrug regimen, it is sometimes better to take blood samples at times other than in the morning. This tactic is rarely necessary, however, because the levels determined from the morning samples will usually indicate which drug is present in the blood at a high level (Porter, 1984).

Finally, one must consider that non-compliance is a major cause of uncontrolled seizures. Poor compliance with the physician's instructions regarding medication is not a problem unique to epilepsy; it is a difficulty encountered in the therapy of any chronic disease for which daily therapy is indicated. The typical patient with infrequent seizures forgets to take his medications for a myriad of reasons, and continues to have seizures. Observing neither toxic effects nor seizure control, the frustrated doctor prescribes higher and higher doses of drugs. Then, if the patient suddenly becomes compliant, toxicity occurs swiftly; the doctor is dumbfounded, and the patient disillusioned. It is an even more difficult problem if the patient has intractable seizures or deliberately omits medication. Furthermore, poor compliance is by no means limited to patients of lower socioeconomic backgrounds. Children from socioeconomically advantaged families may resist compliance in spite of logical explanations and emotional cajoling. Sometimes such forgetfulness can be detected by the pattern of the plasma drug levels (*Figure 7.2*) (Porter, 1984). A specific plan for dealing with non-compliance has been outlined in detail (Porter, 1984).

THE USE OF INTENSIVE MONITORING IN THE CLINICAL CARE OF PATIENTS WITH EPILEPSY

Establishment of the seizure diagnosis by intensive monitoring

Among the uses of intensive monitoring are (1) establishment of the seizure diagnosis; (2) differentiation of non-epileptic attacks from epileptic attacks; and (3) improved therapy of the patient. The most important of these uses is the establishment of the seizure diagnosis.

At a fundamental level, the *etiological diagnosis* involves identification of the cause of the epileptic seizures. At a more superficial, yet therapeutically important level, the *seizure diagnosis* is based on the nature of the seizure type. The search for both diagnoses is necessary for the proper care of the patient with epilepsy. Failure to establish the etiological diagnosis means that some patients will continue to have seizures because of, for example, undiagnosed tumors; or because absence attacks have been treated as complex partial seizures. This is not to say that there is no relationship between the etiological diagnosis, which is often unknown, and the seizure diagnosis, which can almost always be determined. There usually is such a relationship, and knowledge of one may lead to an understanding of the other (Porter, 1984). Intensive monitoring may play an important role in establishing the seizure diagnosis.

The kind of seizures that a patient has determines the correct medication or other therapy. This highly empirical approach still predominates in spite of continuing efforts to establish more basic and more rational diagnostic methods. The likelihood that basic neuroscience will contribute to the precise diagnosis of epilepsy still seems many years away. We do know, however, that the antiepileptic drugs now available are often considerably specific for various types of epileptic seizures and that proper seizure classification is crucial to appropriate therapy.

When the data on seizure characteristics are inadequate, the seizure diagnosis will be in doubt. If the physician is thereby forced to make a tentative diagnosis, an erroneous decision can result in inappropriate therapy. Even if the seizure diagnosis is correct, multiple medications may be unnecessarily prescribed or plasma drug levels may be inadequate. Intensive monitoring is an extension of the physician's usual skills; it allows more rational diagnostic and therapeutic decisions in the approximately 5% of patients with epilepsy who fail to respond to conventional approaches (Penry and Porter, 1977).

The seizure diagnosis which is established should approximate that given by the International Classification of Epileptic Seizures (ICES) (1981); such classification will allow the physician to make rational therapeutic decisions. The use of this classification and the therapy of the various seizure types is reviewed elsewhere in this volume (Chapters 6 and 9 to 11).

Differentiation of non-epileptic attacks from epilepsy

Intensive video and EEG monitoring are usually effective in establishing whether or not attacks of altered behavior are epileptic or non-epileptic. Such differentiation is only possible if the attacks can be recorded; if they are either infrequent or they cannot be precipitated at the time of the recording then no attack may be recorded and intensive monitoring is a failure.

Many patients with paroxysmal attacks which resemble epilepsy do not have this disorder. They have non-epileptic attacks which do not arise from abnormal neuronal discharge. If the word 'seizure' is used in its broadest sense to include any

Table 7.1 Some conditions associated with seizure or seizure-like phenomena (from Porter (1984); modified and expanded from Mattson, 1980)

Organic conditions	*Non-organic conditions*
Epileptic	Psychogenic
Cardiovascular	(hysterical,
aortic stenosis	conversion,
arrhythmias	functional,
vasovagal	pseudoseizures)
orthostatic hypotension	Other psychiatric
Transient cerebral ischemia	disorders (such as
Movement disorders	schizophrenia)
Toxic or metabolic disorders	Sleep disorders
hypoglycemia	Malingering
drug toxicity	
'Headache'	

paroxysmal attacks with apparent alteration of responsiveness, and/or motor, sensory, or autonomic dysfunction, then it is possible to construct a logical sequence of restrictive terms to describe these phenomena (*Table 7.1*). Epileptic seizures are most commonly encountered and are, by definition, caused by abnormal neuronal discharge. Other organic seizures involve other systems, such as the cardiovascular system. Metabolic disorders may also be associated with seizures. An overlap between epileptic and other organic seizures is apparent (Desai, Porter and Penry, 1982). Non-organic seizures are those in which no clear anatomic pathological change can be correlated with the disorder; sleep disorders such as narcolepsy and cataplexy are arbitrarily included in this category even though a physiological abnormality is likely.

Intensive monitoring of patients with intractable seizures has uncovered a remarkably high incidence of psychogenic attacks, 'pseudoseizures'. Since these patients naturally tend to be refractory to therapy, they often gravitate to specialized centers; many such facilities have monitoring units that establish the diagnosis of psychogenic seizures in patients who may or may not have associated epileptic attacks. The criteria for psychogenic seizures have gradually become more sophisticated as we learn more about the characteristics of these attacks as well as the characteristics of epileptic attacks themselves. Criteria to differentiate psychogenic seizures from specific seizure types are especially important. Generalized tonic-clonic seizures and complex partial seizures are the two epileptic attacks most likely to be confused with pseudoseizures. Some criteria are more important than others. A tabular description of such differentiating criteria is presented in *Tables 7.2, 7.3* and *7.4*.

Table 7.2 Major criteria: useful for diagnosing epileptic or psychogenic seizures (from Desai *et al.*, 1982)

	Epileptic seizures		*Non-epileptic seizures*
Characteristics	*Generalized tonic-clonic seizures*	*Complex partial seizures*	*Psychogenic seizures*
Comparison of questionable seizure with known seizure types	Relatively little variation in events	Wide range of events, but most common are well described	Extremely wide range of events with bizarre and unusual behavior
EEG during seizure	Abnormal and changed from preictal	Almost always abnormal and changed from preictal	Usually normal and unchanged from preictal
EEG immediately after seizure	Almost always abnormal and changed from preictal	Frequently abnormal and changed from preictal	Usually normal and unchanged from preictal
Relation of attacks to medication regimen	Prominent, especially in severely affected patients	Usually related	Usually unrelated

Table 7.3 Minor criteria: primarily useful for diagnosing suspected psychogenic seizures (from Desai *et al.*, 1982)

	Epileptic seizures		*Non-epileptic seizures*
Characteristics	*Generalized tonic-clonic seizures*	*Complex partial seizures*	*Psychogenic seizures*
Onset	Usually paroxysmal, but may be preceded by seizure of different type	Usually paroxysmal, but may be preceded by aura of only few seconds	Often gradual, prolonged non-specific warning period may occur
Primary or secondary gain	Rare; a few patients use seizures for secondary gain	Unusual, but a few patients use seizures for secondary gain	Common
Postictal confusion, lethargy, sleepiness	Prominent	Almost always present and often prominent but may be mild	Often conspicuously absent; patient may be normal immediately after attack
Postictal subjective complaints	Prominent if aroused	Usually prominent; patient rarely feels well	May be smiling or laughing after seizure
Suggestibility	None	Rare	Occasionally
Recollection of events during attack	None	Usually scant and most often none	Sometimes detailed
Violent behavior	None	Rare; virtually always in response to restraint and not highly directed	Rare, though may be highly directed

Unfortunately, the positive diagnosis of psychogenic seizures is rarely possible, and no single criterion should be singled out as diagnostic. The diagnosis remains one of exclusion of other conditions. Also, the separation of hysteria from malingering is often impossible. The coexistence of epileptic and psychogenic seizures in the same patient is not infrequent (Porter, 1984).

Several kinds of non-epileptic attacks other than psychogenic attacks can be confused with epilepsy. As with pseudoseizures, intensive monitoring provides a useful tool in the diagnosis of these other non-epileptic attacks. Acute anxiety attacks, for example, may take many forms, but the common feature is an overwhelming sense of fear or panic. The fear may be either 'free floating' or directed, and although often related to interpersonal encounters, attacks may also occur when the patient is completely alone. Patients are especially vulnerable 'when unaccompanied in the street, in crowds, buses, shops, and particularly when inactive or compelled to wait, as in cinemas or queues' (Harper and Roth, 1962).

The diagnosis of acute anxiety attacks usually rests on three factors. First, the duration of some of the attacks is quite prolonged, up to 15–30 min or more – much

Table 7.4 Minor criteria: primarily useful for diagnosing suspected epileptic seizures (from Desai *et al.*, 1982)

Characteristics	*Epileptic seizures* *Generalized tonic-clonic seizures*	*Complex partial seizures*	*Non-epileptic seizures* *Psychogenic seizures*
Age	Any, past infancy	Any, usually > 3 years	Usually older child or adult
Gross tonic-clonic motor phenomena	Always	Rare; seen only in secondarily generalized attacks	None, but resemblance is related to sophistication of mimicry
Tongue biting	Frequent	Rare	Rare
Urinary incontinence	Frequent	Unusual, but not rare	Rare
Abnormal neurological signs during seizure	May be present	May be present	None
Nocturnal occurrence	Common	May occur	Rare
Injuries sustained as a result of event	Common	Common	Rare, but occasionally occur
Stereotypy of attacks	Relatively little variation	Attacks may or may not be varied, but usually have some consistent patterns	Attacks may or may not be varied; patterns may occasionally be widely divergent

longer than most epileptic seizures. Second, consciousness is usually not altered during the attack; even though the patient may feel strange, appropriate interaction with the environment is still possible. The patient can almost always recite in detail the events and his or her own actions. Hyperventilation may be a prominent feature. Third, the EEG usually does not show epileptiform abnormalities, and the results are often completely normal (Porter, 1984).

Certain other psychiatric conditions are sometimes confused with epilepsy, especially psychogenic amnesia, psychogenic fugue, multiple personalities, and depersonalization (American Psychiatric Association, 1980). In the latter, certain symptoms are actually more common in the phobic-anxiety syndrome than in epilepsy, and the use of psychic symptoms to make the diagnosis of epilepsy is unwise unless accompanied by other signs and symptoms which are more definitive. In general, the more complicated and intricate the performance of the patient during the attack, the less likely the event will prove to be epileptic. If the attack can be recorded by intensive monitoring, the correct diagnosis can usually be established.

Another symptom which is often difficult to differentiate from epilepsy is syncope, usually defined as an alteration of normal brain function caused by paroxysmal cerebral hypoxia. In most patients, the hypoxia is caused by decreased blood flow to the brain. The various syncopal syndromes have been subdivided into three major and two minor categories by Riley (1982), who has organized a comprehensive list of the etiologies of syncope.

The differential diagnosis of epilepsy and syncope is highly dependent on an adequate medical history. The setting of the attacks may be an important clue to their etiology. Some patients have stereotyped emotional causes of their attacks; association with venepuncture is common. Many of the psychologically stressful environments associated with acute anxiety attacks are also implicated in syncope and in psychogenic attacks, including hyperventilation. Syncope is also precipitated in some patients by non-anxiety-related events, such as micturition and coughing. Patients with syncope often have a prolonged prodrome; the aura in epileptic attacks is usually only a few seconds. Although tonic extension occasionally occurs in syncope and a few clonic jerks are common, the classic sequence of the generalized tonic-clonic epileptic seizure is rare. The diagnosis can be difficult to establish if the attacks are infrequent. If the spells are frequent or precipitable, monitoring and simultaneous recording of the EEG and ECG can be definitive (Goldstein *et al.*, 1982). The use of the ambulatory EEG monitor is beneficial when one lead is used to record the ECG (Lai and Ziegler, 1981).

Therapeutic uses of monitoring

Since the early 1960s the use of plasma concentrations in monitoring the efficacy and toxicity of antiepileptic drugs has contributed greatly to improved care of patients with epilepsy. Widespread usage of such levels occurred, however, only after the introduction of gas-liquid chromatographic methods for simultaneous determinations of multiple antiepileptic drugs in the late 1960s. Even more widespread and convenient levels can be determined using newer immunoassay techniques.

In the early 1970s studies appeared which documented the usefulness of blood level measurement in clinical control of seizures. Sherwin, Robb and Lechter (1973) studied 70 patients with absence (petit mal) seizures: in 37 patients with uncontrolled attacks; 14 had plasma ethosuximide levels below the 95% tolerance limits. Adjustment of plasma levels of this drug resulted in reduction of seizures in 48% of the previously uncontrolled patients, as well as some improvement in less severe cases. They concluded that 'monitoring of plasma ethosuximide increases the effectiveness of therapy by recognition of noncompliance and the individualization of drug requirements'. Likewise, Lund (1974) published convincing data for the use of phenytoin levels in patients with grand mal seizures. Over a 3-year period, the average plasma level increased from 6.1 to 15.0 μg/ml. Many patients had optimal control at levels of 20 μg/ml or greater, substantiating the view that individualization of therapy can be efficacious. During the 3-year period, the annual mean number of grand mal seizures decreased from 5.8 to 1.6.

Until 1977, however, there had been no efforts to use simultaneously a combination of video monitoring, long-term EEG recording, and plasma concentrations of antiepileptic drugs in the treatment of seizure disorders. The reasons why these techniques had not been combined include: (1) lack of resources, equipment, personnel, or interested and qualified investigators; and (2) failure to understand the usefulness of the techniques. The results of the study by Porter, Penry and Lacy (1977) suggest that the benefits of video recordings, prolonged, telemetered EEGs, and frequent plasma antiepileptic drug determinations are enhanced by their simultaneous application, especially in patients with intractable seizures. In this study, patients were monitored in the hospital for an average of eight weeks and after discharge were followed for an average of eight months. At follow-up, 70% of the patients continued to have improved seizure control as compared with baseline studies; 83% had decreased toxicity, and about half had made gains in social adjustment.

In addition to the general improvement gained by establishing the correct diagnosis and by optimizing blood levels, intensive monitoring has allowed new insights into specific choices of drugs within the antiepileptic armamentarium. Since the development of phenytoin in the late 1930s, scientists and clinicians have recognized that an antiepileptic drug need not be sedative. Although the often dramatic and sometimes paradoxical effects of barbiturates and benzodiazepines have long been recognized, the more subtle effects of these drugs are only recently becoming apparent. The optimal use of non-sedative drugs such as phenytoin, carbamazepine, ethosuximide, and valproic acid has been shown, in studies using intensive monitoring, to be sufficient to obtain maximal seizure control (Theodore and Porter, 1983a and b). Furthermore, in a study by Vining *et al.* (1982), the deleterious effects of phenobarbital on performance tests were documented in a double-blind study with valproate. Intensive monitoring, therefore, not only provides the environment for improving the therapy of individual patients but also for challenging current concepts of appropriate medications.

THE IMPORTANCE OF MONITORING IN EPILEPSY RESEARCH

Intensive monitoring in clinical trials

The technique of intensive monitoring is important in two ways in the clinical evaluation of new therapies, especially new antiepileptic drug therapies. First, the nature of the seizures to be studied must be determined before the trial begins in order to permit some semblance of homogeneity in the group under investigation. Each patient must conform to these predetermined criteria; the most effective means of determining the seizure type in each individual patient is by intensive monitoring. In the very best centers, a majority of the uncontrolled patients who are entered into a clinical trial will have their seizure type documented by monitoring, usually at a previous admission.

The second use of intensive monitoring in clinical trials is highly specialized. Although most seizure types are not associated with characteristic EEG changes that allow quantification of seizure frequency by use of the EEG alone, absence seizures are characteristically associated with generalized, high voltage, spike-and-wave discharges in the EEG; these abnormal waveforms usually occur at 2.5–3.5 Hz. A large number of behavioral measures, reviewed by Penry (1973), have shown that performance is decreased during the spike-and-wave discharge. In these and later studies, using a simple amplitude detector on one channel of the

EEG machine, the abnormal EEG discharge triggered a reaction-time stimulus (Porter, Penry and Dreifuss, 1973). These studies, which were extended by Browne *et al.* (1974), allow several important observations regarding absence seizures. Most important, generalized spike-and-wave paroxysms in the EEG are highly correlated with a decrement in consciousness. The generalized spike-and-wave abnormality, therefore, unlike most electrographic abnormalities, correlates directly with the seizure itself, and obviously the number of generalized spike-and-wave paroxysms will give an excellent estimate of the seizure frequency. A decrement in consciousness occurs even if the paroxysm is brief (that is, lasts less than 2–3 s). Although efforts have been made to automate the counting of such events (Ehrenberg and Penry, 1976), most studies have utilized hand counting of the discharges. For the doctor treating a patient with absence seizures, a long-term EEG recording before and after each medication change will help to assess the effectiveness of therapy. For the clinical investigator, the availability of an objective and recordable method for determining seizure frequency is extremely useful (Porter, 1984). This technique was used, for example, in studies which documented the efficacy of valproic acid in the absence seizure (Sato *et al.*, 1982).

The use of intensive monitoring to further our knowledge of seizure types and improve classification

Inherent in any effort to describe the various seizure types is a classification of these seizures. The most important step forward in this regard was the classification of epileptic seizures published in 1970 by Gastaut, which divided seizures into two fundamental groups – partial and generalized. Following adoption of the 1970 classification, the methods of intensive monitoring allowed objective methods for studying seizures, and a gradual effort was undertaken to improve this classification using data generated from monitoring units around the world. Workshops were held, first in Bethesda in 1975, then in Berlin in 1977, and finally again in Bethesda in 1979, under the auspices of the Commission on Classification and Terminology of the International League Against Epilepsy. The commission was tirelessly led, first by the late Jerome K. Merlis of Baltimore and later by Fritz E. Dreifuss of Charlottesville. The work of the Commission was possible because of the data made available from monitoring units throughout the world. The resulting classification departs from the previous one, but more in emphasis than in substance; it alleviates, for example, the difficult classification problems related to the consciousness of the patient during the seizure, but retains the overall division of partial and generalized attacks. Furthermore, new emphasis is placed on seizure progression (Commission on Classification and Terminology of the ILAE, 1981). That the classification must continue to be modified as new data become available is apparent; further studies, for example, using data from an intensive monitoring unit have expanded our concepts of seizure progression and secondary generalization (Porter and Sato, 1982).

Intensive monitoring is a technique which extends the ability of the physician in the diagnosis and therapy of seizures. The discussion and the examples given in this chapter, while not exhaustive, document the efficacy of the technique for patients with epilepsy.

References

AMERICAN PSYCHIATRIC ASSOCIATION (1980) *Diagnostic and Statistical Manual of Mental Disorders,* 3rd edn., pp. 253–260. Washington, DC: APA

BROWNE, T. R., PENRY, J. K., PORTER, R., J., and DREIFUSS, F. E. (1974) Responsiveness before, during, and after spike-wave paroxyms. *Neurology,* **24,** 659–665

COMMISSION ON CLASSIFICATION AND TERMINOLOGY OF THE INTERNATIONAL LEAGUE AGAINST EPILEPSY (ILAE) (1981) Proposal for revised clinical and electroencephalographic classification of epileptic seizures. *Epilepsia,* **19,** 447–452

DESAI, B. T., PORTER, R. J. and PENRY, J. K. (1982) Psychogenic seizures: a study of 42 attacks in six patients, with intensive monitoring. *Archives of Neurology,* **39,** 202–209

EHRENBERG, B. L. and PENRY, J. K. (1976) Computer recognition of generalized spike-wave discharges. *Electroencephalography and Clinical Neurophysiology,* **41,** 25–36

GASTAUT, H. (1970) Clinical and electroencephalographic classification of epileptic seizures. *Epilepsia,* **11,** 102–113

GOLDSTEIN, D. S., SPANARKEL, M., PITTERMAN, A. *et al.* (1982) Circulatory control mechanisms in vasodepressor syncope. *American Heart Journal,* **104,** 1071–1075

HARPER, M. and ROTH, M. (1962) Temporal lobe epilepsy and the phobic anxiety depersonalization syndrome. Part I: a comparative study. *Comprehensive Psychiatry,* **3,** 129–151

IVES, J. R., THOMPSON, C. J. and GLOOR, P. (1976) Seizure monitoring: a new tool in electroencephalography. *Electroencephalography and Clinical Neurophysiology,* **41,** 422–427

LAI, C. and ZIEGLER, D. K. (1981) Syncope problem solved by continuous ambulatory simultaneous EEG/ECG recording. *Neurology,* **31,** 1152–1154

LUND, L. (1974) Anticonvulsant effect of diphenylhydantoin relative to plasma levels. *Archives of Neurology,* **31,** 289–294

MATTSON, R. H. (1980) Value of intensive monitoring. In *Advances in Epileptology: The Xth Epilepsy International Symposium*, edited by J. A. Wada and J. K. Penry, pp. 43–51. New York: Raven Press

PENRY, J. K. (1973) Behavioral correlates of generalized spike-wave discharge in the electroencephalogram. In *Epilepsy: Its Phenomena in Man*, edited by M. A. B. Brazier, pp. 171–188. New York: Academic Press

PENRY, J. K. and PORTER, R. J. (1977) Intensive monitoring of patients with intractable seizures. In *Epilepsy: The Eighth International Symposium*, edited by J. K. Penry, pp. 95–101. New York: Raven Press

PORTER, R. J. (1980) Methodology of continuous monitoring with videotape recording and electroencephalography. In *Advances in Epileptology: The Xth Epilepsy International Symposium*, edited by J. A. Wada and J. K. Penry, pp. 35–42. New York: Raven Press

PORTER, R. J. (1983) Efficacy of antiepileptic drugs. In *Epilepsy*, edited by A. A. Ward, Jr., J. K. Penry, and D. Purpura, pp. 225–237. New York: Raven Press

PORTER, R. J. (1984) *Epilepsy: 100 Elementary Principles.* London: Saunders

PORTER, R. J. and LAYZER, R. B. (1975) Plasma albumin concentration and diphenylhydantoin binding in man. *Archives of Neurology,* **32,** 298–303

PORTER, R. J., PENRY, J. K. and DREIFUSS, F. E. (1973) Responsiveness at the onset of spike-wave bursts. *Electroencephalography and Clinical Neurophysiology,* **34,** 239–245

PORTER, R. J., PENRY, J. K. and LACY, J. R. (1977) Diagnostic and therapeutic reevaluation of patients with intractable epilepsy. *Neurology,* **27,** 1006–1011

PORTER, R. J., PENRY, J. K. and WOLF, A. A. JR (1976) Simultaneous documentation of clinical and electroencephalographic manifestations of epileptic seizures. In *Quantitative Analytic Studies in Epilepsy*, edited by P. Kellaway and I. Petersen, pp. 253–268. New York: Raven Press

PORTER, R. and SATO, S. (1982) Secondary generalization of epileptic seizures. In *Advances in Epileptology: XIIIth Epilepsy International Symposium*, edited by H. Akimoto, H. Kazamatsuri, M. Seino and A. A. Ward Jr, pp. 47–48. New York: Raven Press

PORTER, R. J., SCHULMAN, E. A. and PENRY, J. K. (1980) Phenytoin monotherapy in intractable epilepsy. In *Advances in Epileptology: XIth Epilepsy International Symposium*, edited by R. Canger, F. Angeleri and J. K. Penry, pp. 419–422. New York: Raven Press

PORTER, R. J., WOLF, A. A., JR. and PENRY, J. K. (1971) Human electroencephalographic telemetry: a review of systems and their applications and a new receiving system. *American Journal of Electroencephalographic Technology,* **11,** 145–159

RILEY, T. L. (1982) Syncope and hyperventilation. In *Pseudoseizures,* edited by T. L. Riley and A. Roy, pp. 34–61. Baltimore: Williams and Wilkins

SATO, S., WHITE, B. G., PENRY, J. K., DREIFUSS, F. E., SACKELLARES, J. C. and KUPFERBERG, H. J. (1982) Valproic acid versus ethosuximide in the treatment of absence seizures. *Neurology,* **32,** 157–163

SHERWIN, A. L., ROBB, J. P. and LECHTER, M. (1973) Improved control of epilepsy by monitoring plasma ethosuximide. *Archives of Neurology,* **28,** 178–181

THEODORE, W. H. and PORTER, R. J. (1983a) Removal of sedative-hypnotic antiepileptic drugs from the regimens of patients with intractable epilepsy. *Annals of Neurology,* **13,** 320–324

THEODORE, W. H. and PORTER, R. J. (1983b) Withdrawal of sedative-hypnotic antiepileptic drugs from outpatients. In *The Rational Prescription of Antiepileptic Drugs*, edited by S. Shorvon and G. Birdwood. Berne: Hans Huber

VINING, E. P. G., MELLITS, E. D., CATALDO, M. F., DORSEN, M. M., SPIELBERG, S. P. and FREEMAN, J. M. (1982) Effects of phenobarbital and sodium valproate on neuropsychological function. In *Abstracts of Joint Annual Meeting of the American Electroencephalographic Society and American Epilepsy Society,* (Phoenix, 1982), p. 50

8
The electroencephalogram in the routine evaluation of patients with epilepsy

Dudley S. Dinner and Hans Lüders

NEURAL BASIS OF THE EEG

Richard Caton in 1875 was the first to record visually evoked and spontaneous brain wave activity in experiments on rabbits and monkeys describing them as 'feeble currents of the brain' (Caton, 1875). However, Hans Berger made the first recordings of the electroencephalogram (EEG) in man in 1924 (Berger, 1929). By recording simultaneously from the scalp and cortical surface he demonstrated that the potentials originated in the brain and in 1931, comparing recordings from grey and white matter, he demonstrated that these potentials were cortical in origin (Berger, 1931). In studies of the cat's neocortex, it was observed that the duration of the action potentials was 1 ms, while that of the EEG waves was 77–125 ms and had characteristics similar to those of postsynaptic potentials (Li and Jasper, 1953). On this basis they postulated that the EEG waves may be the summation of temporally dispersed postsynaptic potentials. A similar concept had been previously proposed based on studies of the cortical response to direct stimulation (Eccles, 1951). It is now widely accepted that the EEG activity is generated by postsynaptic potentials in the vertically oriented pyramidal neurons with their apical dendrites extending toward the surface and branching horizontally in the superficial layers (*Figure 8.1*). The dendritic and somatic portions are supplied with thousands of excitatory (depolarizing) and inhibitory (hyperpolarizing) synaptic endings. In the resting state both the somatic and dendtritic portions of the neuronal membrane are similar, 70 mV negative on the inside with respect to the outside.

If a presynaptic fiber is activated and terminates in an excitatory synapse on the dendrite, the membrane potential at the dendrite is temporarily decreased, for example to 60 mV, while the somatic membrane potential is unchanged. Current then flows between these two points, creating an electrical field surrounding the neuron (*see Figure 8.1*). Activation of an inhibitory synapse terminating on the soma will result in a temporary hyperpolarization of this membrane potential, for example to 80 mV, with a similar current flow from the soma to dendrite. Activation of an inhibitory synapse on the dendrite or excitatory synapse on the soma will result in local current flow in the opposite direction with a corresponding surrounding electrical field. It is the fluctuations in these postsynaptic potentials with the resultant flow of local currents between the somas and apical dendrites of

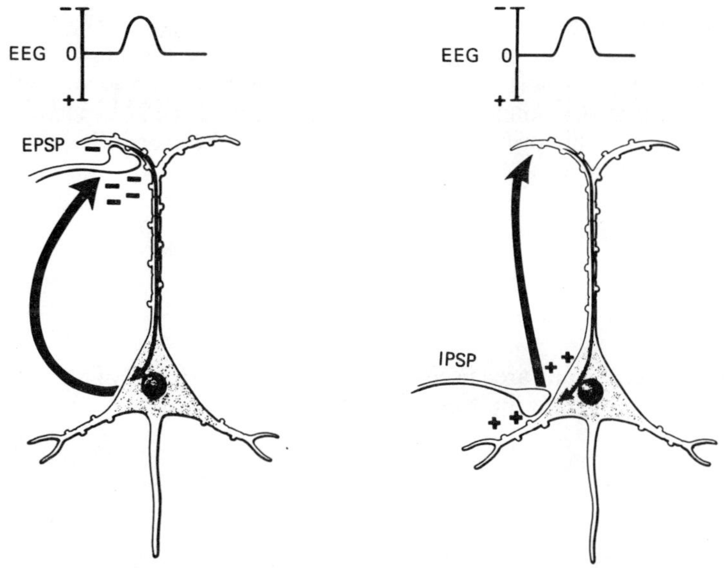

Figure 8.1 Illustrates why superficial excitatory post-synaptic potentials (EPSPs) and deep inhibitory post-synaptic potentials (IPSPs) produce the same current flow, hence deflections of the same polarity when recorded by the surface EEG

the pyramidal cells which act as the generators of the electrical activity which is detected by the scalp surface electroencephalogram.

The role of the thalamus as a pacemaker was first recognized by Berger in 1933 and in 1936 Bishop introduced his theory of corticothalamic reverberating circuits (Bishop, 1936). Andersen and Andersson (1976), based on the similarity of barbiturate spindle activity in animals and human alpha activity, formulated a hypothesis of thalamic control of EEG activity. This hypothesis postulates that the primary driving force for the normal alpha rhythm is in the thalamic nuclei. When an impulse activates the somatic portion of the thalamic neuron it depolarizes, and this in turn via its axon and excitatory synapse activates the cortical neuron and can be recorded with the EEG. A recurrent collateral branch of the thalamic neuron activates an inhibitory interneuron which in turn hyperpolarizes the soma of the thalamic neuron. This is followed by a rebound or postinhibitory excitation which in turn generates an action potential in its axon activating the cortex and also the recurrent inhibitory neuron. This system continues to oscillate indefinitely, giving rise to the rhythmicity of the EEG activity. The physiological basis of the epileptiform discharge will not be discussed here as it has already been reviewed in Chapter 2.

OPTIMAL DISPLAY OF EPILEPTIFORM ACTIVITY

There are certain principles that should be obeyed in the recording of the EEG and are well summarized in the guidelines of the American EEG Society (1980). At least 21 electrodes should be applied routinely to the head, according to the 10–20 International System (Jasper, 1958), to sample adequately activity from all areas accessible by scalp recordings. The exception to this rule is in neonates, particularly prematures, whose heads may be too small to apply 21 electrodes. Sixteen channels of simultaneous recording should be strongly encouraged to define adequately the distribution of EEG activity. Using fewer channels may result in erroneous distributions when attempts are made to map the activity. This is especially important with regard to epileptiform activity. During the recording the technologist should pay particular attention to symmetry of the recorded rhythms and if necessary check the symmetry of electrode placement, as this may result in a false interpretation of the EEG.

ACTIVATION PROCEDURES

Certain techniques of activation are used in the routine EEG looking for epileptiform activity. These include the following:

(1) Sleep
(2) Sleep deprivation
(3) Hyperventilation
(4) Sensory input
(5) Drug withdrawal
(6) Chemical activation.

Sleep

Sleep is an important and effective activator of epileptiform activity and should be obtained in routine EEGs in epilepsy especially if no abnormality is detected in the awake recording. Medication may be necessary to induce sleep in the laboratory. Barbiturates were the first medication to be used and are still used in many laboratories. However, the enhancement of beta-activity by barbiturates can make interpretation of the EEG more difficult. Chloral hydrate has less tendency to increase the amount of beta-activity and is thus an ideal alternate hypnotic. In 1947 one study (Gibbs and Gibbs, 1947) found that in a group of 174 patients 19% had epileptiform activity awake, while 63% had epileptiform activity asleep. Subsequent studies have found sleep necessary to define epileptiform activity in one-third of 667 (Silverman, 1956), in 23 of 36 (White *et al.*, 1962), in 30 of 89 (Mattson *et al.*, 1965), and in 23 of 73 patients (Niedermeyer and Rocca, 1972). In our study of 30 patients with complex partial seizures (CPS), in the first available EEG, epileptiform activity was seen in 16 during the waking record but increased in amount in 14 during sleep, and in an additional eight patients epileptiform discharges occurred in sleep only (Dinner *et al.*, 1984). Frequently sharp waves or spikes are present both awake and asleep, but increased markedly in sleep. This is particularly frequent in benign focal epilepsy of childhood (Blom, 1975) and in partial seizure disorders.

Sleep deprivation

Sleep deprivation increases the chance of obtaining a spontaneous sleep recording during the routine EEG and thus activating epileptiform activity. However, sleep deprivation may increase the yield of epileptiform activity even if the patient does not sleep during the recording. Two studies have found this technique to yield epileptiform abnormalities in a second EEG with sleep deprivation compared with a normal first EEG in 47 of 114 and 31 of 42 patients respectively (Pratt *et al.*, 1968; Scollo-Lavizzarri, Pralle and Radue, 1977). However, this increase in rate of abnormalities may be in part due to the increase in recording time. This question has been studied by various groups. Such sampling effect was calculated by Pratt (1968) to be 18%. Similar to sleep, sleep deprivation involves no risk and can be of significant diagnostic assistance in patients with or suspected of epilepsy.

Hyperventilation

In 1926 Foerster was the first to report that hyperventilation could provoke seizures (Bostem, 1976). The efficacy of hyperventilation in producing epileptiform activity both ictal and interictal is highest in petit mal. Although this technique is of less use for producing interictal focal epileptiform activity, hyperventilation may occasionally precipitate a partial seizure. Eleven of 225 patients with complex partial seizures experienced clinical seizures during hyperventilation in the series of Miley and Forster (1977). One must pay special attention to differentiate the physiological effects of the hyperventilation from epileptiform activity. Generalized rhythmical slowing is a physiological response to hyperventilation, most

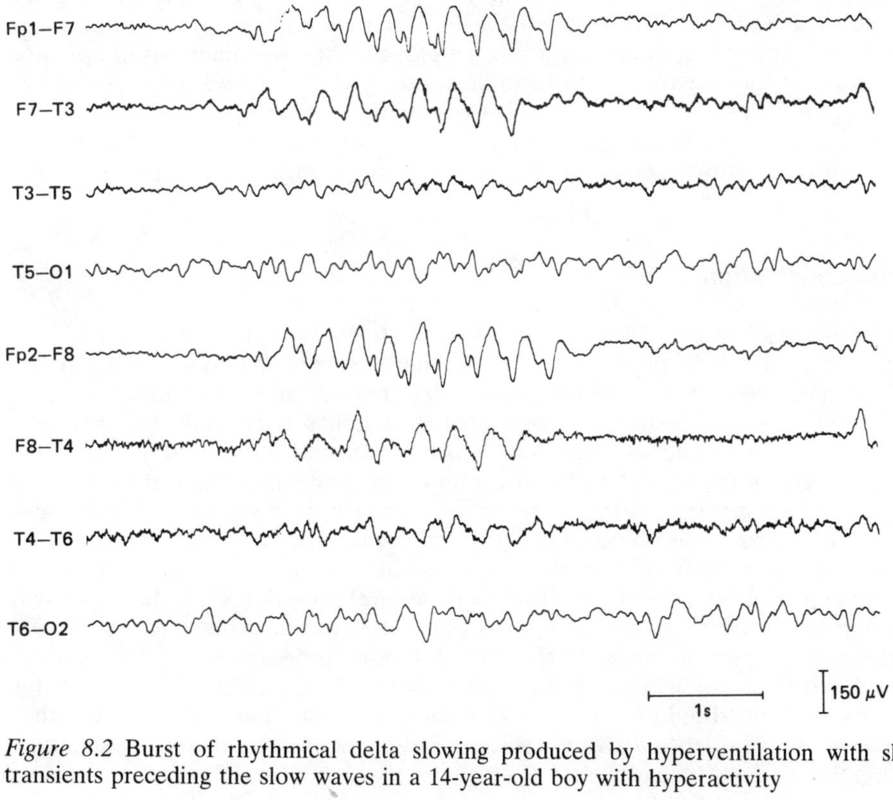

Figure 8.2 Burst of rhythmical delta slowing produced by hyperventilation with sharp transients preceding the slow waves in a 14-year-old boy with hyperactivity

prominent in young children. Sharp transients may also appear preceding the slow waves (*Figure 8.2*). This combination may be misinterpreted as spike and slow wave complexes and a misdiagnosis of a generalized seizure disorder. One must be aware of this possibility and avoid making this error.

Sensory stimulation

Various environmental factors have been reported to produce seizures in susceptible subjects, including light flicker, touch, visual patterns, specific musical passages, movement, eating, higher cognitive function (Forster, 1977; Klass and Fischer-Williams, 1976) and even arcade games (Rushton, 1981). Testing the patient with the specific activating factor during the EEG recording may establish the diagnosis. Photic stimulation with a strobe light is routinely used in the EEG laboratory. It is most likely to yield epileptiform abnormality in generalized seizure disorders. Moreover, self-induced seizures by hand waving in front of or blinking at a light source are seen not infrequently (Newmark and Penry, 1979).

Drug withdrawal

Anticonvulsants not infrequently may 'mask' the occurrence of epileptiform activity during EEG recordings (Ramani *et al.*, 1980). Withdrawal of anticonvulsants is a technique used to increase the chance of recording epileptiform activity both interictal and ictal. This technique is not usually used in the routine follow-up of diagnosed epileptics, but is frequently employed when the diagnosis of epilepsy is uncertain or in patients with intractable seizures where one wants to define the epileptogenic focus. Although there is a possibility that abrupt withdrawal might activate areas not previously epileptogenic, a recent study found that the results after abrupt withdrawal were similar to those prior to withdrawal (Spencer *et al.*, 1981).

Chemical activation

Pentylenetetrazol (Metrazol®) is a stimulant at all levels of the cerebrospinal axis but the cerebral cortex appears to be the major site of action resulting in the production of epileptiform activity and seizures. This chemical is of no value in the routine evaluation and diagnosis of epilepsy as it has been shown to produce epileptiform activity and seizures in normals (Baker and Klass, 1965). However, pentylenetetrazol may be of value in carefully selected cases of focal epilepsy in their evaluation prior to surgical resection, when it is necessary to document carefully the exact localization of onset of the focal seizures if these could not be recorded spontaneously or with the other activating techniques discussed above. Pentylenetetrazol was used in 11 of 163 awake recordings at the Montreal Neurological Institute to localize the origin of seizures (Gloor *et al.*, 1967). However, discrepancies between the localization of spontaneous and chemically induced seizures has also been reported (Wieser *et al.*, 1979). Therefore, this activation method should be restricted to cases of partial epilepsy where all other procedures have failed to activate a seizure and the activated seizure was identical to the patient's habitual seizures.

RECOGNITION OF ARTIFACTS

It is essential both for the EEG technologist and the electroencephalographer to recognize common artifacts which may mimic electroencephalographic abnormalities. It is important so that the technologist can make the necessary adjustments in his or her recording technique to get rid of the artifact if it is being produced by a technical factor such as a loose electrode producing a 'rhythmic slow activity' or when there is poor electrode–skin contact with resultant high impedance and subsequent production of 'electrode pop' artifacts which could be interpreted as epileptiform activity. It is equally important for the technologist to recognize physiological artifacts produced by non-cerebral generators such as eye movement and muscle activity. It is imperative for the electroencephalographer to recognize these artifacts so as not to misinterpret the activity as pathological with subsequent consequences for the diagnosis of the patient's condition.

The artifacts discussed here, however, are only those that may be mistaken for epileptiform activity.

Physiological

Eye movement

The eye movement artifact that appears routinely in the waking record of the EEG is produced by saccadic eye movements and by eyelid movement. The characteristic of this artifact is that it is bilateral. If it is in the vertical direction then the eye movement classically is localized maximally to the frontopolar electrodes located close to the eyes, with dramatic fall-off of activity at electrodes located more distant from the eyes. The purely horizontal saccadic eye movements will effect mainly F7 and F8 electrodes with opposite polarity at each of the two electrodes. Oblique eye movement produces a combination of component activities of horizontal and vertical eye movement. These and their respective distributions should be second nature to the electroencephalographer.

Muscle artifact

Repetitive electromyographic activity is not difficult to recognize. However, it is the isolated muscle spicule which can occasionally be a problem and simulate an epileptiform discharge (*Figure 8.3*). One such example is the muscle spicule produced by the lateral rectus muscles, best seen at electrodes F7 and F8, which immediately precedes saccadic lateral eye movement. It is often well seen with nystagmus or reading. When associated with nystagmus it occurs with the quick phase of the eye movement. Isolated muscle spicules may occur in other distributions but frequently occur at the electrodes where muscle activity is maximally distributed at other times during the EEG, in the temporal and frontal regions. This is not infrequent in sleep, particularly in REM sleep.

Electrocardiogram (ECG)

ECG artifact can be detected fairly frequently in the routine EEG. The ECG may appear as a sharp transient which tends to appear in a periodic fashion at

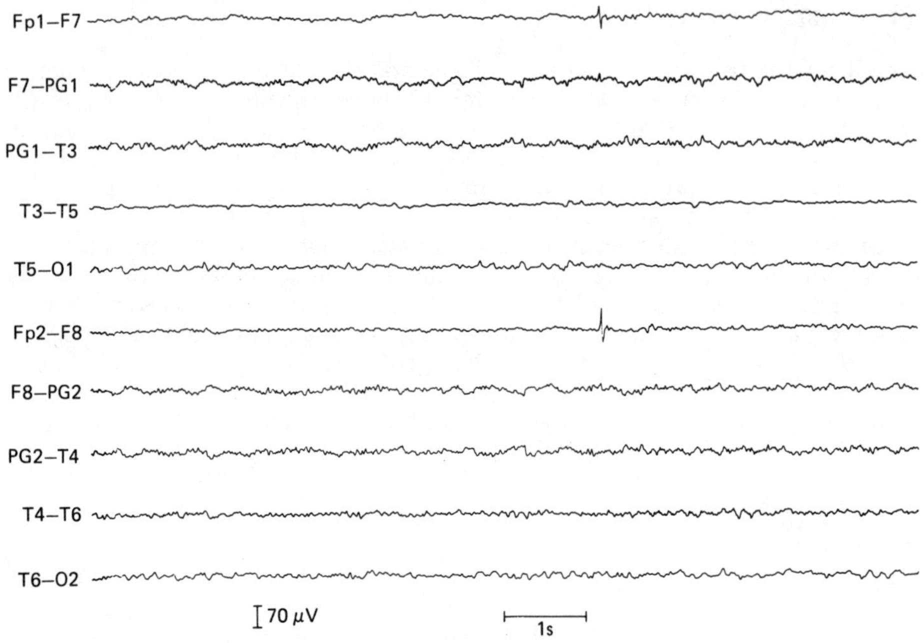

Figure 8.3 Muscle spicule in channels 1 and 6

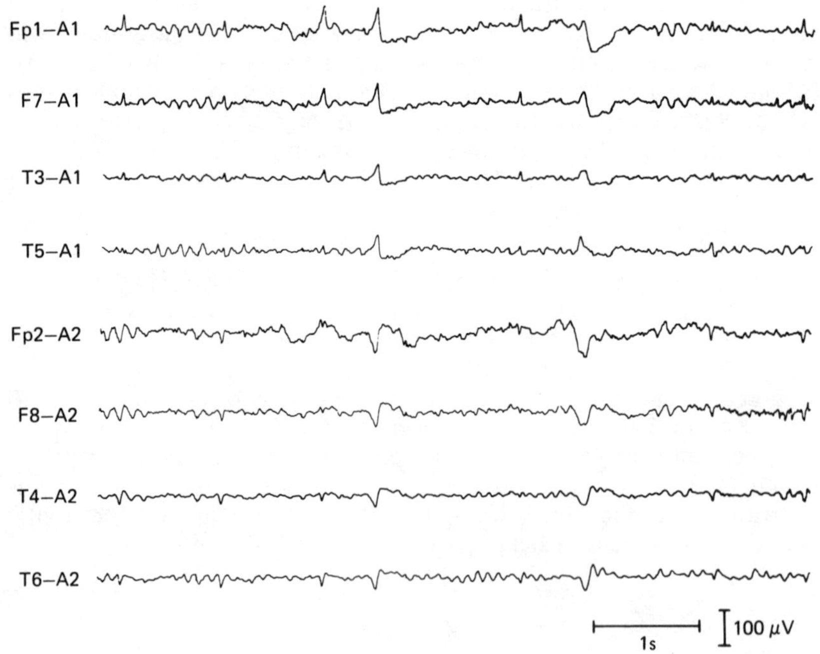

Figure 8.4 Periodic sharp transients produced by ECG artifact with two ectopic beats which appear more prominently

approximately 1 Hz (*Figure 8.4*). The interval between the transients is usually very stable but may vary slightly due to the phenomenon of sinus arrhythmia. The distribution of the ECG vector over the head is diagonal with maximum electronegativity in the right anterior quadrant and maximum electropositivity in the left posterior head region. Thus the ECG artifact is likely to be most prominent when using a montage which links the interhemispheric electrodes, for example A1–A2. One may easily recognize the ECG artifact due to a normal sinus rhythm. However, with ventricular ectopic beats one may find a transient which is occurring with a different distribution to the sinus rhythm and also occurring prematurely with respect to the regular periodicity of the sinus rhythm (*see Figure 8.4*). This must not be mistaken for epileptiform activity. If one is using one of the EEG channels for monitoring ECG one will be able to recognize easily the transients produced by ECG artifact. The artifact due to a cardiac pacemaker strictly speaking should be discussed under technical artifacts. It is characterized by a very short duration spike recognized by its periodicity of 70/minute.

Technical

Electrode artifacts are common. The characteristic 'electrode pop' is due to a sudden change in the impedance due to the poor skin–electrode contact which results in identical upward or downward deflections in all the derivations in which the involved electrode is represented (*Figure 8.5*). This may simulate an epileptiform sharp wave. However, the distribution localizing it to only one electrode is against this transient being epileptogenic and more likely due to artifact, whereas electrical biological activity including artifacts like ECG, EMG and eye movement are almost always seen involving more than one electrode.

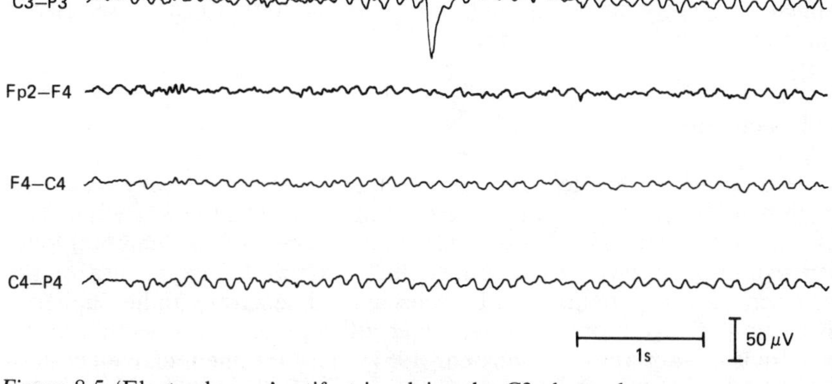

Figure 8.5 'Electrode pop' artifact involving the C3 electrode

Another clue is that the polarity of this activity may change. If this is suspected by the technologist the impedance should be checked and the electrode rescratched, more contact solution administered or the electrode replaced.

SPECIAL ELECTRODES

There are several additional electrodes that can be used to try to optimize the display of epileptiform activity.

Anterior temporal electrode

The best known of the special electrodes is the anterior temporal electrode (Silverman, 1960) which is placed 1 cm above a point one-third the distance from the external auditory meatus to the external canthus. This point is relatively distant from the standard electrode placements and approximately overlies the anterior temporal region.

Nasopharyngeal electrodes

In 1949 MacClean described a nasopharyngeal lead for recording electrical potentials at the base of the brain (MacClean, 1949). The electrode was inserted through the nose to rest against the posterior lateral nasopharynx. Variations of this electrode are the ones in use today. Gloor *et al.* (1957) pointed out that they use nasopharyngeal electrodes routinely in the evaluation of patients with complex partial seizures and noted that accurate localization of the seizure focus was only possible when using these leads in 71 of 177 patients who later underwent temporal lobectomy. We also use nasopharyngeal leads routinely in evaluation of patients suspected of having complex partial seizures. In our experience it is very unusual to see epileptiform discharges only at the nasopharyngeal lead. However, not infrequently the abnormality is much better defined at the nasopharyngeal lead, thus clarifying the nature of discharges which may be poorly defined with routine scalp electrodes (*Figure 8.6*). Respiration and pulse are frequent artifacts producing repetitive rhythmic slow activity in derivations with these electrodes. These artifacts can easily be recognized and if very abundant can be selectively filtered out using a low linear frequency of 5 Hz.

Sphenoidal electrodes

In 1951 Jones described a needle electrode which was inserted laterally under the zygomatic arch to lie in the region of the foramen ovale (Jones, 1951). This electrode facilitated recordings from the mesial basal aspect of the temporal lobe. The Montreal group in 1961 first described their experience in the use of the sphenoidal electrodes in patients with complex partial seizures, finding epileptiform activity in patients previously not detected with use of nasopharyngeal electrodes (Rovit, Gloor and Rasmussen, 1961). Using sphenoidal electrodes Kristensen and Sindrup (1978) found sharp waves in 16% of 294 patients with

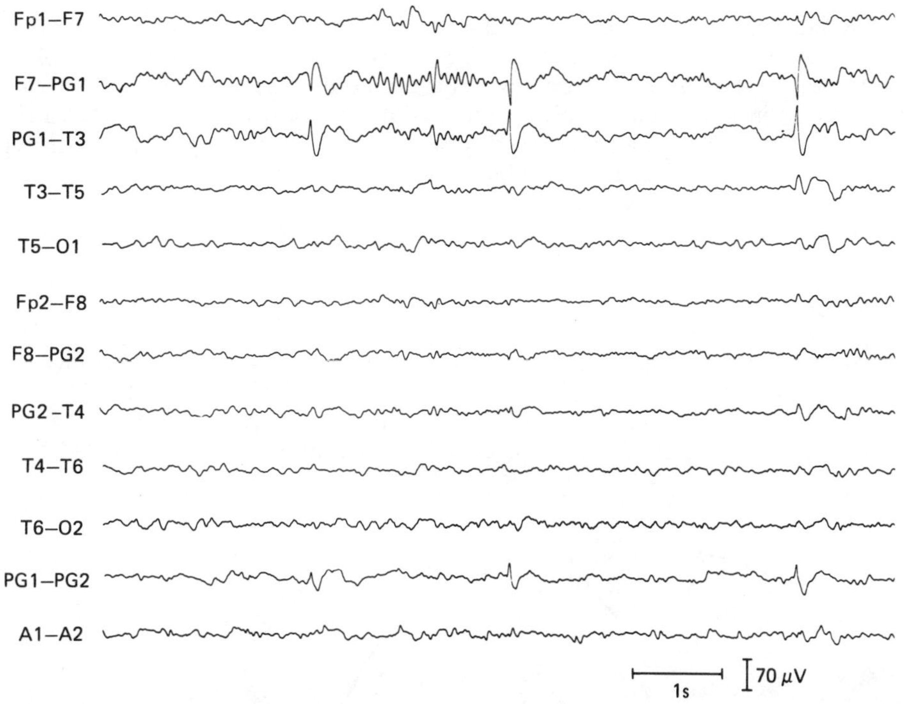

Figure 8.6 Sharp waves in left temporal region maximum at the nasopharyngeal electrode, in a 20-year-old woman with complex partial seizures

complex partial seizures who had no epileptiform activity recorded by surface electrodes. Ying-K'un, Ching-Chin and Tan-Hua (1981) described a technique using acupuncture needles as sphenoidal electrodes. In 55 patients with definite psychomotor epilepsy, epileptic discharges were found in 14 with scalp electrodes and in an additional 31 with sphenoidal electrodes. Initially the type of sphenoidal electrodes used were usually needles. The main disadvantage is that they could not be left in place for a very prolonged period and there was also the risk of the patient sustaining an injury during a seizure. Rovit, Gloor and Henderson (1960) devised a method to replace the needle electrodes by wire electrodes which overcame the disadvantages mentioned above. However, these wires were very susceptible to artifact, especially movement. Ives and Gloor (1977) improved upon Rovit's wire electrodes with a multistranded, teflon-coated silver wire with chloride at the tip. They have left this electrode in place for as long as five days without difficulty.

Ethmoidal electrodes

In 1970 Lehtinen and Bergström described the use of an electrode for recording electrical activity from the inferior surface of the frontal lobe, inserting the electrode through the nose into the ethmoid sinus to rest against the lamina cribrosa of the ethmoid. We have used this technique in three patients with partial seizures whose focus was suspected to be in the basal frontal lobe. We initially used a thin flexible wire with a silver ball tip but have since modified the electrode and use now a multistranded silver wire, teflon-coated, which is inserted with a stainless steel cannula which is subsequently withdrawn. We have left this electrode in place for up to seven days without problems. There is no discomfort to the patient with the electrode in place similar to the sphenoidal electrode, and in contrast to the nasopharyngeal electrode no problem while eating or drinking. The recording characteristics of this electrode have been excellent and we have found no artifacts such as from respiration or pulse.

Closely spaced scalp electrodes

We frequently place additional closely spaced scalp electrodes in positions midway between the 10–20 electrode placements (nomenclature devised by Dr G Chatrain) (*Figure 8.7*). The additional electrodes in the B line are midway between FP and F line of electrodes. Similarly, we have designated additional lines of electrodes, D

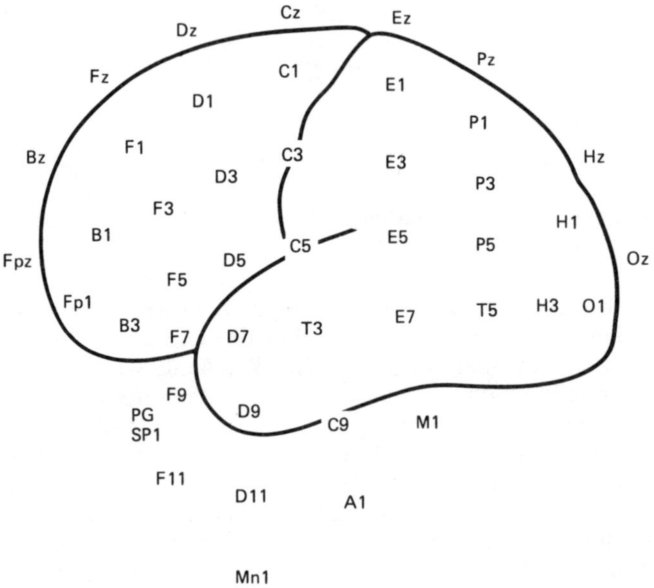

Figure 8.7 Closely spaced additional electrodes in addition to the electrodes of the standard 10–20 system

line, E line and H line. In any particular line the designation of the number affixed to the letter designating the line denotes the distance from the midline. F1 is midway between Fz and F3, F5 midway between F3 and F7. The placement of additional electrodes along the side of the face may be added F10, F12, by measuring out identical interelectrode distances to define their precise location. The additional closely spaced electrodes are placed only in the particular region of interest, for example the left temporal region (*Figure 8.8*). Thus a few additional closely spaced electrodes may prove useful in the routine EEG of patients with partial epilepsy. We utilize this technique of additional electrodes frequently in our

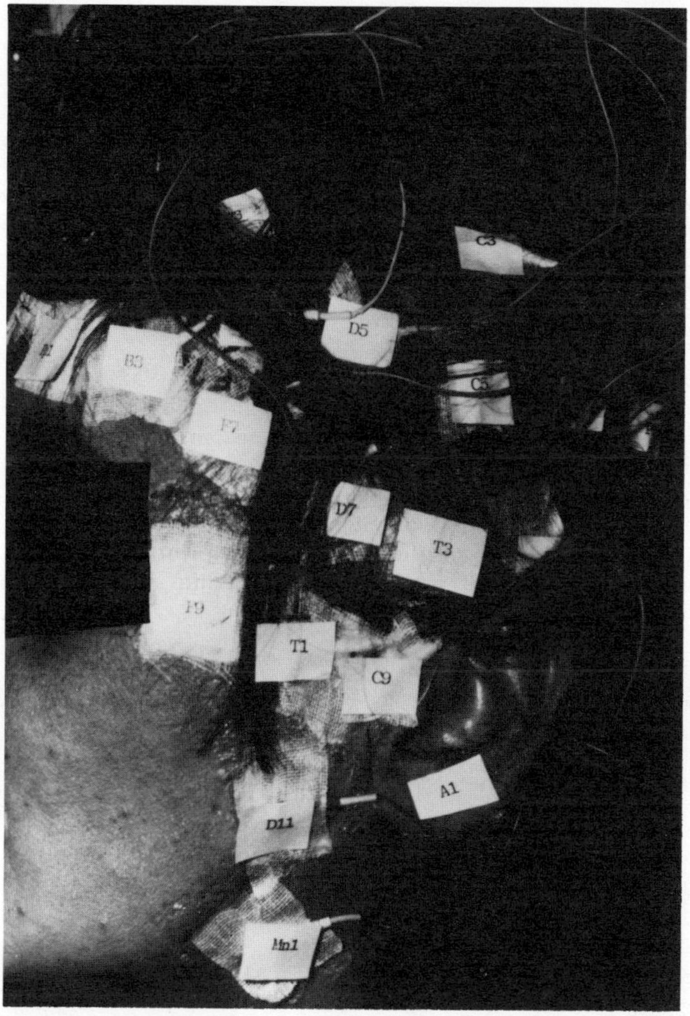

Figure 8.8 Additional closely spaced electrodes in a 34-year-old with complex partial seizures from a left temporal epileptogenic focus

more prolonged evaluations of patients with partial epilepsy. The relationship of these electrodes to the underlying brain can be defined with a lateral skull X-ray. This is useful because of the variation in skull shapes; we have found prominent interindividual differences in electrode placements in relation to the underlying brain. In a series of 27 patients with complex partial seizures (Morris *et al.*, 1983) we found that the maximum activity was located at one of the additional closely spaced electrodes (not included in the 10–20 system) 31% of the time. We believe that additional electrodes, closely spaced and nasopharyngeal, have been extremely helpful in localizing more precisely epileptiform activity and gave essential information to plan further surgical workup of patients with partial epilepsy. Additional electrodes are also of help in clarifying further the location of ambiguously distributed foci, for example inferior frontal *vs.* anterior temporal.

NORMAL EEG

Normal variants confused with epileptiform activity

In the EEG of normal controls there are frequently sharp transients which are of no clinical significance but may be confused with epileptiform activity. It is extremely important to recognize these and not misinterpret them as epileptiform activity which can result in the misdiagnosis of epilepsy.

Small sharp spikes

Small sharp spikes (SSS) were first described by Gibbs and Gibbs (1952). Initially these sharp transients were interpreted as indicative of an epileptic disorder. However, subsequent studies have determined that these transients are of doubtful clinical significance (Reiher and Klass, 1968; White, Langston and Pedley, 1977). The incidence of this type of pattern was described to be between 6–8% in normal adults (Gibbs and Gibbs, 1952), as 3.7% in a psychiatric population (Small, 1970), and 1.36% in a population of epileptics and non-epileptics referred to the EEG laboratory (Kashino and Niedermeyer, 1975). In the study by White, Langston and

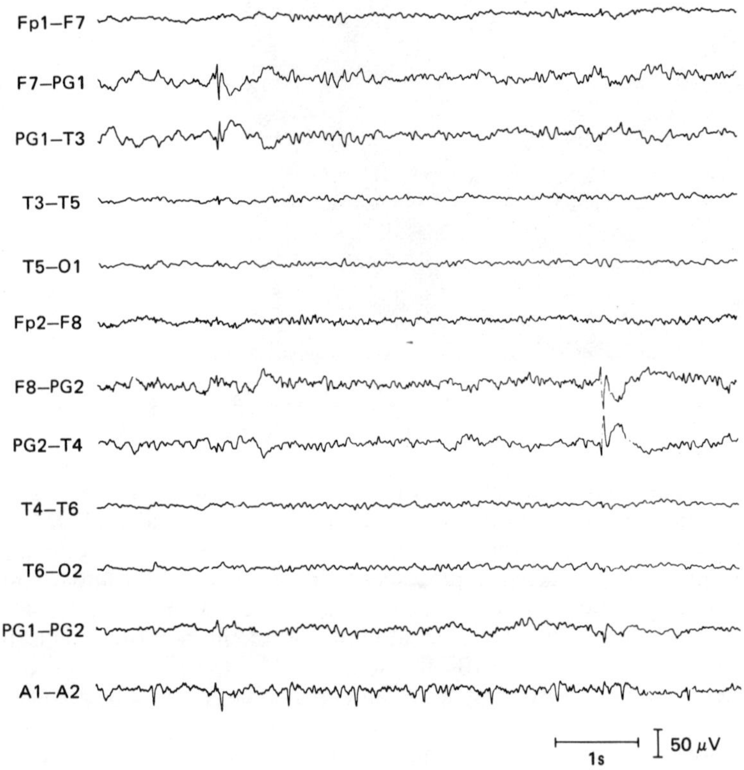

Figure 8.9 Small sharp spikes independently in the left and right temporal regions in a man with headaches and nocturnal seizures

Pedley (1977) the incidence in a population of normal volunteers was shown to be 24%, 20% in unselected patients referred to the EEG lab and in 14% of patients with complex partial seizures. The morphology of this sharp transient is remarkably constant, typically monophasic or diphasic (*Figure 8.9*). Characteristically the decline after the first negative peak is extremely steep and the transient has a short duration of 35–90 ms. The amplitude may vary considerably, less than 50 or as high as 135 μV. The amplitude is greatly increased by long interelectrode distances such as with use of the scalp–ear and scalp–nasopharyngeal derivations. The most prominent deflection of the transient is usually negative in polarity. Small sharp spikes may be confused with temporal spikes of complex partial seizures. Small sharp spikes are frequently sporadic, bilateral and independent, with a broad distribution, consistent morphology, and occur in stage 1 and 2 of non-REM sleep. In contrast, epileptiform temporal spikes are frequently repetitive in runs and bursts, usually unilateral, with a more focal distribution, non-stereotyped morphology and occur awake and increased in sleep.

Positive spikes (6 and 14 Hz)

In 1951 Gibbs and Gibbs reported their findings of 14 and 6 Hz positive spikes in the EEGs of 6% of 5000 epileptic patients and in 2% of 300 normals. The positive spikes occurred predominantly during sleep, only 3% during wakefulness. Of the patients that they had classified as epileptic they found that many had episodic symptomatology of rage, flushing, headache, nausea and vomiting. The Gibbs' initially hypothesized that the positive spikes originated in the thalamus and hypothalamus and are an expression of a type of epilepsy producing the above-mentioned symptomatology. Following this initial report subsequent authors attempted to associate this type of EEG pattern with paroxysmal symptomatology and epilepsy (Grossman, 1954; Kellaway, Crawley and Kagawa, 1959; Nidermeyer and Croft, 1961; Weir and Anderson, 1958). However, subsequent controlled studies have failed to demonstrate any association of this pattern with consistent clinical symptomatology. The first controlled prospective study was performed in a group of 74 children aged 5–20 years referred for EEGs (Walter *et al.*, 1960). They concluded that there was no difference in the different clinical subgroups with reference to the presence of positive spikes in EEG. Wiener *et al.* (1966) looked at the EEGs of 150 healthy male subjects age 13–18 years, 80 of whom had been judged delinquent by the courts, and the rest volunteers from the local community. Excluded were any patients with organic brain disease or mental retardation. The incidence of positive spikes in the two groups was similar at 13%. In another study of 212 normal male subjects this pattern was found in 58% of the records in which sleep was obtained (Lombroso *et al.*, 1966). Today it is well accepted that 14 Hz and 6 Hz positive spikes are of no clinical significance and not associated with the diagnosis of epilepsy. The recording of the 6 Hz and 14 Hz activity varies with age. The 6 Hz positive spikes appear to be more common in children less than 1 year of age and thereafter 14 Hz positive spikes rather than, or in combination with, 6 Hz spikes are common until the age of 40 when the 6 Hz positive spikes again become more prominent (Gibbs and Gibbs, 1963). The sharp transients usually appear in short runs lasting less than two seconds and may occur unilaterally or bilaterally synchronously or independently (*Figure 8.10*). The morphology of the transients consist of a sharply peaked positive spike alternating with a rounded negative

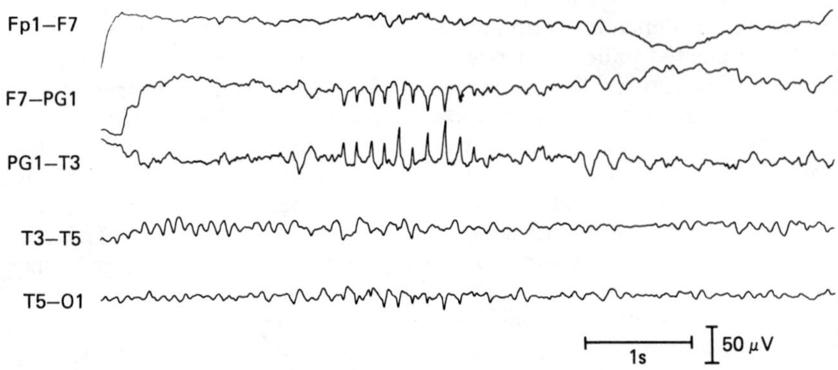

Figure 8.10 Burst of 6 Hz and 14 Hz positive spikes in the left temporal region in 19-year-old man with behavior disorder

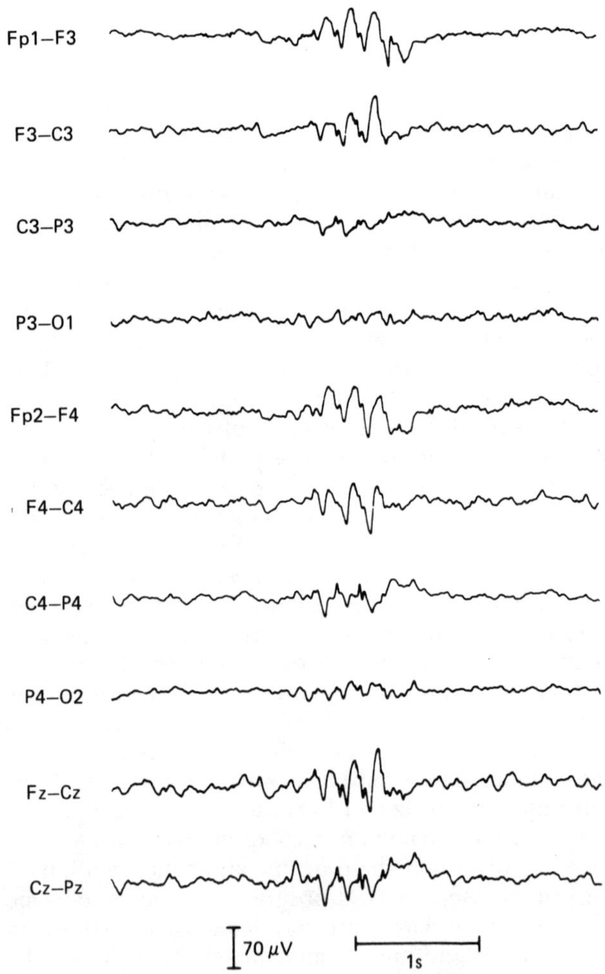

Figure 8.11 Burst of 6 Hz phantom spike and wave in a diffuse distribution in a 14-year-old boy with headaches and dizziness

component with amplitudes varying from 20–60 μV. The spikes are usually distributed maximally in the posterior temporal region. The polarity and typical frequency are the two main distinguishing features from temporal spikes.

Phantom spike and wave (6 Hz)

This entity was first described by Walter (1950). In many of the earlier studies, the phantom spike and wave pattern was frequently associated with various kinds of seizure disorders. Marshall (1955) found an association with seizures in 45% and syncope in 45% of a group of patients. Thomas (1957) found an association with seizures in 59% of patients, and Hughes, Schlagenhauff and Magoss (1965) 62% in their patients. However, it is important to remember that the majority of these studies lacked the proper controls and as a result the findings are likely to be skewed. In contrast to this, subsequent studies have failed to show the association of this pattern with any specific clinical symptomatology and in particular with epilepsy. In a subsequent group of patients studied by Thomas and Klass (1968) there was no statistical significant difference of this pattern in a group of patients with epilepsy compared with age-matched controls. Similarly in a study in patients with acute psychiatric disorders, these patients did not differ significantly from the control group with regard to the incidence of seizures, syncope, head injuries and emotional disturbances (Small, 1968). The overall incidence of this EEG pattern ranges from 0.4 (Hughes, Schlagenhauff and Magoss, 1965) to 4.5% (Small, Sharpley and Small, 1968). The pattern consists of small diphasic spikes with an amplitude of less than 20 μV and duration of less than 30 ms followed by high amplitude slow waves of up to 100 μV at a frequency of approximately 6 Hz (*Figure 8.11*). The burst of the spike and wave pattern is usually less than 1 s, although occasionally it may be as long as 2–3 s in duration. The distribution of the pattern is usually diffuse, bisynchronous and bilaterally symmetrical.

Psychomotor variant

This pattern was again first described by Gibbs and Gibbs (1952) and termed psychomotor variant because of its resemblance to discharges seen in patients with psychomotor epilepsy. Early investigators frequently considered the psychomotor variant to be a seizure disorder, primarily because of its paroxysmal nature and characteristic pattern. Gibbs' data described a high incidence of various episodic disorders, including headache, nausea, vomiting, and dizziness in patients with the psychomotor variant pattern, and anecdotal evidence for improvement with anticonvulsants led to support for this opinion. However, later a review of 1000 consecutive EEGs of patients in a psychiatric setting could document no significant correlation between this pattern and autonomical behavioral dysfunction or seizures (Small, Sharpley and Small, 1968). The incidence of this pattern is variable but most commonly occurs in young adults and adolescents. The incidence is 0.5–1.5% in this population. It usually occurs with equal frequency on both sides of the head and can be precipitated by photic stimulation or hyperventilation. However, it is most evident during drowsiness. The frequency of the pattern is 4–7 Hz, most usually 5–6 Hz. The bursts may appear for 1–10 sec in duration and not infrequently longer. The morphology is characterized by notched or

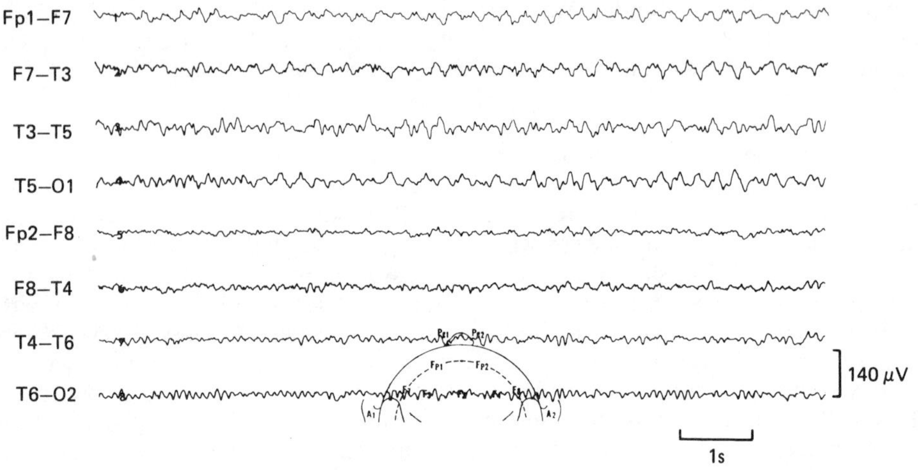

Figure 8.12 Psychomotor variant pattern in left temporal region; the patient had a history of generalized tonic-clonic and absence seizures with 3 Hz spike and wave complexes

sawtoothed waves of medium to high amplitude (*Figure 8.12*). The pattern is usually maximal in the mid-temporal region and may occur unilaterally (27%) or bilaterally (73%), occurring independently with various degrees of synchrony.

Wicket spikes

This is another rhythm which may on occasion be confused with epileptiform activity which is, however, of no clinical significance. It was initially described to occur in 39 of a total of 4458 EEGs performed in their laboratory (Reiher and Lebel, 1977). This pattern is characterized by transients of 60-100 μV in amplitude found both in the awake and sleep states occurring in intermittent bursts in the mid-temporal region (*Figure 8.13*). The transients are of surface negative polarity and on occasion may occur as single sharp transients which may be difficult to distinguish from anterior or mid-temporal spikes. The frequency of the transients is 6–11 Hz and they appear to be monophasic in morphology, not followed by any slow wave. They are characteristically recorded over the temporal regions, usually bilaterally and independently. Their stereotyped monophasic morphology and lack of associated slow waves help differentiate these transients from temporal sharp waves of complex partial seizures.

Subclinical rhythmic EEG discharges of adults (SREDA)

This is a distinctive EEG pattern which closely resembles an EEG seizure pattern but is not associated with any clinical manifestations. In a group of 65 patients described by Westmoreland and Klass (1981) the pattern occurred in patients with diverse clinical complaints. There was a low incidence of any history of seizures and seizures did not develop in patients followed for up to 12 years.

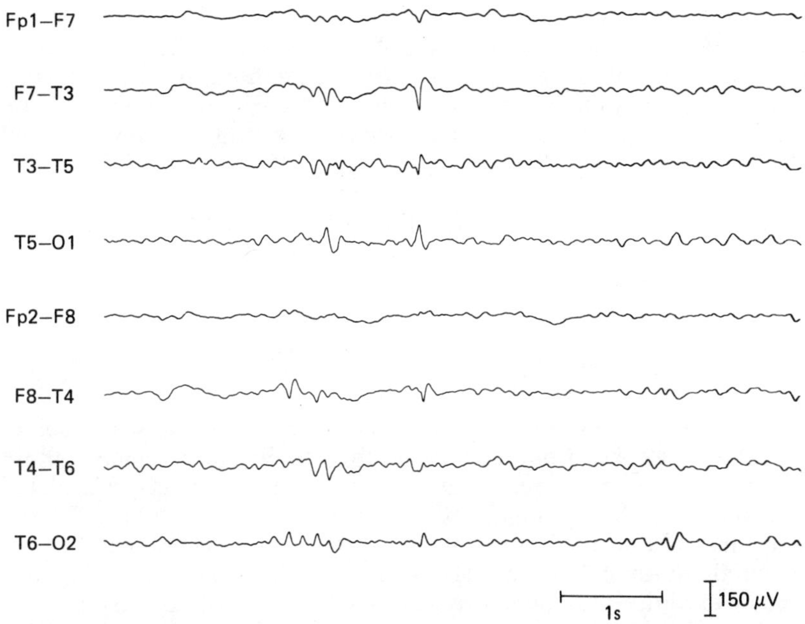

Figure 8.13 Wicket spike in left temporal region in a 36-year-old woman with generalized tonic-clonic seizures; the EEG also showed generalized slow spike and wave complexes

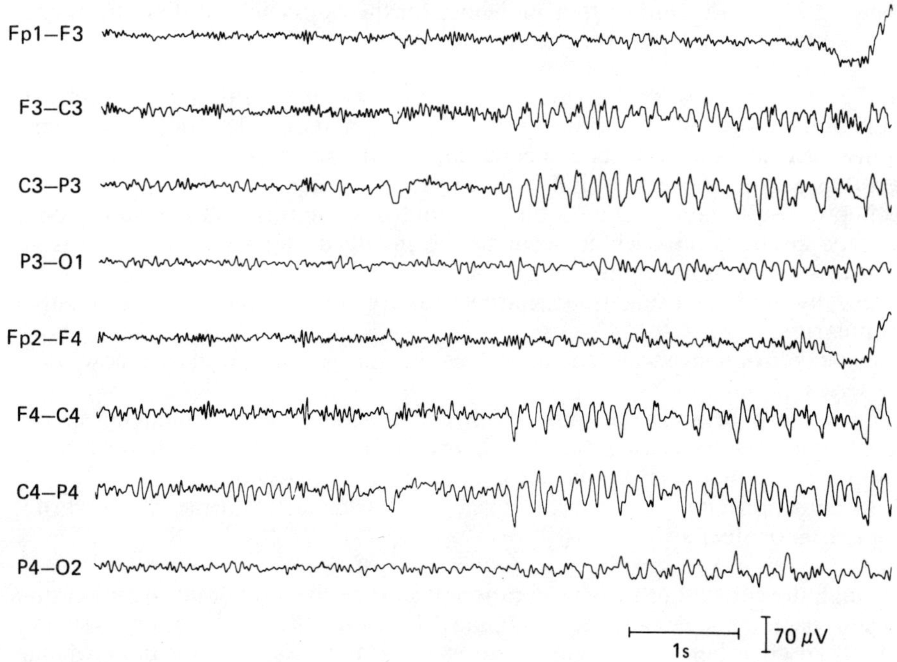

Figure 8.14 Onset of subclinical rhythmic EEG discharge of adults in a 65-year-old woman with a history of generalized seizures

The EEG pattern was fairly stereotyped in a particular patient. The EEG pattern has an abrupt onset with an average duration of 40–80 s (*Figure 8.14*). The usual frequency of the sustained discharges is 5–6 Hz with an amplitude of 40–100 μV in a diffuse distribution over both hemispheres maximum posteriorly. The termination of the pattern is abrupt or gradual. Various activities such as eye opening and closing, hyperventilation and mental activity have little effect on the discharges.

All of the above sharp transients are well accepted as transients of no clinical significance and in particular are not epileptiform in nature. It is important to recognize these and not to misinterpret these as epileptiform transients supporting a clinical diagnosis of epilepsy.

EPILEPTIFORM ABNORMALITIES

Epileptiform activity is an interpretative term which is applied to transients, spikes and sharp waves, distinguished from the background activity and resembling those recorded in a proportion of patients with epilepsy. A transient is any isolated waveform or complex which is distinguished from the background activity. A spike is defined as a transient clearly distinguished from the background activity, with a pointed peak and duration of 20–70 ms. The main component is generally negative in polarity and is of variable amplitude (Chatrian *et al.*, 1974). A sharp wave is defined similarly but its duration is 70-200 msec. Spikes and sharp waves occurring interictally may give evidence to support a clinical diagnosis of epilepsy. However, there may be difficulty distinguishing specific epileptiform activity from the non-epileptiform sharp transients which have been discussed in the section above. Maulsby (1971) set forward certain guidelines for the assessment of sharp transients in deciding what is epileptiform and what is not.

(1) Spikes and sharp waves of cerebral origin always have a definable electrical field and thus should be seen to involve more than one electrode. Any sharp transient which only affects one electrode should be regarded as an artifact. If one has reason to suspect that such a transient is cerebral in origin, possibly epileptiform in nature, one should set about proving this by adding additional closely spaced electrodes adjacent to the involved electrode to demonstrate that it is cerebral in origin.
(2) Clinically significant spikes and sharp waves are almost always surface negative in polarity.
(3) Most spikes or sharp waves of clinical significance are followed by a slow wave or series of slow waves.
(4) Ignore sharp or spikey events which can be logically explained by simple alterations in voltages of existing background rhythms or by superimposition of several components in the background activity of the record.
(5) Recognize phsyiological sharp transients, particularly during sleep–vertex transients of sleep.

Although the concept of the classification of seizures into generalized and partial may date back to the time of Hughlings Jackson, the terminology was not commonly used when describing seizures until the first classification of the International League Against Epilepsy (ILAE) in 1969 (Gastaut, 1970). In partial seizures only a localized part of the brain is epileptogenic, whereas in generalized seizures the entire brain is diffusely epileptogenic. The EEG will demonstrate similarly epileptiform activity which is focal in distribution or generalized. Focal seizures tend to trigger secondary generalized seizures and differentiation clinically may be very difficult when the focal component at the onset is of short duration. In some patients all clinical seizures may appear generalized from the onset and their focal nature may only be detected by the EEG. In patients with two epileptogenic foci and a marked tendency to secondary generalization, the differentiation between partial and generalized seizures is usually impossible. Multiple (three or more) epileptogenic foci almost invariably result in secondary generalization and these cases are usually classified as generalized seizures.

Epileptiform activity thus can be discussed as generalized or focal.

Correlation with generalized seizures

Generalized epileptiform activity is the only EEG abnormality that supports the diagnosis of generalized seizures. This activity is usually in the form of spike and wave (*Figure 8.15*) or sharp and wave complexes. Less frequently, polyspikes (*Figure 8.16*) or polysharp waves, paroxysmal beta or alpha are seen. Once the epileptiform nature of the activity is established, the distribution is more important than the waveform. In generalized seizures the discharges tend to be diffuse but are not of equal amplitude at all electrodes. Usually the maximum occurs at the

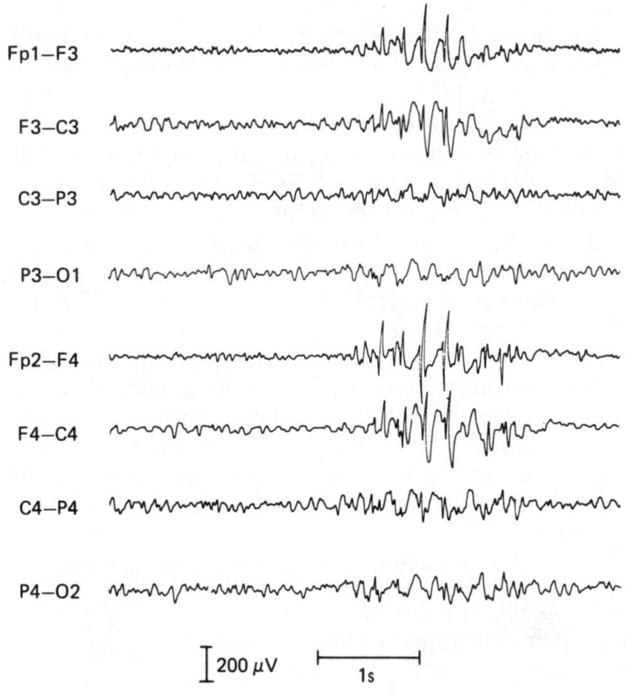

Figure 8.15 Burst of generalized spike and wave complexes in a 25-year-old woman with generalized tonic-clonic seizures

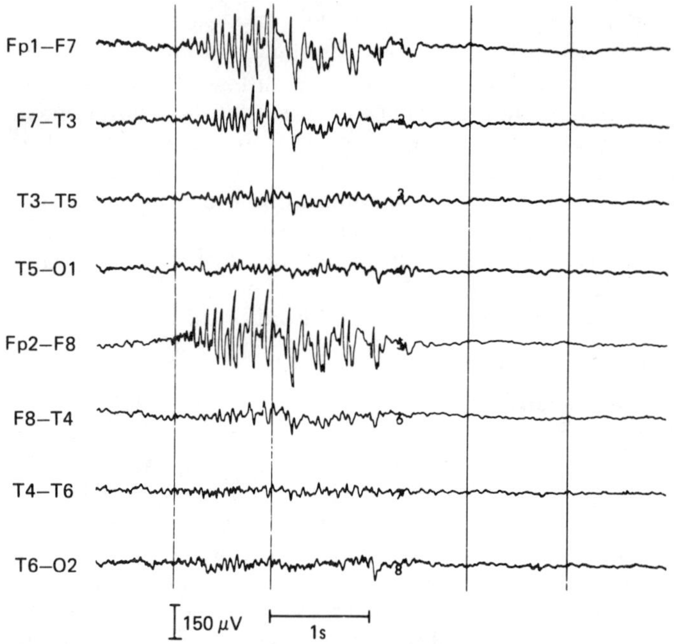

Figure 8.16 Burst of polyspikes during sleep in a patient with absence seizures

superior frontal or central electrodes, with a marked fall-off posteriorly and laterally. Sometimes this fall-off of activity posteriorly and laterally is so pronounced that the discharges appear as bifrontal or bicentral spikes rather than generalized spike and wave complexes. Frequently in generalized seizures, unilateral focal spikes that shift from side to side may occur in the frontal or central region. In cases with infrequent discharges, a routine EEG sample of only 20–30 minutes may demonstrate focal discharges on one side only. Additional recordings would be necessary to differentiate between a focal and a generalized seizure disorder with an interictal focal discharge. In other words, in a generalized seizure disorder, the EEG frequently may show focal epileptiform abnormalities of shifting lateralization and/or localization. Besides, the generalized discharges are usually asymmetric but the maximum shifts from side to side. In addition all transition forms along the following continuum may be seen: (a) strictly unilateral focal spikes, (b) bifrontal maximum left or right hemisphere, (c) generalized maximum left or right hemisphere, (d) generalized bilateral symmetrical. In our laboratory, all these more or less focal or lateralized epileptiform focal discharges are described in the body of the report but not in the classification and impression if consistent with a generalized seizure disorder.

The following generalized EEG patterns have definite clinical correlations:

(1) 3 Hz spike and wave complex: generalized absence.
(2) Slow spike and wave complex: minor motor seizures.
(3) Hypsarrhythmia: infantile spasm.
(4) Multifocal independent spikes: minor motor seizures (tonic, atonic, atypical absence or infantile spasms).
(5) Polyspike and wave complex: myoclonic seizures.

Spike and wave complexes (3 Hz)

The definitive pattern consists of bursts of spike and wave complexes lasting at least 3 s, at a repetition rate of approximately 3 Hz with a short, spike component (50–80 ms) (*Figure 8.17*). Spike and wave complexes tend to have a faster repetition rate at the beginning (4–5 Hz), then stabilize at around 3 Hz (always more than 2.5 Hz) during the main part of the burst, finally slowing down at the end. The bursts have a clearly defined onset and an abrupt cessation. Frequently, shifting asymmetries occur at the beginning of the burst. The bursts occur most frequently in the waking and the REM sleep stage and are activated by hyperventilation. The most characteristic feature is the association with clinical or subclinical unresponsiveness. This is easily tested with a clicker (*see below*). Bursts of spike and wave complexes with some atypical features should be thus classified as 3 Hz spike and wave complexes only if associated with relative unresponsiveness. Otherwise they are simply called generalized spike and wave complexes. Conservative labelling of the 3 Hz spike and wave pattern will significantly increase its specific correlation with clinical absences. It is important to remember that an EEG pattern classified as generalized spike and wave complexes strongly supports the diagnosis of generalized epilepsy and is certainly compatible with clinical absences even if not specific for this type of epilepsy.

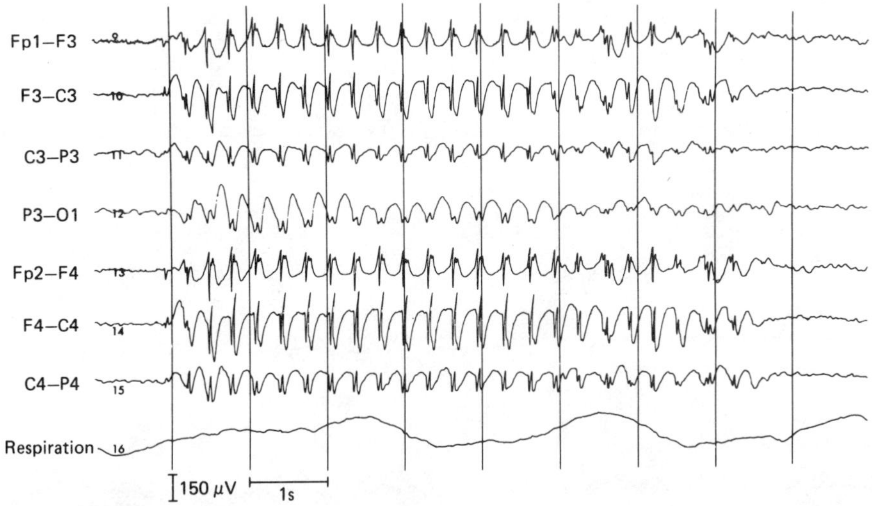

Figure 8.17 Burst of 3 Hz spike and wave complexes in a patient with absence seizures

In addition to the typical 3 Hz spike and wave complexes, focal left or right frontal spikes, atypical short bursts of spike and wave complexes and irregular bursts of polyspikes and waves may occur. The last two patterns are most frequent in slow-wave sleep when the long bursts are replaced by progressively more frequent bursts of shorter duration, irregular repetition rate, and the appearance of polyspikes. It is not infrequent that a patient with absence seizures may only show atypical bursts of generalized spike and wave complexes during sleep. This often occurs when the patient is clinically asymptomatic or exhibits only generalized tonic-clonic seizures at the time of the test.

Slow spike and wave complexes

The characteristic pattern consists of bursts of spike and wave complexes of at least 3 s, repeating at less than 2.5 Hz (*Figure 8.18*). The 'spike' component of the spike and wave complexes is actually a sharp wave with a relatively long duration of more than 80 ms. Frequently, a significant proportion of the record is occupied by slow sharp and wave complexes in bursts of variable duration. Only rarely can one

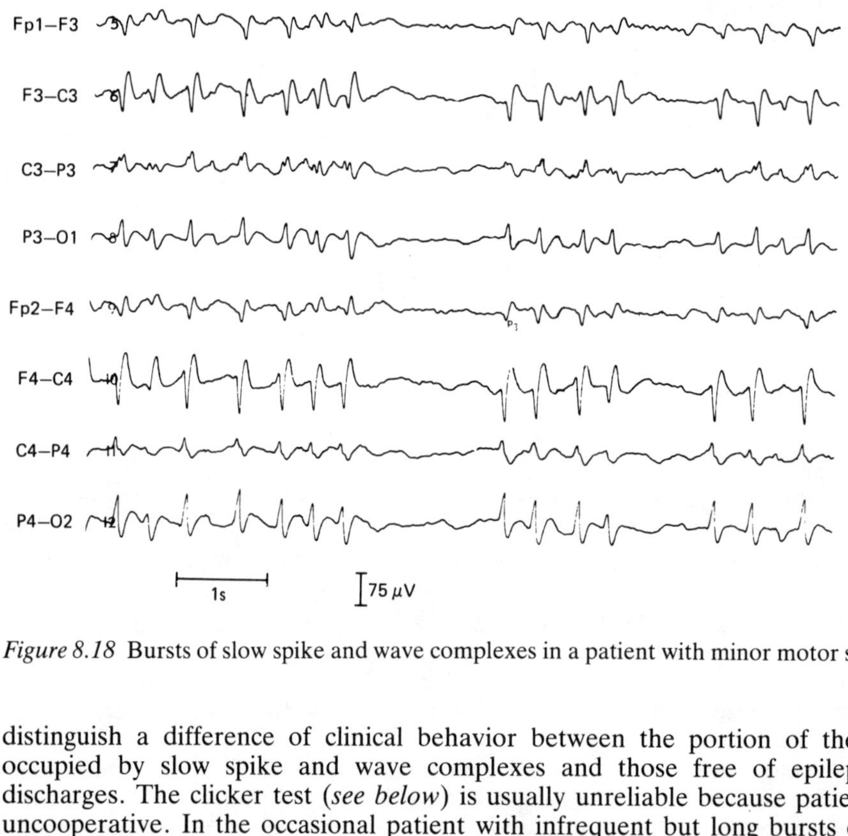

Figure 8.18 Bursts of slow spike and wave complexes in a patient with minor motor seizures

distinguish a difference of clinical behavior between the portion of the EEG occupied by slow spike and wave complexes and those free of epileptiform discharges. The clicker test (*see below*) is usually unreliable because patients are uncooperative. In the occasional patient with infrequent but long bursts of slow spike and wave complexes, a behavior change can be correlated with each burst (relative unresponsiveness, complex automatisms). Frequently, the background rhythm of patients with slow spike and wave complexes is relatively slow for the age of the patient. Almost always, one sees other epileptiform discharges, such as generalized atypical spike and wave complexes, focal left or right frontal spikes, and occasionally in more atypical locations, particularly in the occipital areas. Irregular, short bursts of polyspikes and wave complexes during sleep are also noticed. A fairly characteristic feature is the occurrence of electrodecremental episodes, frequently with superimposed paroxysmal fast activity. These episodes vary between 1 and 10 s and are most frequent during sleep. Longer episodes are typically associated with either tonic, akinetic or atonic seizures or their combination.

Hypsarrhythmia

The characteristic pattern for this EEG classification consists of continuous multifocal independent spikes superimposed on a slow background in the delta range, which has an average amplitude of at least 300 μV (*Figure 8.19*). During sleep, the epileptiform discharges are more prominent and tend to group in 1–10 s bursts of slow waves with superimposed multifocal spikes. These bursts are

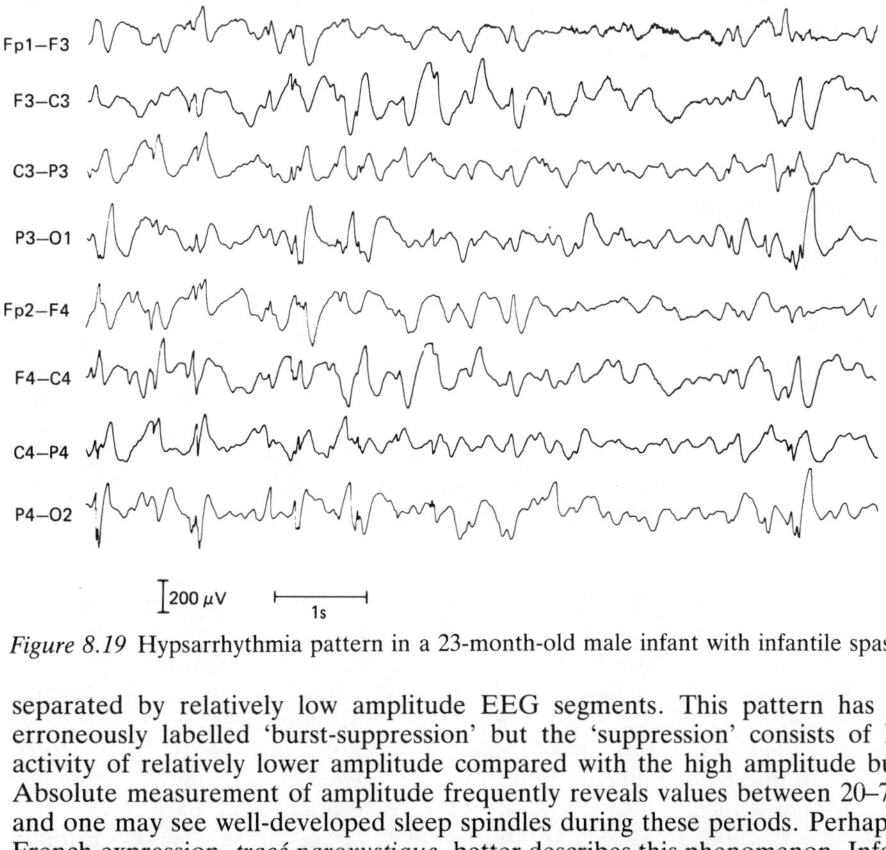

Figure 8.19 Hypsarrhythmia pattern in a 23-month-old male infant with infantile spasms

separated by relatively low amplitude EEG segments. This pattern has been erroneously labelled 'burst-suppression' but the 'suppression' consists of EEG activity of relatively lower amplitude compared with the high amplitude bursts. Absolute measurement of amplitude frequently reveals values between 20–70 μV and one may see well-developed sleep spindles during these periods. Perhaps the French expression, *tracé paroxystique*, better describes this phenomenon. Infantile spasms are typically associated with 5–10 second electrodecremental patterns, which may be associated with low amplitude paroxysmal beta or alpha waves, particularly at the end. The pattern is frequently inconspicuous and can be easily missed. Careful clinical observation by the technologist and the corresponding notations on the record are extremely helpful for correct identification of the ictal nature of this pattern. As in all other typical patterns, one may see generalized spike and wave, or polyspike and wave complexes.

Multifocal independent spikes

This pattern is very similar to hypsarrhythmia except that the background is not in the delta range and/or is of less than 300 μV amplitude. The ictal patterns are identical to slow spike and wave complexes, or hypsarrhythmia. It is important to differentiate the multifocal independent spike pattern from the multifocal independent sharp waves frequently seen in benign focal epilepsy of childhood.

Polyspike and slow wave complexes

Polyspike and slow wave complexes are frequently seen during sleep in association with any of the above patterns. In addition, it is not infrequent to see spike and wave complexes with two or three spikes preceding the slow wave in patients who do not have myoclonic epilepsy. Therefore, this pattern is of very limited specificity and is of diagnostic value only in the awake tracing with a prominent polyspike component.

Correlation with partial seizures

Focal epileptiform activity

Only focal epileptiform activity supports the diagnosis of partial seizures. There is obviously a correlation between the location of the epileptogenic focus and the manifestation of the clinical seizure. The close relationship between anterior temporal spikes and complex partial seizures was first recognized by Gibbs, Gibbs and Fuster (1948). They found that 90% of the cases with anterior temporal spikes had complex partial seizures. Similarly, spikes in the primary motor cortex are associated with partial motor seizures; spikes in the occiptal region with visual seizures and similar electroclinical correlations can be found according to the location of the epileptogenic activity. The presence of focal epileptiform activity must be closely correlated with the clinical symptomatology, as occasionally spikes may occur in normal subjects without seizures. In a study of 1000 normal children, focal spikes were found in 1.5% (Petersen, Eeg-Olofsson and Sellden, 1968), and in a similar study Eeg-Olofsson, Petersen and Sellden (1971) reported 1.9%.

The morphology of specific epileptiform activity has been studied in complex partial seizures (*see Figure 8.6*). There is general agreement that from scalp electrodes spikes are recorded less frequently than sharp waves (Gastaut, 1950; Jasper, Pertuisset and Flanigin, 1951). The only exception is one report which found a higher incidence of spikes: 47% had spikes as opposed to sharp waves, 31% (Wada and Lennox, 1954). Sharp waves may be generated by the primary epileptogenic focus but frequently represent evoked potentials conducted from a distant source (Penfield and Jasper, 1954). Conduction to relatively distant scalp electrodes would produce temporal dispersion of the spike so that its duration would increase.

Analysis of spike foci by electrocorticography usually reveals involvement of an extensive cortical area (10 cm^2 or more) with numerous spike foci firing independently. It is when these small spike foci fire synchronously that discharges can be detected at the scalp.

Benign focal epileptiform discharges of childhood

Benign focal epilepsy of childhood is the term suggested by Blom (Blom, Heijbel and Bergfors, 1972) and refers to a distinctive clinical and electrical syndrome. The seizures usually have a good prognosis and are associated with epileptiform discharges with specific features in the central-temporal-parietal regions which are frequently mutlifocal and independent. The main characteristics of these discharges are as follows (*Figure 8.20*):

(1) The posterior background rhythm is within normal limits for its age group.
(2) The discharges are sharp waves (duration longer than 70 msec).
(3) The sharp waves are followed by predominantly positive slow waves, with a negative phase of usually lower amplitude than the preceding sharp wave.
(4) The sharp waves are of extremely stereotyped waveform, even if varied in amplitude.

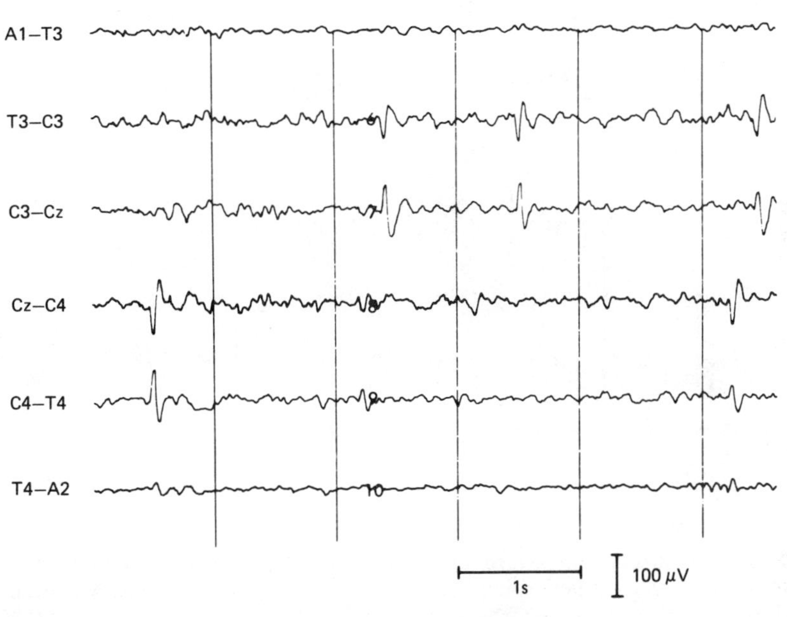

Figure 8.20 Benign focal epileptiform discharges of childhood occurring bifocally and independently in the left and right central regions in an 11-year-old boy with a 2-year history of migraine but no seizures

(5) Horizontal dipoles are characteristic, even if not always present.
(6) The discharges are inhibited by mental activation, hyperventilation, photic stimulation, and increased markedly by sleep. Not infrequently the pattern is present only during sleep.
(7) Usually there are only three to four discrete foci which fire independently or one will trigger the other.
(8) The discharges are not associated with generalized spike and wave complexes. This type of epilepsy is common in children, 16% in one series of childhood epileptics (Blom, Heijbel and Bergfors, 1972), and the prognosis is excellent. One study found 100% of the patients seizure-free by age 15 (Lerman and Kivity, 1975) and another 95% seizure free (Blom, Heijbel and Bergors, 1972).

Periodic lateralizing epileptiform discharges (PLEDs)

PLEDs are sharp waves which appear in a periodic or semiperiodic fashion and have a generalized but clearly lateralized distribution or a focal distribution (*Figure 8.21*). PLEDs may appear bilaterally and independently in each hemisphere (Smith 1975). PLEDs usually occur in association with a slow background activity related

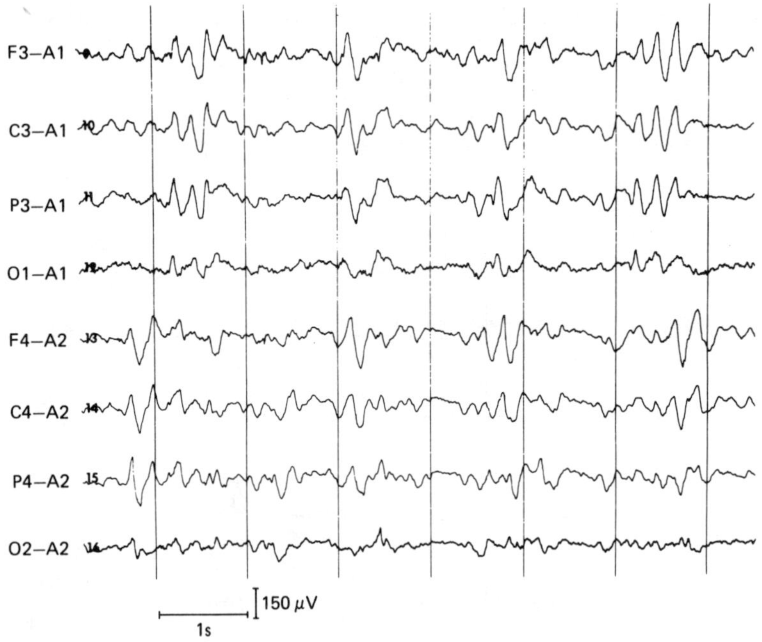

Figure 8.21 Periodic lateralizing epileptiform discharges (PLEDs) occurring bilaterally and independently in the left and right hemispheres in a 53-year-old woman with biopsy-proven herpes encephalitis

to the obtundation which is frequently a prominent clinical manifestation in the patient demonstrating this abnormality. PLEDs are seen in: (a) acute or subacute, severe focal destructive lesions (most often cerebrovascular accident or fast growing tumors); or (b) focal epileptogenic lesions not necessarily associated with significant underlying structural pathology. In both cases the patient presents focal clinical seizures at least during one stage of the illness. Nevertheless only infrequently each discharge is accompanied by clinical motor manifestations (epilepsia partialis continua). When associated with acute structural lesions, PLEDs tend to occur only for a few days or weeks in the acute stage of the illness. The prognosis of the associated seizures is good, ceasing spontaneously after 3–10 days. The incidence of PLEDs appears to be low, 0.4% in one series (Chatrian, Shaw and Leffman, 1964).

THE ROLE OF EEG IN THE DIAGNOSIS OF EPILEPSY

The EEG is only diagnostic of epilepsy when ictal epileptiform activity is recorded in association with a clinical seizure. The recording of interictal epileptiform activity provides strong supportive evidence for epilepsy if there is an appropriate clinical history of a seizure. The distribution of the epileptiform activity may provide important information as to the type of seizure disorder. On occasion it is difficult to differentiate if absence seizures or complex partial seizures are responsible for recurrent episodes of staring, unresponsiveness and automatisms in a particular patient. The EEG besides supporting the diagnosis of a seizure disorder in such a case will distinguish these two types of epilepsy.

The frequency of epileptiform discharges varies in the different types of epilepsy. In patients with frequent absence seizures virtually 100% will demonstrate 3 Hz spike and wave complexes in their EEGs with hyperventilation or sleep. In patients with rare seizures it is more frequent to find a normal than an epileptiform EEG. However, the presence of frequent seizures in association with an EEG or repeated EEGs devoid of epileptiform activity may occasionally occur. The studies of incidence of EEG abnormalities in complex partial seizures report a significant proportion of patients who have no EEG abnormality. Normal EEGs were reported in 18% of Christian's (1962) series and 10% of Gastaut's (1953) series. In patients with fairly frequent seizures, the absence of specific epileptiform discharges makes us consider the possibility that the patient's symptomatology is not of an epileptic nature. Additional recording should be obtained and is frequently associated with anticonvulsant withdrawal to optimize the chance of recording interictal epileptiform activity and seizures. The recording of clinical 'seizures' without associated change in the EEG activity is consistent with psychogenic seizures.

On the other hand the presence of epileptiform activity is not diagnostic of epilepsy. In children with benign focal epileptiform discharges not all have epilepsy. The incidence of seizures in one series was 85% (Beaussart, 1972).

THE ROLE OF EEG IN THE TREATMENT OF EPILEPSY

The EEG helps firstly to support the diagnosis and also to define the type of epilepsy. The EEG is extremely important in the differentiation of epileptic and psychogenic seizures, thus allowing specific appropriate treatment to be instituted, psychotherapy for psychogenic seizures and anticonvulsants for epileptic seizures.

The choice of medication appropriate to the type of epilepsy can then be made. This is important as the patient with staring spells and a diagnosis of absence seizures will be treated with ethosuximide; whereas if the diagnosis is complex partial seizures carbamazepine may be the drug of choice. The EEG may be used for the evaluation of the response to treatment. Hyperventilation is an extremely effective activator of 3 Hz spike and wave complexes in absence seizures. This method can thus be used in patients treated for absence as one of the parameters to follow their progress. In general one would expect that the epileptiform activity would be suppressed when the seizure disorder is being treated with an appropriate and effective anticonvulsant. However, occasionally one sees EEGs of patients whose seizures are well controlled that demonstrate frequent interictal epileptiform activity. Such is the case of benign focal epilepsy of childhood. On the other hand, one also may see patients with medically intractable seizures whose EEGs may show no interictal epileptiform activity. Thus there is a certain limitation of the use of the EEG in the routine follow-up of patients with epilepsy. Thus we do not use periodic EEGs in the routine follow-up of patients with epilepsy.

Patients who have had their epilepsy controlled with anticonvulsants for a period of years are candidates for withdrawal of their medication. However, in two recent series the recurrence of seizures after medication withdrawal was significant, 28% (Thurston *et al.*, 1982) and 31% (Emerson *et al.*, 1981). EEG is one of the tests used to predict the possibility of recurrence. The above two recent studies have addressed this issue. Emerson's study indicates that the EEG is of benefit in predicting which patients can be withdrawn from medication, but according to Thurston's study the EEG is of no prognostic value. We think that the EEG is of value in this respect and have used it routinely for this purpose.

THE FUTURE OF NON-INVASIVE TECHNIQUES OF EEG

The EEG provides the only technique for the specific objective diagnosis of epilepsy, by recording the interictal and ictal electrophysiological manifestations of seizures, and it will continue to do so. In recent years computer systems have been developed for the automatic recognition of interictal spikes and sharp waves, their quantification and distribution (Gotman and Gloor, 1976) and automatic recognition of epileptic seizures (Gotman, 1982). Such systems have been put into practical use with prolonged EEG monitoring of patients who are being evaluated for surgery of epilepsy, as at the Montreal Neurological Institute. This system has the advantages of: (a) reducing the amount of EEG paper to be reviewed; (b) assisting in the quantification and distribution of interictal epileptiform activity; (c) automatically recognizing and storing seizures which facilitates easy review by the electroencephalographer. However, in these systems artifacts, both biological (eye movement and muscle activity) and technical (electrode pops) remain a major source of difficulty for automatic detection methods. The use of computer systems in the routine EEG to our knowledge are currently not in use for evaluation of patients with epilepsy. However, in the future one can anticipate that computer programs will become available to eliminate effectively some of the artifacts that presently pervade the current systems and the introduction of low-priced computers will allow these systems to be introduced to the routine EEG laboratory on a broad scale and be used in the routine evaluation of epilepsy.

MAGNETOENCEPHALOGRAPHY (MEG)

In addition to the electrical potentials which can be recorded on the scalp, there is also a magnetic field that can be recorded over the head. Magnetoencephalography is the recording of magnetic fields associated with current flow within the human brain. The study of the electrophysiological properties of the brain with magnetoencephalography is still in its infancy and its current applicability is mainly as a research tool. So far the best results with magnetoencephalography have been obtained in cases with focal activity localized to the lateral cortex. In cases of medial or basal cortical foci the magnetoencephalography activity is greatly reduced or absent even in the presence of significant EEG abnormalities. Further improvement in the technology of magnetoencephalography is necessary in order for this to become a clinically useful laboratory test. It seems unlikely that the magnetoencephalography will displace the EEG as the primary tool in the routine diagnosis of epilepsy.

References

AMERICAN EEG SOCIETY (1980) *Guidelines in EEG*

ANDERSEN, P. and ANDERSSON, S. A. (1976) Thalamic origin of cortical rhythmic activity. In *The Neuronal Generation of the EEG,* edited by O. Creutzfeldt. *Handbook of Electroencephalography and Clinical Neurophysiology,* **2C,** 90-118

BAKER, R. N. and KLASS, D. W. (1965) The metrazol activation of the normal brain. *Bulletin of the Los Angeles Neurological Societies,* **30,** 201–209

BEAUSSART, M. (1972) Benign epilepsy of children with Rolandic (centro-temporal) paroxysmal foci. *Epilepsia,* **13,** 794–811

BERGER, H. (1929) Über das Elektrenkephalogramm des Menschen. *Archiv für Psychiatrie,* **87,** 527–570

BERGER, H. (1931) Über das Elektrenkephalogramm des Menschen. *Arhiv für Psychiatrie,* **94,** 16–60

BISHOP, G. H. (1936) The interpretation of cortical potentials. *Cold Springs Harbor Symposia on Quantitative Biology,* **4,** 305–319

BLOM, S., HEIJBEL, J. and BERGFORS, P. G. (1972) Benign epilepsy of children with centro-temporal EEG foci. *Epilepsia,* **13,** 609–619

BLOM, S. (1975) Benign focal epilepsy of childhood with centro-temporal EEG foci: discharge rate during sleep. *Epilepsia,* **16,** 133–140

BOSTEM, F. (1976) Hyperventilation. In *Activation and Provocation Methods in Clinical Neurophysiology,* edited by R. Naquet. *Handbook of Electroencephalography and Clinical Neurophysiology,* **3D,** 74–88

CATON, R. (1875) The electrical currents of the brain. *British Medical Journal,* **2,** 278

CHATRIAN, G. E., SHAW, C. M. and LEFFMAN, H. (1964) Significance of periodic lateralized epileptiform discharges in EEG: an electrographic, clinical and pathological study. *Electroencephalography and Clinical Neurophysiology,* **17,** 177–193

CHATRIAN, G. E., BERGRAMINI, L., DONDEY, M., KLASS, D. W., LENNOX-BUCHTAL, M. and PETERSEN, I. (1974) A glossary of terms most commonly used by clinical electroencephalographers. *Electroencephalography and Clinical Neurophysiology,* **37,** 538–548

CHRISTIAN, W. (1962) EEG-Veränderungen bei der psychomotrischen Epilepsie. *Deutsche Zeitschrift für Nervenheilkunde,* **183,** 218–244

DINNER, D. S., LÜDERS, H., ROTHNER, A. D., and ERENBERG, G. E. (1984) Childhood onset CPS: a clinical and EEG study. *Cleveland Clinic Quarterly,* **51,** 287–291

ECCLES, J. C. (1951) Interpretation of action potentials evoked in the cerebral cortex. *Electroencephalography and Clinical Neurophysiology,* **3,** 449–464

EEG-OLOFSON, O., PETERSEN, I. and SELLDEN, U. (1971) The development of the EEG in normal children from the age of 1 to 15 years: paroxysmal activity. *Neuropädiatrie,* **4,** 375–404

EMERSON, R., D'SOUZA, B. J., VINING, E. P., HOLDEN, R. R., MELLITS, E. D. and FREEMAN, J. (1981) Stopping medication in children with epilepsy. *New England Journal of Medicine,* **304,** 1125–1129

FORSTER, F. M. (Ed.) (1977) *Reflex Epilepsy, Behavioral Therapy and Conditional Reflexes.* Springfield, Ill.: Charles C. Thomas

GASTAUT, H. (1950) Étude electroencephalographique du lobe temporal. *Revue d'Oto-Neuro-Ophtalmolosie,* **22,** 219–328

GASTAUT, H. (1953) So called 'psychomotor' and 'temporal' epilepsy: a critical study. *Epilepsia,* **2,** 59–76

GASTAUT, H. (1970) Clinical and EEG classification of epileptic seizures. *Epilepsia,* **11,** 102–110

GIBBS, E. L. and GIBBS, F. A. (1947) Diagnostic and localizing value of electroencephalographic studies in sleep. *Research Publications Association for Research in Nervous and Mental Disorders,* **23,** 366–376

GIBBS, E. L., GIBBS, F. A. and FUSTER, B. (1948) Psychomotor epilepsy. *Archives of Neurology and Psychiatry,* **60,** 331–339

GIBBS, E. L. and GIBBS, F. A. (1951) Electroencephalographic evidence of thalamic and hypothalamic epilepsy. *Neurology,* **1,** 136–144

GIBBS, F. A. and GIBBS, E. L. (1952) *Atlas of Electroencephalography,* pp. 346–358. 2nd ed. Vol. 2. Cambridge, Mass.: Addison-Wesley

GIBBS, F. A. and GIBBS, E. L. (1963) Fourteen and six per second positive spikes. *Electroencephalography and Clinical Neurophysiology,* **15,** 553–558

GLOOR, P., TSAI, C., HADDAD, F. and JASPER, H. H. (1957) The lack of necessity for sleep in the EEG or ECG diagnosis of temporal seizures. *Electroencephalography of Clinical Neurophysiology,* **9,** 379–380

GOTMAN, J. and GLOOR, P. (1976) Automatic recognition and quantification of interictal epileptic activity in the human scalp EEG. *Electroencephalography and Clinical Neurophysiology,* **41,** 513–529

GOTMAN, J. (1982) Automatic recognition of epileptic seizures in the EEG. *Electroencephalography and Clinical Neurophysiology,* **54,** 530–540

GROSSMAN, C. (1954) Laminar cortical blocking and its relation to episodic aggressive outbursts. *Archives of Neurology and Psychiatry (Chicago),* **71,** 576–587

HUGHES, J. R., SCHLAGENHAUFF, R. E. and MAGOSS, M. (1965) Electroclinical correlations in the six per second spike and wave complex. *Electroencephalography and Clinical Neurophysiology,* **18,** 71–75

IVES, J. R. and GLOOR, P. (1977) New sphenoidal electrode assembly to permit long-term monitoring of the patients ictal or interictal EEG. *Electroencephalography and Clinical Neurophysiology,* **42,** 575–580

JASPER, J., PERTUISSET, B. and FLANIGIN, H. (1951) EEG and cortical electrograms in patients with temporal lobe seizures. *Archives of Neurology and Psychiatry,* **65,** 272–290

JASPER, H. H. (1958) Report on the committee on methods of clinical examination in electroencephalography. *Electroencephalography and Clinical Neurophysiology,* **10,** 370–375

JONES, D. P. (1951) Recording of the basal electroencephalogram with sphenoidal needle electrodes. *Electroencephalography and Clinical Neurophysiology,* **3,** 100

KASHINO, Y. and NIEDERMEYER, E. (1975) The clinical significance of small sharp spikes in the electroencephalogram. *Clinical Electroencephalography,* **6,** 131–140

KELLAWAY, P., CRAWLEY, J. W., and KAGAWA, N. A. (1959) A specific electroencephalographic correlate of convulsive equivalent disorders in children. *Journal of Pediatrics,* **55,** 582–592

KLASS, D. W. and FISCHER-WILLIAMS, M. (1976) Sensory stimulation, sleep and sleep deprivation. In *Activation and Provocation Methods in Clinical Neurophysiology,* edited by R. Naquet. *Handbook of Electroencephalography and Clinical Neurophysiology,* **3D,** 5–73

KRISTENSEN, O. and SINDRUP, E. H. (1978) Sphenoidal electrodes, their use in the electroencephalographic investigation of complex partial epilepsy. *Acta Neurologica Scandinavica,* **58,** 157–166

LEHTINEN, L. O. J. and BERGSTRÖM, L. (1970) Naso-ethomoidal electrode for recording the electrical activity of the inferior surface of the frontal lobe. *Electroencephalography and Clinical Neurophysiology,* **29,** 303–305

LERMAN, P. and KIVITY, S. (1975) Benign focal epilepsy of childhood. *Archives of Neurology,* **32,** 261–264

LI, C. L. and JASPER, H. (1953) Microelectrode studies of the electrical activity of the cerebral cortex in the cat. *Journal of Physiology (London),* **121,** 117–140

LOMBROSO, C. T., SCHWARTZ, I. H., CLARK, D. M., MUENCH, H. and BARRY, J. (1966) Ctenoids in healthy adults. *Neurology,* **16,** 1152–1158

MACCLEAN, P. D. (1949) A new nasopharyngeal lead. *Electroencephalography and Clinical Neurophysiology,* **1,** 110–112

MARSHALL, C. (1955) Some clinical correlates of the wave and spike phantom. *Electroencephalography and Clinical Neurophysiology,* **7,** 633–663

MATTSON, R. H., PRATT, K. L. and CALVERLEY, J. R. (1965) Electroencephalograms of epileptics following sleep deprivation. *Archives of Neurology,* **13,** 310–315

MAULSBY, R. L. (1971) Some guidelines for assessment of spikes and sharp waves in EEG tracings. *American Journal of EEG Technology,* **1,** 3–16

MILEY, C. E. and FORSTER, F. M. (1977) Activation of complex partial seizures by hyperventilation. *Archives of Neurology,* **34,** 371–373

MORRIS, H. H., LUDERS, H., LESSER, R. P. and DINNER, D. S. (1983) Value of multiple electrodes in addition to standard 10/20 system electrodes localizing epileptiform foci. *Epilepsy International XV Meeting,* Washington, DC (abstract)

NEWMARK, M. E. and PENRY, J. K. (1979) *Photosensitivity and Epilepsy: A Review.* New York: Raven Press

NIEDERMEYER, E., ROCCA, U. (1972) The diagnostic significance of sleep electroencephalograms in temporal lobe epilepsy. *European Neurology,* **7,** 119–129

NIEDERMEYER, E. and CROFT, J. R. (1961) Über die bedeutung der 14 und 6 per sec positiven spitzen im EEG. *Archiv für Psychiatrie und Nervenkrankeiter (Berlin),* **202,** 266–280

PENFIELD, W. and JASPER, H. (1954) *Epilepsy and the Functional Anatomy of the Human Brain.* Boston: Little, Brown.

PETERSEN, I., EEG-OLOFSSON, O. and SELLDEN, U. (1968) Paroxysmal activity in EEG of normal children. In *Clinical Electroencephalography in Children,* edited by P. Kellaway and I. Petersen, pp. 167–187. Stockholm: Almqvist and Wiskell

PRATT, K. L., MATTSON, R. H., WEIKERS, N. J. and WILLIAMS, R. (1968) EEG activation of epileptics following sleep deprivation: a prospective study of 114 cases. *Electroencephalography and Clinical Neurophysiology,* **24,** 11–15

RAMANI, S. V., QUESNEY, L. F., OLSON, D. and GUMNIT, R. J. (1980) Diagnosis of hysterical seizures in epileptic patients. *American Journal of Psychiatry,* **137,** 705–709

REIHER, J. and KLASS, D. W. (1968) Two common EEG patterns of doubtful clinical significance. *Medical Clinics of North America,* **4,** 933–940

REIHER, J. and LEBEL, M. (1977) Wicket spikes: clinical correlates of a previously undescribed EEG pattern. *Canadian Journal of Neurological Sciences,* **4,** 39–47

ROVIT, R. L., GLOOR, P. and HENDERSON, L. R. (1960) Temporal lobe epilepsy – a study using multiple basal electrodes. I. Description of method. *Neurochirurgia,* **3,** 6–19

ROVIT, R. L., GLOOR, P. and RASMUSSEN, T. (1961) Sphenoidal electrodes in the electroencephalographic study of patients with temporal lobe epilepsy. *Journal of Neurosurgery,* **18,** 151–158

RUSHTON, D. N. (1981) 'Space Invader' epilepsy. *Lancet,* **1,** 50

SCOLLO-LAVIZZARRI, G., PRALLE, W. and RADUE, E. W. (1977) Comparative study of efficacy of waking and sleep recordings following sleep deprivation as an activation method in the diagnosis of epilepsy. *European Neurology,* **15,** 121–123

SILVERMAN, D. (1956) Sleep as a general activation procedure in electroencephalography. *Electroencephalography and Clinical Neurophysiology,* **8,** 317–324

SILVERMAN, D. (1960) The anterior temporal electrode and the ten-twenty system. *Electroencephalography and Clinical Neurophysiology,* **12,** 735–737

SMALL, J. G. (1968) The six per second spike and wave – a psychiatric population study. *Electroencephalography and Clinical Neurophysiology,* **24,** 561–568

SMALL, J. G. (1970) Small sharp spikes in a psychiatric population. *Archives of General Psychiatry,* **22,** 270–284

SMALL, J. G., SHARPLEY, P. and SMALL, I. F. (1968) Positive spikes, spike-wave phantoms, and psychomotor variants. *Archives of General Psychiatry,* **18,** 232–238

SMITH, J. B. (1975) A distinctive clinical EEG profile in herpes simplex encephalitis. *Mayo Clinic Proceedings,* **50,** 469–474

SPENCER, S. S., SPENCER, D. D., WILLIAMSON, P. D. and MATTSON, R. H. (1981) Ictal effects of anticonvulsant medication withdrawal in epileptic patients. *Epilepsia,* **22,** 297–307

THOMAS, J. E. (1957) A rare electroencephalographic pattern: the six per second spike and wave discharge. *Neurology,* **7,** 438–442

THOMAS, J. and KLASS, D. W. (1968) Six per second spike and wave pattern in the electroencephalogram. *Neurology,* **18,** 587–593

THURSTON, J. H., THURSTON, D. L., HIXOM, B. B. and KELLER, A. J. (1982) Prognosis in childhood epilepsy. *New England Journal of Medicine,* **306,** 831–836

WADA, T. and LENNOX, W. G. (1954) So-called 'temporal' epilepsy. The clinical and interseizure EEG findings. *Folia Psychiatrica et Neurologica Japonica (Niigata),* **8,** 294–301

WALTER, R. D., COLBERT, E. G., KOEGLER, R. R., PALMER, J. D. and BOND, P. M. (1960) A controlled study of fourteen and six per second EEG pattern. *Archives of General Psychiatry,* **2,** 559–566

WALTER, W. G. (1950) Epilepsy. In *Electroencephalography*, edited by D. Hill and G. Parr, pp. 228–272. New York: Macmillan

WEIR, H. F. and ANDERSON, R. L. (1958) Organic and organizational aspects of school adjustment problems. *Journal of the American Medical Association,* **166,** 1708–1710

WESTMORELAND, B. F. and KLASS, D. W. (1981) A distinctive rhythmic EEG discharge of adults. *Electroencephalography and Clinical Neurophysiology,* **51,** 186–191

WHITE, J. C., LANGSTON, J. W. and PEDLEY, T. A. (1977) Benign epileptiform transients of sleep: classification of the small sharp spike controversy. *Neurology,* **27,** 1061–1068

WHITE, P., DYKEN, M., GRANT, P. and JACKSON, L. (1962) Electroencephalographic abnormalities during sleep as related to the temporal distribution of seizures. *Epilepsia,* **3,** 167–176

WIENER, J. M., DELANO, J. G. and KLASS, D. W. (1966) An EEG study of delinquent and nondelinquent adolescents. *Archives of General Psychiatry,* **15,** 144–150

WIESER, H. G., BANCAUD, J., TALAIRACH, J., BONIS, A. and SZIKLA, G. (1979) Comparative value of spontaneous and chemically and electrically induced seizures in establishing the lateralization of temporal lobe seizures. *Epilepsia,* **20,** 47–59

YING-K'UN, F., CHING-CHIN, H. and TAN-HUA, K. (1981) The use of acupuncture needles as sphenoidal electrodes. A report of observations on 648 cases. *Clinical and Experimental Neurology,* **17,** 39–45

9
The medical management of partial and generalized tonic-clonic seizures

Fritz E. Dreifuss

INTRODUCTION

The goals of epilepsy management include the elimination of seizures, and prevention of seizures.

The elimination of seizures

The most effective means of eliminating seizures are those which eliminate the underlying cause. Such treatments include reversal of hypoglycemia, the correction of amino-acid metabolic disturbances, removal of tumors, clots, abscesses, and the treatment of inflammatory lesions, the elimination of toxins and restoration of energy equilibrium. In most instances epilepsy must still be treated symptomatically and the mainstay of therapy will continue to be the administration of anticonvulsant medications.

Uncontrolled seizures may be responsible for further neuronal impairment and may ultimately lead to intractability by virtue of exciting the mechanism of kindling. They will also excite physical, social, psychological, vocational and recational impairment in the quality of life. Distinctions in severity have to be made between different seizure types. On this distinction will be predicated the choice of antiepileptic drug, the vigor and urgency in the prosecution of therapy and the duration. Thus, a potentially benign, self-limited childhood rolandic seizure has a different connotation from frequent bouts of generalized tonic-clonic seizures and episodes associated with prolonged periods of confusion.

Prevention of seizures

The goal of prevention includes prevention of epilepsy by avoidance of potentially preventable head injuries, vigorous management of treatable inflammatory diseases, prevention of birth trauma, attention to the health of mothers and infants at high risk and, possibly, by the use of prophylactic anticonvulsant medications after head trauma.

The prevention of seizures is accomplished by the institution of appropriate anticonvulsant drugs, the avoidance of precipitating factors such as sleep deprivation and exposure to stimuli producing reflex seizures.

The prevention of complications of seizures includes the early termination of prolonged seizures to prevent further neuronal impairment, the avoidance of intolerable drug-induced side-effects and the curtailment of psychosocial consequences.

PRINCIPLES OF ANTICONVULSANT DRUG MANAGEMENT

Because the epilepsies are etiologically diverse, and different types of seizures involve different mechanisms of propagation and excitation, and because the development of antiepileptic drugs has been towards more specific drugs for specific seizure types, accurate identification and classification of the convulsant disorders has assumed an importance transcending taxonomy and leading from empiricism towards application of neurophysiological principles. Nowhere is the need for accurate diagnosis more evident than in the distinction between absence seizures and complex partial seizures (Penry *et al.*, 1975) or between primary generalized epilepsies and those due to cerebral lesions. Accurate history taking and accurate seizure recording is a *sine qua non* for the initiation of appropriate therapy. Occasionally it may be decided not to treat an individual seizure, for example, in selected first seizures or the first febrile seizure, or instances where recurrences may not occur, where the decision not to treat may be sustained by weighing the statistical chances of recurrence of seizures against the potential deleterious consequences of long-term therapy. Moreover, a seizure may have been triggered in a predisposed individual by the administration of certain medications such as phenothiazines and though this might indicate a lower threshold, the option of no specific treatment might well be justified (Dreifuss, 1983a).

The choice of the specific drug to be used will be determined not only by its potential efficacy but by its relative freedom from side-effects which would limit its use in specific instances. Thus, phenytoin may be the drug of choice where infrequent dosing is a major objective and where its cosmetic side-effects are deemed relatively unimportant, whereas carbamazepine may be the drug of choice in a similar seizure type where its relative freedom from impairment of cognitive function and cosmetic side-effects outweigh some other disadvantages. Whichever drug is used, the patient must be educated to understand the need for compliance, the concept of the therapeutic blood level range, and the recognition of both dose-related and idiosyncratic side-effects. The gradual introduction of a drug usually lessens the incidence of side-effects although the severity of the seizures may mandate immediate attainment of the therapeutic range.

Monotherapy should be a therapeutic aim, but the substitution of another drug may be mandated by failure of the first drug to control seizures. Under these circumstances, the first drug is slowly withdrawn as the second drug is introduced. If seizures continue to be refractory, a second drug is added to the regimen and several combinations of drugs may have to be applied before an effective regimen is accomplished. With multiple drug therapy, knowledge of potential drug interactions is essential. Some drug interactions will result in increased blood levels and at other times in diminished blood levels, depending on whether there is enzyme competition or induction. Drugs which are highly protein bound may interact by altering the free blood level of one or other of the drugs.

As important as the institution and maintenance of therapy is consideration for its termination after an appropriate seizure-free period (Emerson *et al.*, 1981). Discontinuation of therapy will, to some extent, depend on the nature of the underlying epilepsy and its prognosis, the duration of the seizure-free period, and the consideration of extraneous factors such as a desire for pregnancy, intercurrent physical or social events which alter the risk–benefit ratio either in the direction of maintenance therapy or its curtailment. In the case of a woman desiring pregnancy, one might consider discontinuation of medication before one otherwise would, because the risk of seizures may not be sufficient to counterbalance the risk of potential teratogenicity. On the other hand, after a similar seizure-free period, if the patient is a teenager about to obtain a driver's licence or to leave home to live in a college dormitory, one might decide that the potential social risk of a recurrent seizure outweighs the disadvantages of continuing anticonvulsant therapy for a longer period of time.

When seizures fail to respond to appropriate therapy, detailed re-evaluation is in order in a search for factors which may have been overlooked or for incorrect initial clinical impressions. Erroneous diagnosis of seizure type with inappropriate drug choice, subtherapeutic blood levels due to poor compliance, poor absorption or drug interaction, the presence of pseudoseizures or the presence of underlying neurological disorders such as tumors, progressive metabolic or degenerative disorders as a cause for the seizures, may all contribute to their intractability.

Principles of management, further, must include attention to social, vocational and educational factors and these must complement the attention to medical therapeutic management.

PARTIAL SEIZURES

Partial seizures are defined as simple partial seizures, in which consciousness is maintained, and complex partial seizures in which consciousness is impaired (Commission on Classification and Terminology, ILAE, 1981). If a simple partial seizure begins to involve those structures on which integrity of the state of consciousness depends, consciousness will be impaired and the seizure will become a complex partial seizure. At any time, a simple partial seizure may become a generalized tonic-clonic seizure or may arrive at that state via sufficient limbic participation to define a complex partial seizure. Simple partial seizures may have motor, sensory, special sensory, autonomic, cognitive or affective manifestations which are predicated on the specific area of cortex involved in the abnormal discharge. From the point of view of pharmacological management, the choice of drug and the prognosis for improvement of this type of seizure will depend more on the specific epileptic syndrome of which the partial seizure is a manifestation than upon the location of the seizure focus responsible for its manifestations. Benign focal epilepsy (rolandic seizures, benign mid-temporal spike epilepsy of childhood) (Beaussart, 1972; Lombroso, 1967) carries a vastly different prognosis from the epileptic aphasic syndrome of Landau and Kleffner (1957), unilateral seizures in infancy (Gastaut *et al.*, 1974), infantile hemiplegia, Sturge–Weber disease, inflammatory conditions such as cysticercosis or seizures secondary to head trauma. This consideration, as much as attention to seizure type and phenomenology, must contribute to decisions regarding medical management both as guide to choice of drug and such factors as duration of treatment and ancillary therapeutic endeavors.

COMPLEX PARTIAL SEIZURES

Complex partial seizures are separated from simple partial seizures by impairment, distortion, or loss of the conscious state, and while there may be impairment of consciousness only, associated psychic phenomena including distortion or memory, emotion and visual sensation are frequently experienced (Daly, 1975). Automatic behavior (psychomotor automatisms) usually occurs and may be oroalimentary, automatisms of mimicry, gestural, verbal or ambulatory (Gastaut, 1973). While the majority of patients with complex partial seizures harbor a temporal lobe etiology, similar psychomotor symptoms may proceed from a frontal focus. As in simple partial seizures, complex partial seizures may become secondarily generalized with supervention of tonic-clonic seizures.

Both simple partial seizures and complex partial seizures may occur in status form. In the former, the result is epilepsia partialis continua, and in the latter a prolonged confusional state (Ellis and Lee, 1978).

As in the case of simple partial seizures, the prognosis of medical management will largely depend on the underlying etiology and may be adversely affected by such factors as the presence of 'alien tissue'.

GENERALIZED TONIC-CLONIC SEIZURES (GRAND MAL)

Generalized tonic-clonic seizures are characterized by loss of consciousness, sharp tonic contractions of muscles, the assumption of a rigid, and frequently a opisthotonic, posture followed by clonic convulsive movements lasting for a variable period of time. Cyanosis, salivation, tongue biting and incontinence are frequent and the postictal stage includes a variable period of unconsciousness.

Both clinically and electroencephalographically there are two main varieties of generalized tonic seizures: (a) primarily generalized seizures due to paroxysmal instability of the corticoreticular system and generalized from the beginning; and (b) clinical or electroencephalographic asymmetries with focal discharge and representing secondarily generalized seizures from a focus. This distinction may be critical in the choice of medication and the assignment of prognosis. Generalized tonic-clonic seizures as representative of primary generalized epilepsy, and including febrile seizures and reflex-induced seizures, are generally considerably more responsive to treatment than generalized tonic-clonic seizures representing secondary or lesional epilepsy (Dreifuss, 1982, 1983b).

From the point of view of management, reflex-induced seizures including photically induced, startle epilepsy, noise-induced and movement-induced epilepsy, should be distinguished because of the desirability of eliminating precipitating factors as an adjunct to seizure management. The management of febrile seizures is considered in detail in Chapter 11.

DRUGS USED IN THE MANAGEMENT OF PARTIAL AND GENERALIZED TONIC-CLONIC SEIZURES

Carbamazepine

Carbamazepine (Tegretol) was introduced in 1962 and is an iminostilbene derivative. The drug is relatively slowly and irregularly absorbed and reaches peak

Table 9.1 Drugs used in the management of seizures

Drug	*Dosage* *Starting*	*Maintenance*	*Blood level*	*Side-effects*	*Precautions*
Carbamazepine	Child 5 mg/kg/day Adult 5–10 mg/kg/ day	10–25 mg/kg/day up to 160 mg/day	5–12 μg/ml	*Dose-related* Diplopia, drowsiness, vertigo, headache, diarrhea, inappropriate ADH, leucopenia, *Idiosyncratic* Aplastic anemia, hepatotoxicity, arrhythmia	Blood counts and SGOT monthly for 6 months then every 4 months
Phenytoin	Child 4–8 mg/kg/ day; adult 4–8 mg/ kg/day In status epilepticus child 20 mg/kg at 1–3 mg/kg/min; adult 20 mg/kg at 50 mg/min	4–8 mg/kg/day maximum 300 mg 4–8 mg/kg/day max 600 mg	10–20 μg/ml	*Dose-related* Dizziness, ataxia, diplopia athetosis, gingival hyperplasia, hirsutism, coarse facies, folate deficiency, vitamin D deficiency, cerebellar dysfunction. *Idiosyncratic* Skin rashes, erythema multiforme, SLE, pseudolymphoma, teratogenicity	Annual blood counts, oral hygiene; avoid in pregnancy if possible, warn re possible effect on birth control medication
Primidone	Child 1–2 mg/kg/ day; adult 250 mg/ day increasing q. 3–7 day	10–25 mg/kg/day 750–1000 mg/day		*Dose-related* Sedation, vertigo, behavior disturbances *Idiosyncratic* Skin rashes, fever	Begin with very small dose; avoid in school age if possible

Table 9.1 (Continued)

Drug	*Dosage*		*Blood level*	*Side-effects*	*Precautions*
	Starting	*Maintenance*			
Phenobarbital	Neonate 10–20 mg/kg i.v.; child 3–4 mg/kg/day; adult 3–5 mg/kg/day In status epilepticus child 20 mg/kg i.v.; adult up to 1 g i.v.	3–4 mg/kg 5 mg/kg	10–30 μg/ml	*Dose-related* Sedation, hyperactivity, irritability *Idiosyncratic* Skin rash, exfoliative dermatitis, fever	
Valproate*	Children 15 mg/kg/day; adults 15 mg/kg/day	up to 60mg/kg/day up to 4 g/day	50–120 μg/ml trough level	Drowsiness, gastrointestinal dusturbance, alopecia, weight gain, tremor, SGOT elevation *Idiosyncratic* Leucopenia, thrombocytopenia, hepatitis, pancreatitis, teratogenicity	CBC, platelets, SGOT, SGPT every 2 weeks for 2 months then every month for 1 year
Clorazepate dipotassium**	3.75 mg i.d.	up to 45 mg/day	0.4–1.5 μg/ml	Drowsiness, depression	

* Valproate is not yet FDA approved for seizure types under discussion in this chapter.
** Adjunctive for complex partial seizures in adults

plasma levels approximately 6–18 hours after dosing. The elimination half-life is approximately 9–15 hours. The short half-life indicates that 2–4 days are required for the serum levels to reach a steady state, and suggests that two to three doses per day are required to avoid undue serum level fluctuations.

Carbamazepine is approximately 70% bound to serum proteins. It is excreted in the urine as carbamazepine-10,11-epoxide, carbamazepine-10, 11-dihydroxide oxide and iminostilbene. There is some evidence that the epoxide may also possess anticonvulsant properties.

Carbamazepine is administered orally in doses of approximately 10–30 mg/kg/day. Adults will usually require a dose of between 600 and 1600 mg/day. The therapeutic blood level range is between 4 and 12 μg/ml, and above this level toxic symptoms (see below) are likely to be encountered. It is usual to obtain trough blood levels for day-to-day management. Should toxic symptoms occur, it is usual to obtain blood levels at the height of the symptoms, as symptoms may occur at different levels in different people.

It is usual to begin dosing at a low level. Children usually tolerate 50–100 mg/day and this may be gradually increased by 50–100 mg increments every other day until an effective dose range is reached. In adults the initial dose is 200 mg/day with gradual increases in dose every other day until the serum concentration is in the therapeutic range. If the serum level reaches 12 μg/ml, any further increases in dose should be carefully monitored until the patient becomes seizure free or toxic symptoms develop. Carbamazepine induces enzymes for its own metabolism so that the steady state serum level after three weeks' therapy will be less than initially attained and the dose has to be adjusted at about this time (Bertilsson *et al.*, 1980).

Carbamazepine interacts with phenytoin, valproic acid and clonazepam, usually resulting in lowering of steady state blood levels of these drugs. Phenytoin, phenobarbital and primidone may lower carbamazepine blood levels presumably by increasing the metabolism of these drugs. In order to avoid drug interactions, monotherapy is desirable but if the use of more than one drug is unavoidable, blood levels of all drugs should be checked whenever the dose of any one of the drugs is changed.

Adverse effects of carbamazepine

TOXIC EFFECTS

Toxic effects which are the results of overdose include diplopia, drowsiness, vertigo, blurred vision, and dryness of the mouth. These effects usually occur at the height of the post-dosing blood level and respond to either reducing the dose or spreading it out more evenly through the day.

UNWANTED SIDE-EFFECTS

Unwanted side-effects which may accompany doses in the therapeutic range include inappropriate ADH secretion, which may lead to water retention and hyponatremia; there may be headache, diarrhea, constipation, paresthesiae, and occasionally cardiac arrhythmias. Carbamazepine may reduce the free thyroxine levels in blood probably due to an effect on the thyroxine binding. Frank hypothyroidism does not occur (Fichsel and Knopfle, 1978; Strandjord *et al.*, 1981). Neurological side-effects are rare with carbamazepine though dystonia has been reported (Corsley and Swendler, 1979; Joyce and Gunderson, 1980). Effects on learning and cognitive function are less with carbamazepine than with other anticonvulsant drugs (Trimble and Thompson, 1983) which together with the absence of behavioral changes makes this a popular drug in the pediatric age group.

Transient leukopenia is frequently seen with carbamazepine and usually does not require termination of therapy. It is usually not severe, and is self-limited though it may require temporary dose reduction.

SPECIFIC ORGAN EFFECTS

Specific organ effects may occur and these include idiosyncratic reactions, among which are skin rashes that are relatively uncommon with carbamazepine, and blood dyscrasias (Pisciotta, 1975; Veall and Hogarth, 1975). To detect bone marrow depression early, it is often recommended that blood counts be performed at monthly intervals with the recommendation that dosage be reduced or the drug discontinued should the total white count fall below 3500 or the proportion of granulocytes below 25% of the total white count. Prescribing physicians are advised to observe patients for the development of fever, sore throat, cutaneous and other hemorrhages. It is now generally recommended that after six months blood counts be checked approximately every 4–6 months in patients on carbamazepine. Hepatic dysfunction has been reported (Levander, 1980; Zucker, Daum and Cohen, 1977).

Phenytoin

Phenytoin has been used extensively since 1938 but its mode of action is still under discussion. It is absorbed slowly and somewhat variably from the gastrointestinal tract and reaches a peak level approximately 8–12 hours after dosing. Its half-life varies but averages 24 hours, ranging from 10 to 36 hours. The hydroxylated metabolic product which has no anticonvulsant activity is excreted in the bile, reabsorbed in the intestine and excreted principally in the urine. Phenytoin is rapidly bound to protein to the extent of about 90%. Factors that interfere with the metabolism of the drug include rare genetic factors such as the inability of the liver to hydroxylate it and common drug interactions with enzyme induction such as are seen with phenobarbital. The long half-life indicates that the steady state is achieved after about four days although this can be shortened by giving an initial loading dose of three times the daily maintenance dose at the beginning of treatment. There is considerable individual variation in blood levels from a standard dose and blood level determinations are, therefore, necessary for monitoring the drug. The therapeutic blood level range of phenytoin is 10–20 μg/ml. Because of the long half-life it is unnecessary to prescribe phenytoin in divided daily doses and one daily dose will usually suffice. The recommended dose is 5–20 mg/kg/day in children and in adults is usually 300–400 mg/day. Because the capacity of the liver to metabolize the drug is limited, the kinetics of phenytoin elimination are exponential at low doses and are linear at higher doses. When this condition is reached, small increases in dose are accompanied by large increases of serum level, and once the therapeutic range is reached further increases in dose should be small to avoid toxicity at this stage. When it is decided to obtain therapeutic levels quickly as in status epilepticus, the intravenous route is better. Intravenously administered phenytoin has a half-life approximately half of that achieved with oral administration.

Drug-to-drug interactions involving phenytoin result in lowering of carbamazepine and primidone levels. Phenytoin levels are lowered by the simultaneous administration of carbamazepine and phenobarbital due to increased metabolism of the drug. Free levels of phenytoin are increased by the simultaneous administration of valproate due to interference with protein binding. When other drugs are simultaneously administered, blood levels should be monitored of all the antiepileptic drugs. An important interaction is interference with birth control efficacy by induction of estrogen metabolism.

Adverse effects of phenytoin include those which are dose-related and consist of drowsiness, ataxia, diplopia, nystagmus, gastrointestinal complaints. Side-effects which may accompany a dose in the therapeutic range include gingival hyperplasia, hypertrichosis, coarsening of facies due to connective tissue effects (Falconer and Davidson, 1973; Hassell, 1981). Dupuytren's contracture may occur (Critchley *et al.*, 1976). Folate deficiency (Reynolds, 1976) and interference with vitamin D metabolism may be seen (Bell *et al.*, 1979; Kruse, 1968). Neurological side-effects include interference with cognitive ability (Trimble and Thompson, 1983). A progressive encephalopathy has been described (Vallarta, Bell and Reichert, 1974), as have abnormal movements (Ahmed *et al.*, 1975, Chadwick, Reynolds and Marsden, 1976; Chalhub *et al.*, 1976; Logan and Freeman, 1969). The drug appears to have a deleterious effect on Purkinje cells (Ghatak, Santoso and McKinney, 1976; Haberland, 1962; Iivanainen, Viukari and Helle, 1977; McLain, Martin and Allen, 1980). Chronic cerebellar dysfunction may thus result. Endocrinological effects include influence on thyroid function (Fichsel and Knopfle, 1978; Strandjord *et al.*, 1981). Plasma cortisol levels may be elevated (Choy *et al.*, 1971; Meikle *et al.*, 1969; Gallagher, 1976). Phenytoin has been implicated in the reduction of IgA in serum in saliva (Aarli, 1976; Fontana *et al.*, 1976).

Idiosyncratic side-effects include skin rashes, either morbilliform or exfoliative, erythema multiforme and Stevens-Johnson's syndrome (Pollack, Burke and Nathanson, 1979). Systemic lupus erythematosus (Benton *et al.*, 1962; Singsen, Fishman and Hansen, 1976) may occur and blood dyscrasias due to bone marrow depression (Parker and Gumnit, 1974; Tsan *et al.*, 1976) have occurred. A mononucleosis-like syndrome with fever, skin rash, hepatosplenomegaly and even jaundice (Chaiken, Goldberg and Segal, 1950) may occur and a pseudolymphoma suggesting Hodgkin's disease is not unusual (Charlesworth, 1977; Halevy and Feuerman, 1977).

While the extent of possible side-effects has not yet been elucidated and studies are continuing, there would seem to be increased teratogenesis when mothers are taking phenytoin and this is expressed as cleft lip, cleft palate, congenital heart disease and the so-called fetal phenytoin syndrome that is characterized by mental retardation, hypoplastic fingernails and hypertelorism. It is generally believed at this time, however, that the teratogenetic risks are lower than the risks from uncontrolled seizures during pregnancy.

Towards the end of pregnancy the mother should receive vitamin K-1 oxide to guard against hemorrhagic disease of the newborn, which may be induced by phenytoin.

Phenobarbital

Since its introduction in 1912 phenobarbital has been one of the most widely used anticonvulsants. Its precursor is barbituric acid which is formed from urea and malonic acid. Phenobarbital results from a replacement of two hydrogen atoms of barbituric acid with an ethyl and phenyl group. The latter has anticonvulsant properties, particularly against the tonic components of major seizures.

Phenobarbital is well absorbed from the gastrointestinal tract and its lipid solubility assures it an affinity for the central nervous system. Peak blood and brain levels are achieved within 1–3 hours. The drug has a long half-life of around 100 hours. In neonates, the half-life is longer, about 150 hours, and low maintenance doses of 3–4 mg/kg are sufficient. The administration of successive doses before complete elimination of the previous dose leads to accumulation, and the concentration in the blood rises until a plateau is reached at a stage when intake and elimination are equal. This 'steady state' is reached after about three-and-a-half times the biological half-life. Final blood levels are thus not obtained for a long time unless a loading dose is given at the beginning of treatment. Sufficient variation in relationship of dose to blood level occurs so that the latter cannot be predicted reliably from the dose administered. The therapeutic blood level range lies between 10 and 30 μg/ml, above which toxic side-effects might be expected.

Phenobarbital is predominantly excreted through the kidney where 30% of the administered dose appears unchanged. In the liver the drug is metabolized into inactive compounds by hydroxylation and glucuronic acid conjugation. Particular care should be taken when the drug is administered to patients with renal disease but it is the anticonvulsant of choice in patients with severe hepatic dysfunction because of the relative insignificance of the hepatic metabolic pathway. About 50% of the drug is protein bound.

Habituation of phenobarbital depends on the activation of metabolizing enzymes in the liver and the adaptation of the nervous system to the presence of phenobarbital. Acute withdrawal often precipitates seizures. The drug has the ability to increase the synthesis and concentration of a variety of enzymes which are responsible for metabolism of bilirubin and steroids as well as other drugs, including phenytoin and beta-hydroxy-coumarin. The simultaneous administration of sodium valproate leads to an increased level of phenobarbital presumably by interference with its metabolism.

In adults, the tolerated dose ranges from 120 to 200 mg/day. It may be prescribed in one daily dose because of its long half-life, but divided doses are usually recommended. Children tolerate 4–5 mg/kg.

Phenobarbital continues to be the drug of first choice in the treatment of seizures in the neonate. Here a loading dose of between 15 and 20 mg/kg is recommended to produce therapeutic blood levels, followed by a maintenance dose of 3–4 mg/kg which will maintain serum concentrations of approximately 20 μg/ml during the course of therapy. With increasing age, the half-life of phenobarbital changes and this in turn mandates a modification of the dosage schedule. During the stabilization period blood level estimations are recommended.

Drug-to-drug interactions

Because of increasing microsomal enzyme production with consequent increases in metabolism, simultaneously administered carbamazepine or phenytoin will have decreased serum levels. Because of metabolic interference, simultaneously administered valproate will lead to an increase in the phenobarbital blood level.

Side-effects

Side-effects include: (a) toxic effects which are the result of overdose and include sedation behavior disturbances and ataxia; (b) unwanted side-effects which may accompany doses in the therapeutic range and include difficulty with concentration, deficit in cognitive function (Trimble and Thompson, 1983), behavior disturbances in children with hyperactivity (Wolf and Forsythe, 1978); (c) specific organ effects which include skin eruptions such as a fixed drug eruption and occasionally even exfoliative dermatitis. Major idiosyncratic reactions, however, are extremely uncommon with phenobarbital. The drug should be avoided, as should most antiepileptic drugs, in cases of acute intermittent porphyria which is exacerbated by the increased production of cytochrome P_{450} and ALAS by antiepileptic drugs, particularly barbiturates.

Primidone

Primidone (Mysoline) has been used since 1952. Like phenobarbital, it is rapidly absorbed from the gastrointestinal tract. It is metabolized to phenobarbital and phenyl-ethyl-malonimide (PEMA). The drug is not significantly protein bound and has a half-life of about 12 hours. Phenobarbital derived from the metabolism of primidone has its characteristic half-life, and PEMA, which is also somewhat active as an anticonvulsant agent, has a half-life of 24 hours. Primidone is administered in low dose initially and is gradually increased to approximately 25 mg/kg. The starting dose should not exceed 100 mg/day to begin with and this may be increased every 2–3 days until a therapeutic dose is reached or until toxic symptoms occur. Adults usually tolerate approximately 750 mg/day. The therapeutic blood level is approximately 5–10 μg/ml. Drug interactions include a lowering of simultaneously administered phenytoin due to microsomal enzyme induction by derived phenobarbital.

The side-effects are those encountered with phenobarbital, though behavioral disturbances and difficulty with learning appear to be more pronounced with primidone than with phenobarbital.

In pregnant women, as with phenytoin, the administration of vitamin K-1 oxide at delivery is recommended because of occasional recurrence of postpartum hemorrhagic disease of the newborn (Waltl, Mitterstieler and Schwingshackl, 1974).

Sodium valproate, valproic acid

While valproate is currently approved in the United States in the treatment of absence seizures, favorable responses have been reported with other generalized seizure types, particularly generalized tonic-clonic seizures (Bruni and Wilder, 1979; Mattson, 1979; Simon and Penry, 1975). Some have reported significant seizure reduction in complex partial seizures (Pinder *et al.*, 1977; Simon and Penry, 1975; Turnbull *et al.*, 1982). Valproic acid is a branched-chain carboxylic acid, is a weak acid, hygroscopic and soluble in water, methanol and ethanol.

When given by mouth it is rapidly and completely absorbed from an empty stomach. Peak blood levels are achieved in 1–4 hours. The elimination half-life in patients varies between 6 and 18 hours but it is not certain what this means in terms of long-term dosing because the drug appears to have a dual effect – an immediate one which is blood level-related and a delayed effect. It appears to be metabolized chiefly by beta and omega oxidation as well as by conjugation to a glucuronide.

The drug is administered initially at 10–15 mg/kg and this may be increased gradually as tolerated to as high a dose as 60 mg/kg (though therapeutic effect is usually achieved at 30–40 mg/kg) for a maximal dose of 4 g in an adult. Because of the relatively short half-life, several doses per day are administered and the drug is better tolerated in divided doses. The therapeutic blood level range is between 50 and 120 μg/ml. Because of large fluctuations in blood level, the value of blood level estimations is under debate. In any event, trough blood levels should be obtained. Valproate is 90% protein bound and when administered with other highly protein bound drugs, free blood levels are useful in clinical management. Because of frequent gastrointestinal side-effects with valproic acid, an enteric absorbed preparation, divalproex sodium, has been developed. The drug has to be given for two weeks before the full therapeutic effect is achieved.

Drug–drug interactions

Valproic acid displaces phenytoin from its binding and a steady state level of phenytoin will fall when valproate is added. However, because a great portion of this lower total serum level of phenytoin is unbound, therapeutic efficacy may not be affected. An interaction with phenobarbital results in a decreased clearance of phenobarbital with increased blood levels.

Adverse effects

Toxic effects which are dose related include drowsiness, nausea, and vomiting. Skin rashes are rare but alopecia has been reported but is not severe and usually spontaneously reversible (Jeavons, Clark, and Maheshwari, 1977). Tremor is common as a dose-related effect and usually responds to dosage diminution. Ankle swelling has been reported, as has amenorrhea (Margraf and Dreifuss, 1981) and hyperammonemia (Coulter and Allen, 1981; Murphy, Marquardt and Swick, 1981). In combination with other drugs, unexplained stupor has also been seen (Sackellares, Lee and Dreifuss, 1981). Specific organ or idiosyncratic effects include neutropenia (Jaeken *et al.*, 1979) and hepatic dysfunction. The latter is valproate's most significant side-effect and has resulted in more than 60 fatalities. This condition does not appear to be dose-related though it does appear to be somewhat more frequent in patients receiving large doses. Most cases have appeared before the end of six months of therapy and few warning symptoms or signs occur. Elevation of SGOT and SGPT are frequently observed in patients receiving valproic acid and usually rapidly reverse with reduction in dosage. Several instances of acute pancreatitis have been reported.

Teratogenicity of valproate includes an increased incidence of myelomeningocele in children born of epileptic mothers taking valproate (Bjerkedal *et al.*, 1982; Robert and Guibaud, 1982).

TREATMENT OF INDIVIDUAL SEIZURE TYPES

Partial seizures

The drugs of choice in the treatment of partial seizures, both simple partial seizures and complex partial seizures, include carbamazepine, phenytoin, phenobarbital and primidone. Until recently, carbamazepine was used predominantly as adjunctive therapy but it is evident that that drug is effective as monotherapy in most forms of partial seizures, particularly those of the complex partial variety (Cereghino, *et al.*, 1974; Troupin, 1978). Serious side-effects are relatively infrequent and carbamazepine is a relatively benign drug, particularly in relation to central nervous system toxicity. Primidone is a drug useful in the treatment of most seizure types other than absence, but the side-effects are sufficiently troublesome to reduce the popularity of this drug, particularly in young people.

Phenytoin continues to be one of the most popular drugs in the treatment of most types of seizures including partial seizures, though it is being superseded by carbamazepine because of the prevalence of troublesome side-effects during long-term therapy. It has the great advantatages of only only having to be administered once daily which frequently improves compliance and that it is relatively inexpensive, which is an important economic consideration.

Phenytoin is one of the drugs of choice for treatment of status epilepticus because of the effectiveness of intravenous administration and its relatively high safety margin.

Phenobarbital, after 70 years, continues to be a popular drug, a sentiment supported by its effectiveness, but its overt and insidious effect on cognitive function is relegating its role to a secondary one in children. It is the drug of choice in the treatment of seizures in infancy, and by the intravenous route is popular in the treatment of status epilepticus and serial seizures.

Valproate has been recommended in the treatment of complex partial seizures where it has been said to reduce attacks by as much as 60% compared with placebo in various studies. It is used primarily as adjunctive therapy.

Clorazepate (Troupin *et al.*, 1980) has been found to be somewhat effective in the treatment of complex partial seizures and has been used as adjunctive therapy in the dose of 3.75–7.5 mg two or three times a day. The drug is usually given with carbamazepine in this setting.

Generalized tonic-clonic seizures

All the drugs used in the treatment of partial seizures are also the drugs generally employed in the management of generalized tonic-clonic seizures. The order in which the drugs are used may depend upon the setting in which generalized tonic-clonic seizures occur. For example, if these are seen in the setting of concomitant absence seizure valproic acid would be the treatment of choice as one would be dealing with a primary generalized epilepsy. Under other circumstances, carbamazepine, phenytoin or phenobarbital might be preferred, particularly if there is evidence that one is dealing with secondarily generalized seizures.

In the treatment of generalized tonic-clonic seizures several anticonvulsant drugs are thus effective, and under different circumstances any of the drugs mentioned may be the drug of choice. The chance of successful control is good. However, when the seizure is secondarily generalized, when there is evidence of other neurological dysfunction such as intellectual impairment or the presence of abnormal neurological signs, and when other seizure types are present, the prognosis becomes considerably less favorable and it is here that control with the use of a single drug is considerably less predictable as is the prognosis for cessation of seizure with cerebral maturation. Here more than one drug may have to be administered, leading to the potential complications inherent in drug interactions.

THE PHARMACOLOGICAL MANAGEMENT OF STATUS EPILEPTICUS

The rapid succession of convulsions or status epilepticus is a life-threatening emergency in the case of generalized tonic-clonic seizures. In the case of partial seizures, status epilepticus is less ominous but may be relatively intractable.

An aim in the treatment of status epilepticus is termination of seizures as rapidly as possible with minimal suppression of consciousness and cardiopulmonary function. After appropriate support of vital functions and assurance of an adequate airway, circulation, blood pressure, rapid evaluation and management of the underlying cause, an intravenous line is secured, glucose administered as 50% dextrose in water, 1 g/kg to children and 25 g to adults in the course of one minute. Pharmacological management consists of the administration of a benzodiazepine drug and/or phenytoin or phenobarbital intravenously. The benzodiazepine may be diazepam administered as follows: in children 0.25–0.4 mg/kg over two minutes with a maximum injection of 5–10 mg; in adults 5–10 mg over 5–10 minutes which may be repeated at 15-minute intervals for a total of not more than 30 mg. The duration of action of diazepam is short and this drug is usually followed by a longer acting anticonvulsant.

In the case of lorazepam, experience with children is limited and the recommended dose would be 0.05–0.2 mg/kg, and in adults 4–8 mg over two minutes. Again this is followed by a longer acting drug such as phenytoin, which is given as follows: in children about 20 mg/kg intravenously at a rate of 1–3 mg/kg/min; in adults 20 mg/kg intravenously with a maximum infusion rate of 50 mg/min. This drug should be administered with caution in the face of severe arteriosclerotic heart disease, congestive heart failure, heart block, bradycardia or history of idiosyncratic reaction to this drug. Alternatively, phenobarbital may be administered as follows: in children, 5–10 mg/kg at 30 mg/min; in adults 9 mg/kg at 50 mg/min, which may be repeated in 20 minutes if necessary up to a total dose of 1 g.

Partial status may be treated similarly but constitutes considerably less of an emergency. Complex partial seizure status usually responds rapidly to intravenous phenytoin. Simple partial seizure status or epilepsia partialis continua usually represents the expression of a severe focal underlying lesion and management should be directed towards the underlying cause and the realization that unduly vigorous anticonvulsant drug treatment may further jeopardize the patient's predicament.

References

AARLI, J. A. (1976) Drug-induced IgA deficiency in epileptic patients. *Archives of Neurology,* **76,** 296–299

AHMED, S., LAIDLAW, J., HOUGHTON, G. W. and RICHENS, A. (1975) Involuntary movements caused by phenytoin intoxication in epileptic patients. *Journal of Neurology, Neurosurgery and Psychiatry,* **38,** 225–231

BEAUSSART, M. (1972) Benign epilepsy of children with rolandic paroxysmal foci: a clinical entity. Study of 221 cases. *Epilepsia,* **13,** 793–796

BELL, R. D., PAK, C. Y., ZERWEKH, J., BARILLA, D. E. and VASKO, M. (1979) Effect of phenytoin on bone and vitamin D metabolism. *Annals of Neurology,* **5,** 374–378

BENTON, J. W., TYNES, B., REGISTER, H. B. JR, ALFORD, C. and HOLLEY, H. L. (1962) Systemic lupus erythematosus occurring during anticonvulsive drug therapy. *Journal of the American Medical Association,* **180,** 115–118

BERTILSSON, L., HOJER, B., TYBRING, G., OSTERLOH, J. and RANE, A. (1980) Autoinduction of carbamazepine metabolism in children examined by a stable isotope technique. *Clinical Pharmacology and Therapy,* **27,** 83–88

BJERKEDAL, T. *et al.* (1982) Valproic acid and spina bifida. *Lancet,* **2,** 1096

BRUNI, J., WILDER, B. J., WILLMORE, L. J., VILLAREAL, J. H., THOMAS, M. and CRAWFORD, L. E. M. (1978) Clinical efficacy of valproic acid in relation to plasma levels. *Canadian Journal of Neurological Science,* **5,** 385–387

BRUNI, J. and WILDER, B. J. (1979) Valproic acid: reveiw of a new antiepileptic drug. *Archives of Neurology,* **36,** 393–398

CEREGHINO, J. J., BROCK, J. T., VANMETER, J. C., PENRY, J. K., SMITH, L. D. and WHITE, B. G. (1974) Carbamazepine for epilepsy. A controlled prospective evaluation. *Neurology,* **24,** 401–410

CHADWICK, D., REYNOLDS, E. H. and MARSDEN, C. D. (1976) Anticonvulsant-induced dyskinesias: a comparison with dyskinesias induced by neuroleptics. *Journal of Neurology, Neurosurgery and Psychiatry,* **39,** 1210–1218

CHAIKEN, B. H., GOLDBERG, J. P. and SEGAL, J. P. (1950) Dilantin sensitivity: report of a case of hepatitis with jaundice, pyrexia and exfoliative dermatitis. *New England Journal of Medicine,* **242,** 897–898

CHALHUB, E. G., DE VIVO, D. C. and VOLPE, J. J. (1976) Phenytoin-induced dystonia and choreathetosis in two retarded epileptic children. *Neurology,* **26,** 494–498

CHARLESWORTH, E. N. (1977) Phenytoin-induced pseudolymphoma syndrome: an immunologic study. *Archives of Dermatology,* **113,** 447–480

CHOY, Y., THRASHER, K., WERK, E. E., SHOLITON, L. J. AND OLINGER, C. (1971) Effect of diphenylhydantoin on cortisol kinetics in humans. *Journal of Pharmacology and Experimental Therapy,* **175,** 27–34

COMMISSION ON CLASSIFICATION AND TERMINOLOGY, ILAE (1981) Proposal for revised clinical and electroencephalographic classification of epileptic seizures. *Epilepsia,* **22,** 489–501

CORSLEY, C. J. and SWENDER, P. T. (1979) Dystonia associated with carbamazepine administration: experience in brain-damaged children. *Pediatrics,* **63,** 612–615

COULTER, D. L. and ALLEN, R. J. (1981) Hyperammonemia with valproic acid therapy. *Journal of Pediatrics,* **99,** 317–319

CRITCHLEY, E. M., VAKIL, S. K., HAYWARD, H. W. and OWEN, V. M. (1976) Dupuytren's disease in epilepsy: a result of prolonged administration of anticonvulsants. *Journal of Neurology, Neurosurgery and Psychiatry,* **39,** 498–503

DALY, D. D. (1975) Ictal manifestations of complex partial seizures. In *Advances in Neurology,* Vol. II, edited by J. K. Penry and D. D. Daly. New York: Raven Press

DREIFUSS, F. E. (1982) Classification of epileptic seizures and the epilepsies. In *Advances in Epileptology,* Vol. XIII, edited by Akimoto *et al.* New York: Raven Press

DREIFUSS, F. E. (1983a) *Pediatric Epileptology,* Littleton, Mass.: Wright PSG

DREIFUSS, F. E. (1983b) Generalized tonic-clonic seizures. In *Acute Epileptic Drug Therapy in Pediatrics,* edited by P. Morselli, C. E. Pippenger and J. K. Penry. New York: Raven Press

DREIFUSS, F. E. (1983c) Adverse effects of antiepileptic drugs. In *Epilepsy,* edited by A. A. Ward, J. K. Penry and D. Purpura. New York: Raven Press

ELLIS, J. M. and LEE, S. I. (1978) Acute prolonged confusion in later life as an ictal state. *Epilepsia,* **19,** 119–128

EMERSON, R., D'SOUZA, B. J., VINING, E. R., HOLDEN, K. R., MERRITS, E. D. and FREEMAN, J. JR (1981) Stopping medication in children with epilepsy. *New England Journal of Medicine,* **304,** 1125–1129

FALCONER, M. A. and DAVIDSON, S. (1973) Coarse features in epilepsy as a consequence of anticonvulsant therapy. *Lancet,* **2,** 1112

FICHSEL, H. and KNOPFLE, G. (1978) Effects of anticonvulsant drugs on thyroid hormones in epileptic children. *Epilepsia,* **19,** 323–336

FONTANA, A., GROB, P. J., SAUTER, R. and JOLLER, H. (1976) IgA deficiency, epilepsy, and hydantoin medication. *Lancet,* **2,** 228–230

GALLAGHER, B. B. (1976) Adrenal hyperplasia in epileptic patients. In *Quantitative Analytic Studies in Epilepsy,* edited by P. Kellaway and I. Petersen. New York: Raven Press

GASTAUT, H., BROUGHTON, R., TASSINARI, C. A. *et al.* (1974) Unilateral epileptic seizures. In *Handbook of Clinical Neurology*, edited by P. J. Vinken and G. W. Bruyn, pp. 235–245. Amsterdam: North Holland Publishing Co.

GASTAUT, H. (1973) *Dictionary of Epilepsy. Part 1: Definitions.* Geneva: World Health Organization

GHATAK, N. R., SANTOSO, R. A. and MCKINNEY, W. M. (1976) Cerebellar degeneration following long-term phenytoin therapy. *Neurology,* **26,** 818–820

HABERLAND, C. (1962) Cerebellar degeneration with clinical manifestation in chronic epileptic patients. *Psychiatrica Neurologica (Basel),* **143,** 29–44

HALEVY, S. and FEUERMAN, E. J. (1977) Pseudolymphoma syndrome. *Dermatologica,* **155,** 321–327

HASSELL, T. M. (1981) Epilepsy and the oral manifestations of phenytoin therapy. Basel: S. Karger

IIVANAINEN, M., VIUKARI, M. and HELLE, E. P. (1977) Cerebellar atrophy in phenytoin-treated mentally retarded epileptics. *Epilepsia,* **18,** 375–386

JAEKEN, J., VAN GOETHEM, C., CAESAR, P., DEVLIEGER, H. and EGGÉRMONT, E. (1979) Neutropenia during sodium valproate treatment. *Archives of Diseases of Children,* **54,** 985–986

JEAVONS, P. M., CLARK, J. E. and MAHESHWARI, M. C. (1977) Treatment of generalized epilepsies of childhood and adolescence with sodium valproate (Epilim). *Developmental Medicine and Child Neurology,* **19,** 9–25

JOYCE, R. P. and GUNDERSON, C. H. (1980) Carbamazepine-induced oro-facial dyskinesia. *Neurology,* **30,** 1333–1334

KRUSE, R. (1968) Osteopathien bei antiepileptischer Lanzeittherapie. *Monatsschrift für Kinderheilkunde,* **116,** 378–381

LANDAU, W. M. and KLEFFNER, F. R. (1957) Syndrome of acquired aphasia with convulsive disorder in children. *Neurology,* **7,** 523–530

LEVANDER, H. G. (1980) Granulomatous hepatitis in a patient receiving carbamazepine. *Acta Medica Scandinavica,* **208,** 333–335

LOGAN, W. J. and FREEMAN, J. M. (1969) Pseudodegenerative disease due to diphenylhydantoin intoxication. *Archives of Neurology,* **21,** 631–637

LOMBROSO, C. J. (1967) Sylvian seizures and mid-temporal spike foci in children. *Archives of Neurology,* **17,** 52–59

MARGRAF, J. and DREIFUSS, F. E. (1981) Amenorrhea following treatment with valproic acid. *Neurology,* **31,** 159

MCLAIN, L. W. JR, MARTIN, J. T. and ALLEN, J. H. (1980) Cerebellar degeneration due to chronic phenytoin therapy. *Annals of Neurology,* **7,** 18–23

MATTSON, R. H. (1979) Valproate and the management of seizures. In *Current Neurology*, edited by H. R. Tyler and D. M. Dawson. Boston: Houghton-Mifflin

MEIKLE, A. W., JUBIZ, W., MATSUKURA, S., WEST, C. D. and TYLER, F. H. (1969) Effect of diphenylhydantoin on the metabolism of metapyrone and release of ACTH in man. *Journal of Clinical Endocrinology,* **29,** 1553–1558

MURPHY, J. V., MARQUARDT, K. and SWICK, H. M. (1981) Hyperammonemia in children receiving valproic acid. *Neurology,* **31,** 142

PARKER, W. A. and GUMNIT, R. J. (1974) Diphenylhydantoin toxicity: dose-dependent blood dyscrasia. *Neurology,* **24,** 1178–1180

PENRY, J. K., PORTER, R. J. and DREIFUSS, F. E. (1975) Simultaneous recording of absence seizures with videotape and electroencephalography: a study of 374 seizures in 48 patients. *Brain,* **98,** 427–440

PINDER, R. M., BROGDEN, R. N., SPEIGHT, T. M. and AVERY, G. S. (1977) Sodium valproate: a review of its pharmacological properties and therapeutic efficacy in epilepsy. *Drugs,* **13,** 81–123

PISCIOTTA, A. V. (1975) Hematologic toxicity of carbamazepine. In *Advances in Neurology,* Vol. 11, edited by J. K. Penry and D. D. Daly. New York: Raven Press

POLLACK, M. A., BURK, P. G. and NATHANSON, G. (1979) Mucocutaneous eruptions due to antiepileptic drug therapy in children. *Annals of Neurology,* **5,** 262–267

REYNOLDS, E. H. (1976) Neurological aspects of folate and vitamin B-12 metabolism. *Clinical Haematology,* **5,** 661–695

ROBERTS, E. and GUIBAUD, P. (1982) Maternal valproic acid and congenital neural tube defects. *Lancet,* **2,** 937

SACKELLARES, J. C., LEE, S. I. and DREIFUSS, F. E. (1979) Stupor following the administration of valproic acid to patients receiving other antiepileptic drugs. *Epilepsia,* **20,** 697–703

SIMON, D. and PENRY, J. K. (1975) Sodium di-n-propylacetate (DPA) in the treatment of epilepsy. *Epilepsia,* **16,** 549–573

SINGSEN, B. H., FISHMAN, L. and HANSON, V. (1976) Antinuclear antibodies and lupus-like syndromes in children receiving anticonvulsants. *Pediatrics,* **57,** 529–534

STRANDJORD, R. E., AANDERUD, S., KYKING, O. L. and JOHANNESSEN, S. I. (1981) Influence of carbamazepine on serum thyroxine and triiodothyronine in patients with epilepsy. *Acta Neurology Scandinavica,* **63,** 111–121

TRIMBLE, M. R. and THOMPSON, P. (1983) Anticonvulsant drugs, cognitive function and behavior. *Epilepsia,* **24** (Suppl. 1), S55–S63

TROUPIN, A. S. (1978) Carbamazepine in epilepsy. In *Clinical Neuropharmacology,* Vol. 3, pp. 15–40, edited by H. L. Klawans. New York: Raven Press

TROUPIN, A. S., WILENSKY, A. J., FRIEL, P., LEAL, K. and OJEMANN, L. M. (1980) Clorazepate as an anticonvulsant. In *Antiepileptic Therapy: Advances in Drug Monitoring,* edited by S. I. Johannessen, P. L. Morselli, C. E. Pippenger, A. Richens, D. Schmidt and H. Meinardi, pp. 291–298. New York: Raven Press

TSAN, M.-F., MEHLMAN, D. J., GREEN, R. S. and BELL, W. R. (1976) Dilantin, agranulocytosis and phagocytic marrow histiocytes. *Annals of Internal Medicine,* **84,** 710

TURNBULL, D. M., RAWLINS, M. D., WEIGHTMAN, D. and CHADWICK, D. W. (1982) A comparison of phenytoin and valproate in previously untreated adult epileptic patients. *Journal of Neurology, Neurosurgery and Psychiatry,* **45,** 55–59

VALLARTA, J. M., BELL, D. B. and REICHERT, A. (1974) A progressive encephalopathy due to chronic hydantoin intoxication. *American Journal of Diseases of Children,* **128,** 27–34

VEALL, R. M. and HOGARTH, N. C. (1975) Thrombocytopenia during treatment with clonazepam. *British Medical Journal,* **4,** 462

WALTL, H., MITTERSTEILER, G. and SCHWINGSCHACKL, A. (1974) Haemorrhagische Diathese bein einem Neugeborenen einer Mutter mit antiepileptischer Therapie. *Deutsche Medizinische Wochenschrift,* **99,** 1315–1317

WOLF, S. M. and FORSYTHE, J. (1978) Behavior disturbance, phenobarbital and febrile seizures. *Pediatrics,* **61,** 728–731

ZUCKER, P., DAUM, F. and COHEN, M. I. (1977) Fatal carbamazepine hepatitis. *Journal of Pediatrics,* **91,** 667–668

10
Medical management of absence, atonic, and myoclonic seizures

Susumu Sato

INTRODUCTION

Absence, myoclonic, and atonic seizures are classified as generalized seizures (Commission on Classification and Terminology, ILAE, 1981). Absence seizures are characterized by interruption of activity, a blank stare, and unresponsiveness. Their EEG manifestations are generalized 2–4 Hz spike-and-wave complexes. In atonic seizures the sudden occurrence of muscle tone diminution may be fragmentary, leading to head drop with slackening of the jaw, dropping of a limb, or loss of all muscle tone with slumping to the ground. Atonic seizures are also known as 'drop attacks'. Electrographically, polyspikes and waves, flattening, or low-voltage fast activity may be associated with these episodes. Myoclonic jerks (single or multiple) are sudden, brief, shock-like muscle contractions. The jerks may be generalized or confined to the face and trunk or to one or more extremities and even to individual muscles or groups of muscles. The EEG may show bursts of polyspike-and-wave complexes, spike-and-wave complexes, or sharp and slow waves. Myoclonic seizures may be associated with absence or atonic seizures.

Patients with absence, atonic, or myoclonic seizures may have more than one of these seizure types, or they may have other types of seizures as well. In the latter situation the coexistence of tonic seizures, particularly, may be an important factor, and treatment with phenytoin is recommended (Erba and Browne, 1983).

ABSENCE SEIZURES

Clinical manifestations

The international classification of epileptic seizures (Commission on Classification and Terminology, ILAE, 1981) describes six types of absence seizures:

(1) absence with impairment of consciousness only
(2) absence with mild clonic components
(3) absence with tonic components
(4) absence with atonic components
(5) absence with automatisms
(6) absence with autonomic components.

The 374 absence seizures studied by Penry, Porter and Dreifuss (1975) lasted from 1 to 45 s (mean, 10.5 s; median, 9.0 s). Absence with impairment of consciousness only (35 seizures) constituted only 9.4% of the seizures, and complex absence seizures accounted for 90.6%. Automatisms were observed in 63.1% and mild clonic components in 45.5% of the seizures. Decreased postural tone occurred in 22.5%, but increased tone was seen in only 4.5%. Although the occurrence of two components in the same seizure was not uncommon (34.8%), the occurrence of three or more components in the same seizure was infrequent (5.1%). Individual patients tended to have seizures of the same kind on different occasions, but some patients had different types of absence seizures at different times.

Incidence

Absence seizures are a relatively uncommon type of epileptic disorder; their incidence ranges from 2% to 11% (Blom, Heijbel and Bergfous, 1978), and they are associated with other types of seizures in 5–20% (median 11%) of the cases (Commission for the Control of Epilepsy and its Consequences, 1978). Absence seizures occur in 6–12% of children with seizures. The number of new cases each year is approximately 6000 (Kurland, 1959–60). The incidence of absence seizures is highest in the first ten years of life and then falls to a negligible level (Hauser and Kurland, 1975).

Genetic and other etiological factors

A significant number (13.3%) of probands with absence attacks have a family history of epilepsy involving either the siblings or parents (Matthes, 1969; Matthes and Weber, 1968). A family history of seizure disorders has been noted in 19–39.6% of patients with absence seizures (Gibberd, 1966; Sato, Dreifuss and Penry, 1976). It has been proposed that the major gene in centrencephalic epilepsy is an irregular, autosomal dominant gene with an age-dependent expression (Metrakos and Metrakos, 1961). Other studies, however, suggest that several genetic factors are responsible for absence seizures, some mutually independent and some either reinforcing or inhibiting the others (Doose *et al.*, 1973).

It has been said that brain damage is not an important pathogenic factor in the causation of absence seizures, although it may act as a trigger mechanism when other factors of heredity, age, and sex are present (Dalby, 1968; Silverman, 1954). Focal and diffuse EEG abnormalities may be seen in up to one-third of patients with absence seizures (O'Brien, Goldensohn and Hoefer, 1959).

Sex

The ratio of males to females ranges from 1:1.1 to 1:1.8 among patients with absence seizures (Gibberd 1966; Sato, Dreifuss and Penry, 1976).

Age at onset

Absence seizures begin most commonly between the ages of 5 and 15 years; they occur infrequently in children younger than 5 years of age, and rarely in those older than 15 years of age (Gibberd, 1966; Sato, Dreifuss and Penry, 1976). Mild non-progressive neurological abnormalities, such as corticospinal tract signs and mental retardation, have been noted in 5.1–24% of patients with absence seizures (Dalby, 1968; Dreifuss, 1972; Holowach, Thurston and O'Leary, 1962; Lennox and Lennox, 1960; Sato, Dreifuss and Penry, 1976).

Intelligence quotient

Patients with absence seizures are said to be of average or above average intelligence (Lennox and Lennox, 1960). However, IQ <90 has been noted in 20–24% (Holowach, Thurston and O'Leary, 1962; Hertoft, 1963) and up to 52% (Sato, Dreifuss and Penry, 1976) of absence seizure patients, and IQ scores of <80 have been noted in 30% of such patients (Charlton and Yahr, 1967).

Associated seizures

Generalized tonic-clonic seizures have been found in 38–59% of patients with absence seizures (Charlton and Yahr, 1967; Currier, Kooi and Saidman, 1963; Gibberd, 1972; Sato, Dreifuss and Penry, 1976). Generalized tonic-clonic seizures may precede or follow the onset of absence seizures and may continue even if absence seizures stop.

Environmental, educational, and social factors

The environment influences seizure frequency, and emotional stress or sleep deprivation may trigger clinical seizures, but more focused attention or activity, such as speech, tends to reduce the paroxysms. Frequent seizures interfere with school performance. Children who have frequent seizures are often thought to be daydreaming, lazy, depressed, or learning-disabled, and this is the complaint that may lead the parents to seek medical help for the child.

Patients with absence seizures should be treated as healthy subjects and encouraged to participate in various sports activities. The only restrictions are horseback riding, climbing to heights, swimming alone, or driving a vehicle until seizures are judged to have ceased.

Diagnosis

The diagnosis of absence seizures can usually be made without difficulty. A good history of a sudden onset and cessation of the ictus is generally diagnostic, but witnessing actual seizures during the neurological examination is confirmatory. An EEG examination documenting bursts of generalized 3 Hz spike-and-wave discharges with ictal manifestations offers further confirmation.

Other tests, such as CT scan, brain scan, blood chemistry and urinalysis are not helpful in establishing the diagnosis of absence seizures. Skull X-ray films are usually normal (Sato, Dreifuss and Penry, 1976) and rarely some abnormalities can be seen in neuroradiographic examination (Hertoft, 1963). The CT scan may show atrophic or non-progressive lesions in some patients with absence seizures (Gastaut and Gastaut, 1977; Lagenstein *et al.*, 1979; Sato *et al.*, 1983).

EEG findings

The spike-and-wave discharge is generalized and appears and disappears suddenly. The discharges have the onset of phase reversal in the midfrontal area, where the maximal voltage occurs in most patients with true absence seizures. In rare cases, the discharges may appear first in the parieto-occipital region, spreading with extreme rapidity to involve the frontal region. The most constant component is the regular series of rounded waves, but the spike component is highly variable and may in fact disappear for a time during the course of a seizure. The spikes appear between the slow waves, or on the descending or ascending limbs of the slow waves. The discharge seldom varies from 3 Hz by more than 0.2 Hz, slowing down a bit toward the end of a long series of waves (Jasper and Droogleever-Fortuyn, 1946).

Frontal polyspikes or spikes and waves are occasionally seen (Gianturco, Wilson and Harris, 1968; O'Brien, Goldensohn and Hoefer, 1959). During sleep the spike-and-wave discharges undergo changes in frequency and morphology (Niedermeyer, 1965; Sato, Dreifuss and Penry, 1973). The background activity is usually normal for the patient's age.

Hyperventilation and photic stimulation are well known to induce absence seizures. Sleep and sleep deprivation are also effective methods of activating EEG discharges.

Differential diagnosis

Absence seizures are most often confused with complex partial seizures, but it should be possible to differentiate nearly all absence seizures on the basis of seizure duration, presence or absence of an aura, rate of mental clearing following the seizure, and presence or absence of *de novo* ambulatory automatisms and complex bilateral motor symptoms (Escueta, Bacsal and Treiman, 1982). The important differentiating features are summarized in *Table 10.1*. Other differential diagnoses

Table 10.1 Differential diagnosis between absence seizures and complex partial seizures

Characteristics	*Absence seizures*	*Complex partial seizures*
Age	Childhood	Any age, though rare in childhood
Predisposition	None	Febrile convulsion
Aura	None	In the majority
Onset	Instantaneous	Commonly preceded by aura
Automatisms	Seen in longer seizures, somewhat simpler	Almost always, more complex
Duration	Majority 10 s or less	Almost always longer than 10 s, often longer than 30 s
Postictal recovery	Immediately with resumption of activity	Slowly (many seconds to minutes), confused
Hyperventilation	A great precipitant	Occasional precipitant
Photic	Frequent precipitant	Almost nil
EEG	Generalized spike–wave	Focal spikes

include Lennox–Gastaut syndrome, hypoglycemia, fainting, micturition, syncope, cataplexy, transient global amnesia, transient cerebral ischemia, cardiac causes of syncope and psychological causes.

Absence status

During absence status the patient may be stuporous, confused, dazed, groggy, respond slowly or incompletely, wander, have automatisms, or be in a catatonic state. Such behavior may last for hours to several days. The EEG during such episodes reveals almost continuous spike-and-wave activity with only occasional brief episodes of normal activity. During absence status the patient may be confused or stuporous but follow simple commands, which often have to be repeated. All movements are slow. Speech consists of simple responses such as yes or no.

Absence status may terminate in generalized tonic-clonic seizures. Physical examination during the ictus may show dull facies with twitching around the eyes or mouth and local or generalized myoclonic jerks.

Absence status must be differentiated from complex partial status epilepticus. Although it may be difficult clinically to distinguish between the two conditions, they can be differentiated on the EEG. Absence status is often clinically misdiagnosed as a functional disorder of psychotic disease.

Course and prognosis

The prognosis is good for patients with absence seizures only, but is less favorable for patients with supervening generalized tonic-clonic seizures. Absence seizures of late onset are more likely to be complicated by generalized tonic-clonic seizures, but the prognosis is slightly better when the seizures commence before the age of ten years. Absence seizures are not transformed into complex partial seizures.

The prognostic importance of immediate, energetic treatment is emphasized. Absence seizures occasionally continue into adulthood (Crews and Sidell, 1973; Gibberd, 1972). Early cessation of seizures is more frequent in males than in females, but the prognosis is the same for each group. The absence of neurological abnormalities and normal EEG background activity favor a better outcome. In one study nearly 90% of patients with a negative history of generalized tonic-clonic seizures, normal or higher IQ, and a negative family history of epilepsy ceased having seizures (Sato, Dreifuss and Penry, 1976; Sato *et al.*, 1983). The overall remission rate ranges from 37.5% to 57.8% (Currier, Kooi and Saidman, 1963; Dalby, 1968; Hertoft, 1963; Lees and Liversedge, 1962; Sato, Dreifuss and Penry, 1976). The relapse rate for absence seizures after withdrawal of medication is 12% (Thurston *et al.*, 1982).

MYOCLONIC SEIZURES

Although the World Health Organization (Gastaut, 1973) offers different definitions of myoclonus and myoclonic jerks, these terms are often used interchangeably. As to the definition of myoclonic seizures, there is even more confusion and usually no statement as to what constitutes epilepsy. However, some investigators state that myoclonic seizures are a cortical event associated with EEG abnormalities (Erba and Browne, 1983; Halliday, 1975; Swanson, Luttrell and Magladery, 1962). Myoclonus may or may not be epileptic in origin.

Myoclonic jerks may be rapidly repetitive or relatively isolated. They may occur predominantly around the onset of sleep or upon awakening from sleep. They may be exacerbated by volitional movement (action myoclonus). At times they may be regularly repetitive.

Myoclonic seizures with associated EEG spikes are seen in progressive myoclonic epilepsy with or without Lafora bodies, cerebral lipidosis, infantile hemiplegia, viral encephalitis, hypoxic encephalopathy, and epilepsy.

Myoclonic epilepsy is uncommon and the reported incidence ranges from 0.3% to 3.8% among all forms of epilepsy (Gastaut *et al.*, 1973; Harper, 1968). Jeavons (1982b) has stated that the international classification of myoclonic epilepsy is inadequate and that it is difficult to classify myoclonic epilepsy. Several classifications of myoclonic seizures have been described (Aicardi, 1979; De Vivo, 1983; Dreifuss, 1983a; Jeavons, 1982b), but the practical classification seems to be a modification of De Vivo's classification (*Table 10.2*).

Table 10.2 Classification of myoclonic seizures

(1) Myoclonic seizures with demonstrable neurological signs, as in
  (a) progressive encephalopathy
  (b) static encephalopathy

(2) Myoclonic seizures without demonstrable neurological signs, as in
  (a) absence seizures
  (b) petit mal variant (Lennox–Gastaut syndrome)
  (c) generalized tonic-clonic seizures
  (d) myoclonic epilepsy

The group of progressive encephalopathies includes a variety of progressive nervous system disorders: metabolic-based disorders such as lipidosis, leukodystrophies, Lafora body disease, non-ketotic hyperglycemia; degenerative processes such as Unverricht–Lundborg syndrome, Ramsey–Hunt syndrome, juvenile neuroaxonal dystrophy, infantile poliodystrophies (Alper's disease), and myoclonus associated with spinocerebellar degeneration; and disorders with infectious etiologies such as subacute sclerosing panencephalitis and Creutzfeldt–Jakob disease. Non-progressive, static encephalopathies may be of either anoxic or obscure origin. They are associated with pyramidal tract signs and mental retardation.

Myoclonic seizures may be associated with other seizure types such as absence seizures, Lennox–Gastaut syndrome, or generalized tonic–clonic seizures. In this case, myoclonus occurs as part of the ictal manifestation. In absence seizures, for example, myoclonus may involve the eyelids, facial muscles, head, neck, or extremities in association with generalized 2–4 Hz spike-wave complexes on the EEG. In Lennox–Gastaut syndrome myoclonic seizures occur in addition to other more common types of seizures such as tonic, atonic, or atypical absence seizures, and are associated with slow spike-wave complexes and mental retardation.

Myoclonus in generalized tonic-clonic seizures constitutes part of the ictal event, particularly at the beginning or toward the end of the clonic phase or during the postictal phase.

Myoclonic epilepsy is represented by juvenile myoclonic epilepsy (Delgado-Escueta, Treiman and Walsh, 1983), which occurs in at least 4% of patients with epilepsy and affects children and adolescents of normal intelligence. It is extremely sensitive to valproic acid and has an excellent prognosis. This myoclonus occurs in patients who frequently have generalized clonic and/or tonic–clonic seizures; 37% of patients also have absence seizures. At first, the attacks occur predominantly upon waking in the morning, and consist of a sudden shock-like contraction, mainly of the shoulder girdles and upper extremities, often with preserved consciousness. If an attack occurs while the patient is standing, the patient may be flung to the floor, often resulting in injury. A jerk may be single or multiple.

The EEG during such an attack is characterized by sudden, bilateral, synchronous, multiple, spike–wave complexes (Dreifuss, 1983a) or by rapid, diffuse spikes at 16–24 Hz (Delgado-Escueta, Treiman and Walsh, 1983). The interictal EEG finding consists of fast spike–wave complexes or 4–6 Hz multispike-and-wave complexes. The EEG findings may persist until the sixth decade of life. The attack lasts for a fraction of a second to a few seconds. Sometimes the jerks may lead to generalized tonic-clonic seizures. There is frequently a family history of similar attacks, suggesting a polygenic mode of inheritance (Delgado-Escueta, Treiman and Walsh, 1983). The prognosis is often for a favorable outcome with increasing age (Dreifuss, 1983a).

Primary generalized myoclonic astatic epilepsy (Doose *et al.*, 1970) has been described as a separate entity (Delgado-Escueta, Treiman and Walsh, 1983). This is a rare form of epilepsy and has a genetic predisposition in which boys are affected three times more often than girls. The age at the onset is between 1 and 5 years, and affected children have normal intelligence. The seizures occur as myoclonic, atonic, absence or tonic-clonic seizures, and are accompanied by bilateral, synchronous, irregular 2–3 Hz and 4–6 Hz multispike-and-wave complexes.

ATONIC SEIZURES

The World Health Organization (Gastaut, 1973) defines atonic seizures as generalized epileptic seizures whose essential symptom is a decrease or abolition of postural tone, causing the subject to fall to the ground. When the loss of tone is very brief (a fraction of a second), the seizure is called an epileptic drop attack. When the loss of tone is of longer duration (usually 1–3 s), it is said to be atonic absence. When the loss of tone is of long duration and the subject remains unconscious on the ground in a complete state of relaxation for one or more minutes, this is called a true atonic epileptic seizure; in such cases the EEG consists of a mixture of rapid rhythms and slow waves, producing more or less regular and rhythmic spike-and-wave complexes of various frequency.

Atonic seizures, however, usually occur as a manifestation of absence or atypical absence seizures and are commonly seen in children. The sudden loss of postural tone in the head, trunk, or legs may manifest as head nodding or sagging of the body or legs, and may result in a fall to the floor if standing, leading to injury. The face is particularly vulnerable to injury. Sudden forward slumping when seated at the table, for example, can injure the nose and teeth by impact with the table.

In the case of more prolonged atonic attacks the slumping may occur progressively in a rhythmic, successive relaxation manner. If consciousness is lost, it is extremely brief. There is usually no detectable change in consciousness during the ictal or postictal phase. The patient usually picks himself up immediately and resumes what he was doing. No tongue biting or urinary incontinence is associated with atonic seizures.

Such attacks may occur spontaneously, but are more commonly provoked by photic stimulation (Gastaut *et al.*, 1974), auditory stimulation (Lance, 1968; Lennox and Lennox, 1960), startle (Lance, 1968) or light touch or tapping the skin (Calderon-Gonzalez and McLean, 1966). They may occur in young children with fever (Gastaut *et al.*, 1974) or emotional stress, fright, or surprise (Kirstein and Silverskield, 1958). At times, intense postural hypotonia may follow one or several myoclonic jerks (Gastaut, 1974). The attacks usually last 3–4 seconds.

Electrographically, the episodes are associated with spike-and-wave complexes, polyspike-and-wave complexes followed by diffuse generalized slow waves, rhythmic slow waves, fast recruiting activity (Lombroso and Erba, 1979), or even a generalized electrodecremental event (Fariello, Doro and Forster, 1979). The interictal EEG may show background slowing with slow, irregular spike–wave discharges, polyspikes-and-waves, spikes, or sharp waves.

The differential diagnosis of atonic seizures, which includes absence seizures, cataplexy, syncope and pseudoseizures, is described extensively elsewhere (Erba and Browne, 1983).

TREATMENT OF ABSENCE, MYOCLONIC, AND ATONIC SEIZURES

From psychological, social, and economic viewpoints, the goal of therapy in all of these seizure types is complete seizure control. Early and adequate treatment is recommended. Treatment should begin with the administration of one drug, the dosage being adjusted until an effective plasma drug concentration is achieved and maintained. If there is no improvement, another drug may be tried after the first drug is discontinued. If there is partial improvement, a second drug should be added and the effect on seizures observed when effective plasma concentrations of both drugs are maintained.

Absence seizures

Four drugs are indicated for the treatment of absence seizures. Ethosuximide is the drug of choice, followed by valproic acid, then clonazepam, and then possibly trimethadione. Ethosuximide is recommended for patients with absence seizures only, but valproic acid is recommended for those who have both absence and generalized tonic-clonic seizures (Sherwin, 1983). Trimethadione is effective, but it produces serious side-effects and is not currently used as often as it was in the past. A combination of ethosuximide and valproic acid may be beneficial in patients with refractory absence seizures (Dreifuss, 1983b; Rowan *et al.*, 1983). The combination of anti-absence drugs and other anti-epileptic drugs for possible complications of generalized tonic-clonic seizures (Livingston *et al.*, 1965) is not recommended.

Intravenously administered diazepam is the drug of choice for absence status. The initial maximum dosage is 10 mg. The most serious complication is respiratory arrest due to excessive doses. Respiratory arrest is particularly likely to occur when diazepam is used immediately after intravenous administration of phenobarbital. Ethosuximide, nitrazepam and clonazepam are also noted to be effective.

Ethosuximide

Ethosuximide [2-ethyl-2-methylsuccinimide; Zarontin] is supplied as 250 mg capsules or flavored syrup, both of which have equal bioavailability. The starting dose is 250 mg/day, and the daily maintenance dose is 15–25 mg/kg. Incremental increases of 250 mg can be made at intervals of 3–7 days, up to a daily dose of 40 mg/kg, aiming at a plasma ethosuximide level of 40–100 μg/ml. Some patients may require a plasma drug level of up to 150 μg/ml to achieve seizure control. Ethosuximide is rapidly absorbed (the peak plasma level occurs within 1–4 hours) and it is not protein bound. The half-life of ethosuximide is 30 hours in children and 60 hours in adults, so that it can be given once a day, but it is wise to give it twice a day to avoid gastrointestinal discomfort.

The side-effects of ethosuximide have been extensively reviewed elsewhere (Dreifuss, 1982). The dose-related adverse reactions are nausea, gastrointestinal discomfort, drowsiness, dizziness, anorexia, headache and fatigue. These reactions are common, relatively trival, and usually respond to dosage reduction. Side-effects not related to the dose include exacerbation of various types of seizures and behavioral changes such as transient psychoses and interference with cognitive function. Delayed specific organ sensitivities, including hematological (leukopenia, pancytopenia), dermatological (skin rashes), and immunological (lupus-like syndrome), represent the most serious and potentially lethal complication, requiring immediate discontinuation of the drug. Ethosuximide rarely interacts with other drugs, although modest elevation in the plasma ethosuximide level has been noted in patients taking valproic acid.

Valproic acid

Valproic acid [2-propylpentanoic acid; Depakene] is as effective as ethosuximide for the treatment of absence seizures (Sato *et al.*, 1982). In patients with gastrointestinal intolerance, enteric-coated divalproex sodium can be tried. Although the absorption of divalproex sodium is delayed, the bioavailability of valproic acid capsules and divalproex sodium tablets is equivalent (Wilder *et al.*, 1983a), and the latter can be substituted for valproic acid without breakthrough seizures (Wilder *et al.*, 1983b).

The initial daily dose is 15 mg/kg. With increments of 125 mg every 3–5 days, the daily dose can be increased to a range of 30–60 mg/kg in children. Both valproic acid and sodium valproate are rapidly absorbed; their peak plasma levels occur within two hours following ingestion (Wilder and Karas, 1982). The peak plasma level of divalproex sodium occurs within three hours. Valproate is 90% protein bound. The half-life of valproic acid is 8–15 hours in children and 9–17 hours in adults. A dosing schedule of four times a day has been recommended because of this relatively short half-life, but administration twice a day, or even once a day, without breakthrough seizures has been described (Wilder *et al.*, 1983b). The effective plasma levels of valproic acid range from 50 to 100 μg/ml, but some patients may require a higher plasma level (up to 150–200 μg/ml). The 'trough' plasma level has been found most useful in managing valproic acid treatment, but seizure control in some patients may be independent of the plasma drug concentration.

The side-effects of valproate or valproic acid have been extensively reviewed elsewhere (Jeavons, 1982a, 1983). Adverse reactions are rare when valproate is given as the sole antiepileptic drug. Anorexia, indigestion, heartburn, and nausea are more common than vomiting and are usually temporary. They may be avoided or reduced by taking the drug with or after meals. Increased appetite and increased body weight may occur. Pancreatitis is a rare complication. Drowsiness is uncommon in patients who take only valproate, but common in patients taking valproate and other drugs. A stuporous condition and profound sedation have been noted in patients taking valproate in addition to phenobarbital or clonazepam. Absence status has been seen in patients taking valproate and clonazepam. Worsened behavior and hyperactivity are rare. Tremor is fairly common and more likely to occur with high dosage of the drug. Temporary thinning of the hair may occur. Hematological toxicity includes neutropenia, fibrinogen depletion, abnormalities in the erythrocyte sedimentation rate, and thrombocytopenia, which is rare, often asymptomatic, and which is most likely to occur and cause symptoms if the daily dosage exceeds 50 mg/kg.

The most serious complication of valproate therapy is hepatic involvement, which manifests as elevation of serum glutamic oxalacetic transaminase (SGOT) and serum glutamic pyruvic transminase (SGPT). These elevations are usually transient and respond to reduction in valproate dosage. A recent review lists 52 fatal cases of hepatic failure following valproate administration (Jeavons, 1983). The recommendations are as follows: if the patient has clinical symptoms and the results of liver function tests (especially SGOT) are abnormal, valproate should be withdrawn immediately. Jeavons states that clinical monitoring is more important than laboratory tests, and that patients taking valproate should be reviewed every two weeks for the first two months and every month for the next four months.

There have been no reports of human fetal or reproductive abnormalities related to valproate, although teratogenic effects have occurred with extremely high doses in animals. Irregular menses and secondary amenorrhea have been noted.

Valproate has many important interactions with other drugs (Mattson, 1982). The effects of valproate on other drugs include rise in plasma phenobarbital level by slowing hydroxylation and elimination of phenobarbital, and initial lowering of plasma phenytoin level by competitive displacement with later return to pre-valproate or higher level. Valproate increases the ethosuximide level slightly, but produces no change in the clonazepam level. Interaction with carbamazepine is not known, although concomitant administration of valproate and carbamazepine is known to cause sedation, nausea, diplopia and/or a confusional state. Phenytoin and phenobarbital are known to lower the valproate level. Salicylic acid displaces valproate from protein, resulting in higher free levels of the drug.

Clonazepam

Clonazepam [5-(2-chlorophenyl)-1,3-dihydro-7-nitro-2H-1, 4-benzodiazepin-2-one; Clonopin] is extremely effective for the treatment of absence seizures. It is superior to ethosuximide in the normalization of the EEG (Dreifuss *et al.*, 1975), but adverse side-effects and the development of tolerance greatly reduce this advantage (Sato *et al.*, 1977). The details of its usefulness are described elsewhere (Dreifuss and Sato, 1982).

The initial daily dose of clonazepam is 0.5 mg or 0.01–0.03 mg/kg (not more than 0.05 mg/kg). This dose is slowly increased at a rate of 0.25–0.5 mg/week up to a maximum daily dose of 8–10 mg, or sometimes even higher (Browne, 1978). The daily maintenance dose is 0.1–0.2 mg/kg.

Clonazepam appears to be well absorbed; the peak plasma level occurs within one to four hours after oral administration. Clonazepam is 82% protein bound, and its half-life is 22–33 hours in children with absence seizures (Dreifuss *et al.*, 1975). Plasma clonazepam levels of 13–72 ng/ml reduce the frequency of absence seizures (Dreifuss *et al.*, 1975).

The incidence of adverse reactions is very high, often leading to eventual discontinuation of clonazepam. Drowsiness and ataxia usually appear a few hours after administration in the early treatment and improve with adjustment of the dosage. Significant behavioral and personality changes, such as hyperactivity, restlessness, short attention span, irritability, disruptiveness and aggressiveness commonly occur in children and occasionally in adults. Other side-effects include nystagmus, dizziness, dysarthria and hypotonia, and, less commonly, blurred vision, diplopia and psychotic reactions. The frequency of various types of seizures may increase, or different types of seizures may emerge. Slight weight gain is also a fairly common problem. Hypersecretion and hypersalivation may be troublesome in children and infants. Leukopenia or thrombocytopenic purpura is rare. Skin pigmentation, transient hair loss, and extensive skin rashes have been described but are rare. Hepatic or renal complications have not been observed. Clonazepam must be withdrawn cautiously, tapering the dose very slowly; for example, 0.25 mg per week.

Trimethadione

Trimethadione [3,5,5-trimethyl-oxazolidine-2,4-dione; Tridione] is no longer the drug of choice for the treatment of absence seizures because effective and safer agents have become available. The trend favoring use of the drug was established before the pharmacokinetics of trimethadione were studied (Booker, 1982). In healthy volunteers, the peak plasma trimethadione level occurred at 30–60 min after a single oral dose and the average half-life was 16 hours. Trimethadione is metabolized to dimethadione in the body. The half-life of dimethadione is not known but has been estimated at around 10 days or more. The trimethadione level fluctuates considerably during the day, whereas the dimethadione level is very stable. Trimethadione is not protein bound. Each mg/kg of trimethadione seems to give an average plasma trimethadione level of 0.6 μg/ml, and dimethadione levels average 20 times the trimethadione levels. The recommended daily dose is 30 mg/kg. Seizure control seems to be associated with plasma dimethadione levels of 700 μg/ml or more.

Common dose-dependent side-effects include hemeralopia (day blindness) and photophobia, sedation, fatigue, lack of concentration, dizziness, ataxia, insomnia, restlessness, and infrequently confusion and hallucinatory psychosis. Side-effects not related to the dose include erythema multiforme and exfoliative dermatitis, and bone marrow depression (neutropenia, pancytopenia), which necessitate withdrawal of the drug. Relatively benign side-effects are morbilliform or acneiform rashes. Side-effects involving the autoimmune system include nephrotic syndrome, which is usually reversible if the drug is withdrawn, and myasthenic syndrome. Fetal malformations due to trimethadione have been noted.

Although no longer the drug of choice, trimethadione remains an effective drug for the control of absence seizures and should be reserved for patients who do not respond to or cannot safely take the other anti-absence drugs (Booker, 1982).

Myoclonic seizures

The drug of choice for myoclonic seizures is valproate, which can be given alone or in combination with other drugs (Chayasirisobhon and Russel, 1983; Jeavons, 1982b; Lance and Anthony, 1977). Clonazepam has been found effective (Mikkelsen, Birket-Smith and Brandt, 1976; Lance and Anthony, 1977), and trimethadione is also beneficial (Davies and Spillane, 1949). Primary generalized myoclonic astatic epilepsy is said to be responsive to valproate (Delgado-Escueta, Treiman and Walsh, 1983).

Atonic seizures

Atonic seizures are relatively intractable to medical treatment and are often associated with other types of seizures. Valproate is the drug of choice for atonic seizures and can be added to other drug therapy (Chayasirisobhon and Russel, 1983; Lance and Anthony, 1977). Clonazepam is also effective (Mikkelsen, Birket-Smith and Brandt, 1976). Carbamazepine may be used, although its efficacy is uncertain. Phenytoin is usually not successful and may exacerbate seizures, and phenobarbital causes drowsiness and consequent seizure exacerbation (Dreifuss, 1983a).

Acknowledgement

The editorial assistance of B. J. Hessie is gratefully acknowledged.

References

AICARDI, J. (1979) Mycolonic epilepsies. In *Aspects of Epilepsy* (Proceedings of the Oxford Scientific Meeting of the International League Against Epilepsy–British Branch), edited by M. J. Parsonage. Tunbridge Wells: MCS Consultants

BLOM, S., HEIJBEL, J. and BERGFOUS, P. G. (1978) Incidence of epilepsy in children: a follow-up study three years after first seizures. *Epilepsia,* **19,** 343–350

BOOKER, H. E. (1982) Trimethadione: relation of plasma concentration to seizure control. In *Antiepileptic Drugs,* 2nd Edition, edited by D. M. Woodbury, J. K. Penry and C. E. Pippenger, pp. 697–699. New York: Raven Press

BROWNE, T. R. (1978) Clonazepam. *New England Journal of Medicine,* **299,** 812–816

CALDERON-GONZALEZ, R. and MCLEAN, W. (1966) Tap seizures: a form of sensory precipitation epilepsy. *Journal of the American Medical Association,* **198,** 521–523

CHARLTON, M. H. and YAHR, M. D. (1967) Long-term follow-up of patients with petit mal. *Archives of Neurology,* **16,** 595–598

CHAYASIRISOBHON, S. and RUSSEL, M. (1983) Valproic acid and intractable seizures in severely brain damaged patients. *Neurology (New York),* **33,** 99–101

COMMISSION FOR THE CONTROL OF EPILEPSY AND ITS CONSEQUENCES (1978) *Plan for Nationwide Action on Epilepsy,* Vol. I. DHEW Publication No. (NIH) 78–276. Bethesda, Md.: National Institute of Health

COMMISSION ON CLASSIFICATION AND TERMINOLOGY OF THE INTERNATIONAL LEAGUE AGAINST EPILEPSY (1981) Proposal for revised clinical and electroencephalographic classification of epileptic seizures. *Epilepsia,* **22,** 489–501

CREWS, R. D. and SIDELL, A. D. (1973) The clinical significance of spike and wave abnormalities in the adult. *Bulletin of the Los Angeles Neurological Societies,* **38,** 60–68

CURRIER, R. D., KOOI, K. A. and SAIDMAN, L. J. (1963) Prognosis of 'pure' petit mal. A follow-up study. *Neurology (Minneapolis),* **13,** 959–967

DALBY, M. A. (1968) The duration of bilaterally synchronous 3/sec spike-wave rhythms. *Electroencephalography and Clinical Neurophysiology,* **24,** 87

DAVIES, G. R. and SPILLANE, J. D. (1949) Tridione therapy in minor epilepsy. *Brain,* **72,** 140–149

DELGADO-ESCUETA, A. V., TREIMAN, D. M. and WALSH, G. O. (1983) The treatable epilepsies. *New England Journal of Medicine,* **308,** 1508–1514

DE VIVO, D. C. (1983) Myoclonic seizures. In *Antiepileptic Drug Therapy in Pediatrics,* edited by P. L. Morselli, C. E. Pippenger and J. K. Penry, pp. 37–143. New York: Raven Press

DOOSE, H., GERKEN, H., LEONHARDT, R., VOLZKE, E. and VOLZ, C. (1970) Centrencephalic-astatic petit mal: clinical and genetic investigations. *Neuropädiatrie,* **2,** 59–78

DOOSE, H., GERKEN, T., HORSTMANN, T. and VOLZKE, E. (1973) Genetic factors in spike-wave absences. *Epilepsia,* **14,** 57–75

DREIFUSS, F. E. (1972) The prognosis of petit mal epilepsy. In *The Epidemiology of Epilepsy: A Workshop.* NINCDS Monograph No. 14, pp. 120–131. Washington: US Government Printing Office

DREIFUSS, F. E. (1982) Ethosuximide. Toxicity. In *Antiepileptic Drugs,* 2nd Edition, edited by D. M. Woodbury, J. K. Penry and C. E. Pippenger, pp. 647–653. New York: Raven Press

DREIFUSS, F. E. (1983a) Treatment of the nonconvulsive epilepsies. *Epilepsia,* **24,** 945–954

DREIFUSS, F. E. (1983b) How to use valproate. In *Antiepileptic Drug Therapy in Pediatrics*, edited by P. L. Morselli, C. E. Pippenger, and J. K. Penry, pp. 219–227. New York: Raven Press

DREIFUSS, F. E., PENRY, J. K., ROSE, S. W., KUPFERBERG, H. J., DYKEN, P. and SATO, S. (1975) Serum clonazepam concentrations in children with absence seizures. *Neurology (Minneapolis),* **23,** 255–258

DREIFUSS, F. E. and SATO, S. (1982) Benzodiazepines. Clonazepam. In *Antiepileptic Drugs,* 2nd Edition, edited by D. M. Woodbury, J. K. Penry and C. E. Pippenger, pp. 737–752. New York: Raven Press

ERBA, G. and BROWNE, T. R. (1983) Atypical absence, myoclonic, atonic and tonic seizures, and the 'Lennox–Gastaut syndrome'. In *Epilepsy: Diagnosis and Management*, edited by T. R. Browne and R. G. Feldman, pp. 75–94. Boston: Little, Brown

ESCUETA, A. V. D., BACSAL, F. E. and TREIMAN, D. M. (1982) Complex partial seizures on closed circuit television and EEG. A study of 619 attacks in 79 patients. *Annals of Neurology,* **11,** 292–300

FAIRELLO, R. G., DORO, J. M. and FORSTER, F. M. (1979) Generalized cortical electrodecremental event: clinical and neurophysiological observations in patients with dystonic seizures. *Archives of Neurology,* **36,** 285–291

GASTAUT, H. (1973) *Dictionary of Epilepsy. Part I: Definitions.* Geneva: World Health Organization

GASTAUT, H., BROUGHTON, R., ROGER, J. and TASSINARI, C. A. (1974) Generalized nonconvulsive seizures without local onset. In *Handbook of Clinical Neurology,* Vol. 15, edited by P. J. Vinken and G. W. Bruyn, pp. 130–144. New York: American Elsevier Publishing Company

GASTAUT, H. and GASTAUT, J. (1977) Computerized axial tomography in epilepsy. In *Epilepsy, The Eighth International Symposium,* edited by J. K. Penry, pp. 5–15. New York: Raven Press

GASTAUT, H., GASTAUT, J. L., GONCALVES, E., SILVA, G. E. and FERNANDEZ-SANCHEZ, G. R. (1973) Relative frequency of different types of epilepsy: a study employing the classification of the International League Against Epilepsy. *Epilepsia,* **16,** 457–461

GIANTURCO, D. T., WILSON, W. P. and HARRIS, B. S. (1968) Interictal focal or lateralized discharges occurring in the electroencephalograms of patients suffering from centrencephalic epilepsy. *Confinia Neurologica,* **30,** 368–374

GIBBERD, F. B. (1966) The clinical features of petit mal. *Acta Neurologica Scandinavica,* **42,** 176–190

GIBBERD, F. B. (1972) The prognosis of petit mal in adults. *Epilepsia,* **13,** 171–175

HALLIDAY, A. M. (1975) The neurophysiology of myoclonic jerking – a reappraisal. In *Myoclonic Seizures,* edited by M. H. Charlton, pp. 1–29. Amsterdam: Excerpta Medica

HARPER, J. R. (1968) True myoclonic epilepsy in children. *Archives of Disease in Childhood,* **43,** 28

HAUSER, W. A. and KURLAND, L. T. (1975) The epidemiology of epilepsy in Rochester, Minnesota, 1935 through 1967. *Epilepsia,* **16,** 1–66

HERTOFT, P. (1963) The clinical, electroencephalographic and social prognosis in petit mal epilepsy. *Epilepsia,* **4,** 298–314

HOLOWACH, J., THURSTON, D. L. and O'LEARY, L. (1962) Petit mal epilepsy. *Pediatrics,* **30,** 893–901

JASPER, H. H. and DROOGLEEVER-FORTUYN, J. (1946) Experimental studies on the functional anatomy of petit mal epilepsy. *Research Publications—Association for Research in Nervous and Mental Disease,* **26,** 272–298

JEAVONS, P. M. (1982a) Valproate. Toxicity. In *Antiepileptic Drugs,* 2nd Edition, edited by D. M. Woodbury, J. K. Penry and C. E. Pippenger, pp. 601–610. New York: Raven Press

JEAVONS, P. M. (1982b) Myoclonic epilepsies: therapy and prognosis. *Advances in Epileptology,* **13,** 141–144

JEAVONS, P. M. (1983) Hepatotoxicity of antiepileptic drugs. In *Chronic Toxicity of Antiepileptic Drugs,* edited by J. Oxley, D. Janz and H. Meinardi, pp. 1–45. New York: Raven Press

KIRSTEIN, L. and SILVERSKIELD, B. P. (1958) A family with emotionally precipitated 'drop seizures'. *Acta Psychiatrica Scandinavica,* **33,** 471–476

KURLAND, L. T. (1959–60) The incidence and prevalence of convulsive disorders in a small urban community. *Epilepsia,* **1,** 143–161

LAGENSTEIN, I., KUHNE, D., STERNOWSKY, H. J. and ROTHE, M. (1979) Computerized cranial transverse axial tomography (CTAT) in 145 patients with primary and secondary generalized epilepsies, West syndrome, myoclonic-astatic petit mal, absence epilepsy. *Neuropädiatrie,* **10,** 15–28

LANCE, J. W. (1968) Myoclonic jerks and falls: aetiology, classification and treatment. *Medical Journal of Australia,* **1,** 113–120

LANCE, J. W. and ANTHONY, M. (1977) Sodium valproate and clonazepam in the treatment of intractable epilepsy. *Archives of Neurology,* **34,** 14–17

LEES, F. and LIVERSEDGE, L. A. (1962) The prognosis of 'petit mal' and minor epilepsy. *Lancet,* **2,** 797–799

LENNOX, W. G. and LENNOX, M. A. (1960) *Epilepsy and Related Disorders.* Boston: Little, Brown

LIVINGSTON, S., TORRES, I., PAULI, L. L. and RIDER, R. W. (1965) Petit mal epilepsy. Results of a prolonged follow-up study of 117 patients. *Journal of the American Medical Association,* **194,** 113–118

LOMBROSO, C. T. and ERBA, G. (1979) Drop seizures: atonic, tonic, myoclonic components. Clinical electrophysiological correlates. *Electroencephalography and Clinical Neurophysiology,* **46,** 12P

MATTHES, A. and WEBER, H. (1968) Klinische und elektroencephalographische Familien untersuchungen bei Pyknolepsein. *Deutsche Medizinische Wochenschrift,* **93,** 429–435

MATTHES, A. (1969) Genetic studies in epilepsy. In *The Physiopathogenesis of the Epilepsies,* edited by H. Gastaut *et al.*, pp. 26–30. Springfield, Ill.: Charles C. Thomas

MATTSON, R. H. (1982) Valproate: interactions with other drugs. In *Antiepileptic Drugs,* 2nd Edition, edited by D. M. Woodbury, J. K. Penry and C. E. Pippenger, pp. 579–589. New York: Raven Press

METRAKOS, K. and METRAKOS, J. D. (1961) Genetics of convulsive disorders. Part 2: Genetic and electroencephalographic studies in centrencephalic epilepsy. *Neurology (Minneapolis),* **11,** 464–483

MIKKELSEN, B., BIRKET-SMITH, F. and BRANDT, S. (1976) Clonazepam in the treatment of epilepsy: a controlled clinical trial in simple absences, bilateral massive epileptic myoclonus and atonic seizures. *Archives of Neurology,* **33,** 322–325

NIEDERMEYER, E. (1965) Sleep electroencephalograms in petit mal. *Archives of Neurology,* **12,** 625–630

O'BRIEN, J. L., GOLDENSOHN, E. S. and HOEFER, P. E. A. (1959) Electroencephalographic abnormalities in addition to bilaterally synchronous 3 per second spike and wave activity in petit mal. *Electroencephalography and Clinical Neurophysiology,* **11,** 747–761

PENRY, J. K., PORTER, R. J. and DREIFUSS, F. E. (1975) Simultaneous recording of absence seizures with video tape and electroencephalography. A study of 374 seizures in 48 patients. *Brain,* **98,** 427–440

ROWAN, A. J., MEIJER, J. W. A., DE BEER-PAWLIKOWSKI, N., VANDER GERST, H. and MEINARDI, H. (1983) Valproate-ethosuximide combination therapy for refractory absence seizures. *Archives of Neurology,* **40,** 797–802

SATO, S., DREIFUSS, F. E. and PENRY, J. K. (1973) The effect of sleep on spike-wave discharges in absence seizures. *Neurology (Minneapolis),* **23,** 1135–1345

SATO, S., DREIFUSS, F. E. and PENRY, J. K. (1976) Prognostic factors in absence seizures. *Neurology (Minneapolis),* **26,** 778–796

SATO, S., DREIFUSS, F. E., PENRY, J. K., KIRBY, D. D. and PALESCH, Y. (1983) Long-term follow-up of absence seizures. *Neurology (Cleveland),* **33,** 1590–1595

SATO, S., PENRY, J. K., DREIFUSS, F. E. and DYKEN, P. R. (1977) Clonazepam in the treatment of absence seizures: a double-blind clinical trial. *Neurology (Minneapolis),* **27,** 371

SATO, S., WHITE, B. G., PENRY, J. K., DREIFUSS, F. E., SACKELLARES, J. C. and KUPFERBERG, J. H. (1982) Valproic acid versus ethosuximide in the treatment of absence seizures. *Neurology (Minneapolis),* **32,** 157–163

SHERWIN, A. L. (1983) How to use ethosuximide. In *Antiepileptic Drug Therapy in Pediatrics,* edited by P. L. Morselli, C. E. Pippenger and J. K. Penry, pp. 220–236. New York: Raven Press

SILVERMAN, D. (1954) Clinical correlates of the spike and wave complex. *Electroencephalography and Clinical Neurophysiology,* **6,** 663

SWANSON, P. D., LUTTRELL, C. N. and MAGLADERY, J. W. (1962) Myoclonus—a report of 76 cases and review of the literature. *Medicine (Baltimore),* **41,** 339

THURSTON, J. H., THURSTON, D. L., HIXON, B. B. and KELLER, A. J. (1982) Prognosis in childhood epilepsy. Additional follow-up of 148 children 15 to 23 years after withdrawal of anticonvulsant therapy. *New England Journal of Medicine,* **306,** 832–836

WILDER, B. J. and KARAS, B. J. (1982) Valproate: relation of plasma concentration to seizure control. In *Antiepileptic Drugs,* 2nd Edition, edited by D. M. Woodbury, J. K. Penry and C. E. Pippenger, pp. 591–599. New York: Raven Press

WILDER, B. J., KARAS, B. J., PENRY, J. K. and ASCONAGE, J. (1983a) Gastrointestinal tolerance of divalproate sodium. *Neurology (Cleveland),* **33,** 808–811

WILDER, B. J., KARAS, B. J., HAMMOND, E. J. and PERCHALSKI, R. J. (1983b) Twice-daily dosing of valproate with divalproex. *Clinical Pharmacology and Therapeutics,* **34,** 501–504

11

The medical management of neonatal and infantile seizures and of febrile seizures

Jean Aicardi

The therapeutic problems posed by neonatal and infantile seizures are different from those in other age groups for several reasons. First, many seizures which occur before two years of age are age-specific responses of the brain to structural or metabolic changes that are unlikely to last more than a few weeks (for example, neonatal seizures) or a few years (for example, febrile convulsions). Secondly, certain seizure disorders, in particular infantile spasms, behave quite differently from most other types of fits in their response to drugs. Thirdly, the metabolism of anticonvulsant drugs is highly age-dependent and changes very rapidly during the first 2–4 years of life. This chapter deals with neonatal seizures, infantile spasms and febrile convulsions.

NEONATAL SEIZURES

Seizures occurring in infants less than 28 days of age (or up to 44 weeks of conceptional age) are usually the result of an acute lesional or metabolic process and they tend to occur serially over a short period. Neonatal seizures occur in 4.2–12 per 1000 newborn infants (Brown and Minns, 1980; Lombroso, 1983).

Clinical features and causes of neonatal seizures

Seizure patterns in the neonate differ considerably from those in older patients. Generalized tonic-clonic seizures are exceptional and most convulsions are focal or fragmentary ones. Four main types of neonatal convulsions are commonly recognized (*Table 11.1*).

In general, the more organized seizure types (clonic convulsions) are seen in full-term infants, are associated with well-formed slow spikes or sharp waves in the ictal EEG and are less likely to be associated with severe brain damage. They were often observed with late onset hypocalcaemia and are consequently becoming less common. However, they are still seen with subarachnoid haemorrhage (Volpe, 1981) or in seizures of unknown origin. Their occurrence does not imply the presence of a localized brain damage, even when the jerks remain confined to a

Table 11.1 Main types of neonatal convulsions

(1) Clonic seizures (primarily full-term infants)
    Focal (do not necessarily imply a localized brain lesion)
    Multifocal or erratic: clonias migrating from one segment to another in disorderly fashion; may involve different segments at same time or in succession; may remain *unilateral* or involve both sides asynchronously
(2) Tonic seizures (primarily premature babies)
    Localized to one segment (minor posturing)
    Generalized, resembling decerebrate or decorticate posturing
(3) Subtle (minimal or fragmentary) seizures (premature and full-term infants,
    Orobuccal-lingual movements; eye opening, deviation or staring; abnormal repetitive limb movements; grimacing; respiratory (apnoeas) or other autonomic phenomena
(4) Myoclonic seizures (premature and full-term babies)
    Include early infantile spasms and massive or erratic myoclonus

single body area. In this case, however, they may be related to a structural lesion, especially an ischaemic or haemorrhagic one. Multifocal clonic seizures are considered by some authors (Lombroso, 1974, 1978) as an intermediate type between unifocal and subtle seizures. However, they are frequently observed in patients with metabolic disturbances as well as in cases of unknown aetiology and favourable prognosis. Subtle seizures most commonly supervene in infants with severe brain insults, especially anoxic-ischaemic encephalopathy, and are accompanied by atypical ictal EEG activity such as rhythmic theta (θ) or delta (δ) waves or a localized alpha-like pattern (Lombroso, 1978; Volpe, 1981). Tonic seizures occur mainly in premature infants, especially with subependymal-ventricular haemorrhage. Their epileptic nature is dubious in many cases because similar fits may be due to release phenomena and because the EEG displays flattening of the record more often than typical paroxysmal activity. The presence of eye deviation and/or orobuccal–lingual movements is a strong argument in favour of an epileptic nature. Massive myoclonic seizures may resemble infantile spasms. They may be associated with erratic myoclonus.

The differential diagnosis of neonatal seizures is of variable difficulty. Clonic seizures should be distinguished from jitteriness and tremor which are periodic oscillatory movements that are induced by positioning or moving the limbs and can be suppressed by immobilizing the limbs in a position of relaxation. Subtle seizures, a very common type, may easily go unrecognized or may be difficult to identify as epileptic seizures, so that a simultaneous EEG recording is often necessary to categorize them properly. The same applies to ictal apnoeas which are much rarer than the common non-epileptic apnoeas, especially in premature infants (Watanabe *et al.*, 1982). Ictal apnoeas, however, are usually accompanied by one or another of the subtle manifestations listed in *Table 11.1*. In the rare patient, definite seizures occur without EEG concomitants, especially at a late stage of serial seizures (Dreyfus-Brisac and Monod, 1972). Abnormal movements, such as boxing or pedalling, commonly observed in metabolic disorders, are most often unassociated with paroxysmal EEG activity and are probably of a non-epileptic nature.

The main causes of neonatal seizures are listed in *Table 11.2*. More detailed studies can be found elsewhere (Lombroso, 1978; Volpe, 1981). Although some of the aetiological factors may be effective in isolation (such as late hypocalcaemia or intoxications) in most patients several factors are at play at the same time. For example, early hypocalcaemia occurs in a context of prematurity, dysmaturity or other neonatal difficulties, and in association with hypoxia, hypoglycaemia or other disturbances which are of greater prognostic significance than the low calcium level itself. One should therefore try to establish a hierarchy of the causes, giving priority

Table 11.2 Main causes of neonatal seizures

(1) Metabolic causes
- Hypocalcaemia (early type in association with other aetiologic factors; late type after five days of age)
- Hypomagnesaemia (usually associated with hypocalcaemia)
- Hypoglycaemia
- Hyponatraemia and water intoxication
- Hyperammonaemia, disorders of organic acids and amino acids
- Pyridoxine dependency

(2) Toxic causes
- Local anaesthetic intoxication
- Drug withdrawal (narcotic-analgesics or sedative-hypnotics)

(3) Hypoxic-ischaemic encephalopathy

(4) Intracranial haemorrhage
- Intraventricular (preterm infants)
- Subarachnoid
- Intraparenchymal

(5) Infections
- Bacterial meningitis
- Intrauterine infections

(6) Vascular causes
- Neonatal strokes

(7) Brain dysplasias

(8) Unknown causes
- Genetic origin (benign familial neonatal seizures)
- Non-genetic (including 'fifth day fits')

to treatable causes. Seizures of unknown cause represent a significant proportion of the patients (from 10 to 25%). They tend to occur relatively late – after the third day of life – in contrast to convulsions of hypoxic–ischaemic origin which arise mainly within the first 24 hours. A small proportion of them may be familial. Some authors distinguish a subgroup of 'fifth day fits' (Dehan *et al.*, 1977; Pryor, Don and Macourt, 1981) characterized by repeated clonic fits, a relatively normal interictal EEG with episodic bursts of sharp theta rhythm, and a consistently favourable course. This syndrome has not been encountered by all investigators and its incidence has varied considerably in the same location (Pryor, Don and Macourt, 1981). Its definitive characterization must await further studies.

Management of neonatal seizures

General management

A newborn with seizures is easier to nurse in an incubator without clothes so that fits are easily observed and recorded. Monitoring of respiration and heart rate is essential and EEG recording is highly desirable if it can be obtained without delaying therapeutic measures. A secure intravenous line should be established and fluids administered but the quantity should be restricted to 75% of the normally required amount to avoid dilutional hyponatraemia. Control of body temperature is essential, so a thermocouple feedback to the incubator may be necessary. Assisted ventilation may be required although neonatal seizures rarely interfere severely with vital functions. Urine should be collected and tested for reducing substances and ketone bodies and blood drawn for glucose, electrolytes, CO_2 and pH determinations. A lumbar puncture is imperative. An ultrasound examination is essential whenever there is a suspicion of intracranial haemorrhage or of any structural abnormality but CT scan is best postponed until the infant has recovered. Although some workers advise treatment of 'cerebral oedema' with dexamethasone (Brown and Minns, 1980), the evidence for such a treatment is far from compelling in true epileptic seizures.

Specific treatment

Whenever a treatable cause to the seizures can be identified, specific therapy is immediately indicated. If hypoglycaemia is present, 2–4 ml/kg of a 20–30% solution of glucose is administered intravenously. This initial loading dose is followed by an infusion of up to 0.5 g/kg per hour depending upon blood glucose levels. If hypocalcaemia is found, a slow intravenous injection of 2.5–5% calcium gluconate solution is given at doses of 5–20 ml under electrocardiographic monitoring. Magnesium sulphate (2–3% solution) can be injected at doses of 2–8 ml if there is associated hypomagnesaemia. Intramuscular injection of 0.2 ml/kg of 50% solution of magnesium sulphate is an alternative method. Pyridoxine should be tried in all patients prior to administration of anticonvulsant drugs so that its effect, if any, can be evaluated without ambiguity. Although pyridoxine dependency is a rare cause of neonatal seizures, it must be recognized early if mental sequelae are to be avoided or limited. Other specific therapies (such as of meningitis) should be applied according to the usual techniques in appropriate cases.

Non-specific treatment of seizures

Anticonulvsant drug treatment of neonatal seizures is indicated in infants whose seizures are not accessible to specific therapy and as an adjunct to the latter if it does not control the fits immediately. Although the main predictor of prognosis is the cause of the seizures, there is some suggestion that neonatal seizures may produce brain damage, either by indirect mechanisms such as hypercapnia with increased brain lactate and consequent increase in cerebral blood flow with the attendant risk of haemorrhage (Lou and Friis-Hansen, 1979), or directly, by decreasing brain ATP and phosphocreatinine concentrations despite the delivery to the brain of an increased supply of substrates (Meldrum, 1978). The synthesis of protein in the brain is also decreased in experimental animals with neonatal convulsions (Wasterlain, 1976).

Although all authors agree that early treatment is imperative, there is no consensus regarding its modalities. While some authors (*see* Volpe, 1981) recommend immediate therapy with large doses of long-acting drugs, others (Lombroso, 1978, 1983) favour the initial administration of the short-acting agent diazepam in doses of 0.8–1.2 mg/kg (total dose). The dose is given either as a slow injection of a solution containing 1 mg/ml or as a bolus of 0.2–1.0 mg as total dose for babies weighing 1.5–3.0 kg. Rectal diazepam may also be used at slightly higher dosages as it is rapidly absorbed as a solution, but not as suppositories (Dulac *et al.*, 1978; Knudsen, 1977). A second dose of diazepam can be administered after about 20 min but repeated doses produce considerable accumulation and are better avoided, even though respiratory arrest is rare (Aicardi, 1983). Despite the variability in active dose and the very rapid clearance from the brain, diazepam is useful when employed only as an initial drug or for relatively mild cases (such as newborns with late seizures of unknown origin) and not for frequently repeated convulsions, as it avoids the systematic administration of massive doses of anticonvulsant drugs.

In the case of repeated seizures, or systematically from onset for those workers who do not use diazepam, long-acting anticonvulsant drugs are used. Phenobarbital is generally considered as the drug of first choice, phenytoin being reserved for resistant cases. For both drugs (especially phenytoin), absorption by the oral route is unreliable, and the same applies to the intramuscular route for phenytoin, which should be given only intravenously (Painter *et al.*, 1981).

The apparent elimination half-life of both drugs is much longer in the first 7–14 days than at any other period. The average elimination half-life of phenobarbital is 100 h or more (range 40–200 h) and that of phenytoin is also quite long (range 4–140 h). These half-lives rapidly decline over the next few weeks to levels two to three times shorter than in adults, and apparent half-lives of 20–70 h for phenobarbital and of 7–20 h for phenytoin have been measured in postneonatal infants (Painter *et al.*, 1978, 1981; Pitlick, Painter and Pippenger, 1978). There is thus a need for careful monitoring of blood levels and for rapid dosage adjustment if treatment is maintained beyond the early neonatal period. As a result of these kinetic properties, conventional methods of giving anticonvulsants produce low blood concentrations for several days with later accumulation. Because neonates tend to convulse serially during the first days of life, conventional schedules do not give protection at the time of maximum seizure activity, while they may produce toxicity when the fits tend to remit. The use of loading doses permits one to achieve rapidly concentrations of 20–40 μg/ml, levels which are considered adequate (Aicardi, 1983; Pippenger and Rosen, 1975; Volpe, 1981) but without exceeding these concentrations in succeeding days. Most workers use doses of 15–20 mg/kg or even of up to 40 mg/kg of phenobarbital (Fisher *et al.*, 1981; Gal *et al.*, 1982; Lockman *et al.*, 1979; Painter *et al.*, 1978). These doses can be used regardless of birth weight and gestational age. The distribution of phenytoin and phenobarbital to the brain in neonates is similar to that in adults and also independent of both gestational age and weight (Gold *et al.*, 1979; Painter *et al.*, 1981). The loading doses should be administered slowly, especially phenytoin, at a rate not exceeding 50 mg/min. In fact, slower administration by pump infusion over 30–45 min seems better tolerated. Infusion by umbilical catheter should be avoided as necrosis may occur.

Phenobarbital, administered first, controls the seizures in 32–39% of the cases at blood levels of 20 mg/l (Lockman *et al.*, 1979; Painter *et al.*, 1978). Gal *et al.* (1982) have obtained a control rate of up to 85% with blood levels in excess of 30 mg/l in 12% of their patients. Phenytoin has produced control in 32% of 25 infants who continued to exhibit seizures after receiving adequate doses of phenobarbital (Painter *et al.*, 1981). Maintenance dosages of both drugs are between 2.5 and 4.0 mg/kg per day. Fisher *et al.* (1981) advise monitoring plasma concentrations after loading until a decrease is apparent, and only then starting maintenance treatment. The optimal duration of maintenance therapy is not known. Some discontinue therapy only when all neurological signs have cleared (Volpe, 1981). Others suggest discontinuation a week or so after the seizures have stopped (Sun *et al.*, 1981) or at one month of age (Brown and Minns, 1980).

Convulsions which do not abate with phenobarbital or phenytoin are generally due to severe brain damage and are difficult to treat. Painter (1983) has used primidone in 16 infants as a loading dose of 15–25 mg/kg, with a maintenance dose of 10–20 mg/kg in three divided doses. Eleven of these infants stopped having fits but an indirect effect of raising the concentration of phenobarbital cannot be excluded. Paraldehyde is regarded as very effective by some (Brown and Minns, 1980) but only moderately so by others (Painter *et al.*, 1981; Volpe, 1981). It can be given intramuscularly (but not in the buttock) at a dose of 0.2 ml/kg, or rectally at a dose of 0.5 ml to a maximum of 3 ml, mixed with 2.3 ml of mineral oil as a retention enema (Lombroso, 1983). Lignocaine (lidocaine) administered as a constant-rate intravenous infusion at an initial rate of 4–10 mg/kg per h for 24 hours slowly discontinued over the subsequent 48 hours has been advocated (Browne, 1983).

Prognosis of neonatal seizures

The outlook for patients with neonatal seizures is globally severe. The average figure for mortality is about 15% and mental and neurological sequelae are observed in 30–35% of the patients (Lombroso, 1978, 1983; Volpe, 1981). Subsequent seizures occur in about 20% of the cases. The outcome of neonatal seizures is mainly dependent on their cause (*Table 11.3*). Other unfavourable

Table 11.3 Prognosis of neonatal seizures in relation to aetiology. Data from Lombroso (1978, 1983), Volpe (1981), Kellaway and Hrachovy (1983)

	Normal development (%)
Hypoxic–ischaemic encephalopathy	16–50
Haemorrhage	
Intraventricular	0–10
Subarachnoid	85–90
Bacterial meningitis	25–65
Developmental defect	0–5
Hypocalcaemia	
Early onset	42–50
Late onset	94–100
Hypoglycaemia	25–50
Unknown	55–62

factors include: (1) a seizure pattern of subtle, tonic or myoclonic fits; (2) certain EEG patterns such as inactive or paroxysmal tracings (Lombroso, 1974, 1978; Dreyfus-Brisac, 1979); (3) a profound compromise at neurological examination including a low Apgar score (Nelson and Ellenberg, 1981). Also indicative of a poor prognosis is long duration and frequent repetition of the seizures (Dreyfus-Brisac and Monod, 1972), and an onset of seizures before 24 or 48 hours of age. Conversely, an onset after 120 hours of age, a normal neurological examination at the time of discharge from the newborn unit, and brief seizures are associated with a favourable outcome (Dennis, 1978), as is a normal or mildly abnormal EEG.

INFANTILE SPASMS

Clinical features and causes of infantile spasms (IS)

Infantile spasms are one type of epileptic seizure in infants. The spasms consist of an abrupt initial contraction, lasting less than 2 s, at times followed by a more sustained (2–10 s) tonic phase (Kellaway *et al.*, 1979). The muscle contraction is bilateral and usually symmetrical and produces either flexion of the trunk, neck and limbs (flexor spasms), a mixture of flexion of the trunk and upper limbs with extension of the lower limbs (mixed type), or, less often, a generalized extension. The spasms usually occur in series of a few seizures to several dozens at intervals of 5–30 s.

Although the spasms are a distinctive type of seizure, they are classified as a syndrome because they are regularly associated with a remarkable EEG tracing termed hypsarrhythmia and with mental retardation and/or regression (Kellaway, Frost and Hrachovy, 1983; Lombroso, 1983).

The hypsarrhythmic EEG in the waking state consists of a chaotic mixture of high-voltage slow waves, interspersed with randomly occurring, asynchronous sharpwaves or spikes. During slow sleep this tracing tends to be replaced by bursts of polyspike–wave complexes separated by intervals of low-amplitude activity. Mental retardation may antedate the onset of spasms but a sudden behavioural deterioration may be observed in infants with previously normal development.

The syndrome has its onset between birth and one year of age with a peak incidence between four and seven months. It may be atypical or incomplete: mental retardation may be absent or mild; the hypsarrhythmia may be atypical ('modified') in up to 40% of the patients (Jeavons and Bower, 1974), and the spasms may be unilateral or otherwise atypical.

Table 11.4 Known aetiological factors of infantile spasms

Neurocutaneous syndromes (especially tuberous sclerosis)
Brain malformations (especially agenesis of corpus callosum, lissencephaly, holoprosencephaly)
Intrauterine infections
Metabolic disorders (phenylketonuria and non-ketotic hyperglycinaemia)
Anoxic–ischaemic brain damage of prenatal or perinatal origin (including prenatal deprivation in small-for-dates infants)
Acquired brain damage of any cause

The syndrome of infantile spasms has many causes, the main categories being shown in *Table 11.4*. Boys are more commonly affected than girls and a family history of epilepsy is uncommon (Aicardi and Chevrie, 1978; Gastaut *et al.*, 1964; Kurakawa *et al.*, 1980; Riikonen and Donner, 1979). A distinction of practical importance is between symptomatic and cryptogenic or idiopathic spasms. However, these terms are not used synonymously by all authors: some regard as cryptogenic all cases in which no definite cause can be found (Kellaway, Frost and Hrachovy, 1983; Kurakawa *et al.*, 1980). Other include only those cases without known cause in which the development of the infant had been normal prior to the onset of spasms (Aicardi and Chevrie, 1978; Lombroso, 1983). These differences in definition have consequences on the evaluation of the results of any form of treatment.

Management of infantile spasms

Anticonvulsant drugs

Infantile spasms are notoriously resistant to most anticonvulsant drugs. Only the benzodiazepines and sodium valproate or valproic acid have been used with some success, but no controlled studies are available. Benzodiazepines, especially nitrazepam, at dosages of 0.6–1.0 mg/kg per day (Hanson and Menkes, 1972; Jan *et al.*, 1971; Völzke, Doose and Stephan, 1967) have been found to control the spasms in up to half the patients studied. The improvement in the EEG tends to be less striking than that obtained with hormonal therapy and the development of tolerance is common after 6–8 weeks of treatment. The effect on mental development has not been evaluated (Lacy and Penry, 1976). Clonazepam has been found as effective as nitrazepam by some (O'Donohoe, 1980; Vassella *et al.*, 1973) but other investigators (Hanson and Menkes, 1972) have less favourable results. Diazepam is thought to be less effective than the other benzodiazepines (Gibbs and Anderson, 1965). No comparative study of the benzodiazepines versus hormonal therapy has been reported. However, the current trend is clearly in favour of hormonal therapy (Kellaway, Frost and Hrachovy, 1983, Lerman and Kivity, 1982; Riikonen, 1982; Singer, Rabe and Haller, 1980; Snead, Benton and Myers, 1983).

Sodium valproate, at dosages of 15–60 mg/kg per day in three divided doses, has been found to control the spasms in four out of 18 patients of Pavone *et al.* (1981) and in eight out of the 19 patients of Bachman (1982). Both studies emphasize the relative lack of side-effects of valproate as compared with hormonal treatment, but the results seem less favourable than in most series using steroids or ACTH. Further study of this drug is indicated. The ketogenic diet has been used in classical or modified forms (Huttenlocher, 1976; Schwartz *et al.*, 1983) for infantile spasm patients. Although good results have been reported, these are impossible to evaluate, due to the small size and mixed composition of the treated series which include patients with both infantile spasms and myoclonic epilepsy or Lennox syndrome.

Corticotropin and corticosteroid treatment

The efficacy of corticotropin for infantile spasms has long been recognized (*see* Kellaway, Frost and Hrachovy, 1983). Both natural ACTH and tretracosactrin, usually in long-acting forms, have been used successfully. Corticosteroids are also effective, whether in the form of hydrocortisone, prednisolone or dexamethasone. However, the ways of using these drugs are so varied (singly or in succession, at different dosages, for various durations, associated or not with conventional anticonvulsants) and the criteria of judgement so diverse that no comparison is possible between the many therapeutic schemes proposed. Recommended dosages of ACTH have varied from 10 to 120–160 IU/24 h, those of tetracosactrin from 0.25 to 1.0 mg/day. No precise correspondence has been established between doses of corticotropin and of corticosteroids or between various steroids. Doses of 2–10 mg/kg per day for prednisolone, of 0.3–1.0 mg/kg per day for dexamethasone, and of 5–20 mg/kg per day for hydrocortisone are commonly used. Aicardi *et al.* (1967) found that the mean daily cortisol output of the adrenals of infants receiving 40 IU of ACTH for the treatment of infantile spasms (approximately 100 mg) corresponded roughly to the administration of about 15 mg/kg per day of hydrocortisone. However, the doses of synthetic steroids necessary to obtain a similar effect on infantile spasms are not determined. It is not known whether ACTH acts entirely by stimulating cortisol secretion or independently by a direct influence on the nervous system, perhaps related to its peptidic nature (Strand *et al.*, 1973–74). However, a few trials of ACTH fragments devoid of corticotropic effect have given rather disappointing results (Pentella, Bachman and Sandman, 1982; Willig and Lagenstein, 1982). The proposed durations of hormonal therapy have been no less variable. Some authors favour relatively short courses of 4–8 weeks (Aicardi and Chevrie, 1978; Riikonen, 1982), while others advocate administration of ACTH over 12–16 weeks or longer (Lombroso, 1983; Singer, Rabe and Haller, 1980), at times followed by a more or less prolonged course of steroids. Similar differences exist regarding the association of anticonvulsant drugs (Lacy and Penry, 1976).

The evaluation of the therapeutic results of these various schemes is also difficult because the groups treated are not comparable. In particular, the proportions of symptomatic and of cryptogenic cases vary from one series to another and this is likely to be reflected in the long-term outcome and, to a lesser extent, in the short-term results of treatment. These proportions are difficult to determine in any individual series because the definition of cryptogenic cases is not the same in all studies. A stringent definition of the cryptogenic cases will produce a low proportion of such cases but these are then likely to have a more favourable outcome than if looser criteria are used. In other words, the outcome in series of treated infantile spasms may reflect the composition of the initial series and the criteria for selecting patients as much as the effect of therapy itself, and claims for superiority of one treatment scheme over another (Lerman and Lombroso, 1983; Singer, Rabe and Haller, 1980), should be received with great reservations because they are not based on controlled studies.

The short-term effects of hormonal therapy on the seizures and on the EEG are relatively consistent. Complete control is obtained in 60–70% of cases, a reduction in frequency in another 20%, while in 10% there is no effect at all (Aicardi, 1980; Jeavons, Bower and Dimitrakoudi, 1973; Kellaway, Frost and Hrachovy, 1983). Disappearance of hypsarrhythmia is observed in 60–90% of cases, although Lacy and Penry (1976) computed from several published series a mean figure of only 13% of excellent EEG results, and of 43% for less marked EEG improvement. Marked flattening of the EEG tracing is common and may last for several days after discontinuation of hormonal therapy. Persistence of some residual abnormalities, especially focal spikes, is common (Gastaut *et al.*, 1964; Riikonen, 1982). Relapses occur in about 30% of cases, so that complete cure is obtained following a first course of hormones in only 32–41% of all cases (Jeavons and Bower, 1974; Riikonen, 1982). Some authors, using high-dosage (80–120 IU), prolonged (3–10 months) ACTH therapy, have reported control of the spasms in 75–100% of their patients (Lerman and Kivity, 1982; Singer, Rabe and Haller, 1980; Snead, Benton and Myers, 1983) as well as a low relapse rate, 67% of the patients being cured after the initial treatment course (Singer, Rabe and Haller, 1980). Hrachovy *et al.* (1983) in a prospective, controlled study, found no significant difference in short-term effects between 12 patients receiving 20 IU ACTH/day and 12 given 2 mg/kg per day of prednisone. Although this study demonstrates that both drugs are effective and that either one may be active when the other has failed, its design permitted only the detection of a difference of 50% or more in favour of either treatment, and smaller differences (30%, for example) would obviously be of clinical importance. Further studies are needed, therefore. Whatever the exact figures, the remarkable fact remains that a significant proportion of the patients seem to be definitively 'cured' by courses of ACTH or steroid treatment as brief as two weeks, as opposed to what is observed with antiepileptic drugs in the other epileptic syndromes (Hrachovy *et al.*, 1983).

The long-term effects of hormonal treatment are far less dramatic. The mortality rate remains around 15–20%. The rate of residual epilepsy may be reduced from 45–60% to 35% (Lombroso, 1983) although this point has been little studied. The effect on mental development remains controversial. As shown in *Table 11.5*, 6–29% of treated infants have a normal mental development while the remaining patients are moderately or, in a majority, severely retarded. These results are not strikingly different from the spontaneous cure rate which averages 11% in five series (Chevrie, personal communication). Global figures, however, are of limited significance, since several variables other than treatment have been found to profoundly affect the outcome (Chevrie and Aicardi, 1971; Jeavons and Bower, 1974; Lombroso, 1983). The major variable is the symptomatic or cryptogenic character of the spasms. Only 4%, on an average, of the symptomatic cases are mentally normal at end of follow-up, while 21–58% of the patients with cryptogenic spasms have a normal mental level (average 37%). Other variables unfavourably affecting the mental outlook include an early age of onset of the spasms (before three months), the occurrence of other types of seizures before the onset of spasms (Chevrie and Aicardi, 1971; Jeavons and Bower, 1974; Jeavons, Bower and Dimitrakoudi, 1973), and neuroradiological evidence of brain atrophy before treatment (Singer *et al.*, 1982). These variables are closely linked with a symptomatic origin of the spasms. The occurrence of relapses after a first cure is of unfavourable significance although Riikonen (1982) and Hrachovy *et al.* (1983) found that a second course of treatment could be effective. On the contrary, a relatively good mental status at onset of treatment and a rapid response to therapy may indicate a more favourable prognosis. The prognostic significance, if any, of the initial EEG characteristics is uncertain. Unilateral and grossly asymmetrical tracings predict an unfavourable outcome, while a typical hypsarrhythmic pattern may be associated with a more favourable prognosis. Riikonen (1982) found that the persistence of focal abnormalities after disappearance of the hypsarrhythmia had no prognostic significance. The influence of the modalities of hormonal treatment on mental outcome is debated. Some workers (Lerman and Kivity, 1982; Lombroso, 1983) state that ACTH or tetracosactrin in high dosages (110–150

U/m^2/day or up to 160 IU/day) and for long periods (12 weeks to several months) is the most effective therapy. However, the proportions of mentally normal patients in these series are not impressively higher than those obtained by workers who use less massive doses (*see Table 11.5*), and Riikonen (1982) found that large doses (120–160 IU/day) did not give better results than conventional (20–40 IU/day) doses. The less favourable effect of prednisone, as compared with ACTH, which has been found by some investigators (Lombroso, 1983; Snead, Benton and Myers, 1983), may be related to a dose effect or to methodological differences, since these studies were uncontrolled. Minimizing the delay between onset of spasms and initiation of treatment may increase the rate of favourable mental outcomes (Jeavons, Bower and Dimitrakoudi, 1973; Riikonen, 1982; Singer, Rabe and Haller, 1980; Snyder, 1967). Lerman and Kivity (1982) reported a success rate of 85% for patients treated within one month of onset. The relationship between early treatment and favourable outcome, however, is not necessarily a causal one. Chevrie and Aicardi (1971) showed that cryptogenic cases are treated earlier, on an average, than symptomatic ones, probably because behavioural deterioration rapidly calls the attention of parents and physicians. The best cases may thus receive earlier treatment, making the effect of treatment itself difficult to evaluate. However, the advantage of early therapy may not be entirely explained by the selection of more favourable cases (Chevrie and Aicardi, 1971; Riikonen, 1982) and rapid initiation of treatment is, therefore, recommended.

Side-effects of hormonal therapy include irritability or depression, hirsutism, Cushingoid features and arterial hypertension. Blood electrolytes and serum protein disturbances have been reported with tetracosactrin (Cret *et al.*, 1976). Infectious complications (gastroenteritis, pneumonia, sepsis, meningitis) are the most frequent causes of death related to treatment; they were responsible for four out of six deaths among the 90 infants reported by Pinsard *et al.* (1976), of six of the eight deaths in the 214 cases reviewed by Riikonen and Donner (1980), and of three out of seven deaths in the 124 patients of Chevrie and Aicardi (1978). However, some series do not include fatalities (Singer, Rabe and Haller, 1980). The consequences of treatment on brain growth have not been fully assessed. The widening of the sulci and ventricular cavities noted in patients receiving ACTH is usually rapidly reversible (Hrachovy *et al.*, 1983) although it may exceptionally persist.

Summary

To summarize the present situation:

(1) Hormonal therapy is effective for the spasms and for the EEG abnormalities; its effectiveness is probably greater than that of anticonvulsant drugs, including the benzodiazepines and sodium valproate.
(2) The long-term efficacy on mental development and on later epilepsy has not been conclusively established; this possibility rests on clinical impressions and on indirect evidence.
(3) The selection of patients to be treated depends on an evaluation of risks and benefits which remains imprecise, due to the lack of prospective studies. We

Table 11.5 Course of cases of West's syndrome with hormonal treatment

Authors	*Normal mental level*						*Duration of follow-up*
	All cases		*Cryptogenic*		*Symptomatic*		
Snyder (1967)	8/28	29%	8/18	44%	0/10	0%	2 months–8 years
Chevrie and Aicardi (1971)	11/78	14%	11/40	28%	0/38	0%	1–7 years
Jeavons, Bover and Dimitrakoudi (1973)	18/105	17%	18/55	33%	0/50	0%	2–12 years
Pinsard *et al*. (1976)	16/90	18%	16/28	58%	0/62	0%	1–15 years
O'Donohoe (1976)	21/100	21%	21/44	48%	0/56	0%	5–15 years
Gibbs and Gibbs (1976)	42/240	18%	27/129	21%	15/111	14%	1 month–13 years
Chevrie and Aicardi (1978)	30/124	24%	25/60	42%	5/64	8%	1–11 years
Matsumoto *et al*. (1981)*	32/139	23%		(40%)		(9.4%)	> 5 years
Singer *et al*. (1982)**	8/71	11%	8/20***	40%	0/51	0%	14–207 months
Riikonen (1982)	21/162	13%	11/25	44%	10:137	7%	3–19 years
Lerman and Kivity (1982)+			24/25	56%			?
Lombroso (1983)			36/90	40%			≥ 6 years

+ Cryptogenic cases only

* Figures in brackets are derived from the whole seris (n=159) not only from treated cases, the authors state that there was no difference in results whether or not patients were treated with ACTH

** Symptomatic means abnormal at initial presentation; patients may have been normal earlier

*** 12 of these 20 infants had an abnormal neuroradiological examination; all fared poorly

feel that the risks of hormonal therapy are justified only in cryptogenic or in doubtful cases, in view of the uniform failure to improve mental prognosis in symptomatic cases.

(4) The choice between the various modalities of hormonal therapy is very much a matter of personal preference and will remain so until proper comparisons between various drugs and regimens are available.

(5) In the case of failure of hormonal treatment and in obviously symptomatic cases, valproate and/or benzodiazepines are indicated.

FEBRILE SEIZURES

Clinical features and aetiological factors of febrile seizures

Seizures precipitated by fever occur in 2–5% of all children before the age of six years (Hauser, 1981). In this chapter, the term 'febrile convulsions' is used to describe a convulsion that occurs with fever (temperature of 38° or more) not due to an infection which primarily affects brain or meninges. Children below one month or over 6–7 years of age and those who had any afebrile fit prior to their first febrile seizure are not included. Febrile convulsions occur with increased frequency among family members of patients with febrile convulsions (Tsuboi, 1977; Van den Berg, 1974). This suggests that genetic factors are important in that disorder, but there is no agreement regarding the possible mode of inheritance: a dominant (Frantzen *et al.*, 1970) or a polygenic (Tsuboi, 1977) mode are most likely. Acquired factors, especially prenatal or perinatal ones, may play a complementary role both in favouring manifestation of the trait and in modulating the severity of its expression (Chevrie and Aicardi, 1975; Wallace, 1975a). Most febrile convulsions are brief, bilateral clonic or tonic-clonic seizures. However, 7.6% of 1706 children in a recent population study had a convulsion lasting 15 min or more, 4.3% had a fit lasting at least 30 min, and 4.0% had a focal or unilateral seizure. An additional 16% had two or more febrile convulsions during the same febrile episode (Nelson and Ellenberg, 1978). Such seizures are termed 'complex' or 'complicated' febrile convulsions.

Febrile convulsions usually have a benign course. They are infrequent before age six months or after five years, the peak incidence being in the second year; 60–70% of patients will have a single seizure and 30–35% will have two convulsions. Severe febrile convulsions are, in 75% of the cases, the initial seizure and 'complicated' seizures represent only 8% of the recurrences following an initial, simple febrile convulsion (Nelson and Ellenberg, 1978). Intellectual dysfunction and neurological sequelae following febrile convulsions may occur in the case of febrile status epilepticus (Aicardi and Chevrie, 1976). The frequency of such sequelae is low but it is difficult to assess precisely, since at least some cases labelled 'acute febrile neurological disorders' or 'acute acquired hemiplegia' are probably complicated febrile seizures. The risk of late afebrile epilepsy is between 2 and 4% (Annegers *et al.*, 1979; Frantzen, Lennox-Buchtal and Nygaard, 1968; Nelson and Ellenberg, 1976). Factors associated with an increased risk of subsequent epilepsy include neurological abnormalities existing prior to the first febrile convulsion, epilepsy in first-degree relatives and 'complex' seizures. Late epilepsy is associated with an increased risk of mental sequelae (Ellenberg and Nelson, 1978).

Management of the child with febrile convulsions

Investigations in children with febrile convulsions

Cerebrospinal fluid examination should be performed in infants under six months of age (Heijbel, Blom and Bergfors, 1980), and in those who do not show rapid improvement or with signs suggestive of meningitis. In infants under 18 months lumbar puncture is advised by several authors, because, in this age range, meningitis can present as simple febrile convulsions without meningeal signs (Ratcliffe and Wolf, 1977; Rutter and Smales, 1976). Other investigations, including blood sugar, electrolytes and skull X-rays, are generally unhelpful (Nealis, 1981). Blood counts and chest X-rays are indicated according to the nature of the accompanying symptoms and signs. EEG tracings are useless as they do not help predict the occurrence of later epilepsy (Frantzen, Lennox-Buchtal and Nygaard, 1968).

The acute treatment of febrile convulsions

Brief febrile seizures do not necessitate any treatment beyond elementary supportive measures. Prompt lowering of body temperature by sponging, tepid baths or antipyretic drugs is usually advised, although its efficacy has not been proved (Camfield *et al.*, 1980). Prolonged febrile seizures must be treated vigorously since they can produce lasting brain damage. Diazepam is, at present, the drug of first choice by the intravenous or rectal routes but not as suppositories (Knudsen, 1979, 1981). The average doses are 0.25 mg/kg by a slow intravenous 'push' injection or 0.5 mg/kg of the undiluted injectable form by the rectal route. In the latter case, care should be taken to avoid rejection of the drug. These doses may be repeated once, after 20–30 min. Rectal administration is easier than the intravenous route and produces, within minutes, a satisfactory blood level (Dulac *et al.*, 1978; Knudsen, 1977) and positive clinical effects (Franzoni, Carboni and Lambertini, 1983); rectal administration can help avoid the unnecessary delays which may result from difficulties in finding a venous access under unfavourable emergency circumstances (such as an agitated infant at home). Ventura *et al.* (1982) have shown that rectal diazepam can be safely administered at home by parents if precise instructions have been given, and can prevent prolonged seizures. Only eight out of 660 patients whose parents had been instructed to administer 0.5 mg of diazepam rectally in the case of recurrent seizure had a convulsion lasting more than 10 minutes and in six of these the diazepam solution had been rejected or not administered. No severe apnoea has been recorded so far with rectal diazepam, which may thus represent a promising technique for prophylaxis against long convulsions and possible brain damage.

Prophylactic treatment against recurrences

Prevention of recurrences of febrile convulsions is desirable because they are frightening events for the children and their family and because they may occasionally be severe and produce brain damage.

CONTINUOUS PROPHYLAXIS

Several studies (Faerø *et al.*, 1972; Herranz, Armijo and Arteaga, 1984; Thorn, 1975; Wallace, 1975b; Wolf *et al.*, 1977) have demonstrated that the continuous administration of phenobarbital, with maintenance of a serum phenobarbital level of 15 mg/l or above, will reduce the recurrence rate at 6 months by approximately two-thirds (from 30% to 8–12%). This prophylactic effect is obtained not only in simple febrile seizures but also in children with an abnormal development and in those with 'complex' seizures (Wolf *et al.*, 1977). Very similar results have been obtained with sodium valproate (Cavazzuti, 1975; Herranz, Armijo and Arteaga, 1984; Ngwane and Bower, 1980; Wallace and Smith, 1980). Primidone (Wallace, 1975; Herranz, Armijo and Arteaga, 1984) may also be effective but has not been extensively tested. No preventive effect on recurrences has been found using phenytoin (Melchior, Buchtal and Lennox-Buchtal, 1971) and carbamazepine (Camfield, Camfield and Tibbles, 1982).

The therapeutic benefits of phenobarbital and of valproate have to be balanced against the adverse effects of the drug. With phenobarbital, the most obvious side-effects are behaviour disorders which are observed in 20–40% of the children and which lead to discontinuation in 10–30% (Camfield and Camfield, 1981; Heckmatt *et al.*, 1976; Wolf and Forsythe, 1978). Studies in children treated for epilepsy have shown no significant effect of therapeutic doses of phenobarbital on learning and development (Camfield and Camfield, 1981; Wallace and Cull, 1979) although this possibility should be kept in mind. Sodium valproate produces few behavioural changes (Herranz, Armijo and Arteaga, 1984) but the risk of hepatic failure (Jeavons, 1983) and of other potential toxic effects precludes its use as long as the incidence of severe complications is imperfectly known. Monitoring serum levels of phenobarbital after the steady state has been achieved is important, especially to check the compliance of the families. Monitoring of sodium valproate may be less useful because the levels are very variable, due to the short half-life of the drug and because peak and 'trough' levels are achieved at unpredictable times, when enteric-coated preparations are used (Loiseau *et al.*, 1982). The optimal levels of 15–25 mg/l for phenobarbital and of 50–80 mg/l for valproate are generally obtained with dosages of 3–4 mg/kg per day of phenobarbital and of 20–30 mg/kg per day for sodium valproate. It is essential to check blood levels of drugs immediately in the case of a recurrent febrile convulsion.

The balance of the hazards resulting from recurrences of febrile convulsions and the risks attendant with continuous drug prophylaxis are such that it does not seem reasonable to propose continuous prophylaxis for all children who have had a first febrile seizure. This would involve treating 2–4% of all children under five years of age, 70% of whom will not have a recurrence if left untreated. The main rationale for this method is that any febrile seizure may be severe and produce brain damage. This risk is small, however, and can be prevented by prompt treatment of lasting seizures. Most workers presently favour continuous prophylaxis for selected patients (Fishman, 1981; Nelson and Ellenberg, 1978; Wallace, 1975b). These would include children who, at the time of their first febrile seizure, have significant abnormalities on neurological examination or developmental delay by history, who have 'complex' or 'complicated' febrile seizures and those who have a positive family history of epilepsy (Consensus Development Panel, 1981). A young age at the first febrile seizure (less than 12–15 months) is also an indication accepted by several authors, since it is clearly associated with a higher risk of recurrences and with a greater probability of severe recurrences (Lennox-Buchtal, 1973; Van den

Berg and Yerushalmy, 1971). The factors listed above (except for young age) are risk factors for later non-febrile seizures rather than for febrile recurrences or for severe recurrent convulsions. There is no evidence that the treatment of febrile convulsions can prevent later epilepsy (Nelson, 1981) and febrile recurrences constitute the most common hazard and the only one that can be prevented. Since a positive family history of febrile seizures (Frantzen, Lennox-Buchtal and Nygaard, 1968; Lennox-Buchtal, 1973) the female sex and a severe or complicated initial episode (Lennox-Buchtal, 1973; Wallace, 1974) were found to be associated with a higher risk of recurrences in only some studies, the bases for allocating patients to selective prophylaxis are fragile. Moreover, Ellenberg and Nelson (1981) have shown that the assumption that using such factors as criteria for selected prophylaxis would lead to a limitation of prophylactic treatment to a small subgroup of children with febrile seizures is incorrect. In fact, most of the existing selective recommendations would justify chronic therapy for one-third to two-thirds of children with febrile convulsions.

INTERMITTENT PROPHYLAXIS

Considering the drawbacks of continuous prophylaxis, it would seem advantageous to use anticonvulsant drugs intermittently at the onset of a febrile illness. The problems associated with this method are difficult to solve. In the first place the parents and guardians should be able to recognize the onset of illness so that medication may be given early enough to be effective. In the second place they should be able to give the medication in due time without being excessively stressed by the necessity of not doing it too early or too late. Thirdly, the absorption of the drug should be fast and reliable by the oral or the rectal routes. Finally, the drug should gain access to the brain at sufficient concentration, so that a relatively large loading dose must be given initially (Porter, 1981). Phenobarbital is clearly inadequate; diazepam has better prospects. Knudsen and Vestermark (1978) found a recurrence rate of 16% and Thorn (1981) a rate of 12%, well below that expected for an untreated population, in two large groups of patients given 5 mg of diazepam as suppositories every eight hours. Knudsen (1981), using rectal instillation of an injectable solution, achieved a level of recurrences as low as that obtained with continuous phenobarbital prophylaxis. Diazepam given orally (Dianese, 1979) also achieved a high degree of protection against recurrences (4% versus 48% in untreated children). The oral administration of clonazepam has also given encouraging, although uncontrolled, results (Lalande and De Paillerets, 1978).

Despite these favourable results, intermittent prophylaxis remains a complex and unreliable method, and involves the risk of creating neurotic problems in parents as well as that of a seizure occurring as a first manifestation of fever, an event found by Wolf *et al.* (1977) in 25% of infants.

Summary

In summary, the prophylactic treatment of febrile seizures still raises unsolved problems. Continuous prophylaxis in my view is indicated only for young children because the risk of a severe seizure is real in this case. It may also be necessary – even though not desirable – for patients from very anxious families when all efforts at persuasion fail, and for those with multiple recurrences. Intermittent prophylaxis may be satisfactory for patients whose parents or guardians are both calm and able to administer the treatment properly. Whatever the controversies and difficulties, the rapid availability of emergency treatment for promptly interrupting febrile convulsions is essential and every effort should be made, through public health measures and education, to extend such facilities in all areas.

References

AICARDI, J. (1980) Seizures and epilepsy in children under two years of age. In *The Treatment of Epilepsy*, edited by J. H. Tyrer, pp. 203–250. Lancaster: MTP Press

AICARDI, J. (1983) Neonatal and infantile seizures. In *Antiepileptic Drug Therapy in Pediatrics*, edited by P. L. Morselli, C. E. Pippinger and J. K. Penry, pp. 103–113. New York: Raven Press

AICARDI, J. and CHEVRIE, J. J. (1976) Febrile convulsions: neurological sequelae and mental retardation. In *Brain Dysfunction in Infantile Febrile Convulsions*, edited by M. A. B. Brazier and F. Coceani, pp. 247–257. New York: Raven Press

AICARDI, J. and CHEVRIE, J. J. (1978) Les spasmes infantiles. *Archives Françaises de Pédiatrie,* **35,** 1015–1023

AICARDI, J., WEINMAN, S., CHEVRIE, J. J. and THIEFFRY, S. (1967) Les spasmes en flexion du nourrisson. Etude de l'excrétion urinaire des 17-hydroxy-cortico-stéroïdes et du taux de sécrétion du cortisol au cours de leur traitement par l'ACTH. *Archives Françaises de Pédiatrie* **24,** 521–530

ANNEGERS, J. F., HAUSER. W. A., ELVEBACK, L. R. and KURLAND, L. T. (1979) The risk of epilepsy following febrile convulsions. *Neurology,* **29**, 297–303

BACHMAN, D. S. (1982) Use of valproic acid in treatment of infantile spasms. *Archives of Neurology,* **39,** 49–52

BROWN, J. K. and MINNS, R. A. (1980) Epilepsy in neonates. In *The Treatment of Epilepsy*, edited by J. H. Tyrer, pp. 161–202, Lancaster: MTP Press

BROWNE, T. R. (1983) Paraldehyde, chlormethiazole and lidocaine for treatment of status epilepticus. *Advances in Neurology,* **34,** 509–517

CAMFIELD, C. S. and CAMFIELD, P. R. (1981) Behavioral and cognitive effects of phenobarbital in toddlers. In *Febrile Seizures,* edited by K. B. Nelson and J. H. Ellenberg, pp. 203–210. New York: Raven Press

CAMFIELD, P. R., CAMFIELD, C. S., SHAPIRO, S. H. and CUMMINGS, C. (1980). The first febrile seizure – antipyretic instruction plus either phenobarbital or placebo to prevent recurrence. *Journal of Pediatrics,* **97,** 16–21

CAMFIELD, P., CAMFIELD, C. and TIBBLES, J. (1982) Carbamazepine does not prevent febrile seizures in phenobarbital failures. *Neurology (NY),* **32,** 228–229

CAVAZZUTI, G. B. (1975) Prevention of febrile convulsions with dipropylacetate. *Epilepsia,* **16,** 647–648

CHEVRIE, J. J. and AICARDI, J. (1971) Le prnostic psychique des spasmes infantiles traités par l'ACTH ou les corticoïdes. Analyse statistique de 78 cas suivis plus d'un an. *Journal of the Neurological Sciences,* **12,** 351–357

CHEVRIE, J. J. and AICARDI, J. (1975). Duration and lateralization of febrile convulsions. Etiological factors. *Epilepsia,* **16,** 781–789

CHEVRIE, J. J. and AICARDI, J. (1978) Convulsive disorders in the first year of life: mortality, neurological and mental outcome. *Epilepsia,* **19**, 67–74

CONSENSUS DEVELOPMENT PANEL (1980) Febrile seizures: long-term management of children with fever-associated seizures. *Pediatrics,* **66,** 1009–1012

CRET, L., DAVID, M., MACABEO, V., FREDERICH, A. and JEUNE, M. (1976) Maladie des spasmes en flexion; troubles cliniques et métaboliques observés en cours de traitement par le tetracosactide zinc. *Pediatrics,* **31,** 33–48

DEHAN, M., QUILLERON, D., NAVELET, Y. *et al.* (1977) Les convulsions du cinquième jour de vie: un nouveau syndrome? *Archives Françaises de Pédiatrie,* **34,** 730–742

DENNIS, J. (1978) Neonatal convulsions: aetiology, late neonatal status and long-term outcome. *Developmental Medicine and Child Neurology,* **20,** 143–158

DIANESE, G. (1979) Prophylactic diazepam in febrile convulsions. *Archives of Diseases in Childhood,* **54,** 244–245

DREYFUS-BRISAC, C. (1979) Neonatal electroencephalograpy. In *Reviews of Perinatal Medicine,* Vol. 3, edited by E. M. Scarpelli and E. V. Cosmi. New York: Raven Press

DREYFUS-BRISAC, C. and MONOD, N. (1972) Neonatal status epilepticus. *Electroencephalography and Clinical Neurophysiology,* **15,** 38–52

DULAC, O., AICARDI, J., REY, E. and OLIVE, G. (1978) Blood levels of diazepam after single rectal administration to infants and children. *Journal of Pediatrics,* **93,** 1039–1041

ELLENBERG, J. H. and NELSON, K. B. (1978) Febrile seizures and later intellectual performance. *Archives of Neurology,* **35,** 17–21

ELLENBERG, J. H. and NELSON, K. B. (1981) The efficiency of published recommendations for the treatment of febrile seizures. In *Febrile Seizures,* edited by K. B. Nelson and J. H. Ellenberg, pp. 97–102. New York: Raven Press

FAERØ, O., KASTRUP, K. W., LYKKEGAARD NIELSEN, E., MELCHIOR, J. C. and THORN, I. (1972) Successful prophylaxis of febrile convulsions with phenobarbital. *Epilepsia,* **13,** 279–285

FISHER, J., LOCKMAN, L., ZASKE, D. and KRIEL, R. (1981) Phenobarbital maintenance dose requirements in treating neonatal seizures. *Neurology (NY),* **31,** 1042–1044

FISHMAN, M. A. (1981) An approach to the management of children with febrile seizures: a child neurologist's point of view. In *Febrile Seizures,* edited by K. B. Nelson and J. H. Ellenberg, pp. 87–92. New York: Raven Press

FRANTZEN, E., LENNOX-BUCHTAL, M. A. and NYGAARD, A. (1968) Longitudinal EEG and clinical study of children with febrile convulsions. *Electroencephalography and Clinical Neurophysiology,* **24,** 197–212

FRANTZEN, E., LENNOX-BUCHTAL, M. A., NYGAARD, A. and STENE, J. (1970) A genetic study of febrile convulsions, *Neurology,* **20,** 909–917

FRANZONI, E., CARBONI, C. and LAMBERTINI, A. (1983) Rectal diazepam: a clinical and EEG study after a single dose in children. *Epilepsia,* **24,** 35–41

GAL, P., TOBACK, J., BOER, H. R., ERKAN, N. V. and WELLS, T. J. (1982) Efficacy of phenobarbital monotherapy in treatment of neonatal seizures – relationship to blood levels. *Neurology (NY),* **32,** 1401–1404

GASTAUT, H., ROGER, J., SOULAYROL, R. and PINSARD, N. (1964) *L'encéphalopathie myoclonique infantile avec hypsarythmie (Syndrome de West).* Paris: Masson

GIBBS, F. A. and ANDERSON, E. M. (1965) Treatment of hypsarrhythmia and infantile spasms with a librium analogue. *Neurology (Minneapolis),* **15,** 1173–1176

GIBBS, F. A. and GIBBS, E. L. (1976) Follow-up of ACTH-treated and untreated cases of hypsarrhythmia. *Clinical Electroencephalography,* **7,** 149–157

GOLD, R., BOURIN, M., GRANRY, J. C., AMINE, A., BRETEAU, M. and LAUGIER, J. (1979) Intérêt de la voie intraveineuse pour l'utilisation du phénobarbital chez le nouveau-né à terme asphyxié. *Archives Françaises de Pédiatrie,* **36,** 610–616

HANSON, R. A. and MENKES, J. H. (1972) A new anticonvulsant in the management of minor motor seizures. *Developmental Medicine and Child Neurology,* **14,** 3–14

HAUSER, W. A. (1981) The natural history of febrile seizures. In *Febrile Seizures,* edited by K. B. Nelson and J. H. Ellenberg, pp. 5–17. New York: Raven Press

HECKMATT, J., HOUSTON, A., CLOW, D. *et al.* (1976). Failure of phenobarbitone to prevent febrile convulsions. *British Medical Journal,* **1,** 559–561

HEIJBEL, J., BLOM, S. and BERGFORS, P. G. (1980) Simple febrile convulsions. A prospective incidence study and an evaluation of investigations initially needed. *Neuropädiatrie,* **11,** 45–56

HERRANZ, J. L., ARMIJO, J. A. and ARTEAGA, R. (1984) Effectiveness and toxicity of phenobarbital, primidone and sodium valproate in the prevention of febrile convulsions controlled by plasma levels. *Epilepsia,* **25,** 89–95

HRACHOVY, R. A., FROST, J. D., KELLAWAY, P. and ZION, T. E. (1983) Double-blind study of ACTH vs prednisone therapy in infantile spasms. *Journal of Pediatrics,* **103,** 641–645

HUTTENLOCHER, P. R. (1976) Ketonemia and seizures: metabolic and anticonvulsant effects of two ketogenic diets in childhood epilepsy. *Pediatric Research,* **10,** 536–540

JAN, J. E., RIEGL, J. A., CRICHTON, J. U. and DUNN, H. G. (1971) Nitrazepam in the treatment of epilepsy in childhood. *Canadian Medical Association Journal,* **104,** 571–575

JEAVONS, P. M. (1983) Hepatotoxicity of antiepileptic drugs. In *Antiepileptic Therapy: Chronic Toxicity of Antiepileptic Drugs,* edited by J. Oxley *et al.*, pp. 1–45. New York: Raven Press

JEAVONS, P. M. and BOWER, B. D. (1974) Infantile spasms. In *Handbook of Clinical Neurology,* Vol. 15, *The Epilepsies,* edited by P. J. Vinken and G. W. Bruyn. Amsterdam: North-Holland

JEAVONS, P. M., BOWER, B. D. and DIMITRAKOUDI, M. (1973) Long-term prognosis of 150 cases of 'West syndrome'. *Epilepsia,* **14,** 153–164

KELLAWAY, P., FROST, J. D. and HRACHOVY, R. A. (1983) Infantile spasms. In *Antiepileptic Drug Therapy in Pediatrics,* edited by P. L. Morselli, C. E. Pippenger and J. K. Penry, pp. 115–136. New York: Raven Press

KELLAWAY, P. and HRACHOVY, R. A. (1983) Status epilepticus in newborns: a perspective on neonatal seizures. In *Advances in Neurology,* Vol. 34, *Status Epilepticus,* edited by A. V. Delgado-Escueta, C. G. Wasterlain, D. M. Treiman and R. J. Porter, pp. 93–99. New York: Raven Press

KELLAWAY, P., HRACHOVY, R. A., FROST, J. D. and ZION, T. (1979) Precise characterization and quantification of infantile spasms. *Annals of Neurology,* **6,** 214–218

KNUDSEN, F. V. (1977) Plasma diazepam in infants after rectal administration in solution and by suppositories. *Acta Paediatrica Scandinavica,* **67,** 699–704

KNUDSEN, F. V. (1979) Rectal administration of diazepam in solution in the acute treatment of convulsions in infants and children. *Archives of Diseases in Childhood,* **54,** 855–857

KNUDSEN, F. U. (1981) Successful intermittent diazepam prophylaxis in febrile convulsions: preliminary results of a prospective controlled series. In *Advances in Epileptology, the XIth Epilepsy International Symposium,* edited by M. Dam, L. Gram and J. K. Penry, pp. 165–168, New York: Raven Press

KNUDSEN, F. U. and VESTERMARK, S. (1978) Prophylactic diazepam or phenobarbitone in febrile convulsions: a prospective controlled study. *Archives of Diseases in Childhood,* **53,** 660–663

KURAKAWA, T., NAGAHIDE, G., FUKUYAMA, Y., SUZUKI, M., SEKI, T. and OHTAHARA, S. (1980) West syndrome and Lennox-Gastaut syndrome: a survey of natural history. *Pediatrics,* **65,** 81–88

LACY, J. R. and PENRY, J. K. (1976) *Infantile Spasms.* New York: Raven Press

LALANDE, J. and DE PAILLERETS, F. (1978) Prevention of hyperthermic convulsions: utility of discontinuous treatment with clonazepam. In *Advances in Epileptology,* edited by H. Meinardi and A. Rowans, pp. 313–317. Amsterdam: Swets and Zeitlinger

LENNOX-BUCHTAL, M. A. (1973) Febrile convulsions. A reappraisal. *Electroencephalography and Clinical Neurophysiology* (Suppl. 32), 1–132

LERMAN, P. and KIVITY, S. (1982) The efficacy of corticotropin in primary infantile spasms. *Journal of Pediatrics,* **101,** 294–296

LOCKMAN, L. A., KRIEL, R., ZASKE, D., THOMPSON, T. and VIRNIG, N. (1979) Phenobarbital dosage for control of neonatal seizures. *Neurology (NY),* **29,** 1445–1449

LOISEAU, P., LÉVY, R. H., GUYOT, M., MORSELLI, P. and BRACHET-LIERMAIN, A. (1982) Est-il préférable de prescrire une ou trois prises quotidiennes de valproate de sodium. *Nouvelle Presse Médicine,* **11,** 3693–3696

LOMBROSO, C. T. (1974) Seizures in the newborn period. In *Handbook of Clinical Neurology*, Vol. 15, *The Epilepsies,* edited by P. J. Vinken and G. W. Bruyn, pp. 189–218. Amsterdam: North-Holland

LOMBROSO, C. T. (1978) Convulsive disorders in newborns. In *Pediatric Neurology and Neurosurgery*, edited by R. A. Thompson and J. R. Green, pp. 205–239. New York: Spectrum

LOMBROSO, C. T. (1983) A prospective study of infantile spasms: clinical and therapeutic correlations. *Epilepsia,* **24,** 135–158

LOU, H. C. and FRIIS-HANSEN, B. (1979) Arterial blood pressure elevations during motor activity and epileptic seizures in newborn. *Acta Paediatrica Scandinavica,* **68,** 803–806

MATSUMOTO, A., WATANABE, K., NEGORO, T. *et al.* (1981) Long-term prognosis after infantile spasms: a statistical study of prognostic factors in 200 cases. *Developmental Medicine and Child Neurology,* **23,** 51–65

MELCHIOR, J., BUCHTAL, F. and LENNOX-BUCHTAL, M. (1971) The ineffectiveness of diphenylhydantoin in preventing febrile convulsions in the age of greatest risk, under three years. *Epilepsia,* **12,** 55–62

MELDRUM, B. (1978) Physiological changes during prolonged seizures and epileptic brain damage. *Neuropädiatrie,* **9,** 203–212

NEALIS, J. G. T. (1981) Management of febrile seizures by pediatricians in the United States. In *Febrile Seizures,* edited by K. B. Nelson and J. H. Ellenberg, pp. 81–86. New York: Raven Press

NELSON, K. B. (1981) Can treatment of febrile seizures prevent subsequent epilepsy? In *Febrile Seizures,* edited by K. B. Nelson and J. H. Ellenberg, pp. 143–145. New York: Raven Press

NELSON, K. B. and ELLENBERG, J. H. (1976) Predictors of epilepsy in children who have experienced febrile seizures. *New England Journal of Medicine,* **295,** 1029–1033

NELSON, K. B. and ELLENBERG, J. H. (1978) Prognosis in children with febrile seizures. *Pediatrics,* **61,** 720–727

NELSON, K. B. and ELLENBERG, J. H. (1981) Apgar scores as predictors of chronic neurologic disabilities. *Pediatrics,* **68,** 36–44

NGWANE, E. and BOWER, B. (1980) Continuous sodium valproate or phenobarbitone in the prevention of 'simple' febrile convulsions. *Archives of Diseases in Childhood,* **55,** 171–174

O'DONOHOE, N. V. (1976) A 15-year follow-up of 100 children with infantile spasms. *Irish Journal of Medical Science,* **145,** 138–143

O'DONOHOE, N. V. (1980) *Epilepsies in Childhood.* London: Butterworths

O'DONOHOE, N. V. and PAEZ, B. A. (1977) A trial of clonazepam in the treatment of severe epilepsy in infancy and childhood. In *Epilepsy, the Eighth International Symposium,* edited by J. K. Penry, pp. 159–162. New York: Raven Press

PAINTER, M. J. (1983) How to use primidone. In *Antiepileptic Drug Therapy in Pediatrics*, edited by P. L. Morselli, C. E. Pippenger and J. K. Penry, pp. 263–270. New York: Raven Press

PAINTER, M. J., PIPPENGER, C., MACDONALD, H. and PITLICK, W. (1978) Phenobarbital and diphenylhydantoin levels in neonates with seizures. *Journal of Pediatrics,* **92,** 315–319

PAINTER, M. J., PIPPENGER, C., WASTERLAIN, C. *et al.* (1981) Phenobarbital and phenytoin in neonatal seizures. Metabolism and tissue distribution. *Neurology (NY),* **31,** 1107–1112

PAVONE, L., INCORPORA, G., LA ROSA, M., LIVOLTI, S. and MOLLICA, F. (1981) Treatment of infantile spasms with sodium dipropylacetic acid. *Developmental Medicine and Child Neurology,* **23,** 454–461

PENTELLA, K., BACHMAN, D. S. and SANDMAN, C. A. (1982) Trial of an ACTH 4–9 analogue (ORG 2766) in children with intractable seizures. *Neuropediatrics,* **13,** 59–62

PINSARD, N., FERRACCI, J. P., RUFO, M. and BERNARD, R. (1976) Aspects évolutifs du syndrome de West. A propos de 90 observations. *Pédiatrie,* **31,** 92–93

PIPPENGER, C. E., and ROSEN, T. V. (1975) Phenobarbital plasma levels in neonates. *Clinical Perinatology,* **2,** 111–115

PITLICK, W. H., PAINTER, M. J. and PIPPENGER, C. (1978) Phenobarbital pharmacokinetics in neonates. *Clinical Pharmacology and Therapeutics,* **23,** 346–350

PORTER, R. J. (1981) Pharmacokinetic basis of intermittent and chronic anticonvulsant drug therapy in febrile seizures. In *Febrile Seizures*, edited by K. B. Nelson and J. H. Ellenberg, pp. 107–118. New York: Raven Press

PRYOR, D. S., DON, N. and MACOURT, D. C. (1981) Fifth day fits: a syndrome of neonatal convulsions. *Archives of Diseases in Childhood,* **56,** 753 758

RATCLIFFE, J. C. and WOLF, S. M. (1977) Febrile convulsions caused by meningitis in young children. *Annals of Neurology,* **1,** 285–286

RIIKONEN, R. (1982) A long-term follow-up study of 214 children with the syndrome of infantile spasms. *Neuropediatrics,* **13,** 14–23

RIIKONEN, R. and DONNER, M. (1979) Incidence and aetiology of infantile spasms from 1960 to 1976: a population study in Finland. *Developmental Medicine and Child Neurology,* **21,** 333–349

RIIKONEN, R. and DONNER, M. (1980) ACTH therapy in infantile spasms: side-effects. *Archives of Diseases in Childhood,* **55,** 664–672

RUTTER, N. and SMALES, O. R. C. (1977) Role of routine investigations in children presenting with their first febrile convulsion. *Archives of Diseases in Childhood,* **52,** 188–191

SCHWARTZ, R. H., EATON, J., ANSLEY-GREEN, A. and BOWER, B. D. (1983) Ketogenic diets in the management of childhood epilepsy. In *Research Progress in Epilepsy*, edited by F. Clifford Rose, pp. 326–332. London: Pitman

SINGER, W. D., HALLER, J. S., SULLIVAN, L. R., WOLPERT, S., MILLS, C. and RABE, E. F. (1982) The value of neuroradiology in infantile spasms. *Journal of Pediatrics,* **100,** 47–50

SINGER, W. D., RABE, E. F. and HALLER, J. S. (1980) The effect of ACTH therapy upon infantile spasms. *Journal of Pediatrics,* **96,** 485–489

SNEAD, O. C., BENTON, J. W. and MYERS, G. J. (1983) ACTH and prednisone in childhood seizure disorders. *Neurology (Cleveland),* **33,** 966–970

SNYDER, C. H. (1967) Infantile spasms. Favorable response to steroid therapy. *Journal of the American Medical Association,* **201,** 198–201

STRAND, F. L., STOBOY, J. and CAYER, A. (1973–74) A possible direct action of ACTH on nerve and muscle. *Neuroendocrinology,* **13,** 1–5

SUN, S., CASTILLO, M., VANGVANICHYAKORN, K. and KOENIGSBERGER, R. (1981) Long-term follow-up of neonatal seizures due to perinatal asphyxia. *Pediatric Research,* **15,** 712 (abstract)

THORN, I. (1975) A controlled study of prophylactic long-term treatment of febrile convulsions with phenobarbital. *Acta Neurologica Scandinavica* (Suppl. 75), **60,** 67–73

THORN, I. (1981) Prevention of recurrent febrile seizures: intermittent prophylaxis with diazepam compared with continuous treatment with phenobarbital. In *Febrile Seizures,* edited by K. B. Nelson and J. H. Ellenberg, pp. 119–126. New York: Raven Press

TSUBOI, T. (1977) Genetic aspects of febrile convulsions. *Human Genetics,* **38,** 169–173

VAN DEN BERG, B. J. (1974) Studies on convulsive disorders in young children. IV: Incidence of convulsions among siblings. *Developmental Medicine and Child Neurology,* **16,** 457–464

VAN DEN BERG, B. J. and YERUSHALMY, J. (1971) Studies on convulsive disorders in young children. II: Intermittent phenobarbital prophylaxis and recurrence of febrile convulsions. *Journal of Pediatrics,* **78,** 1004–1012

VASSELLA, F., PAVLINCOVA, E., SCHNEIDER, H. J., RUDIN, H. J. and KARBOWSKI, K. (1973) Treatment of infantile spasms and Lennox-Gastaut syndrome with clonazepam (Rivotril). *Epilepsia,* **14,** 165–175

VENTURA, A., BASSO, T., BORTOLAN, A. *et al.* (1982) Home treatment of seizures as a strategy for the long-term management of febrile convulsions in children. *Helvetica Paediatrica Acta,* **37,** 581–587

VÖLZKE, E., DOOSE, H. and STEPHAN, E. (1967) The treatment of infantile spasms and hypsarrhythmia with Mogadon. *Epilepsia,* **8,** 64–70

VOLPE, J. (1981) *Neurology of the Newborn*, pp. 111–137. Philadelphia: Saunders

WALLACE, S. J. (1974) Recurrence of febrile convulsions. *Archives of Diseases in Childhood,* **49,** 763–775

WALLACE, S. J. (1975a) Factors predisposing to a complicated initial febrile convulsion. *Archives of Diseases in Childhood,* **50,** 943–947

WALLACE, S. J. (1975b) Continuous prophylactic anticonvulsants in selected children with febrile convulsions. *Acta Neurologica Scandinavica* (Suppl. 75), **60,** 62–66

WALLACE, S. J. and CULL, A. M. (1979) Long-term psychological outlook for children whose first fit occurs with fever. *Developmental Medicine and Child Neurology,* **21,** 28–40

WALLACE, S. J. and SMITH, J. A. (1980) Successful prophylaxis against febrile convulsions with valproic acid or phenobarbitone. *British Medical Journal,* **280,** 353–354

WASTERLAIN, C. G. (1976) Effects of neonatal status epilepticus on rat brain development. *Neurology (Minneapolis),* **26,** 975–986

WATANABE, K., HARA, K., MIYAZAKI, S., HAKAMADA, S. and KUROYANAGI, M. (1982) Apneic seizures in the newborn. *American Journal of Diseases of Children,* **136,** 980–984

WILLIG, R. P. and LAGENSTEIN, I. (1982) Use of ACTH fragments in children with infantile spasms. *Neuropediatrics,* **13,** 55–58

WOLF, S. M., CARR, A. C., DAVIS, D. C. *et al.* (1977) The value of phenobarbital in the child who has had a single febrile seizure: a controlled prospective study. *Pediatrics,* **59,** 378–395

WOLF, S. M. and FORSYTHE, A. B. (1978) Behavior disturbances, phenobarbital and febrile seizures. *Paediarics,* **61,** 728–731

12
Discontinuation of antiepileptic drugs

Dieter Schmidt

INTRODUCTION

The rationale to discontinue an antiepileptic drug is based on a clinical assessment of the individual risk-to-benefit ratio. The major risk is a severe exacerbation of the epilepsy with an increase in seizure frequency or even the development of status epilepticus, while the major benefit clearly lies in the reduction of preventable drug toxicity and the prospect of leading a life without drugs. The discontinuation may include the total drug intake or may involve a reduction of multiple drug therapy. Even though the discontinuation of antiepileptic drugs is part of the everyday clinical management of patients with epilepsy, there are few systematic studies on its clinical effects. Furthermore, there is new clinical evidence that a reduction of multiple drug therapy may not only be beneficial for clinical drug toxicity but may also improve seizure control. It may therefore be worthwhile to assess the effects of the complete discontinuation of antiepileptic drugs in patients with complete seizure control, to evaluate the reduction of multiple drug therapy in uncontrolled epilepsy, and to suggest clinical guidelines for patient management.

COMPLETE DISCONTINUATION

The effect of the discontinuation of antiepileptic drugs on the natural history of the epilepsy and on drug toxicity has been studied systematically in what can only be a tiny minority of the vast number of patients with epilepsy who undergo discontinuation of drug therapy every day. Furthermore, the studies vary in both clinical characteristics and treatment data. The global results in 2909 patients pooled from 17 studies suggest a rate of relapse of about 50% in adult patients and 25% in children when the drug is discontinued within 1–3 years of complete seizure control. The rate of relapse drops to about 33% in adults when the drug is discontinued later (*Figure 12.1*). The relapse occurs most frequently within the first six months following the complete discontinuation (*Figure 12.2*). The predictors for a seizure relapse can be classified in those related to clinical characteristics including the electroencephalogram and treatment variables.

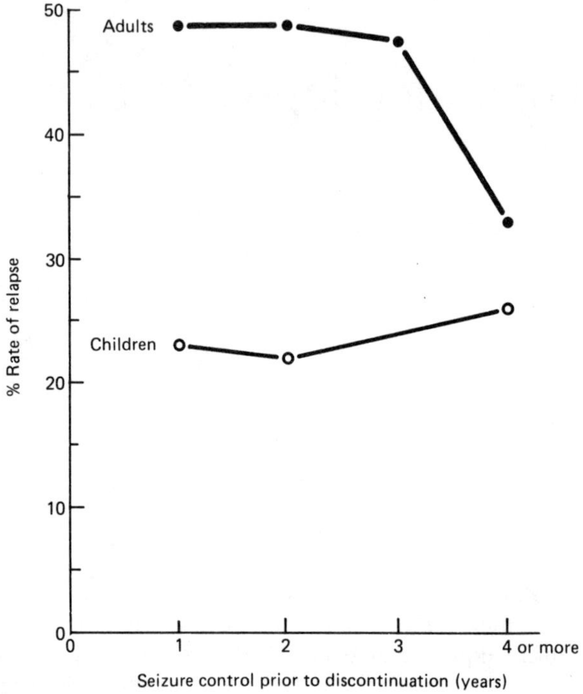

Figure 12.1 Rate of relapse (in %) following the discontinuation of antiepileptic drugs in 2098 adults and 810 children pooled from the data in the literature (Emerson *et al.*, 1981; Förster and Schmidberger, 1978; Heycop ten Ham, 1980; Holowach, Thurston and O'Leary, 1972; Janz and Sommer-Burkhardt, 1976; Janz *et al.*, 1983; Juul-Jensen, 1964, 1968; Loiseau, Henry and Prissard, 1972; Merritt, 1958; Ohtsuka *et al.*, 1982; Oller-Daurella, Oller and Pamies, 1977; Overweg *et al.*, 1981; Strobos, 1959; Tudor *et al.*, 1973; Yahr *et al.*, 1952; Zenker, Groh and Roth, 1957). Each point represents at least the results of two studies

CLINICAL CHARACTERISTICS

The relation between various clinical characteristics and the rate of relapse has been studied in a number of trials. There is no significant difference in the rate of relapse among patients with generalized or partial epilepsy according to Janz *et al.* (1983), while a higher relapse rate has been reported for partial epilepsy by Oller-Daurella, Pamies and Oller (1976). Patients with complex partial seizures have the highest relapse rate among partial epilepsies (*Figure 12.3*). Among the generalized epilepsies the rate of relapse is highest in patients with juvenile myoclonic seizures (impulsive petit mal) and generalized tonic-clonic seizures followed by patients with a combination of absence seizures and generalized tonic-clonic seizures (Janz *et al.*, 1983). The rate of relapse cannot be reliably predicted from the previous seizure prognosis of the individual patient even though Oller-Daurella, Pamies and Oller (1976) reported a low relapse rate in patients whose epilepsy could be controlled easily. Heycop ten Ham (1980) showed that

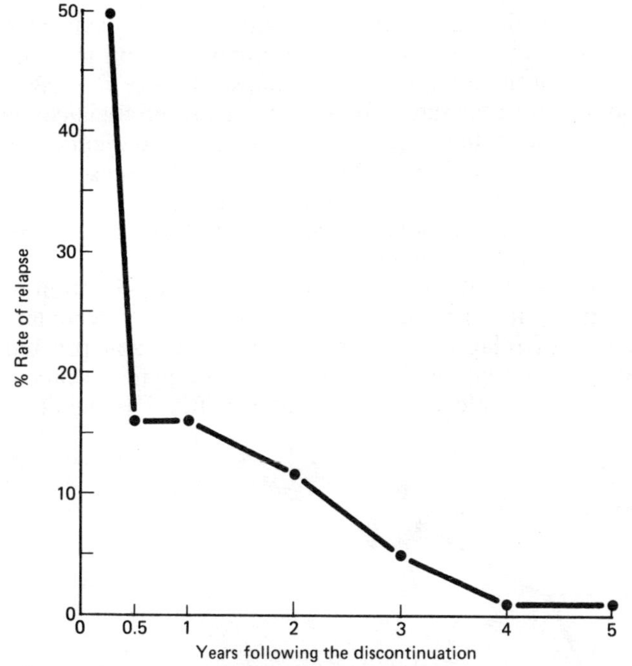

Figure 12.2 Rate of relapse following the discontinuation of antiepileptic drugs (data from Mössinger, 1983)

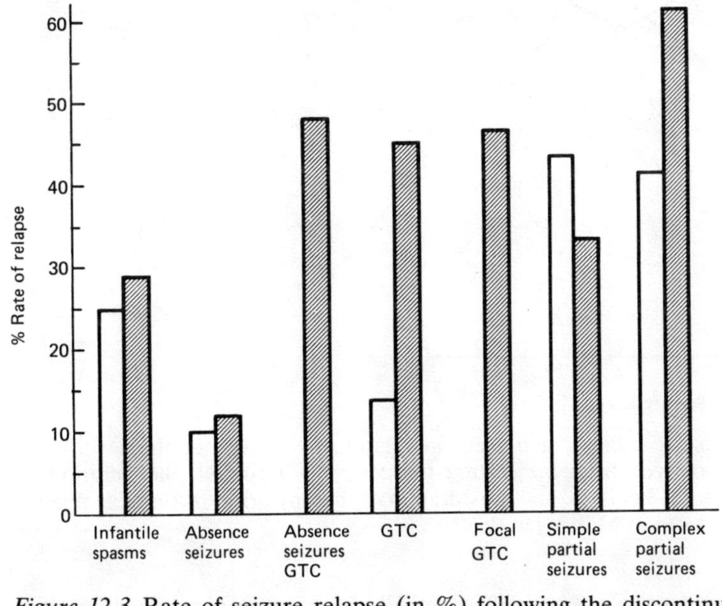

Figure 12.3 Rate of seizure relapse (in %) following the discontinuation of antiepileptic drugs in 674 adults (white bars) and 213 children (dark bars) with various types of seizures pooled from data in the literature (Holowach, Thurston and O'Leary, 1972; Loiseau, Henry and Prissard, 1972; Tudor *et al.*, 1973; Janz and Sommer-Burkhardt, 1976; Oller-Daurella, Oller and Pamies, 1977; Heycop ten Ham, 1980; Janz *et al.*, 1983). GTC: generalized tonic-clonic seizures

secondarily generalized epilepsies with a relatively poor seizure prognosis may have a low relapse rate once they are controlled. Patients with impulsive petit mal and good seizure prognosis have one of the highest rates of relapse (Janz *et al.*, 1983). Biological variables may also influence the rate of relapse. Generalized tonic-clonic seizures on awakening have a higher rate of relapse as compared to patients with seizures occurring mostly during sleep (Janz *et al.*, 1983). The age of onset seems to influence the rate of relapse. Children generally have a lower relapse rate (*see Figures 12.1* and *12.3*). Others, however, found the age at onset of epilepsy not predictive for the relapse rate (Thurston *et al.*, 1982).

The 'severity' of epilepsy assessed by the frequency of seizures, the duration of epilepsy prior to onset of therapy, and the duration of therapy prior to complete control was related to the rate of relapse for primary generalized epilepsy but apparently less so for partial epilepsy (*Figure 12.4*). If it took more than six years to reach complete seizure control, the rate of relapse was significantly higher in

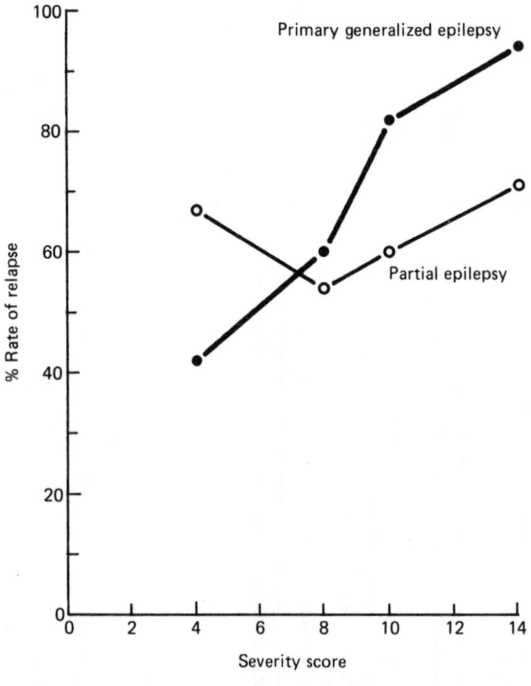

Figure 12.4 Rate of seizure relapse in percent in relation to a score of the severity of epilepsy. The score is derived from the seizure frequency (3–9 points), the duration of epilepsy prior to therapy (3–8 points), and the duration of therapy prior to complete seizure control (3–8 points) (data from Mössinger, 1983)

children as compared to those who were controlled earlier (Holowach, Thurston and O'Leary, 1972). In adults, the rate of relapse increased from 60% to 83% when the epilepsy was completely controlled within 3–5 years as compared to one year (*Figure 12.5*). In a recent prospective study, children were more likely to have a relapse if they were mentally retarded, if their seizures had begun before two years of age, if they had many generalized seizures before control, or if they had had a definitely abnormal electroencephalogram before the drug was discontinued (Emerson *et al.*, 1981). Factors associated with an increased risk of relapse were a long duration of epilepsy before control, neurological dysfunction and Jacksonian seizures or multiple seizure types (Thurston *et al.*, 1982). A family history of epilepsy does not seem to be a good predictor for the relapse rate (Mössinger, 1983; Thurston *et al.*, 1982).

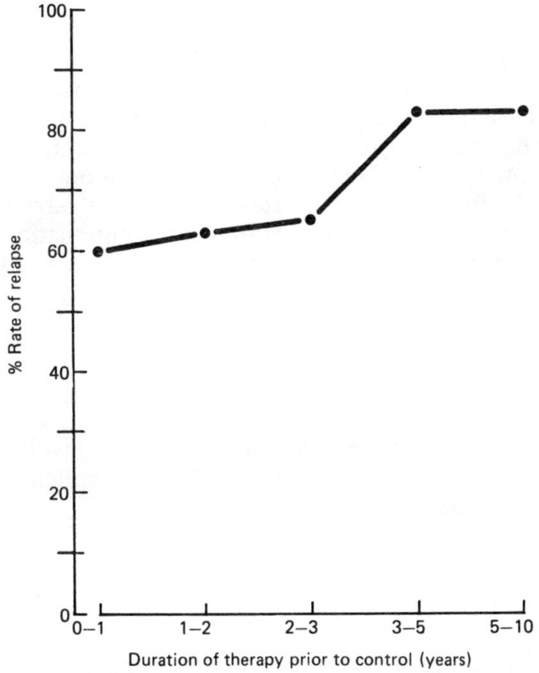

Figure 12.5 Rate of seizure relapse in percent in relation to the duration of drug therapy prior to complete seizure control following the discontinuation of antiepileptic drugs in 228 adult patients (data from Mössinger, 1983)

There seems to be general agreement that the electroencephalographic findings prior to the discontinuation are of little predictive value for the rate of relapse (Förster and Schmidberger, 1979; Janz and Sommer-Burkhardt, 1976; Overweg *et al.*, 1981; Puhlmann, 1982; Thurston *et al.*, 1982). However, a recent prospective study suggested that a definitely abnormal electroencephalogram before medication was discontinued is a good predictor of relapse in children (Emerson *et al.*, 1981). In Juul-Jensen's (1964, 1968) series of 200 patients the relapse rate was higher for patients with slow wave foci. However, an EEG was available prior to reduction in only approximately 50% of the patients and no data are available from the period following the discontinuation of the drug. An increase of paroxysmal spikes or spike and waves following the discontinuation is associated with a higher relapse rate in children (Holowach, Thurston and O'Leary, 1972; Förster and Schmidberger, 1979; Zenker, Groh and Roth, 1957).

TREATMENT VARIABLES

Any effort to investigate the relation between treatment characteristics and the rate of relapse is hampered by the difficulty in comparing various drugs and different dosages. Furthermore, more severe epilepsies may receive a higher daily dosage or a higher number of drugs, thus confounding the relation between drug therapy and rate of relapse. Non-compliance has been shown to be associated with a high rate of relapse in patients with primary generalized epilepsy but not in partial epilepsy (Mössinger, 1983).

Among the treatment variables the duration of seizure control prior to reduction, the dose decrement and the duration until the drug is discontinued completely may influence the rate of relapse. Patients who tolerated a dose reduction without relapse will subsequently be reduced more rapidly, while patients with a relapse will be reduced more slowly. In one large series the rate of relapse seemed to be independent from the dose decrement and the number of years from the onset of dose reduction (Mössinger, 1983). The first step of dose reduction does not carry a higher risk of relapse compared to subsequent and the final step of discontinuation (Mössinger, 1983). Fortunately, in approximately 80% a relapse can be treated successfully with re-administration of the previously effective dose (Todt, 1979).

MECHANISMS OF RELAPSE

The recurrence of a seizure when a drug is discontinued may involve seizure-provoking factors unrelated to drug intake, loss of necessary antiepileptic drug therapy, and finally a withdrawal reaction.

Seizure provocation unrelated to drug intake

Patients who were successfully controlled by a combination of drug therapy and prevention of seizure-provoking factors such as loss of sleep, intake of alcoholic beverages, or sensory stimulation may suffer a relapse if they simultaneously discontinue their medication and expose themselves to seizure-provoking factors which lead to an exacerbation of the epilepsy. Patients who celebrate the day when their medication was stopped with a party which lasts all night may suffer a relapse seizure the following morning.

Loss of necessary drug therapy

The concept to discontinue the antiepileptic drugs in a patient who remained well controlled for several years implies that either the drug therapy or the natural history itself reduced the seizure propensity to a degree that drug therapy is no longer necessary. If one assumes that drug therapy is in fact directly or indirectly responsible for a decrease in the seizure propensity, antiepileptic drug therapy may be seen as 'curing' epilepsy instead of merely suppressing temporarily the recurrence of seizures without any long-lasting effect on the natural history of the disease.

Prior to the introduction of modern antiepileptic drugs in 1912 (Hauptmann, 1912) the long-term seizure control was reported to range from 5% to 12.5% (Habermaas, 1901; Schilling, 1968). If one compares this figure with the percentage of patients who remained seizure-free for at least two years following the discontinuation, which is around 14% (Mössinger, 1983), there is no good clinical evidence that antiepileptic drugs cure epilepsy. Thus we are faced with the somewhat disappointing concept that the seizure control when the drug is discontinued reflects the natural remission of the disease in a subpopulation who become seizure-free.

Withdrawal reaction

Antiepileptic drugs differ in the clinical effects of discontinuation. A transient increase in seizure frequency was seen during removal of primidone, phenobarbital, methobarbital, clonazepam, diazepam, chlordiazepoxide, nitrazepam and sodium bromide from multiple drug therapy in 20 out of 48 patients (42%) and in nine out of 30 outpatients (30%). No episodes of status epilepticus occurred, and only two patients needed temporarily increased doses of barbiturates before withdrawal was completed. The drugs were withdrawn within two weeks in inpatients and within three months in outpatients. The withdrawn drugs were replaced by phenytoin, valproic acid, ethosuximide and carbamazepine (Theodore and Porter, 1983). Withdrawal reactions requiring re-administration of the drug have been observed in 27 out of 137 institutionalized patients (20%) during reduction of multiple drug therapy from valproic acid (four out of 30 patients), carbamazepine (three out of ten patients), clonazepam (three out of 14 patients), and phenobarbital (12 out of 60 patients). A psychotic episode was noted in one patient when clonazepam was discontinued. Three patients developed a status of complex partial seizures and adversive seizures, and a confusional episode during the withdrawal of phenobarbital. No withdrawal seizures were seen when phenytoin and ethosuximide were discontinued (Schobben, 1979). Withdrawal reactions may also be seen in newborns exposed to antiepileptic drugs during the fetal period (Koch *et al.*, 1983). A temporary increase in seizure frequency was also noted during withdrawal of clonazepam (Kruse and Blankenhorn, 1973), carbamazepine and phenytoin (Spencer *et al.*, 1981). Additional withdrawal symptoms include irritability, tremor, sleep disturbances, weight loss, tachycardia, and psychotic episodes. Clinical signs of withdrawal appear within a few days to several weeks following sudden discontinuation of a drug, depending on its individual biological half-life. Phenobarbital, primidone, or clonazepam withdrawal may continue for up to four weeks; for phenytoin it ends within two weeks (Rosenblum, 1971). It is useful to note that primidone withdrawal seizures are not prevented by concomitant phenytoin in plasma concentrations of more than 12 μg/ml (*Figure 12.6*).

One would like to know more about the following clinical aspects of the development of withdrawal: relation to previous development of tolerance and predictors of withdrawal reactions through monitoring of the decay of the plasma concentration, long-term electroencephalographic recordings, and clinical features of the patients and treatment variables. The clinical phenomenology of withdrawal seizures needs further documentation. A recent study on ictal effects of antiepileptic drug withdrawal in epileptic patients found that 'new' clinical seizures

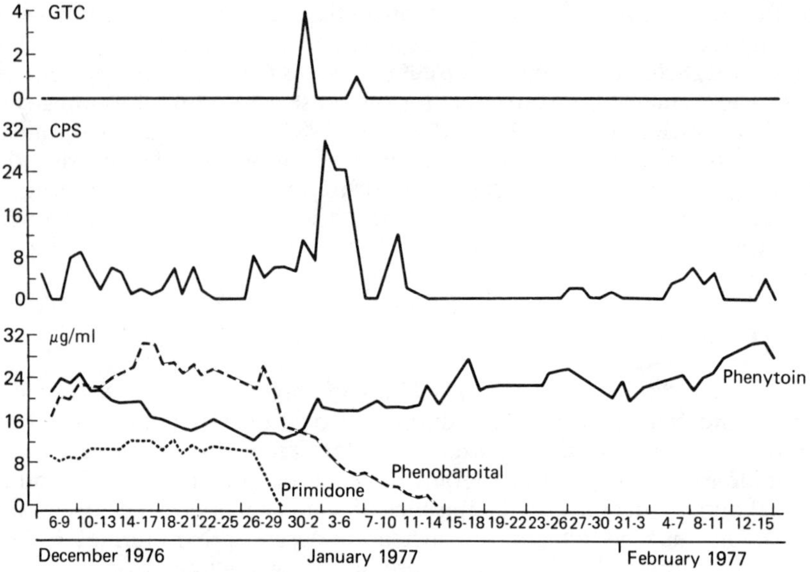

Figure 12.6 Decline of primidone and phenobarbital plasma concentrations and appearance of ictal withdrawal reaction following abrupt discontinuation of primidone in a patient with additional phenytoin treatment. Note that the onset of generalized tonic-clonic seizures (GTC) and the significant increase of complex-partial seizures (CPS) during withdrawal does not occur during the rapid decline of primidone plasma concentration but during the subsequent decrease in the phenobarbital plasma level (from Schmidt and Seldon, 1982)

and/or electroencephalographical abnormalities may occur during withdrawal in patients in whom bilateral or multifocal seizure onset was confirmed electroencephalographically outside the withdrawal period. The withdrawal period was defined in this study as the time after abrupt cessation of medication between one and five half-lives of the drug (Spencer *et al.*, 1981). An earlier study limited itself to the interictal changes in the scalp EEG induced by antiepileptic drug withdrawal in epileptic patients (Ludwig and Marsan, 1975). Furthermore, we are usually inclined to see ictal withdrawal effects as those leading to a recurrence of seizures. However, there is some clinical evidence that withdrawal of one of several drugs in a patient with uncontrolled epilepsy may in fact be beneficial for seizure control (Schmidt, 1983b).

CLINICAL GUIDELINES

The decision when to discontinue antiepileptic drugs depends on the assessment of risk factors for a relapse in the individual patient (*Table 12.1*). Prior to the first reduction step there should be a joint understanding by the patient and the physician on the plan to discontinue the medication. The drug will be reduced after 2–3 years of complete control in low-risk cases defined as in *Table 12.1*. In patients on single-drug therapy the recommended dose decrement is 25% every six months or even longer. Sedative drugs, drugs of second choice, or drugs at very low plasma concentrations are withdrawn first. As the risk of relapse seems to be similar for each step of reduction there is no need for concern to withdraw the last dose for final and complete discontinuation. The risk of relapse will be lowest when the patient is seen before each dose decrement. The patient should be reminded to avoid seizure-provoking factors and the physician may enquire if the patient is in fact taking a lower dosage. There is a surprisingly large number of patients who will

Table 12.1 Assessment of risk for relapse following the discontinuation of antiepileptic drugs

Clinical characteristics		*Risk of relapse*	
	high	*intermediate*	*low*
Seizure control (years)	1–2	2–3	4 or more
Therapy prior to control (years)	more than 5	2–5	1–2
Duration of epilepsy (years)	more than 5	2–5	1–2
Type of seizure	complex partial absence and GTC GTC on awakening	GTC only GTC during sleep	absence only
Multiple types of seizures	+		
High previous seizure frequency	+		
Non-compliance of sleep, intake of alcoholic beverages following discontinuation	+		
Mental retardation	+		
Increase in generalized or focal paroxysmal discharges during reduction or following discontinuation	+		
Patient is not convinced to discontinue	+		
Treatment			
Duration of discontinuation (months)	1–6	6–12	more than 12

continue to take the original daily dose and prefer not to participate in the planned discontinuation, sometimes without telling the physician. The reluctance to discontinue the drug may be caused by the grave social consequences of a seizure recurrence for the individual patient. In that case, the reduction for the individual patient should only be continued if the patient wishes so. Furthermore, the risk of relapse should not be underestimated; after all only about 14% of the patients remain seizure-free. The patient may feel safer if told that a relapse can easily be treated in most cases and is not a major setback in medical terms for the continued good seizure prognosis in case the drug has to be reintroduced.

A re-occurrence of paroxysmal discharges in the EEG during reduction in a patient without a seizure relapse will delay a further reduction and require a re-assessment of the individual risk.

In case of a single seizure recurrence during reduction, close consultation is useful to assess whether the patient has followed the plan of discontinuation or has abruptly stopped taking the drug altogether or if there has been exposure to seizure-provoking factors. The options are: a delay to change medication until a further seizure occurs, an increase to the previous step of reduction, an increase above the daily dose or the plasma concentration at which the patient had the last seizure prior to reduction. If the recurrence was associated with an increase in paroxysmal discharges the EEG may be useful for further monitoring in the individual patient. If the patient develops non-ictal withdrawal reactions, oral diazepam or nitrazepam are helpful to control tremor, anxiety, agitation, and insomnia.

REDUCTION OF MULTIPLE-DRUG THERAPY

Despite the widespread use of multiple drug therapy, especially for intractable epilepsy, there is a surprising lack of evidence that two antiepileptic drugs are better than one drug for chronic uncontrolled epilepsy with partial seizures or generalized tonic-clonic seizures. In fact, a recent prospective trial showed that seizure control improved in only 13% of patients with intractable complex partial seizures when a second drug was added (Schmidt, 1982b). Similar data were reported for newly diagnosed cases with partial seizures or generalized tonic-clonic seizures. Only 15% of the patients who did not respond fully to either phenytoin or carbamazepine did benefit from a multiple drug therapy with both drugs (Hakkarainen, 1981). In addition, single drug therapy with carbamazepine, phenytoin or phenobarbital is successful even in chronic epilepsy (Callaghan *et al.*, 1978; Schmidt, 1983a; Strandjord and Johannessen, 1980). There is no doubt, however, that the incidence and severity of adverse effects is higher during multiple drug therapy (Koch *et al.*, 1983; Kutt *et al.*, 1975; Schmidt and Seldon, 1982). As a result of the concern about adverse effects a transfer from multiple-drug to single-drug therapy is of interest. In recent years several studies have assessed the clinical effects of the discontinuation of one drug in patients uncontrolled by multiple-drug therapy. A reduction of the number of drugs from 2.47 to 2.02 was associated with a decrease of side-effects from 45% to 26% and a reduction of seizure frequency by more than 50% in 45% of the patients (Milano Collaborative Group for Studies on Epilepsy, 1977). Shorvon and Reynolds (1980) were able to reduce multiple-drug therapy in 29 patients; the seizure frequency improved by over 50% in 55% of the patients. In nine patients the number of seizures decreased by more than 80% and six patients became seizure-free. Even in institutionalized patients with severe epilepsy a reduction in the number of drugs from 1.58 to 1.48 was associated with a marked reduction of seizure frequency in 23% (Schobben, 1979). A reduction of polypharmacy in 130 patients resulted in a marked decrease of seizure frequency by more than 80% in 11% of the patients (Maheshwari and Padmini, 1981). A removal of sedative antiepileptic drugs from the regimen of 78 patients with severe epilepsy, 51% showed improvement in both drug toxicity and seizure control, 19% in toxicity alone, 12% in seizure control alone; 16% were unchanged and 2% were worse. Sedative drugs do not seem to be necessary for good seizure control even in intractable epilepsy, and they may safely be withdrawn (Theodore and Porter, 1983). Removal of sedative drugs in patients with intractable epilepsy may, however, require an increase in the dose of the remaining drug with the unfortunate result that the side-effects are not reduced despite a reduction of multiple-drug therapy (Schmidt and Machus, 1980)

The effects of reducing two-drug therapy to single-drug therapy were recently monitored in 36 patients with intractable complex partial seizures (Schmidt, 1983b). In 30 patients (83%) this was possible without an increase in seizure frequency. A slow transfer was not compromised by unwanted withdrawal effects. An improvement in seizure control was noted in 13 patients (36%). Two patients became seizure-free, and one patient had a reduction of seizure frequency by 87%. The number of side-effects was lower during single-drug therapy (*Table 12.2*). In a

Table 12.2 Clinical side-effects encountered in patients with complex partial seizures during a transfer from two-drug to single-drug therapy (from Schmidt, 1983b)

Side-effect	*Two-drug therapy*		*Single-drug therapy*	
	n^a	n^b	n^a	n^c
Nystagmus	16	7	13	4
Sedation	7	2	5	2
Ataxia	8	5	3	1
Diplopia	3	1	1	–
Vertigo	2	2	3	1
Nausea	–	–	2	1
Anxiety	1	–	1	1
Gingival hyperplasia	1	–	–	–
Fever	1	–	–	–
Exanthema	1	–	–	–
Myoclonias	–	–	1	–
Myalgia	–	–	1	–
Tremor	–	–	1	–
Vomiting	1	1	–	–
Total	41	18	31	10

[a] Total number of side-effects during two-drug or single-drug therapy.
[b] Number of side-effects disappearing with the transfer to single-drug therapy.
[c] Number of side-effects occurring with the transfer to single-drug therapy

recent study on the effects of the discontinuation of primidone in three patients with intractable complex partial seizures uncontrolled by high-dose multiple-drug therapy with phenytoin and primidone, the number of seizures and paroxysmal discharges in the EEG disappeared in one patient (*Figure 12.7*). In a Canadian study 72 of 90 patients (80%) were reduced from an average of 2.75 drugs to an average of 1.49 drugs. No change or even an improvement in seizure control was observed and sedative side-effects were reduced in many patients. In 18 patients with mostly multiple seizure types the number of drugs could not be reduced; in ten of these seizure control was inadequate on their existing medication, and a second drug was added. In eight patients an increase in seizure frequency following the

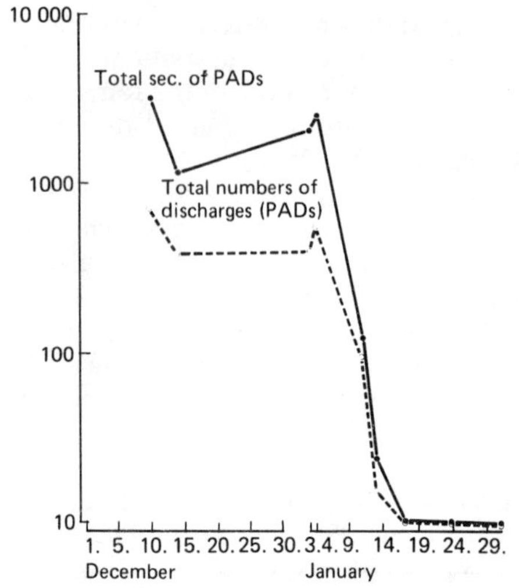

Figure 12.7 The effect of primidone withdrawal on paroxysmal discharges (PAD) in a patient with complex partial seizures. The number and the total duration of paroxysmal abnormal discharges decreased at the 9th day after the withdrawal of primidone in this patient, uncontrolled by combined phenytoin and primidone treatment. At day 22 no more paroxysmal abnormal discharges were detectable in the printout of the telemetered 8 h EEG. Following a temporary increase in seizure frequency the patient became seizure-free following the withdrawal of primidone and has been seizure-free for two years (from Schmidt, 1982a)

discontinuation required a return to the previous drug regimen (Albright and Bruni, 1983). Patients with partial seizures and generalized tonic-clonic seizures (Schmidt, 1980) and a subpopulation of patients with absence seizures may require more than one drug (Rowan *et al.*, 1983). These findings suggest that multiple-drug therapy is unnecessary in a large number of patients exposed to several antiepileptic drugs. From these studies it seems safe to conclude that reduction of multiple-drug therapy is possible without comprising seizure control in about 80% of the patients. However, we have no adequate information of features predictive for patients who can be reduced safely and those who require a return to the previous regimen. There is no valid explanation for the improvement in seizure control associated with a reduction of multiple drug therapy in some patients. The concept that antiepileptic drugs may be epileptogenic possibly in a dose-dependent fashion is not well outlined nor has it been supported by unequivocal clinical evidence (Reynolds and Shorvon, 1981; Schmidt and Seldon, 1982). Clearly, further investigations on this disturbing feature of multiple antiepileptic drug therapy are warranted.

CLINICAL GUIDELINES

Reduction of multiple-drug therapy in an outpatient with uncontrolled seizures is carried out stepwise with a dose decrement of 25% for one drug every two months. Sedative drugs or drugs of second choice or drugs with a low daily dose or a low plasma concentration are reduced first. During the reduction a non-sedative drug of first choice is either introduced or increased in its daily dose for maximum efficacy.

A programme of withdrawal enters its critical phase when a transient increase in seizure frequency occurs. Pressure builds up in both the patient and the relatives to reintroduce the previous regimen in the face of continuing seizures. If the physician can convince the patient and others that persistence is most valuable for long-term result, the programme will be successful in most cases. Emergency treatment of a series of seizures by rectal instillation of 10–20 mg diazepam in an adult patient, or treatment of insomnia with nitrazepam, will rarely be necessary. Status epilepticus seems to be rare, if it occurs at all, during reduction of multiple drug therapy when the non-sedative drug is concomitantly increased in daily dose to maximum efficacy (Schmidt, 1983b; Theodore and Porter, 1983).

If the increase of seizure frequency persists longer than six weeks despite an increase in non-sedative drugs, a readministration of a sedative drug, such as phenobarbital, may be necessary. Before re-administration it may be worthwhile to check whether the patient had a similar increase in seizure frequency in the previous history unrelated to a change in medication. In that case, the re-administration should be delayed as long as possible. Most patients will appreciate the concern of the physician not to choose 'the easy way' and add another drug but rather wait as long as possible for that decision. Frequent consultations and close communication are required during a programme of withdrawal. A successful programme of withdrawal is currently the optimum drug management of a patient unresponsive to standard drug therapy until new and better antiepileptic drugs are available for intractable epilepsy.

References

ALBRIGHT, P. S. and BRUNI, J. (1983) Reduction of polypharmacy in epileptic patients. *Abstract, XVth Epilepsy International Symposium,* Washington, p. 435.

CALLAGHAN, N., O'CALLAGHAN, M., DUGGAN, B. and FEELY, M. (1978) Carbamazepine as a single drug in the treatment of epilepsy. *Journal of Neurology, Neurosurgery and Psychiatry,* **41,** 907–912

EMERSON, R., D'SOUZA, B. J., VINING, E. P., HOLDEN, K. R., MELLITS, E. D. and FREEMAN, J. M. (1981) Stopping medication in children with epilepsy: predictors of outcome. *New England Journal of Medicine,* **304,** 1125–1129

FÖRSTER, C. and SCHMIDBERGER, G. (1979) Prognostische Wertigkeit von EEG—Verlaufsuntersuchungen bei Kindern mit Anfallsrezidiven nach Absetzen der antikonvulsiven Therapie. In *Epilepsie 1978,* edited by H. Doose, G. Gross-Selbeck, pp. 252–255. Stuttgart: Georg Thieme Verlag

HABERMAAS (1901) Über die Prognose der Epilepsie. *Allgemeine Zeitschrift für Psychiatrie,* **58,** 243–253

HAKKARAINEN, H. (1981) Carbamazepine and diphenylhydantoin as monotherapy or in combination in the treatment of adult epilepsy. *Abstract, XIIIth Epilepsy International Symposium,* Kyoto, p. 140

HAUPTMANN, A. (1912) Luminal bei Epilepsie. *Münchner Medizinische Wochenschrift,* **59,** 1907–1909

HEYCOP TEN HAM, M. W. (1980) Complete recovery from epilepsy? Discontinuance of anti-epileptic drugs after five or more seizure-free years. *Huisarts en Wetenschap,* **23,** 309–311

HOLOWACH, J., THURSTON, D. L. and O'LEARY, J. (1972) Prognosis in childhood epilepsy: follow-up study of 148 cases in which therapy had been suspended after prolonged anticonvulsant control. *New England Journal of Medicine,* **286,** 169–174

JANZ, D. and SOMMER-BURKHARDT, E. M. (1976) Discontinuation of antiepileptic drugs in patients with epilepsy who have been seizure-free for more than two years. In *Epileptology*, edited by D. Janz, pp. 228–234. Stuttgart: Georg Thieme Verlag

JANZ, D., KERN, A., MÖSSINGER, H.-J. and PUHLMANN, U. (1983) Rückfall-Prognose nach Reduktion der Medikamente bei Epilepsiebehandlung. *Nervenarzt,* **54,** 525–529

JUUL-JENSEN, P. (1964) Frequency of recurrence after discontinuance of anticonvulsant therapy in patients with epileptic seizures. *Epilepsia,* **5,** 352–363

JUUL-JENSEN, P. (1968) Frequency of recurrence after discontinuance of anticonvulsant therapy in patients with epileptic seizures. *Epilepsia,* **9,** 11–16

KOCH, S., GÖPFERT-GEYER, I., JÄGER-ROMAN, E. *et al.* (1983) Antiepileptika während der Schwangerschaft. *Deutsche Medizinische Wochenschrift,* **108,** 250–257

KRUSE, R. and BLANKENHORN, V. (1973) Zusammenfassender Erfahrungsbericht über die klinische Anwendung und Wirksamkeit von Ro 5–4023 (clonazepam) auf verschiedene Formen epileptischer Anfälle. *Acta Neurologica Scandinavica* (Suppl. 53), 60–71

KUTT, H., SOLOMON, G., WASTERLAIN, C., PETERSON, H., LOUIS, S. and CARRUTHERS, R. (1975) Carbamazepine in difficult to control epileptic outpatients. *Acta Neurologica Scandinavia* (Suppl. 60), 27–32

LOISEAU, P., HENRY, P. and PRISSARD, A. (1972) Considérations sur l'arrêt des traitements antiépileptiques. *Bordeaux Médical,* **19,** 2631–2642

LUDWIG, B. I. and MARSAN, C. A. (1975) EEG changes after withdrawal of medication in epileptic patients. *Electroencephalography and Clinical Neurophysiology,* **39,** 173–181

MAHESHWARI, M. C. and PADMINI, R. (1981) Role of carbamazepine in reducing polypharmacy in epilepsy. *Acta Neurologica Scandinavica,* **64,** 22–28

MERRITT, H. H. (1958) Medical treatment in epilepsy. *British Medical journal,* **1,** 666–669

MILANO COLLABORATIVE GROUP FOR STUDIES ON EPILEPSY (1977) Long-term intensive monitoring in the difficult patient. Preliminary results of 16 months of observations – usefulness and limination. In *Antiepileptic Drug Monitoring,* edited by C. Gardner-Thorpe, D. Janz, H. Meinardi and C. E. Pippenger, pp. 197–213. Kent: Pitman Medical

MÖSSINGER, H. (1983) Rückfallhäufigkeit und Prognose nach Reduktion der Antikonvulsiva in der Epilepsiebehandlung. *Inaugural-Dissertation,* Freie Universität Berlin

OHTSUKA, Y., YAMATOGI, Y., OKA, E. and OHTAHARA, S. (1982) Treatment and discontinuation of antiepileptic drugs in childhood epilepsy. *Folia Psychiatrica et Neurologica Japonica,* **36,** 279–286

OLLER-DAURELLA, L., PAMIES, R. and OLLER, L. (1976) Reduction or discontinuance of antiepileptic drugs in patients seizure-free for more than 5 years. In *Epileptology,* edited by D. Janz, pp. 218–227. Stuttgart: Georg Thieme Verlag

OLLER-DAURELLA, L., OLLER, L. and PAMIES, R. (1977) Clinical, therapeutic, and social status of epileptic patients without seizures for more than five years. In *Epilepsy, The Eighth International Symposium,* edited by J. K. Penry, pp. 69–75. New York: Raven Press

OVERWEG, J., ROWAN, A. J., BINNIE, C. D., OOSTING, J. and NAGELKERGE, N. J. D. (1981) Prediction of seizure recurrence after withdrawal of antiepileptic drugs. In *Advances in Epileptology: XIIth Epilepsy International Symposium*, edited by M. Dam, L. Gram and J. K. Penry, pp. 503–508. New York: Raven Press

PUHLMANN, H.-U. (1982) Über die Bedeutung von EEG-Kriterien für die Therapieprognose bei Epilepsie. *Inaugural-Dissertation,* Freie Unversität Berlin

REYNOLDS, E. H. and SHORVON, S. D. (1981) Monotherapy or polytherapy for epilepsy? *Epilepsia,* **22,** 1–10

ROSENBLUM, J. A. (1971) Diphenylhydantoin sodium (Dilantin) withdrawal in non-epileptics. *Current Therapy and Research,* **13,** 369–373

ROWAN, A. J., MEIJER, J. W. A., BEER-PAWLIKOWSKI, N. DE, VAN DER GEEST, P. and MEINARDI, H. (1983) Valproate–ethosuximide combination therapy for refractory absence seizures. *Archives of Neurology,* **40,** 797–802

SCHILLING, D. (1968) Langzeitresultate ambulanter Epilepsiebehandlung. *Inaugural-Dissertation,* Universität Heidelberg

SCHMIDT. D. (1980) One drug treatment with phenytoin in difficult-to-treat epilepsies with complex partial seizures: a preliminary report of a prospective study. In *Antiepileptic Therapy: Advances in Drug Monitoring*, edited by S. I. Johannessen, P. L. Morselli, C. E. Pippenger, A. Richens, D. Schmidt and H. Meinardi, pp. 221–228. New York: Raven Press

SCHMIDT, D. (1982a) The influence of antiepileptic drugs on the electroencephalogram: a review of controlled clinical trials. *Electroencephalography and Clinical Neurophysiology* (Suppl. 36), 453–466

SCHMIDT, D. (1982b) Two antiepileptic drugs for intractable epilepsy with complex partial seizures. *Journal of Neurology, Neurosurgery and Psychiatry,* **45,** 1119–1124

SCHMIDT, D. (1983a) Single drug therapy for intractable epilepsy. *Journal of Neurology,* **229,** 221–226

SCHMIDT, D. (1983b) Reduction of two-drug therapy in intractable epilepsy. *Epilepsia,* **24,** 368–376

SCHMIDT, D. and MACHUS, B. (1980) The use of blood levels in the treatment of patients with Lennox syndrome. In *Antiepileptic Therapy: Advances in Drug Monitoring*, edited by S. I. Johannessen, P. L. Morselli, C. E. Pippenger, A. Richens, D. Schmidt and H. Meinardi, pp. 279–285. New York: Raven Press

SCHMIDT, D. and SELDON, L. (1982) *Adverse Effects of Antiepileptic Drugs*. New York: Raven Press

SCHOBBEN, F. (1979) *Pharmacokinetics and Therapeutics in Epilepsy*. Nijmegen: Stichting Studentenpers

SHORVON, S. D. and REYNOLDS, E. H. (1980) Reduction in polypharmacy for epilepsy. In *Antiepileptic Therapy: Advances in Drug Monitoring,* edited by S. I. Johannessen, P. L. Morselli, C. E. Pippenger, A. Richens, D. Schmidt and H. Meinardi, pp. 203–209. New York: Raven Press

SPENCER, S. S., SPENCER, D. D., WILLIAMSON, P. D. and MATTSON, R. H. (1981) Ictal effects of anticonvulsant medication withdrawal in epileptic patients. *Epilepsia,* **22,** 297–307

STRANDJORD, R. E. and JOHANNESSEN, S. I. (1980) Carbamazepine as the only drug in patients with epilepsy: serum levels and clinical effect. In *Antiepileptic Therapy: Advances in Drug Monitoring,* edited by S. I. Johannessen, P. L. Morselli, C. E. Pippenger, A. Richens, D. Schmidt and H. Meinardi, pp. 229–233. New York: Raven Press

STROBOS, R. R. J. (1959) Prognosis in convulsive disorders. *Archives of Neurology,* **1,** 216–225

THEODORE, W. H. and PORTER, R. J. (1983) Removal of sedative-hypnotic antiepileptic drugs from the regimens of patients with intractable epilepsy. *Annals of Neurology,* **13,** 320–324

THURSTON, J. H., THURSTON, D. L., HIXON, B. B. and KELLER, A. J. (1982) Prognosis in childhood epilepsy. Additional follow-up of 148 children 15 to 23 years after withdrawal of anticonvulsant therapy. *New England Journal of Medicine,* **306,** 831–836

TODT, H. (1979) Zur Spätprognose kindlicher Epilepsien – Ergebnisse einer prospektiven Längsschnitt-studie. *Inaugural-Dissertation,* Medizinische Akademie Carl Gustav Carus, Dresden

TUDOR, I., MILEA, S., BICESCU, E. and IVANA, D. (1973) Catamnestic study of childhood epilepsy. *Revue Roumania Neurologica,* **10,** 341–352

YAHR, M. D., SCIARRA, D., CARTER, S. and MERRITT, H. H. (1952) Evaluation of standard anticonvulsant therapy in 319 patients. *Journal of American Medical Association,* **150,** 663–667

ZENKER, C., GROH, C. and ROTH, C. (1957) Probleme und Erfahrungen beim Absetzen antikonvulsiver Therapie. *Neue Österreichische Zeitschrift für Kinderheilkunde,* **2,** 152–163

13

Positron emission tomography (PET) in the diagnosis of epilepsy

Jerome Engel, Jr.

INTRODUCTION

Patients with epilepsy may have a variety of underlying diseases and related symptoms. The pathophysiological processes, however, which cause transient, paroxysmal epileptic seizures – the common disabling feature of all epileptic disorders – reflect functional rather than structural changes in the brain. Even when patients with epilepsy have structural abnormalities identifiable by routine radiological studies (Gastaut and Gastaut, 1976), the nature, localization and extent of these abnormalities may not be as important to the ultimate diagnosis and management of the patient as an understanding of the functional disturbances that: (1) occur during the seizure itself, and (2) persist between seizures to some extent. Consequently, diagnosis of epilepsy relies heavily on the EEG as the single routinely available laboratory test for localization of functional abnormalities in patients. Furthermore, the current international classification of epileptic seizures is based entirely on characterization of ictal behavior and patterns of interictal and ictal EEG activity (Commission on Classification and Terminology, ILAE, 1981).

Although the EEG is extremely useful for diagnosis in epilepsy (Engel, 1984a), spatial localization is limited to the lateral surfaces of the hemispheres directly beneath the scalp electrodes, and transients representing a primary epileptogenic lesion cannot be differentiated from transients propagated to the surface from lesions within inaccessible areas of cortex located on the mesial and basal surfaces of the hemispheres. Sphenoidal (Rovit, Gloor and Rasmussen, 1961) and nasopharyngeal (Mavor and Hellen, 1964) electrodes aid in localization to mesial temporal structures, and nasoethmoidal electrodes (Quesney *et al.*, 1981) may provide some information about orbitofrontal EEG activity, but even these techniques are greatly lacking in spatial resolution. Stereotaxic depth electrode EEG (SEEG) evaluation (Crandall, Walter and Rand, 1963; Talairach *et al.*, 1974) can provide more accurate localization when this is required for resective surgical therapy, but this is an invasive technique and also susceptible to error, since only limited areas of the brain can be sampled during this procedure.

In recent years a variety of additional tests have been utilized experimentally to localize cerebral function within the human brain, and these have been applied, on occasion, to studies of epilepsy (Engel, 1983a). Early techniques for determining regional cerebral blood flow required intracarotid injections, were also limited to measurements of the lateral cortex, and could only determine changes in one hemisphere at a time. These techniques were utilized to reveal abnormalities in regional cerebral blood flow (rCBF) in patients with partial epilepsy, but results were contradictory, some indicating an interictal increase in rCBF at the site of the epileptic focus (Hougaard *et al.*, 1976; Sakai *et al.*, 1978), while others indicated a decrease (Ingvar, 1973, 1975; Lavy *et al.*, 1976). With the advent of positron emission tomography (Phelps *et al.*, 1975, Phelps, Mazziotta and Huang, 1982), it is now possible to perform non-invasive studies capable of producing three-dimensional functional images of the entire human brain with excellent spatial resolution. Most commonly, measurements have consisted of local cerebral metabolism for glucose ($LCMRG_{lc}$) and oxygen ($LCMRO_2$), and local cerebral blood flow (LCBF). The word *local* rather than *regional* here refers to the improved spatial resolution that will soon approach 4 mm (Phelps *et al.*, 1982). Applications of PET to epilepsy have been recently reviewed (Engel, 1983b, 1984b; Engel *et al.*, 1985; Mazziotta and Engel, 1984, 1985). PET images of abnormal local cerebral function in patients with epilepsy are already of great diagnostic value for localization of the epileptogenic lesion when resective surgery is considered (Engel *et al.*, 1982b, 1984), and this technique promises to have more general application to the diagnosis of epilepsy in the future.

TECHNICAL CONSIDERATIONS

Methodology

Positron emission tomography utilizes the same mathematical reconstruction technique employed in X-ray CT to obtain cross-sectional images of the brain based on detection of photon emission from positron emitting radioisotopes labeled to various biochemical substrates or tracers of cerebral blood flow. Positron decay is uniquely suited for reconstruction tomography since positrons interact with electrons to produce annihilation radiation consisting of two 511 keV photons that are emitted in opposite directions. Consequently, when radiation detectors are placed in a ring around the source of emission, detection of an event occurring simultaneously at two detectors on opposite sides of the source indicates that the photons originated on a line between the detectors (Phelps *et al.*, 1975). When rings of detectors are placed around the head of a subject who has been intravenously injected with a positron emitting tracer that becomes selectively localized within the brain, collimation based on this *coincidence detection*, and mathematically computed image reconstruction, results in a cross-sectional display of tracer distribution within the brain (*Figure 13.1*). Multiple slices throughout the brain can then be taken with appropriate corrections for photon attenuation in soft tissue and bone, to produce a reliable three-dimensional representation of the entire brain with excellent spatial resolution (Phelps, Mazziotta and Huang, 1982). The Neuro-ECAT used at UCLA presently has a spatial resolution of 8 mm within the plane of section and 12.5 mm in slice thickness (Hoffman *et al.*, 1981). It is anticipated that a new signal amplification technique (SAT) will result in improvement in spatial resolution to approximately 4 mm, within the plane of section (Phelps *et al.*, 1982). A positron tomograph based upon SAT is now under construction (CTI Inc., Knoxville, Tennessee) and is scheduled to be delivered by spring 1984. PET has a theoretical resolution limit of approximately 1 mm.

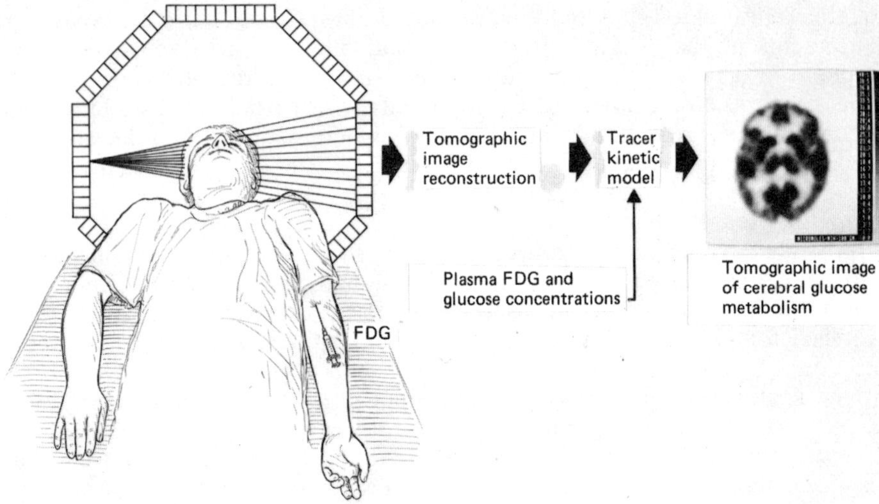

Figure 13.1 Approximately 40 min after intravenous injection of fluorodeoxyglucose, coincidence detectors obtain tomographic data on ^{18}F tissue activity distribution and cross-sectional images are mathematically reconstructed. Plasma fluorodeoxyglucose and glucose concentrations are entered into the computer image of the tomograph that also contains the operational equation of the fluorodeoxyglucose kinetic model. Images are then converted to local cerebral metabolic rate for glucose. Tomographic images are displayed on a television screen with a grey scale in proportion to local cerebral metabolic rate for glucose. Lines through the head show the 180° emission of two photons in positron decay that are recorded by the surrounding ring of detectors (Phelps, Schelbert and Mazziotta (1983), courtesy of the Publisher, *Annals of Internal Medicine*)

The most important positron emitting isotopes have short half-lives, and therefore must be produced in a medical cyclotron located near the PET facility. Positron emitting radioisotopes that are commonly incorporated into biologically active tracers for PET studies, and their half-lives, include: oxygen-15 (123 s), nitrogen-13 (10 min), carbon-11 (20 min), and fluorine-18 (110 min). Because these are common natural elements (fluorine-18 is employed as a substitute for hydrogen), they can be used to label a wide variety of substrates, analogs of substrates or drugs without disrupting their biochemical properties. With appropriate tracer kinetic modeling (Lassen and Perl, 1979), these labeled compounds provide a means for measuring local cerebral oxygen and glucose metabolism, transport, and extraction fraction, as well as local cerebral blood flow, blood volume, amino acid metabolism, protein synthesis, receptor ligand binding, and pharmacokinetics of specific drugs (*see* Phelps, Mazziotta and Huang, 1982; Phelps, Schelbert and Mazziotta, 1983). Although the present equipment and personnel necessary to perform PET studies limit widespread use, the development of small self-shielded laboratory cyclotrons combined with automated chemistry synthetic techniques, all controlled by a small microprocessor-based video terminal used by a single technician, should put PET capabilities within the reach of most large medical centers (Phelps, Mazziotta and Huang, 1982).

The majority of PET studies of epilepsy have been carried out using ^{18}F-fluorodeoxyglucose (FDG) (Barrio *et al.*, 1981; Reivich *et al.*, 1979) based on the tracer kinetic methods used for 2-deoxyglucose (2DG) autoradiography (Sokoloff *et al.*, 1977), modified for the human brain (Phelps *et al.*, 1979b; Huang *et al.*, 1980). Deoxyglucose is taken up by cells in the brain and phosphorylated competitively with glucose, but is not further metabolized to any significant degree. Consequently, when fluorodeoxyglucose is injected intravenously it becomes localized within the brain in proportion to the metabolic rate for glucose, and PET images of fluorodeoxyglucose tissue concentration can be carried out 40–60 min following injection when the majority of fluorine-18 is in the form of FDG-6-PO_4 and free fluorodeoxyglucose has been cleared from the blood. $LCMRG_{lc}$ is calculated with an equation that requires values for plasma fluorodeoxyglucose and glucose concentrations during fluorodeoxyglucose uptake, obtained from 'arterialized' venous blood sampling (Phelps *et al.*, 1979b), and values for local tissue concentration of fluorine-18 in the brain, determined by PET. Once these data are available, the operational equation incorporated in the PET computer is used to generate cross-sectional images of $LCMRG_{lc}$ displayed as μmol or mg/min per 100 g tissue.

This model assumes that steady state conditions of glucose utilization exist throughout the period of fluorodeoxyglucose incorporation into FDG-6-PO_4. Such assumptions apply for interictal studies of epilepsy, but are violated when seizures occur. Therefore, true quantitative determinations of $LCMRG_{lc}$ are not possible with fluorodeoxyglucose studies of transient ictal events. Even though the final image represents a weighted average, predominantly reflecting alterations occurring in the first 5–10 min following fluorodeoxyglucose injection (Huang *et al.*, 1981), seizures usually last less than a minute and ictal fluorodeoxyglucose scans reflect ictal, postical and interictal metabolic activity. Furthermore, the temporal sequence of occurrence of metabolic alterations appearing on the final averaged fluorodeoxyglucose scan cannot be accurately determined, although mathematical solutions to this problem may ultimately be possible (Huang *et al.*, 1981).

Another problem with attempts to perform quantitiative measurements of ictal events arises from the assumption that the lumped constant of the operational equation is the same during seizures as in the normal state. If membrane transport should become rate limiting, the fluorodeoxyglucose method would over-estimate $LCMRG_{lc}$ (Phelps, Mazziotta and Huang, 1982); however, a five-fold increase in glucose transport would be necessary to produce saturation (Raichle *et al.*, 1975), and cerebral blood flow usually increases during seizures, suggesting that a shift to transport limitation during ictal states may not, in fact, occur. Such changes in the lumped constant, if any, that might occur during ictal and postictal events need to be experimentally determined.

Positron emission tomography studies of epilepsy have also been carried out using other positron labeled tracers such as nitrogen-13 labeled ammonia (Kuhl *et al.*, 1980) that can estimate local cerebral blood flow (LCBF) (Phelps, Hoffman and Raybaud, 1977), and oxygen-15 labeled O_2 and water (Bernardi *et al.*, 1983), which can measure oxygen metabolism, oxygen extraction fraction and blood flow (Rhodes *et al.*, 1981). Ammonia does not appear to reliably monitor LCBF at abnormally high and low flow rates (Phelps *et al.*, 1981a) and is no longer used at UCLA for this purpose. A single intravenous injection of $H_2{}^{15}O$ can now be used to reliably determine alterations in LCBF (Huang *et al.*, 1983), and ${}^{15}O_2$ inhalation methods of measuring oxygen metabolism provide complementary information to fluorodeoxyglucose studies that allow aerobic and anaerobic metabolism to be calculated. Oxygen-15 has the added advantage of a much shorter half-life than fluorine-18, which permits repeated administration of isotope and PET measurements at 10 min intervals without contamination from previous administrations. This, combined with the fact that the duration of measurements for oxygen metabolism and blood flow range from 40 s to 2 min, allow for more dynamic studies of transient epileptic events with oxygen-15 than with fluorodeoxyglucose, although temporal resolution is still not sufficient to monitor the sequence of epileptiform events that take seconds, rather than minutes.

Another technique, utilizing carbon-11-labeled carbon monoxide which irreversibly binds to hemoglobin, allows repeated measures of transient changes in blood volume (Phelps *et al.*, 1979a), which can be limited to selected brief periods of time and subsequently averaged (Raichle, 1983). Triggering such brief measurements repeatedly from specific events using a concept similar to obtaining averaged event-related EEG potentials can reveal averaged event-related alterations in blood volume. This technique could theoretically be applied to epilepsy by triggering such measurements from interictal EEG spikes, or brief ictal events, although consequent alterations in blood volume may not be an ideal reflection of spatial or temporal aspects of neuronal function.

Positron labeled substrates for protein synthesis (Bustany *et al.*, 1981; Phelps *et al.*, 1984), and ligands for dopamine (Wagner *et al.*, 1983), opioid peptides (Maziere *et al.*, 1981) and benzodiazepine (Comar *et al.*, 1979) receptors are now being used with PET, but have not yet been applied to studies of epilepsy. Local cerebral pharmacokinetics of drugs, such as phenytoin (Baron *et al.*, 1983), may also prove useful in PET investigations of epileptic patients.

Functional interpretation

There is a tendency to refer to functional imaging of the brain based on PET scans of $LCMRG_{lc}$ or LCBF as though cerebral metabolism or blood flow and cerebral function were synonymous. Measurements of local alterations in metabolism and blood flow provide some information relevant to the specific activity of neurones within the brain area examined, but cannot be simply translated into neurophysiological terms such as excitation and inhibition. Furthermore, simultaneous alterations in measures of electrical activity, blood flow and glucose metabolism can vary independently (Ackermann *et al.*, 1983; Engel *et al.*, 1982c), suggesting that these separate indicators of neuronal function are complementary, and that while each in itself provides an incomplete view, they might be used together to derive reliable neurophysiological information.

There is good correlation between the site of an epileptogenic lesion determined by a variety of electrophysiological techniques and the location of alterations in $LCMRG_{lc}$ observed on fluorodeoxyglucose scans; however, there is no relationship between the degree of metabolic alteration and any parameter of the EEG transients (Engel *et al.*, 1982c). Clearly PET with fluorodeoxyglucose and EEG measure different aspects of cerebral function. The signals recorded by EEG reflect the degree of synchrony of membrane potential changes of neurones induced by synaptic activation, with less regard for the number of neurones involved than for the orientation of the electrical dipole produced by the neurone, the excitatory or inhibitory nature of the synaptic events, and the spatial arrangement of the neurones and their connections with respect to the recording electrode. PET measurements with fluorodeoxyglucose, on the other hand, reflect primarily the energy needs of an area of tissue and are influenced by the number of cells involved regardless of the types of cells, or the particular activities responsible for this glucose consumption. Glucose is the major substrate for ATP production in the brain and ATP is the principal energy source. However, energy is required for many neuronal and non-neuronal functions and there is no way to differentiate these various processes by energy consumption.

In the chronic epileptogenic lesion there may be severe neuronal loss (Babb *et al.*, 1984; Brown, 1973) and other neurones may be inactive during the interictal state (Babb, Carr and Crandall, 1973). Only a few neurones discharging in a hypersynchronous fashion can result in high amplitude interictal EEG spike transients but decreased glucose metabolism. This is the typical interictal finding when EEG and PET with fluorodeoxyglucose are measured concurrently in patients with partial seizures (Engel et al., 1982b and c; Kuhl *et al.*, 1980; Theodore *et al.*, 1984).

Under normal circumstances, cerebral blood flow and metabolism are tightly coupled, and increased energy demands result in increased blood flow to ensure adequate delivery of substrate to the brain. Blood flow and metabolism can become uncoupled under pathological conditions, however, and autoradiographic studies in animals using 2-deoxyglucose to measure glucose metabolism and iodoamphetamine or iodoantipyrine to measure blood flow suggest that this may occur in the hippocampus during seizures, when $LCMRG_{lc}$ is increased but LCBF appears to be reduced (Ackermann *et al.*, 1983). This indicates that conclusions about neuronal metabolism cannot be automatically inferred from studies of blood flow and that both measurements together may provide important insights into fundamental mechanisms, in this case perhaps mechanisms of epilepsy-induced brain damage.

Glucose metabolism and oxygen metabolism also do not provide identical measures of cerebral function since anaerobic glycolysis not only occurs, but requires more glucose to produce the same amount of energy than aerobic glycolysis. Consequently, even if increases in $LCMRG_{lc}$ observed on ictal fluorodeoxyglucose scans accurately reflect the magnitude of increased energy demands, they may not reflect parallel increases in neuronal activity. A large increase in $LCMRG_{lc}$ could accompany conversion to anaerobic glycolysis during only a small increase in neuronal firing. Repeated measures of similar ictal events using both fluorodeoxyglucose and oxygen-15 would be necessary to resolve this issue in a particular patient.

An assumption that is often made when interpreting alterations in $LCMRG_{lc}$ on fluorodeoxyglucose scans is that hypermetabolism indicates neuronal excitation, and hypometabolism indicates neuronal inhibition. This particular issue was specifically examined experimentally by using 2-deoxyglucose autoradiography to determine the metabolic alterations resulting from selectively induced excitatory and inhibitory synaptic activity in the hippocampus of the rat (Ackermann *et al.*, 1984). The results demonstrated, as might have been suspected, that inhibitory and excitatory synaptic activity both require energy, and both can result in increased glucose metabolism. Consequently, areas of increased $LCMRG_{lc}$ observed on fluorodeoxyglucose scans could represent enhanced inhibition, enhanced excitation or both, while zones of hypometabolism might occur when neurones become more energy efficient for some reason, or when synaptic input is decreased, because this input represents projections from areas that have been actively inhibited or damaged.

It is also clear from animal experiments that marked alterations in EEG activity can be seen in a specific brain area, for instance ictal discharges in amygdala, with no clear changes in glucose metabolism measured in the same area by 2-deoxyglucose autoradiography (Engel, Wolfson and Brown, 1978). This could occur if the hypermetabolism and hypometabolism accompanying ictal and postictal states respectively cancelled each other out. It could also be explained if ictal activity involved only a very small proportion of neurones, or if energy-efficient mechanisms of some sort became established with repeated seizures. In any event, simultaneous measurements of electrophysiological and metabolic changes provide more information than either alone, and interpretations concerning neuronal activity should be made using as many simultaneous and independent measures of neuronal function as possible.

Normative data

In order to interpret PET scans of patients with epilepsy, it is important to make comparisons with control populations of healthy subjects. Fluorodeoxyglucose studies carried out for this purpose at UCLA (Phelps *et al.*, 1981b) indicated that changes in $LCMRG_{lc}$ on repeated scans of the same subject vary with a standard deviation of 13%. Variation between contralateral homotopic areas of the same scan is 3% (Mazziotta *et al.*, 1981). This is true only when studies are carried out under similar ambient conditions with eyes and ears open. When subjects were studied with ears plugged and eyes closed, there was more variability, an increase in left–right asymmetry, and a reduction in the anterior–posterior ratio may also occur (Mazziotta *et al.*, 1982a).

For a variety of methodological reasons, it has been difficult to draw conclusions about local alterations in metabolism of fluorodeoxyglucose in patients with partial seizures based on absolute measures of $LCMRG_{lc}$ compared to control data. It has been easier to identify abnormal zones of hypometabolism upon visual analysis, and confirm this using quantitative measures of relative alterations based on ratios (Engel *et al.*, 1982c). When making quantitative measurements by comparing homotopic regions of interest in the two hemispheres, it is important to account for head tilt and make certain that these regions are equivalent on the two sides. Because head tilt may also produce apparent asymmetries on visual inspection, a true zone of hypometabolism must be identified as present on two or more adjacent planes of section. Ideally, a standard head holder should be employed and rectolinear scans should be performed at the time of the PET study to verify head position in the scanner (Mazziotta *et al.*, 1982b). As resolution of PET scanners improves, making smaller structures visible for quantitative measurement, the opportunities increase for errors due to head tilt, partial volume effects on structures adjacent to ventricles and cisterns, and normal variation. Thus adequate control data from healthy subjects, as well as mechanisms for ensuring the reliability of head position within the scanner, become increasingly important.

FLUORODEOXYGLUCOSE STUDIES IN EPILEPTIC PATIENTS

Partial seizure disorders

Well over 100 interictal fluorodeoxyglucose studies have been carried out at UCLA on patients with partial seizure disorders. Results of these studies indicate that

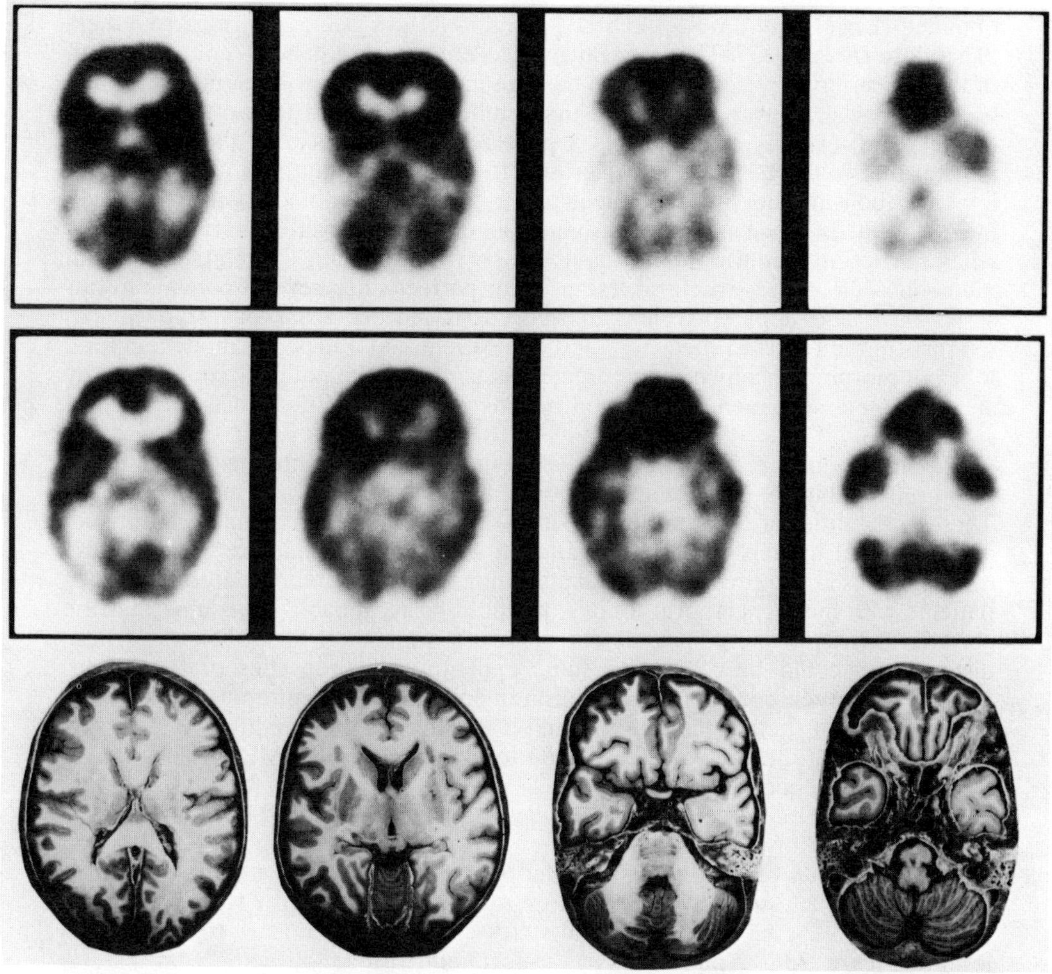

Figure 13.2 Four representative sections of an interictal fluorodeoxyglucose scan from a patient with partial complex seizures (*top*) show a zone of relative hypometabolism in the left temporal lobe. The hypometabolic area can be appreciated on all planes through the temporal lobes. Similar sections from a scan taken from a volunteer subject (*middle*) are normal. Some asymmetry of temporal lobe metabolism is present in the far left section, but since this was seen only in one plane it may reflect head rotation and cannot be considered abnormal. Photographs (*bottom*) show anatomical features included in planes of section more clearly (Engel *et al.*, 1982c, courtesy of the Publishers, *Annals of Neurology*)

approximately 70% show one or more zones of interictal hypometabolism (*Figure 13.2*) (Engel *et al.*, 1982c; Kuhl *et al.*, 1980). There is good correlation between the location of the zone of hypometabolism and the location of the primary epileptic focus as determined by a combination of EEG and SEEG recorded interictal and ictal events, but there is no relationship between the degree of metabolic abnormality in the hypometabolic zone and any feature of the abnormal electrophysiological events recorded at the time the fluorodeoxyglucose scan is obtained (Engel *et al.*, 1982c). These results have now been confirmed by others (Theodore *et al.*, 1983). There is also an excellent correlation between the location of the zone of hypometabolism, and the presence of a structural lesion determined by pathological analysis of resected tissue following anterior temporal lobectomy (Engel *et al.*, 1982a), but there is a poor relationship between the size of the structural lesion determined by microscopic analysis and the size of the zone of hypometabolism. For most patients, the zone of hypometabolism typically includes, but is much more extensive than, the pathological lesion, particularly when this lesion is in the hippocampus (Engel *et al.*, 1982a). Correlation between metabolic defect and structural lesion is not perfect since several patients in our series have had apparently normal fluorodeoxyglucose scans but hippocampal sclerosis in the resected specimen, and one patient had a hypometabolic temporal lobe but morphologically normal resected tissue that could not be accounted for by an incomplete specimen, or a lesion outside the limits of the lobectomy (Engel *et al.*, 1984).

Hypometabolism in areas that appear normal by routine pathological evaluation could reflect abnormalities in synaptic or dendritic structure, or in microperfusion. These possibilities are currently being investigated in resected human brain tissue, and in animal models, using Golgi and ultrastructural techniques. Should these investigations fail to reveal structural alterations in hypometabolic lateral cortex of patients with mesial temporal lesions, it would be reasonable to assume that the chronic interictal metabolic defects indicate functional disturbances. These disturbances could be related to some epileptogenic properties of the lesion. Interictal focal temporal hypometabolism in epilepsy has been reported to resolve when section of the corpus callosum improved the seizure condition (Gur *et al.*, 1982) suggesting that, in some cases, the focal decrease in $LCMRG_{lc}$ does reflect some aspect of epileptogenicity.

Although careful parametric studies have not yet been carried out to determine whether there is any relationship between the degree of focal hypometabolism and either the severity of the seizure disorder or the proximity of the scan to the most recent seizure, transient hypometabolism of the calcarine cortex was observed in one patient following complex partial status epilepticus secondary to an occipital lesion (*Figure 13.3*), and this was associated with a postictal contralateral hemianopia (Engel *et al.*, 1983). One year later, when the postical hemianopia had resolved, the calcarine metabolism was found to be normal (Engel *et al.*, 1983). This observation cannot be interpreted as typical of focal postictal disturbances since both the visual and the metabolic deficit persisted for weeks following status epilepticus, rather than a single seizure, and undoubtedly represented more profound disruption of neuronal function, or even structural changes that were ultimately reversed (Engel, Ludwig and Fetell, 1978).

An interictal increase in $LCMRG_{lc}$ was observed in only one patient in our series (*Figure 13.4*) (Engel *et al.*, 1982c). An interictal scan obtained one year previously had shown a large zone of hypometabolism in the area of the suspected epileptogenic lesion. Two subsequent ictal scans demonstrated increased metabolism in a discrete area within this hypometabolic zone. The final interictal scan showed the previously observed interictal zone of hypometabolism and, within it, small areas of increased metabolic activity. The pattern of increased $LCMRG_{lc}$ did not resemble that of the ictal scans, and simultaneous EEG and behavioral monitoring did not indicate that the patient had had a seizure during the study. The patient subsequently developed hemiatrophy on the side of the lesion and is

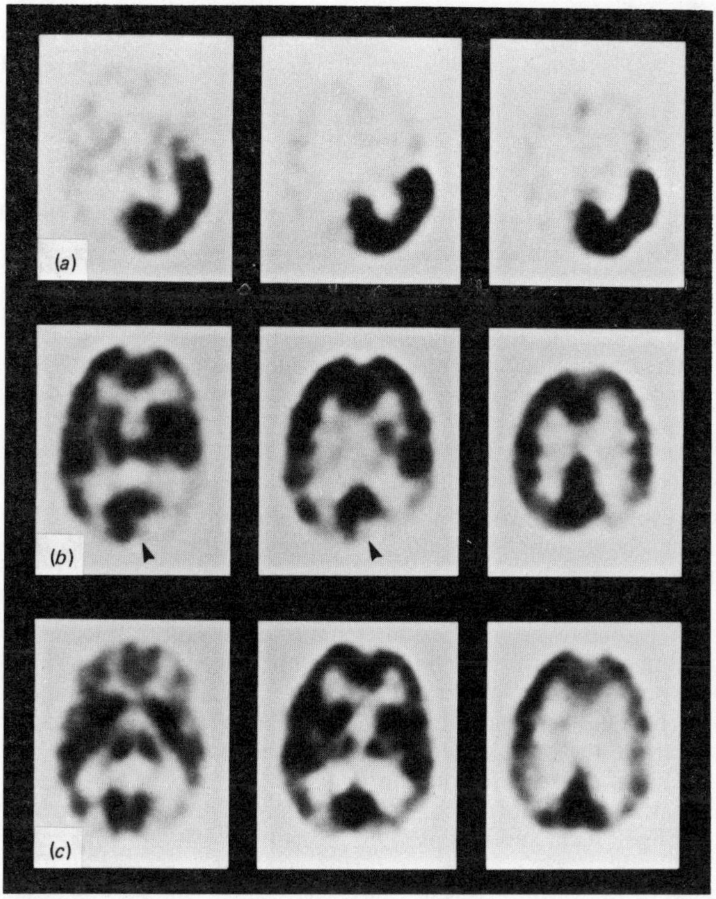

Figure 13.3 Representative sections of an ictal (*a*) and two interictal (*b, c*) fluorodeoxyglucose scans from a patient with complex partial seizures originating in the right occipital lobe. The ictal scan (*a*), obtained when several seizures occurred following fluorodeoxyglucose injection, revealed hypermetabolism of the right occipital and temporal area, and hypometabolism of the remainder of the brain. One month later when the patient still demonstrated a postictal left homonomous hemianopsia, the involved area of the right occipital and temporal lobe are now hypometabolic (*b*), including the right calcarine cortex (*arrows*). One year later, after the visual field deficit had resolved, a small zone of hypometabolism remained at the right occipitotemporal junction, but the right calcarine cortex was metabolically normal (*c*). This demonstrates that seizures can be followed by transient metabolic defects associated with functional disturbances, but the duration of this event was too long to consider it a typical postictal phenomenon (Engel *et al.* (1983), courtesy of the Publishers, *Neurology*)

believed to have a unilateral chronic inflammatory process (Aguilar and Rasmussen, 1960). The cause of this interictal hypermetabolism remains undetermined.

Transient zones of hypometabolism were observed in two of our patients who underwent fluorodeoxyglucose studies while depth electrodes were in place, and

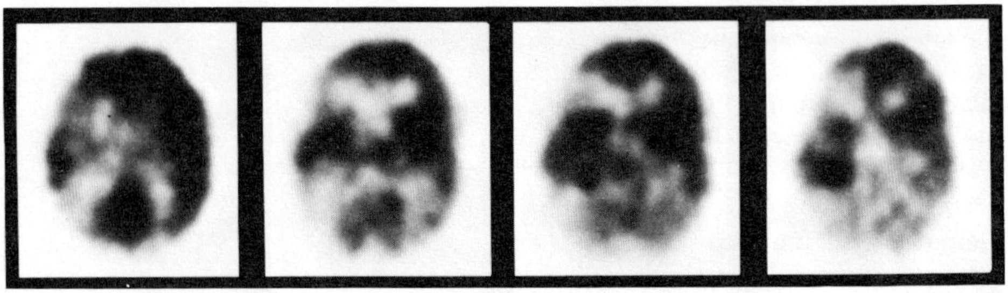

Figure 13.4 Interictal fluorodeoxyglucose scan from a child with frequent partial seizures shows a small area of relative hypermetabolism within a large left hemisphere hypometabolic zone. An earlier interictal scan in this patient showed only the hypometabolic zone, while two ictal scans demonstrated a different pattern of hypermetabolism (*see* Figure *13.5b*). Concurrent EEG recordings and behavioral observations during the uptake of fluorodeoxyglucose for the scan demonstrated here indicated that no seizure occurred (Engel *et al.*, 1982c, courtesy of the Publishers, *Annals of Neurology*)

this hypometabolism resolved following depth electrode removal (Engel *et al.*, 1982a and c). These metabolic deficits did not correlate with the presence of an epileptogenic lesion and were believed to be artificially induced by depth electrodes. Consequently, studies for localizing an epileptogenic lesion in patients who are candidates for resective surgery are no longer performed during depth electrode evaluation. Since structural lesions that are not epileptogenic may be associated with focal hypometabolism on fluorodeoxyglucose scans, this finding on an interictal study does not, in itself, indicate an epileptic focus. EEG continues to be necessary to demonstrate the epileptogenic nature of the lesion.

Ictal fluorodeoxyglucose studies carried out during partial seizures have revealed a variety of metabolic patterns, most often consisting of areas of both increased and decreased $LCMRG_{lc}$ (Engel, Kuhl and Phelps, 1982; Engel *et al.*, 1983; Kuhl *et al.*, 1980; Theodore *et al.*, 1983). In most patients the area of hypermetabolism corresponds to the site of seizure onset, and also areas of propagation. Consequently, metabolism may be increased throughout one hemisphere or bilaterally (*Figure 13.5a* and *b*), extremely focal zones of hypermetabolism may occur when partial seizures are fairly well contained (*Figure 13.5b*), or areas of discrete projection may be demonstrated (*Figure 13.5c*). Often, more diffuse hypometabolism may be superimposed upon the pattern of focal increases in $LCMRG_{lc}$ (*Figure 13.5c*) and, in our series, this has correlated with an alteration in consciousness. Since postictal depression appears to be associated with a decrease in metabolic activity (Engel, Kuhl and Phelps, 1982), it is assumed that the hypometabolism seen on ictal scans represents the postictal contribution to the final averaged values calculated for the entire period of fluorodeoxyglucose uptake. The diffuse hypometabolism observed with partial seizures associated with altered consciousness may reflect the postictal changes consequent upon ictal involvement of more generalized brain areas. As mentioned earlier, however, more careful studies are necessary using mathematical solutions (Huang *et al.*, 1981) that may allow better resolution of the temporal sequence of events, or parallel studies with tracers having shorter half-lives, such as oxygen-15, permitting studies with brief examination time that can be repeated at short intervals (Huang *et al.*, 1983).

One patient in our series experienced a single complex partial seizure induced by electrical stimulation of the hippocampus at the time of fluorodeoxyglucose injection, and the resultant scan revealed a focal decrease in $LCMRG_{lc}$, limited to the lateral temporal lobe, but not including the hippocampus (*Figure 13.5d*). Since the complex partial seizure in this patient was followed by a period of confusion and EEG depression in the temporal lobe, it was assumed that the very brief ictal event did not contribute as heavily to the final measurements as the more prolonged postictal period (Engel, Kuhl and Phelps, 1982; Engel *et al.*, 1983).

Generalized seizures

Ictal studies were performed on patients with petit mal epilepsy during 10 min of hyperventilation when absences occurred frequently, and compared to fluorodeoxyglucose studies carried out following successful medical therapy, during 10 min of hyperventilation that did not produce absences (Engel, Kuhl and Phelps, 1982). In all patients absence seizures were associated with a marked and diffuse increase in metabolism that was greater than any observed for ictal scans of other types of seizures (*Figure 13.5e*). Marked hypermetabolism may be seen on fluorodeoxyglucose scans obtained during petit mal absences because postictal depression does not follow these ictal events. These studies failed to identify any specific area of the brain selectively activated during petit mal absences, and interictal scans were all normal.

In contrast to non-convulsive generalized seizures, tonic-clonic convulsions induced by electroconvulsive shock therapy (ECT) are associated with profound diffuse postictal reduction in $LCMRG_{lc}$ (*Figure 13.5f*) (Engel, Kuhl and Phelps, 1982). Most likely due to the contribution of these alterations to the final averaged measurements, ictal fluorodeoxyglucose scans during ECT show only mild diffuse hypermetabolism (Engel, Kuhl and Phelps, 1982), no changes, or even diffuse hypometabolism (Engel *et al.*, unpublished data).

A number of studies have been carried out at UCLA on patients with secondary generalized seizure disorders of various types, including atypical absences, infantile spasms, Lennox-Gastaut syndrome, and neonatal seizures. As indicated by others (Gur *et al.*, 1982), patients in our series with secondary generalized seizures and normal CT scans often demonstrate focal, multifocal or hemispheric metabolic deficits on interictal fluorodeoxyglucose scans (Chugani *et al.*, 1984). No specific patterns have yet been found to correlate with aspects of the seizure disorder, but this work is currently in progress.

POSITRON EMISSION TOMOGRAPHY STUDIES OF EPILEPSY USING OTHER TRACERS

Early studies of partial epilepsy employed nitrogen-13 labeled ammonia, along with fluorodeoxyglucose, to estimate LCBF in association with $LCMRG_{lc}$ (Kuhl *et al.*, 1980). These studies revealed that interictal zones of hypometabolism were associated with a corresponding decrease in LCBF, while ictal hypermetabolic areas were associated with a corresponding increase in LCBF. Because alterations in ammonia uptake did not faithfully follow high and low blood flow rates, quantitative measurements could not be made, and anatomical information derived from these studies did not add to information already available from fluorodeoxyglucose studies. Consequently, the use of ammonia as a tracer in PET studies of epilepsy has not been continued.

Various methods using oxygen-15 (*see* Huang *et al.*, 1983; Phelps, Mazziotta and Huang, 1982b) are currently employed to quantitatively evaluate LCBF, as well as oxygen metabolism and oxygen extraction fraction. Applications of oxygen-15 methods to studies of patients with presumed temporal lobe epileptogenic lesions (Bernardi *et al.*, 1983) indicated absolute values for oxygen metabolism and LCBF were decreased in both temporal lobes. Bilateral temporal hypometabolism was also found on interictal fluorodeoxyglucose studies of patients with complex partial seizures when absolute measures of $LCMRG_{lc}$ were made (Engel *et al.*, 1982c), but only relative measurements, comparing the area of the apparent zone of hypometabolism to the contralateral homotopic area, resulted in reliable focal quantitative determinations. With less variability in the more recent fluorodeoxyglucose studies, it is likely that quantitative determinations using absolute values of $LCMRG_{lc}$ will also reveal reliable deficits in both temporal lobes.

The oxygen-15 studies did demonstrate one focal change which appeared to be restricted to the area of the epileptogenic lesion; an increase in oxygen extraction fraction (Bernardi *et al.*, 1983). This finding indicates that, despite an interictal decrease in $LCMRO_2$, oxygen demand is relatively greater compared to blood flow on the side of the focus than contralaterally, suggesting a greater compromise of LCBF. Such an apparent abnormal uncoupling is of interest in view of the fact noted earlier that animal autoradiographic experiments have demonstrated a marked uncoupling of blood flow and metabolism in the hippocampus during seizures with decreased LCBF in areas where $LCMRG_{lc}$ is high (Ackermann *et al.*, 1983). A similar mechanism could conceivably result in more permanent changes and play some role in the development of epilepsy-induced brain damage (Meldrum, Horton and Brierley, 1974).

As mentioned previously, oxygen-15 methodologies will make it possible to study local cerebral metabolism and blood flow with a temporal resolution that is considerably better than that provided by the fluorodeoxyglucose technique, and should help to determine the temporal sequence of ictal and postictal events, although studies performed at 10 min intervals will still be unable to achieve truly quantitative measures of these transient events. Combined fluorodeoxyglucose and oxygen-15 studies will also provide information about aerobic and anaerobic glycolysis in epilepsy.

Another application of PET to the study of patients with epilepsy utilized carbon-11 labeled diphenylhydantoin to determine whether regional alterations existed in the cerebral pharmacokinetics of this antiepileptic drug (Baron *et al.*, 1983). This is an interesting and potentially useful approach to clinical neuropharmacology that has yet to be fully exploited.

DIAGNOSTIC APPLICATIONS OF POSITRON EMISSION TOMOGRAPHY

Localization of an epileptogenic lesion for resective surgery

The fluorodeoxyglucose scan has already been proved of clinical value as a confirmatory test to aid in localization of the epileptogenic lesion in patients with partial epilepsy who are candidates for resective surgical therapy (Engel *et al.*, 1981, 1982b, 1984). The success of surgical therapy in partial epilepsy depends upon accurate identification of the epileptogenic lesion, and traditional methods that involve measurements of interictal EEG spike activity, and sites of seizure generation, are subject to error (Ajmone Marsan, 1980; Engel, Crandall and Rausch, 1983a; Gloor, 1975) due to a variety of reasons:

(1) The EEG has limited spatial resolution and records only neuronal activity occurring in neocortex immediately below the scalp electrodes, or close to the tips of sphenoidal or nasopharyngeal electrodes inserted to record from basal structures.
(2) Although SEEG recordings have the ability to monitor activity from deep structures in the brain, the numbers of implantation sites are limited and sampling error can occur if the sites chosen for implantation are not sufficiently close to the epileptogenic lesions.
(3) Electrical epileptiform transients propagate widely, even to the contralateral hemisphere, and there is as yet no adequate method to differentiate EEG or SEEG recorded interictal spikes or ictal discharges that originate in the primary lesion from those that are recorded at a distance from the primary lesion as projected events.
(4) The epileptic brain demonstrates areas of hyperexcitability distant from the primary epileptogenic area that may generate spontaneous interictal spike activity, and even seizures in some provocative situations (Engel and Crandall, 1983; Wieser *et al.*, 1979) even though these areas are ordinarily of no clinical consequence.

In order to reduce the chances of false localization based on measures of focal epileptiform excitability, most pre-surgical evaluation protocols now include additional independent confirmatory tests of focal functional deficit (Engel, Crandall and Rausch, 1983; Engel *et al.*, 1981) such as: intravenous thiopental injection in order to demonstrate focal attenuation of induced EEG fast rhythms (Engel, Driver and Falconer, 1975), intracarotid amytal to identify shifts in hemispheric dominance for language (Rausch and Walsh, 1984; Wada and Rasmussen, 1960) or inability of one temporal lobe to support memory (Milner, Branch and Rasmussen, 1962; Rausch *et al.*, 1984), and standard psychometric batteries. When depth electrodes are implanted, demonstration of focal attenuation of thiopental induced fast rhythms, as well as focal abnormal slow activity, or attenuation of normal fast rhythms, may aid in identification of an epileptogenic lesion (Engel, Crandall and Rausch, 1983; Engel *et al.*, 1981). In addition, focal stimulation of the hippocampus may reveal an elevated afterdischarge threshold when hippocampal sclerosis is present (Cherlow *et al.*, 1977; Engel, Crandall and Rausch, 1983; Engel *et al.*, 1981). These tests of focal functional deficit rarely result in false localization; however, the yield is considerably less than that for tests of epileptiform excitability since results of the former are often non-diagnostic.

The interictal fluorodeoxyglucose scan as a confirmatory test, on the other hand, has identified focal hypometabolism in approximately 70% of patients in our surgical series, a yield which is as high or higher than the true localization achieved by all tests of focal epileptiform excitability at UCLA except ictal onset recorded from depth electrodes (Engel *et al.*, 1984). The high yield with this latter test may not reflect its accuracy as much as the fact that this is still the single most important criterion for surgery at UCLA in patients who undergo depth electrode implantation and, consequently, very few patients receive surgery without this finding (Engel, Crandall and Rausch, 1983). In contrast to tests of epileptiform excitability, false localization with PET has only occurred in two patients and this was transient and felt to be artificially induced by depth electrodes (Engel *et al.*, 1982b and c). As mentioned earlier, fluorodeoxyglucose studies for purposes of localization are no longer performed in patients while depth electrodes are in place.

There is considerable divergence of opinion concerning the amount of information necessary to confidently localize an epileptogenic lesion for surgical resection. Until 1979 the presurgical protocol at UCLA was designed with the view that only SEEG recorded ictal onsets provide such consistently reliable localizing data. Based on the high yield and high reliability of localization of an epileptogenic lesion with the fluorodeoxyglucose scan, specific criteria were established at UCLA in 1979 to carry out anterior temporal lobectomy in some patients without requiring depth electrode evaluation (Engel, Crandall and Rausch, 1983). At the present time, if a patient demonstrates a consistent focal ictal onset from one sphenoidal electrode, there is a preponderance of interictal spikes in that temporal lobe, and fluorodeoxyglucose scan demonstrates a zone of hypometabolism in the same area, and focal dysfunction is confirmed for that temporal lobe by two additional confirmatory tests, anterior temporal lobectomy is recommended. Approximately one-third of the patients who undergo anterior temporal lobectomy at UCLA now do so under these new criteria with excellent results, and are spared the depth electrode implantation procedure (Engel *et al.*, 1982b, 1984).

At the present time the criteria for resective surgery without SEEG evaluation apply specifically to patients with epileptogenic lesions in one temporal lobe since most of the tests of focal functional deficit are particularly sensitive to disturbances of the temporal lobe. This appears to be true of the fluorodeoxyglucose scan as well as the electrophysiological and neuropsychological evaluations. Lesions in

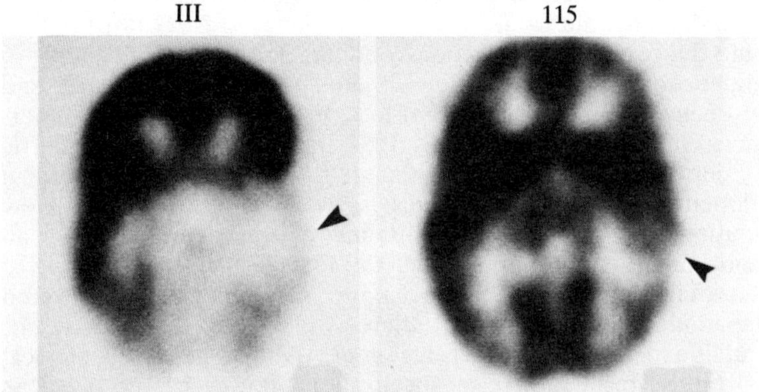

Figure 13.6 Representative sections of two fluorodeoxyglucose scans obtained from two patients with complex partial seizures due to lesions in the right temporal lobe. Patient III underwent a right anterior temporal lobectomy which revealed sclerosis of the hippocampus, subiculum and amygdala, but the fluorodeoxyglucose scan indicated a much more diffuse zone of hypometabolism involving the entire right temporal lobe (*arrow*). Patient 115 also underwent a right anterior temporal lobectomy, which revealed a small tumor in the cortex of the middle temporal gyrus. This fluorodeoxyglucose scan shows only a small lateral zone of hypometabolism conforming to the location of the tumor (*arrow*). Both patients are now seizure free, suggesting that the epileptogenic lesions were removed (adapted from Engel *et al.*, 1982a, courtesy of the Publishers, *Annals of Neurology*)

mesiotemporal structures reduce $LCMRG_{lc}$ over a wide area of temporal lobe, resulting in an easily recognizable zone of hypometabolism. Epileptogenic lesions of the lateral temporal cortex may also be associated with zones of hypometabolism, but these are often much more limited in extent than the mesial temporal lesions (*Figure 13.6*). Well-defined extratemporal areas of focal cortical hypometabolism are rarely seen on fluorodeoxyglucose scans of patients with partial seizure disorders, except when structural lesions are sufficiently large that they also appear on X-ray CT scans as well.

A zone of hypometabolism is indicative of an area of focal functional deficit but the EEG continues to be necessary to demonstrate that an area of dysfunction is epileptogenic. The fluorodeoxyglucose scan is particularly useful to localize the disturbance accurately and, theoretically, distinguish between primary and secondary epileptic foci. Positron emission tomography alone may be sufficient to demonstrate the existence of an epileptogenic lesion when an interictal scan reveals a zone of hypometabolism, and a subsequent ictal scan demonstrates increased $LCMRG_{lc}$. In this case, however, the ictal fluorodeoxyglucose scan can be falsely localizing since it cannot distinguish between the site of ictal onset and sites of subsequent ictal propagation, which may be quite widespread. For this reason, ictal fluorodeoxyglucose scans are of much less localizing value than interictal scans in patients who are candidates for resective surgery.

Future applications of positron emission tomography for surgery of epilepsy

Approximately 30% of patients with partial seizures who ultimately benefit from resective surgery have fluorodeoxyglucose scans that appear to be normal (Engel *et al.*, 1982c). In some of these patients hippocampal sclerosis was observed in the resected temporal lobe specimen (Engel *et al.*, 1984). Consequently, the fluorodeoxyglucose scan does not always identify an epileptogenic lesion when one is present and when its removal might result in seizure relief. In order to increase the yield of fluorodeoxyglucose scans for localization of such lesions, it may be useful to use specific behavioral stimulation, such as verbal and non-verbal continuous performance memory tasks that might selectively activate left and right mesial temporal structures respectively in normals, but fail to activate brain tissue adjacent to an epileptogenic lesion. Attempts to identify such deficits in activation are presently being carried out at UCLA (Halgren, unpublished data).

Patients with secondary generalized seizure disorders may show focal, multifocal or hemispheric metabolic disturbances (Chugani *et al.*, 1984; Gur *et al.*, 1982) that could be useful in identifying candidates for resective surgical procedures, or corpus callosum section. The value of cerebral metabolic patterns for selecting candidates for corpus callosum section is presently being explored at UCLA (Sutherling, unpublished data) and elsewhere (Gur *et al.*, 1982).

Other potential diagnostic applications of positron emission tomography for epilepsy

The classification of epileptic seizures (Commission on Classification and Terminology, ILAE, 1981) is based on behavioral and electrophysiological phenomena and, although diagnosis on the basis of this classification has certain prognostic and therapeutic implications, considerable confusion continues to exist concerning the relationships between various types of seizures. Classification of epileptic disorders is even less well defined. Furthermore, it is not clear whether certain myoclonic phenomena, neonatal seizures, or infantile spasms represent cortical epileptic disturbances, or subcortical dysfunction more related to movement disorders than epilepsy. Perhaps PET will reveal patterns of cerebral metabolism, or specific disturbances related to blood flow, protein synthesis, neurotransmitter activity, or other aspects of cerebral function measurable with positron-labeled tracers that could help to divide seizure disorders into logical categories with even more reliable specific prognostic and therapeutic implications than the present classification. Such studies may also help to diagnose epilepsy-related postictal and interictal behavioral disturbances (Blumer and Benson, 1982; Engel and Caldecott-Hazard, 1984), and eventually provide insights into fundamental mechanisms of epilepsy and other abnormal behaviors that could lead to new treatment approaches (Ackermann, Engel and Phelps, 1985).

It is not known when the fluorodeoxyglucose abnormality develops with respect to the onset of an epileptic disorder but, if it is related to epileptogenicity in some fashion, it may precede the appearance of seizures and could serve as a prognostic sign to identify patients at risk for epilepsy, for instance after head trauma or neonatal injury. The application of a variety of new positron-labeled tracers may be even more useful than fluorodeoxyglucose in this regard and multiple techniques should eventually be used in a complementary fashion in repeated studies.

With the exception of petit mal epilepsy (Kellaway, 1981), the interictal EEG provides little information of value concerning the severity of an epileptic disorder. Consequently, apart from detailed prolonged EEG telemetry, there is no adequate way to quantitatively verify patients' reports concerning the frequency of epileptic seizures. If it can be demonstrated that seizure severity can be reflected by certain aspects of the metabolic alterations observed on interictal FDG scans, or any other feature of PET scans performed with other positron-labeled tracers, this test would become extremely useful for assessing the effects of therapeutic intervention. Attempts to identify a relationship between the degree or extent of hypometabolism and parameters of epileptic severity such as seizure frequency or duration are in progress.

The use of PET with positron-labeled pharmaceuticals (Baron *et al.*, 1983) could prove useful if local cerebral pharmacokinetic measures for specific antiepileptic drugs are found to be unique for different areas of the brain, or for the epileptic focus itself. Such studies could conceivably be used to help understand why specific antiepileptic drugs may be ineffective in certain patients, or certain epileptic disorders, and also to screen antiepileptic drugs in order to determine the most appropriate medication for individual patients.

COMPARISON OF POSITRON EMISSION TOMOGRAPHY TO OTHER METHODS FOR MEASURING CEREBRAL FUNCTION

Spectral nuclear magnetic resonance (NMR) has been used to measure dynamically aspects of cerebral function reflected by alterations in organic phosphate and intracellular pH during epileptic seizures in animals (Petroff *et al.*, 1984). NMR imaging, on the other hand, involves measurements of hydrogen ions, and provides a three-dimensional view of cerebral structure with extremely high resolution

(Brady and Pykett, 1983), but it is unclear whether the different patterns provided by T_1 and T_2 relaxation times and spin echo can provide meaningful insights into cerebral function. No series of epileptic patients studied with NMR has yet been published, although anecdotal reports have appeared (Bydder *et al.*, 1982). There is an immediate functional interpretation that can be made from NMR scans with the present methodology, since blood moving through large vessels of the brain is recorded as a hole in the image. Consequently, measurements can certainly be made of alterations in large vessel cerebral blood volume, and some data regarding cerebral blood flow in these vessels may also be possible (Singer and Crooks, 1983). Otherwise, as a brain-imagining technique, NMR should be viewed as a measure of structure, with excellent spatial resolution, that would complement PET measurements of function but provide little or no information regarding function itself. On the other hand, spectral NMR may soon be applicable to measurements of human cerebral energy metabolism and pH, but with a spatial resolution limited to large areas of the brain, for instance making it possible to compare one hemisphere to the other, or the anterior part of the brain to the posterior part.

X-ray CT was the first three-dimensional brain imaging technique routinely available for diagnostic purposes, and also measures structure. Attempts have been made to take advantage of certain characteristics of X-ray CT to provide information that might indicate alterations in cerebral function. CT scans obtained during xenon inhalation can demonstrate regional changes in cerebral blood flow (Meyer *et al.*, 1981), and subtracting enhanced from non-enhanced scans also theoretically reflects changes in regional cerebral perfusion (Oakley *et al.*, 1979). The latter has been applied to studies of patients with partial epilepsy and findings suggest that this technique may have some value for identifying mesial temporal epileptogenic lesions (Oakley *et al.*, 1979). Others have used X-ray CT combined with subarachnoid contrast injection to better visualize the tentorial notch, and have suggested that patients with complex partial seizures demonstrate evidence of uncal herniation on the side of the epileptogenic lesion (Bolender and Wyler, 1982). Consequently, it is conceivable that clever use of X-ray CT methodology may ultimately provide useful information concerning alterations in local cerebral function in epilepsy, but again this information will provide insights into functions that are different from those measured by PET and should be considered complementary.

Single photon emission computed tomography (SPECT) (Ell and Holman, 1982) using iodine-123 iodoamphetamine (Kuhl *et al.*, 1982; Magistretti *et al.*, 1982) and xenon-133 (Bonte *et al.*, 1983) have been applied to studies of patients with partial seizures in order to measure changes in cerebral blood flow. Interictal studies do demonstrate areas of decreased rCBF in some patients (Bonte *et al.*, 1983, Kuhl *et al.*, 1982), and one ictal study has shown a focal increase in rCBF (Magistretti *et al.*, 1982), but the spatial resolution does not approach that now available with PET. This technique has the advantage that single photon-emitting isotopes have much longer half-lives than positron-emitting isotopes, therefore a nearby cyclotron is not required. Because of the longer half-lived isotopes, however, the studies result in a higher radiation exposure to the patient, and single photon emitting isotopes are also not easily incorporated into biologically active tracers. These problems, in addition to the relatively poor resolution which will make reliable, quantitative measurements difficult in individual patients, account in part for the fact that SPECT has not become generally available. Nevertheless, it appears that the ability of SPECT to localize the epileptogenic lesion in some patients may justify a more general diagnostic application in centers performing resective surgery for epilepsy. If new single photon-emitting isotope labeled tracers and methodologies are developed with SPECT, however, this technique may provide additional diagnostic information that is sufficiently different from that seen with PET to make it useful as a complementary test.

Computer analysis of EEG and evoked potentials have been used to identify areas of focal functional deficit (Gotman *et al.*, 1982), as well as areas of focal epileptiform excitability (Gotman, 1983), and can demonstrate the sequence of epileptiform and epilepsy-related events with a much higher temporal resolution than any of the functional imaging techniques. Because the EEG is a more dynamic procedure, it yields essential diagnostic information in epilepsy. Measurements of abnormal epileptiform transients and slowing in patients with epilepsy indicate that these do not correlate with alterations in metabolism determined by PET with fluorodeoxyglucose (Engel, Kuhl and Phelps, 1982; Engel *et al.*, 1982), but spectral analysis of EEG frequencies in healthy individuals indicates that there may be a relationship between normal EEG frequency and blood flow in other situations (Ingvar, 1967). Topographical maps of EEG spectra and features of evoked potentials can be obtained using computerized extrapolation between electrodes, and this display can easily demonstrate the location of alterations in these electrophysiological parameters in two dimensions over the scalp (Duffy, Burchfiel and Lombroso, 1979; Duffy, Bartels and Burchfiel, 1981). There is reason to believe that this electrical activity mapping technique will provide useful information about cerebral function in patients with epilepsy that will be quite different from, and therefore nicely complement, three-dimensional images of cerebral function provided by PET.

Another new technique that has recently been applied to measurements of abnormal epileptiform events in patients with epilepsy is magnetoencephalography (MEG) (Barth *et al.*, 1982, 1984; Modena *et al.*, 1982). This technique measures the magnetic fields produced by current flow within the brain and characteristics of magnetic fields allow current sources to be accurately located in three dimensions, in contrast to EEG which can only record neocortical activity immediately under the scalp electrodes. In addition, MEG signals are not as attenuated by bony structures as EEG and the direction, as well as the location, of current flow can be determined (Williamson and Kaufman, 1981). MEG measures of interictal EEG spikes in patients with partial seizure disorders have demonstrated the ability of this technique to localize generators of epileptiform events, and single spikes often appear to have multiple sources (Barth *et al.*, 1982, 1984). MEG measurements of epileptiform events clearly provide information different from that seen with scalp EEG and may be equal to, in some respects, measurements made from depth electrode recordings without the limitations imposed by restriction on the number of electrodes that can be implanted. The most reliable MEG measurements require tedious averaging of signals with a single probe to collect data from one point on the scalp at a time. Since these MEG averages are triggered by EEG recorded interictal spikes, they only measure events that can be seen by the EEG. Furthermore, the assumption that events recorded from one point on the scalp at one period in time reflect the same process as events recorded some time later from another point on the scalp may be false.

Improvements in MEG methodology and multiple probe recording devices may eventually allow this technique to be used to identify epileptiform transients that are not visible on routine scalp EEG, over wide areas of the brain simultaneously.

COLOUR PLATE SECTION

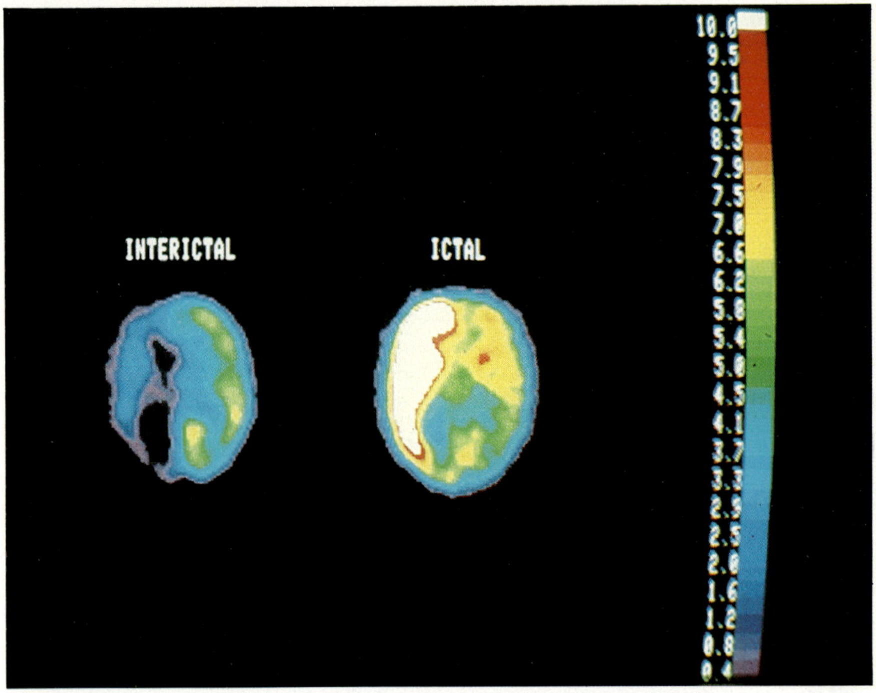

(*a*)

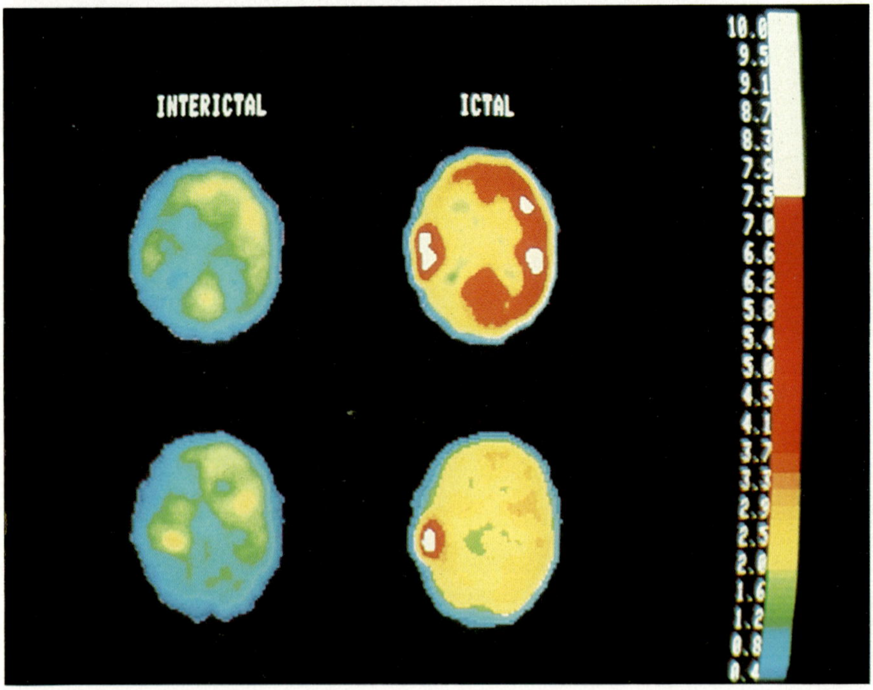

(*b*)

Plate 13.1 Representative sections of interictal and ictal fluorodeoxyglucose scans from four patients with complex partial seizures (*a*)–(*d*), one with petit mal absences (*e*), and one undergoing electroconvulsive therapy (ECT) (*f*). Note that log scales were necessary for some patients in order to better demonstrate patterns for metabolic values, and that the color code used for (*a*)–(*d*) is different from the code used for (*e*) and (*f*). (*a*) In this patient with left hemisphere seizures, the ictal scan demonstrates a global increase in cerebral metabolic rate, which is much more marked for the atrophic left hemisphere. (*b*) In this patient with seizures confined to the left temporal lobe, there is a focal increase in $LCMRG_{lc}$ in this area during the ictal scan, and also a global increase in metabolism, compared to the interictal study.

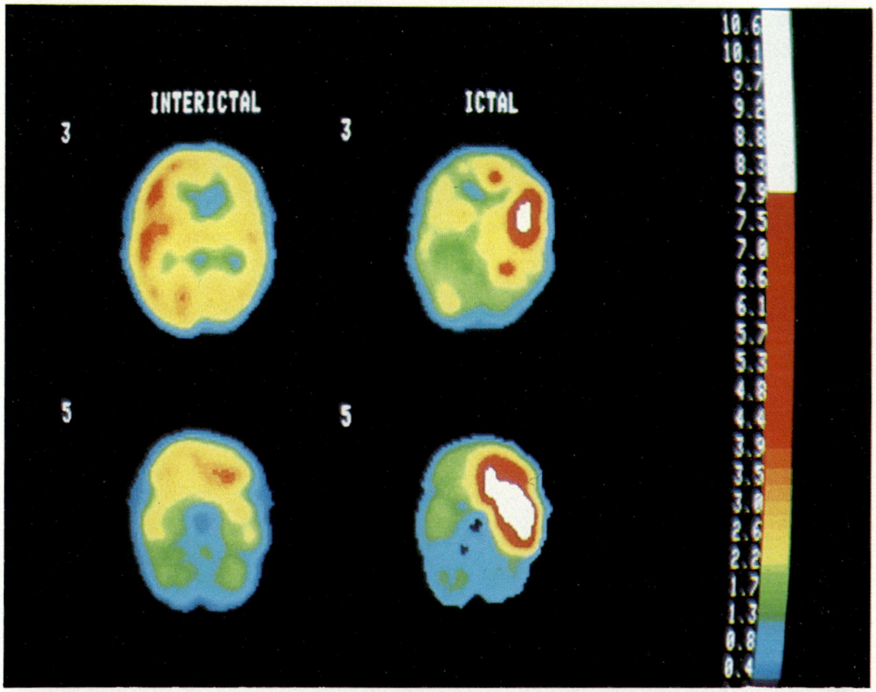

(*c*)

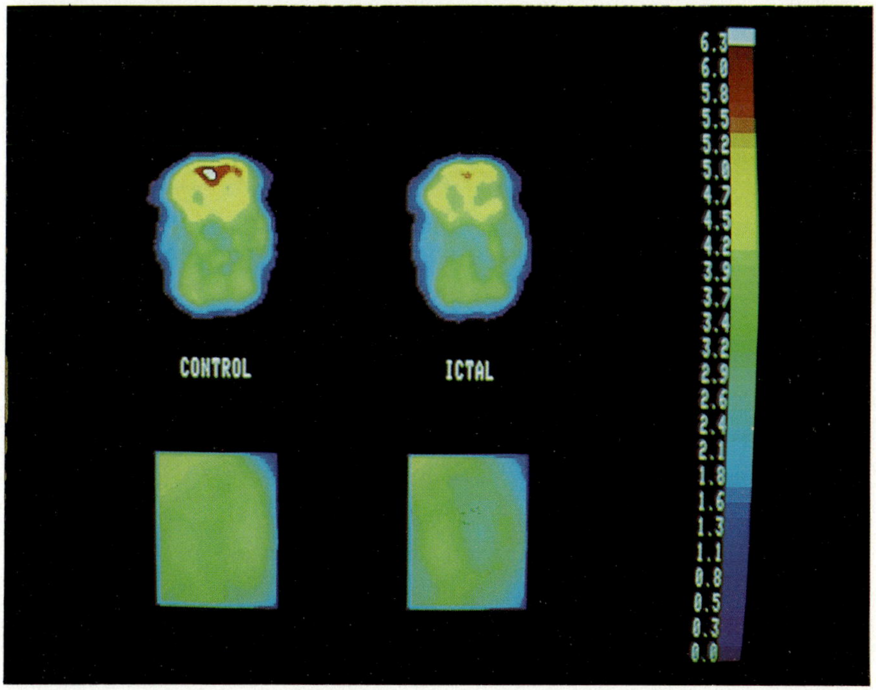

(*d*)

(*c*) On this ictal scan, during seizures of right temporal lobe origin, well-defined zones of hypermetabolism are seen in frontal and temporal lobes, cingulate cortex, and hippocampus on the right, whereas the remainder of the brain is hypometabolic compared with the interictal study. (*d*) The patient had an epileptogenic lesion in the left hippocampus and hypometabolism of the left temporal lobe interictally, but the ictal scan was obtained during a complex partial seizure induced by electrical stimulation of the right hippocampus during depth electrode evaluation. Full sections (*top*) and details of the entire right temporal lobe (*bottom*) demonstrate a decrease in $LCMRG_{lc}$ on the lateral surface of the stimulated right temporal lobe on the ictal scan. (*a*)–(*d*) From Engel *et al.* (1983), courtesy of the Publishers, *Neurology*

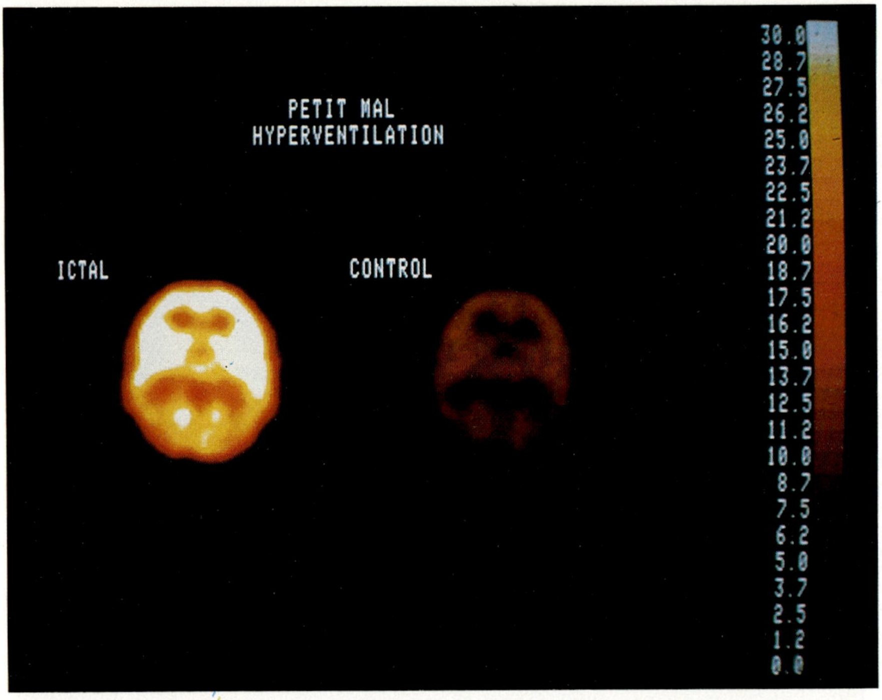

(*e*)

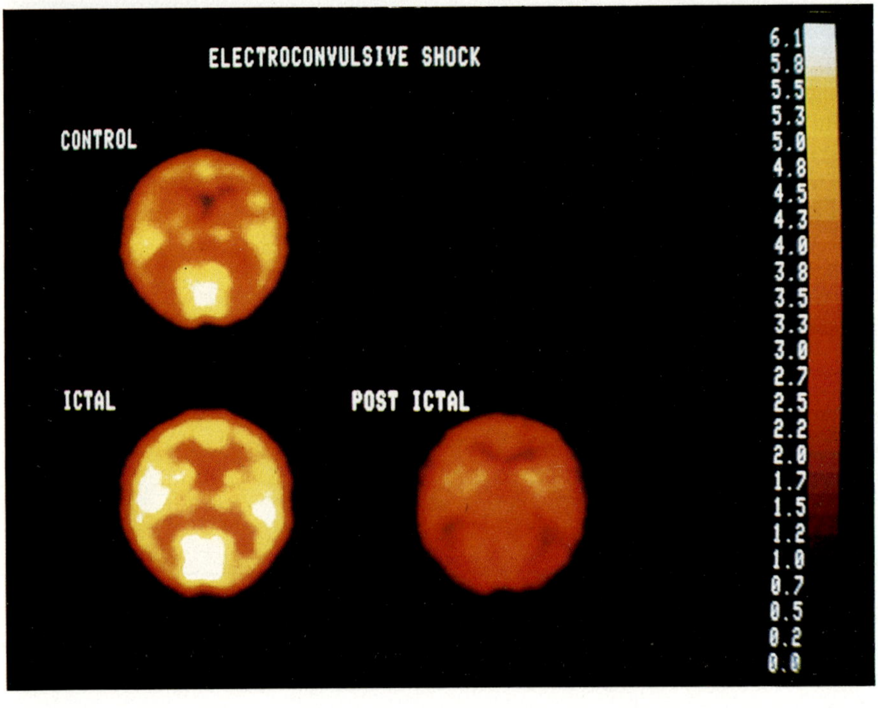

(*f*)

(*e*) This ictal scan was obtained in an untreated patient with petit mal seizures during 10 min of hyperventilation when frequent absences occurred. A diffuse, marked increase in metabolism is seen, compared to the control scan obtained several months later following successful treatment, when 10 min of hyperventilation produced no absences. (*f*) The ictal scan in this patient being treated with ECT was obtained by injecting fluorodeoxyglucose at the time the electroshock was delivered, and shows a diffuse increase in $LCMRG_{lc}$, compared to the control image. The postictal scan was obtained during ECT on a different day, when fluorodeoxyglucose was injected at the end of the convulsion and beginning of postictal depression. This scan demonstrates a diffuse decrease in $LCMRG_{lc}$ compared to control, but with a slightly different pattern of metabolic activity. (*e*) and (*f*) From Engel (1983b), courtesy of the Publishers, John Libbey & Co Ltd

It is anticipated that MEG, like EEG, will provide important information that is complementary to, and not redundant with, the biochemical information obtained by PET.

CONCLUSIONS

Positron emission tomography is a non-invasive technique capable of creating functional images of the entire human brain in three dimensions with excellent spatial resolution. The use of positron-emitting isotopes incorporated into biologically active tracers already allows measurements of local cerebral metabolism and extraction fraction for glucose and oxygen, as well as local cerebral blood flow, blood volume, protein synthesis, specific neurotransmitter activity, and pharmacokinetics of certain drugs. Potential applications for measuring other aspects of cerebral function are great. The requirement of a medical cyclotron close to the PET scan facility, in order to make the positron emitting isotopes readily available at the proper specific activity, is the major disadvantage of PET. Development of small cyclotron-based labeled compound generator systems, however, should place PET technology within the reach of most major medical centers.

SPECT, spectral NMR, NMR imaging, various approaches using X-ray CT, computer analysis of EEG and MEG offer additional promise for improved diagnosis of epilepsy in the future. The information provided from all of these various technologies reveals different and complementary aspects of cerebral function and structure. Consequently, these tests should ideally be used together to derive diagnostic and mechanistic insights into the normal and abnormal human brain from as many perspectives as possible. However, all have strengths and weaknesses that dictate their use in particular situations, and perhaps not in others. Although PET at the present time may have the best potential for producing images of a variety of useful aspects of cerebral function that can be quantitatively displayed with high resolution, this potential will in no way replace the use of existing technologies, or justify abandoning the development of new ones.

Positron emission tomography applications to the study of human epilepsy have mostly utilized fluorodeoxyglucose, and these scans already have great diagnostic value for localizing the epileptogenic lesion in patients with partial seizures who are considered candidates for surgical resection. There is also no doubt, from studies already completed, that PET can reveal patterns of abnormal metabolism that will be useful in differential diagnosis. The possibility that PET with fluorodeoxyglucose, or other tracers, may provide new insights into diagnostic classification that will have specific prognostic and therapeutic implications is anticipated. Parallel studies utilizing autoradiographic techniques in animals and PET in patients, along with complementary investigations of electrical activity and other measures of cerebral function, also promise unique opportunities to study fundamental mechanisms of epileptogenesis, and epilepsy-related disturbances in patients, in a manner that was previously possible only in animals. Undoubtedly, this will also increase the ability of neuroscientists to utilize epileptic patients to study basic mechanisms of normal brain function as well.

Acknowledgements

The UCLA studies discussed here were supported by grants NS-15654, NS-02808, and CA-32855 from the US Public Health Service, and contract DE-AM03-76-SF00012 from the Department of Energy.

References

ACKERMANN, R. F., ENGEL, J. JR and PHELPS, M. E. (1985) Identification of seizure-mediating brain structures with deoxyglucose method: studies of human epilepsy with positron computed tomography, and animal seizure models with contact autoradiography. In *Basic Mechanism of the Epilepsies*, edited by A. V. Delgado-Escueta. New York: Raven Press

ACKERMANN, R. F., CHUGANI, H. T., FINCH, D. M., BABB, T. L., LEAR, J. L. and ENGEL, J. JR (1983) Autoradiographic studies of stimulation-induced changes in rat hippocampal metabolism and blood flow. *Journal of Cerebral Blood Flow Metabolism,* **3,** S238–S239

ACKERMANN, R. F., FINCH, D. M., BABB, T. L. and ENGEL, J. JR (1984) Increased glucose metabolism during long-duration recurrent inhibition of hippocampal pyramidal cells. *Journal of Neuroscience,* **4,** 251–264

AGUILAR, M. J. and RASMUSSEN, T. (1960) Role of encephalitis in pathogenesis of epilepsy. *Archives of Neurology,* **2,** 663–676

AJMONE MARSAN, C. (1980) Depth electrography and electrocorticography. In *Electrodiagnosis in Clinical Neurology,* edited by M. J. Aminoff, pp. 167–196. New York: Churchill Livingstone

BABB, T. L., CARR, E. and CRANDALL, P. H. (1973) Analysis of extracellular firing patterns of deep temporal lobe structures in man. *Electroencephalography and Clinical Neurophysiology,* **34,** 247–257

BABB, T. L., LIEB, J. P., BROWN, W. J., PRETORIUS, J. and CRANDALL, P. H. (1984) Distribution of pyramidal cell density and hyperexcitability in the epileptic human hippocampal formation. *Epilepsia,* **25,** 721–728

BARON, J. C., ROEDA, D., MUNARI, C., CROUZEL, C., CHODKIEWICZ, J. P. and COMAR, D. (1983) Brain regional pharmacokinetics of ^{11}C-labeled diphenylhydantoin: positron emission tomography in humans. *Neurology,* **33,** 580–585

BARRIO, J. R., MACDONALD, N. S., ROBINSON, G. D. JR *et al.* (1981) Remote, semiautomated production of F-18-labeled 2-deoxy-2-fluoro-D-glucose. *Journal of Nuclear Medicine,* **22,** 372–375

BARTH, D. S., SUTHERLING, W., ENGEL, J. JR and BEATTY, J. (1982) Neuromagnetic localization of epileptiform spike activity in the human brain. *Science,* **218,** 891–894

BARTH, D. S., SUTHERLING, W., ENGEL, J. JR and BEATTY, J. (1984) Neuromagnetic evidence of spatially distributed sources underlying epileptiform spikes in the human brain. *Science,* **223,** 293–296

BERNARDI, S., TRIMBLE, M. R., FRACKOWIAK, R. S. J., WISE, R. J. S. and JONES, T. (1983) An interictal study of partial epilepsy using positron emission tomography and the oxygen-15 inhalation technique. *Journal of Neurology, Neurosurgery and Psychiatry,* **46,** 473–477

BLUMER, D. and BENSON, D. F. (1982) Psychiatric manifestations of epilepsy. In *Psychiatric Aspects of Neurological Disease,* Vol. II, edited by D. F. Benson and D. Blumer, pp. 25–48. New York: Grune and Stratton

BOLENDER, N. F. and WYLER, A. R. (1982) CT measurements of mesial temporal lobe herniation in epileptics. *Epilepsia,* **23,** 409–416

BONTE, F. J., STOKELY, E. M., DEVOUS, M. D. JR and HOMAN, R. W. (1983) Single photon tomographic study of regional cerebral blood flow in epilepsy. *Archives of Neurology,* **40,** 267–270

BRADY, T. J. and PYKETT, I. L. (Eds.) (1983) Nuclear magnetic resonance. *Seminars in Nuclear Medicine,* **13,** 305–396

BROWN, W. J. (1973) Structural substrates of seizure foci in the human temporal lobe. In *Epilepsy: Its Phenomena in Man,* edited by M. A. B. Brazier, pp. 339–374. New York: Academic Press

BUSTANY, P., SARGENT, T., SAUDUBAY, J. M., HENRY, J. F. and COMAR, D. (1981) Regional human brain uptake and protein incorporation of ^{11}-C-L-methionine studied *in vivo* with PET. *Journal of Cerebral Blood Flow Metabolism,* **1** (Suppl 1), S17–18

BYDDER, G. M., STEINER, R. E., YOUNG, I. R. *et al.* (1982) Clinical NMR imaging of the brain. *American Journal of Radiology,* **139,** 215–236

CHERLOW, D. G., DYMOND, A. M., CRANDALL, P. H. *et al.* (1977) Evoked response and after-discharge thresholds to electrical stimulation in temporal lobe epileptics. *Archives of Neurology,* **34,** 527–531

CHUGANI, H., ENGEL, J. JR, MAZZIOTTA, J. and PHELPS, M. (1984) ^{18}F-2-fluorodeoxyglucose positron emission tomography in medically refractory childhood epilepsy. *Neurology*, **34** (Suppl.), S107

COMAR, D., MAZIERE, M., GADOT, M. M., BERGER, G. and SOUSSALINE, F. (1979) Visualization of ^{11}C-flunitrazepam displacement in the brain of the live baboon. *Nature,* **280,** 329–331

COMMISSION ON CLASSIFICATION AND TERMINOLOGY OF THE INTERNATIONAL LEAGUE AGAINST EPILEPSY (1981) Proposal for revised clinical and electroencephalographic classification of epileptic seizures. *Epilepsia,* **22,** 489–501

CRANDALL, P. H., WALTER, R. D. and RAND, R. W. (1963) Clinical applications of studies of stereotactically implanted electrodes in temporal lobe epilepsy. *Journal of Neurosurgery,* **20,** 827–840

DUFFY, F. H., BARTELS, P. H. and BURCHFIEL, J. L. (1981) Significance probability mapping: an aid in the topographic analysis of brain electrical activity. *Electroencephalography and Clinical Neurophysiology,* **51,** 455–462

DUFFY, F. H., BURCHFIEL, J. L. and LOMBROSO, C. T. (1979) Brain electrical activity mapping (BEAM): a method for extending the clinical utility of EEG and evoked potential data. *Annals of Neurology,* **5,** 309–321

ELL, P. J. and HOLMAN, B. L. (Eds.) (1982) *Computed Emission Tomography*, Oxford: Oxford University Press

ENGEL, J. JR. (1983a) Functional localization of epileptogenic lesions. *Trends in Neurosciences,* **6,** 60–65

ENGEL, J. JR. (1983b) Metabolic patterns of human epilepsy: clinical observations and possible physiological correlates. In *Current Problems in Epilepsy,* edited by M. Baldy-Moulinier, D. H. Ingvar and B. S. Meldrum, pp. 6–18 London: John Libbey

ENGEL, J. JR. (1984a) A practical guide for routine EEG studies in epilepsy. *Journal of Clinical Neurophysiology*, **1,** 109–142

ENGEL, J. JR. (1984b) The use of PET scanning in epilepsy. *Annals of Neurology*, **15** (Suppl.), S180–S191

ENGEL, J. JR., ACKERMANN, R. F., KUHL, D. E. and PHELPS, M. E. (1985) Brain imaging of glucose utilization in convulsive disorders. *Association for Research into Nervous and Mental Disease Research Publications,* Vol. 63 (in press)

ENGEL, J. JR., BROWN, W. J., KUHL, D. E., PHELPS, M. E., MAZZIOTTA, J. C. and CRANDALL, P. H. (1982a) Pathological findings underlying focal temporal lobe hypometabolism in partial epilepsy. *Annals of Neurology,* **12,** 518–528

ENGEL, J. JR. and CALDECOTT-HAZARD, S. (1984) Altered behavioral states in epilepsy: clinical observations and approaches to basic research. In *Modulation of Sensorimotor Activity During Altered Behavioral States,* edited by R. Bandler, pp. 471–486. New York: Alan R. Liss, Inc.

ENGEL, J. JR. and CRANDALL, P. H. (1983) Falsely localizing ictal onsets with depth EEG telemetry during anticonvulsant withdrawal. *Epilepsia,* **24,** 344–355

ENGEL, J. JR., CRANDALL, P. H. and RAUSCH, R. (1983) The partial epilepsies. In *The Clinical Neurosciences,* Vol. 2, edited by R. N. Rosenberg, R. G. Grossman, S. Schochet, E. R. Heinz and W. D. Willis, pp. 1349–1380. New York: Churchill Livingstone

ENGEL, J. JR., DRIVER, M. V. and FALCONER, M. A. (1975) Electrophysiological correlates of pathology and surgical results in temporal lobe epilepsy. *Brain,* **98,** 129–156

ENGEL, J. JR., KUHL, D. E. and PHELPS, M. E. (1982) Patterns of human local cerebral glucose metabolism during epileptic seizures. *Science,* **218,** 64–66

ENGEL, J. JR., KUHL, D. E., PHELPS, M. E. and CRANDALL, P. H. (1982b) Comparative localization of epileptic foci in partial epilepsy by PCT and EEG. *Annals of Neurology,* **12,** 529–537

ENGEL, J. JR., KUHL, D. E., PHELPS, M. E. and MAZZIOTTA, J. C. (1982c) Interictal cerebral glucose metabolism in partial epilepsy and its relation to EEG changes. *Annals of Neurology,* **12,** 510–517

ENGELS, J. JR., KUHL, D. E., PHELPS, M. E., RAUSCH, R. and NUWER, M. (1983) Local cerebral metabolism during partial seizures. *Neurology,* **33,** 400–413

ENGEL, J. JR., LUDWIG, B. I. and FETELL, M. (1978) Prolonged partial complex status epilepticus: EEG and behavioral observations. *Neurology,* **28,** 863–869

ENGEL, J. JR., RAUSCH, R., LIEB, J. P., KUHL, D. E. and CRANDALL, P. H. (1981) Correlation of criteria used for localizing epileptic foci in patients considered for surgical therapy of epilepsy. *Annals of Neurology,* **9,** 215–224

ENGEL, J. JR., SUTHERLING, W. W., CAHAN, L., CRANDALL, P. H., KUHL, D. E. and PHELPS, M. E. (1984) The role of positron emission tomography in the surgical therapy of epilepsy. In *Advances in Epileptology: Epilepsy International Symposium*, edited by R. J. Porter, R. H. Mattson, A. A. Ward and M. Dam, pp. 427–432. New York: Raven Press

ENGEL, J. JR., LUDWIG, B. I. and FETTEL, M. (1978) Prolonged partial complex status epilepticus: EEG and behavioural observations. *Neurology*, **28,** 863–369

ENGEL, J. JR., WOLFSON, L. and BROWN, L. (1978) Anatomical correlates of electrical and behavioural events related to amydaloid kindling. *Annals of Neurology*, **3,** 538–544

GASTAUT, H. and GASTAUT, J. L. (1976) Computerized transverse axial tomography in epilepsy. *Epilepsia,* **17,** 325–336

GLOOR, P. (1975) Contributions of electroencephalography and electrocorticography to the neurosurgical treatment of the epilepsies. *Advances in Neurology,* **8,** 59–106

GOTMAN, J. (1983) Measurement of small time differences between EEG channels: method and application to epileptic seizure propagation. *Electroencephalography and Clinical Neurophysiology,* **56,** 501–514

GOTMAN, J., GLOOR, P., QUESNEY, L. F. and OLIVIER, A. (1982) Correlations between EEG changes induced by diazepam and the localization of epileptic spikes and seizures. *Electroencephalography and Clinical Neurophysiology,* **54,** 614–621

GUR, R. C., SUSSMAN, N. M., ALAVI, A. *et al.* (1982) Positron emission tomography in two cases of childhood epileptic encephalopathy (Lennox-Gastaut syndrome). *Neurology,* **32,** 1191–1194

HOFFMAN, E. J., PHELPS, M. E., HUANG, S. C. *et al.* (1981) A new tomograph for quantitative emission computed tomography of the brain. *IEEE Transactions of Nuclear Science,* **NS-28**, 99–103

HOUGAARD, K., OIKAWA, T., SVEINSDOTTIR, E. *et al.* (1976) Regional cerebral blood flow in focal cortical epilepsy. *Archives of Neurology,* **33,** 527–535

HUANG, S. C., CARSON, R. E., HOFFMAN, E. J. *et al.* (1983) Quantitative measurement of local cerebral blood flow in humans by positron computed tomography and ^{15}O water. *Journal of Cerebral Blood Flow Metabolism,* **3,** 141–153

HUANG, S. C., PHELPS, M. E., HOFFMAN, E. J. and KUHL, D. E. (1981) Error sensitivity of fluorodeoxyglucose method for measurement of cerebral metabolic rate of glucose. *Journal of Cerebral Blood Flow Metabolism,* **1,** 391–401

HUANG, S. C., PHELPS, M. E., HOFFMAN, E. J., SIDERIS, K., SELIN, C. J. and KUHL, D. E. (1980) Non-invasive determination of local cerebral metabolic rate of glucose in normal man with ^{18}F-2-deoxyglucose and emission computed tomography: theory and results. *American Journal of Physiology,* **238,** E69–E82

INGVAR, D. H. (1967) The pathophysiology of the stroke related to findings in EEG and to measurement of regional cerebral blood flow. In *Stroke. Thule International Symposia (Stockholm),* edited by A. Engel and T. Larsson, pp. 105–122. Stockholm: Nordiska Bokhandelns Forlag

INGVAR, D. H. (1973) Regional cerebral blood flow in focal cortical epilepsy. *Stroke,* **4,** 359–360

INGVAR, D. H. (1975) rCBF in focal cortical epilepsy. In *Cerebral Circulation and Metabolism*, edited by T. W. Langfitt, L. C. McHenry, Jr, M. Reivich and H. Wollman, pp. 361–364. New York: Springer-Verlag

KELLAWAY, P. (1981) The incidence, significance and natural history of spike foci in children. In *Current Clinical Neurophysiology,* edited by C. E. Henry, pp. 151–175. Amsterdam: Elsevier/North-Holland

KUHL, D. E., ENGEL, J. JR, PHELPS, M. E. and SELIN, C. (1980) Epileptic patterns of local cerebral metabolism and perfusion in humans determined by emission computed tomography of ^{18}FDG and $^{13}NH_3$. *Annals of Neurology,* **8,** 348–360

KUHL, D. E., BARRIO, J. R., HUANG, S. C. *et al.* (1982) Quantifying local cerebral blood flow with N-isopropyl-*p*-^{123}I-iodoamphetamine tomography. *Journal of Nuclear Medicine,* **23,** 196–203

LASSEN, N. A. and PERL, W. (1979) *Tracer Kinetic Methods in Medical Physiology.* New York: Raven Press

LAVY, S., MELAMED, E., PORTNOY, Z. *et al.* (1976) Interictal regional cerebral blood flow in patients with partial seizures. *Neurology,* **26,** 418–422

MAGISTRETTI, P., UREN, R., SHOMER, D., BLUME, H., HOLMAN, B. and HILL, T. (1982) Emission tomographic scans of cerebral blood flow using I^{123} iodoamphetamine in epilepsy. In *Nuclear Medicine and Biology. Proceedings of the Third World Congress of Nuclear Medicine and Biology,* edited by C. Raynaud, pp. 139–143. Paris: Pergamon Press

MAVOR, H. and HELLEN, M. K. (1964) Nasopharyngeal electrode recording. *American Journal of EEG Technology,* **4,** 43–50

MAZIERE, M., BERGER, G., GODOT, J. M., PRENANT, C. and COMAR, D. (1981) Etorphine ^{11}C: a new tool for *in vivo* study of brain opiate receptors. *Journal of Labeled Compound Radiopharmaceuticals,* **18,** 15–16

MAZZIOTTA, J. C. and ENGEL, J. JR. (1984) The use and impact of PET scanning in epilepsy. *Epilepsia*, **25,** Supp. 2, S86–S104

MAZZIOTTA, J. C. and ENGEL, J. JR. (1985) Advanced neuro-imaging techniques in the study of human epilepsy: PET, SPECT and NMR-CT. In *Recent Advances in Epilepsy,* Vol. 2, edited by T. Pedley and B. S. Meldrum, pp. 65–99. New York: Churchill Livingstone

MAZZIOTTA, J. C., PHELPS, M. E., MILLER, J. *et al.* (1981) Tomographic mapping of human cerebral metabolism: normal unstimulated state. *Neurology,* **31,** 503–516

MAZZIOTTA, J. C., PHELPS, M. E., CARSON, R. E. and KUHL, D. E. (1982a) Tomographic mapping of human cerebral metabolism: sensory deprivation. *Annals of Neurology,* **12,** 435–444

MAZZIOTTA, J. C., PHELPS, M. E., MEADORS, A. K., RICCI, A., WINTER, J. and BENTSON, J. R. (1982b) Anatomical localization schemes for use in positron computed tomography using a specially designed head holder. *Journal of Computer Assisted Tomography,* **6,** 848–853

MELDRUM, B. S., HORTON, R. W. and BRIERLEY, J. B. (1974) Epileptic brain damage in adolescent baboons following seizures induced by allylglycine. *Brain,* **97,** 407–418

MEYER, J. S., HAYMAN, L. A., AMANO, T. *et al.* (1981) Mapping local blood flow of human brain by CT scanning during stable xenon inhalation. *Stroke,* **12,** 426–436

MILNER, B., BRANCH, C. and RASMUSSEN, T. (1962) Study of short-term memory after intracarotid injection of sodium amytal. *Transactions of the American Neurological Association,* **87,** 224–226

MODENA, I., RICCI, G. B., BARBANERA, S., LEONI, R., ROMANI, G. L. and CARELLI, P. (1982) Biomagnetic measurements of spontaneous brain activity in epileptic patients. *Electroencephalography and Clinical Neurophysiology,* **54,** 622–628

OAKLEY, J., OJEMANN, G. A., OJEMANN, L. M. *et al.* (1979) Identifying epileptic foci on contrast-enhanced computerized tomographic scans. *Archives of Neurology,* **36,** 669–671

PETROFF, O. A. C., PRITCHARD, J. W., BEHAR, K. L., ALGER, J. R. and SHULMAN, R. R. (1984) *In vivo* phosphorus nuclear magnetic resonance spectroscopy in status epilepticus. *Annals of Neurology*, **16,** 169–177

PHELPS, M. E., HOFFMAN, E. J. and RAYBAUD, C. (1977) Factors which affect cerebral uptake and retention of $^{13}NH_3$. *Stroke,* **8,** 694–702

PHELPS, M. E., MAZZIOTTA, J. C. and HUANG, S. C. (1982) Study of cerebral function with positron computed tomography. *Journal of Cerebral Blood Flow Metabolism,* **2,** 113–162

PHELPS, M. E., SCHELBERT, H. R. and MAZZIOTTA, J. C. (1983) Positron computed tomography for studies of myocardial and cerebral function. *Annals of Internal Medicine,* **98,** 339–359

PHELPS, M. E., HOFFMAN, E. J., MULLANI, N. A. and TER-POGOSSIAN, M. M. (1975) Application of annihilation coincidence detection to transaxial reconstruction tomography. *Journal of Nuclear Medicine,* **16,** 210–224

PHELPS, M. E., HUANG, S. C., HOFFMAN, E. J. and KUHL, D. E. (1979a) Validation of tomographic measurement of cerebral blood volume with C-11 labeled carboxyhemoglobin. *Journal of Nuclear Medicine,* **20,** 328–334

PHELPS, M. E., HUANG, S. C., HOFFMAN, E. J., SELIN, C. E., SOKOLOFF, L. and KUHL, D. E. (1979b) Tomographic measurement of local cerebral glucose metabolic rate in humans with (^{18}F) fluorodeoxyglucose: validation of method. *Annals of Neurology,* **6,** 371–388

PHELPS, M. E., HUANG, S. C., KUHL, D. E., HOFFMAN, E. J. and SELIN, C. (1981a) Cerebral extraction of n-13 ammonia: its dependence on cerebral blood flow and capillary permeability. *Stroke,* **12,** 607–619

PHELPS, M. E., MAZZIOTTA, J. C., KUHL, D. E. *et al.* (1981b) Tomographic mapping of human cerebral metabolism: visual stimulation and deprivation. *Neurology,* **31,** 517–529

PHELPS, M. E., HUANG, S. C., HOFFMAN, E. J., PLUMMER, D. and CARSON, R. (1982) An analysis of signal amplification using small detectors in positron emission tomography. *Journal of Computer Assisted Tomography,* **6,** 551–565

PHELPS, M. E., BARRIO, J. R., HUANG, S. C., KEEN, R. E., CHUGANI, M. D. and MAZZIOTTA, J. C. (1984) Criteria for the tracer kinetic measurement of cerebral protein synthesis in humans with positron emission tomography. *Annals of Neurology*, **15** (Suppl.), S192–S202

QUESNEY, L. F., KATSARKAS, A., GLOOR, P. and ANDERMANN, F. (1981) Contribution of naso-ethmoidal electrode recording in the electrographic exploration of frontal and temporal lobe epilepsy. In *Advances in Epileptology,* Vol. XII, edited by M. Dam, L. Gram and J. K. Penry, pp. 293–301. New York: Raven Press

RAICHLE, M. E. (1983) Presented at the Workshop on Positron Emission Tomography, Winter Conference in Brain Research, Keystone, January 1983

RAICHLE, M. E., LARSON, K. B., PHELPS, M. E. *et al.* (1975) *In vivo* measurement of brain glucose transport and metabolism employing glucose-11-C. *American Journal of Physiology,* **228,** 1936–1948

RAUSCH, R., FEDIO, P., ARY, C., ENGEL, J. JR. and CRANDALL, P. H. (1984) Resumption of behavior following intracarotid sodium amobarbital injection. *Annals of Neurology,* **15,** 31–35

RAUSCH, R. and WALSH, G. O. (1984) Right hemisphere language dominance in right-handed patients. *Archives of Neurology*, **14,** 1077–1080

REIVICH, M., KUHL, D. E., WOLF, A. *et al.* (1979) The ^{18}F-fluorodeoxyglucose method for the measurement of local cerebral glucose utilization in man. *Circulation Research,* **44,** 127–137

RHODES, C. G., LENZI, G. L., FRACKOWIAK, R. S. J., JONES, T. and PAZILLI, C. (1981) Measurement of CBF and $CMRO_2$ using the continuous inhalation of $C^{15}O_2$ and $^{15}O_2$. *Journal of Neurological Science,* **50,** 381–389

ROVIT, R. L., GLOOR, P. and RASMUSSEN, T. (1961) Sphenoidal electrodes in the electrographic study of patients with temporal lobe epilepsy. *Journal of Neurosurgery,* **18,** 151–158

SAKAI, F., MEYER, J. S., NARITOMI, H. *et al.* (1978) Regional cerebral blood flow and EEG in patients with epilepsy. *Archives of Neurology,* **35,** 648–657

SINGER, J. R. and CROOKS, L. E. (1983) Nuclear magnetic resonance blood flow measurements in the human brain. *Science,* **221,** 654–656

SOKOLOFF, L., REIVICH, M., KENNEDY, C. *et al.* (1977) The ^{14}C deoxyglucose method for the measurement of local cerebral glucose utilization: theory, procedure and normal values in the conscious and anesthetized albino rat. *Journal of Neurochemistry,* **28,** 897–916

TALAIRACH, J., BANCAUD, J., SZIKLA, G. *et al.* (1974) Approche nouvelle de la neurochirurgie de l'epilepsie. Methodologie stereotaxique et resultats thérapeutiques. *Neurochirurgie,* **20** (Suppl. 1), 240

THEODORE, W. H., BROOKS, R., SATO, S. *et al.*, (1984) The role of positron emission tomography in the evaluation of seizure disorders. *Annals of Neurology*, **15** (Suppl.), 176–179

THEODORE, W. H., NEWMARK, M. E., SATO, S. *et al.* (1983) ^{18}F-fluorodeoxyglucose positron emission tomography in refractory complex partial seizures. *Annals of Neurology,* **14,** 429–437

WADA, J. and RASMUSSEN, T. (1960) Intracarotid injection of sodium amytal for the lateralization of cerebral speech dominance: experimental and clinical observations. *Journal of Neurosurgery,* **17,** 266–282

WAGNER, H. N. JR., BURNS, H. D., DANNALS, R. F. *et al.* (1983) Imaging dopamine receptors in the human brain by positron tomography. *Science,* **221,** 1264–1266

WIESER, H. G., BANCAUD, J., TALAIRACH, J. *et al.* (1979) Comparative value of spontaneous and chemically and electrically induced seizures in establishing the lateralization of temporal lobe seizures. *Epilepsia,* **20,** 47–60

WILLIAMSON, S. J. and KAUFMAN, L. (1981) Biomagnetism. *Journal of Magnetism and Magnetic Materials,* **22,** 129–201

14
The role of stereo-electroencephalography (SEEG) in the evaluation of partial epileptic seizures

C. Munari and J. Bancaud

INTRODUCTION

The first functional stereotaxic investigation in epileptic patients was accomplished by Spiegel and Wycis in 1950, who explored both the thalamus and the hypothalamus in patients with petit mal absences, with the aim of a better understanding of the physiopathology of this seizure type. At that time the partial cortical epilepsies were defined by electrocorticography, the methodology of which had been systematized by Penfield and Jasper (1954).

In 1953 a series of studies, based on the use of chronically implanted 'depth' electrodes in man, was initiated (Ajmone Marsan and Van Buren, 1958; Bickford, Dodge and Sem-Jacobsen, 1953; Brazier, 1956; Dodge *et al.*, 1953; Delgado and Hamelin, 1956; Kelloway, 1956; Walker and Ribstein, 1957). Initially, this new technique was not based on stereotaxic procedures and the implantation, usually of several flexible electrodes, was rather imprecise. Furthermore, when it was first initiated, this investigational method was dependent on the same concepts developed by corticographic investigations. The primary goal of inserting depth electrodes was to record the 'disturbed' electrical activity (essentially stationary spike discharges) of certain cerebral structures.

In subsequent years, as a result both of the availability of atlases providing the spatial coordinates of most cerebral structures (Spiegel and Wycis, 1952; Schaltenbrand and Bailey, 1959; Talairach, de Ajuriaguerra and Davis, 1952; Talairach *et al.* 1947, 1967) and of the development of technical means for reaching such structures, functional stereotaxic investigations became a new methodological approach in partial epilepsies (Bancaud, 1959; Bancaud and Talairach, 1975).

The term 'stereo-electroencephalography' (SEEG) was proposed in 1962 (Bancaud *et al.*, 1962) to emphasize the importance of recording electrical activity from different cerebral structures and to stress the necessity of using stereotaxic procedures for localizing these structures. In the methodology that we utilize for investigating the severe drug-resistant partial epilepsies, the stereo-EEG occupies a most important place in identifying and defining a cortical 'epileptogenic' area (related to a lesion); the technique defines the spatial and temporal organization of the epileptic discharge.

The validity of the stereo-EEG exploration depends on several factors, and ideally it should precisely define the epileptic pattern of each patient. Furthermore, the data obtained by stereo-EEG (and by its interpretation) should be subsequently validated by a correlation with the surgical results (*Figure 14.1*). A methodology is, after all, valuable only if it can be verified, discussed, and subsequently improved.

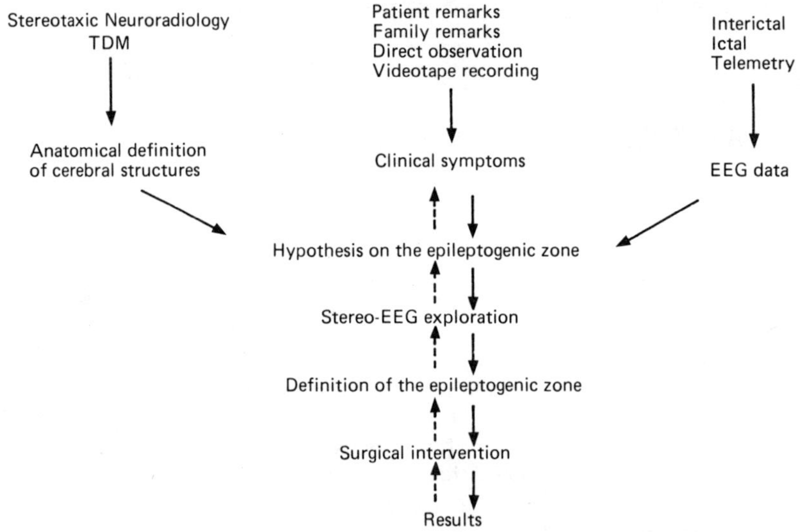

Figure 14.1 The hypothesis on the localization of the epileptogenic area is the result of the study of the clinical symptoms strengthened by the EEG data and by the neuroradiological stereotaxic studies. Good results confirm the validity of the methodology, whereas if the surgical results are poor, the surgical intervention is at least questionable – in such cases (except for cases in which the removal was smaller than it should have been because of functional risks) the definition of the epileptogenic area was incorrect. Thus, the data obtained by the stereo-EEG exploration were at least incomplete (or wrong). The main reasons for poor SEEG results are often that the hypothesis on the localization of the epileptogenic area was wrong. Finally, if the hypothesis is wrong, we were misled by an improper interpretation of preliminary investigations. Arrows indicate that the methodological process should be verified at each step.

The major aim of an SEEG exploration is to suggest to the neurosurgeon an ideal 'model' of cortical resection that he can modulate, taking into account other important factors (anatomical, functional, social, economical, psychological, etc.).

In this review we shall:

(1) Specify precisely the conditions of an SEEG exploration, permitting an evaluation of the seizures as correctly as possible.
(2) Interpret the organization of the discharges in the explored cortical structures and on the scalp.
(3) Propose a schematic definition of the principal types of partial seizures characterizing the paroxysmal disorganization of the cerebral cortex.

GENERAL METHODOLOGY OF INVESTIGATION OF THE SEVERE PARTIAL EPILEPSIES

Preliminary investigations (prior to stereo-EEG explorations)

The importance of the preliminary investigations prior to a SEEG exploration has often been stressed by our group (Bancaud, 1959, 1968, 1969; Bancaud and Talairach, 1970; Bancaud *et al.*, 1965, 1973; Bonis *et al.*, 1981; Talairach and Bancaud, 1963, 1971, 1973; Talairach, Davis and Turnoux, 1958; Talairach *et al.*, 1962, 1974) and can be divided into clinical investigations, electrophysiological and neuroradiological studies.

Clinical investigations

This fundamental preliminary step is to characterize a patient's epilepsy prior to submission to a SEEG exploration.

The investigation consists of a precise and detailed reconstruction of the history of the disease (modalities of occurrence, possible aetiology, possible neurological deficits), of the characteristics of the seizures (especially the stability or instability, the provoking factors, the length and frequency of the attack, and the chronological distribution of the seizures), the associated neurological and/or psychiatric abnormalities, and the psychosocial–professional adaptation.

Electrophysiological investigations

INTERICTAL RECORDING

EEG studies are accomplished under different conditions: waking, night sleep or after sleep deprivation, with the usual medical treatment or during withdrawal, with activating agents (hyperventilation, bemegride (Mesimide) and/or Metrazol) and eventually with different types of stimulations (auditory, visual, proprioceptive, etc.). The validity of such information has been largely discussed elsewhere (Bancaud *et al.*, 1973). The different recordings may be obtained either under standard conditions or with a radiotelemetric system. The electrical activity of the scalp is recorded simultaneously with some neurovegetative parameters and electromyography. The modalities of the EEG investigations are individually defined for each patient as a function of the problems determined by the clinical data.

Interictal abnormalities have relatively poor localizing value and are much less useful than ictal recordings. For example:

(1) Slow waves may be related to a cerebral lesion, but they may also be the result, more or less transitory, of an ictal episode.
(2) Spike frequency, amplitude and, above all, localization may vary with the frequency, the length, and the extent of the seizures; furthermore, the absence of spikes at the scalp does not exclude their existence in deep structures (Abraham and Ajmone Marsan, 1958).
(3) Spikes may be found in non-epileptic patients.

ICTAL RECORDING

The ictal EEG recording of a partial seizure may present with any of the following patterns in the surface EEG:

(1) absence of any perceptible modification;
(2) local flattening (fast activity);
(3) diffuse flattening (fast activity);
(4) localized spikes and/or spikes and waves;
(5) localized (often rhythmic) slow waves;
(6) largely diffuse (bilateral) spikes and/or spikes and waves;
(7) largely diffuse (bilateral) slow waves.

These different surface patterns (and their various successive associations) are linked to the extent and to the duration of the intracerebral ictal discharges. In order to use the ictal EEG findings in the perspective of stereo-EEG investigations one must study very precisely the chronological relationships between the occurrence of the different clinical symptoms and the EEG modifications. Of particular interest and importance are subjective manifestations which are not accompanied by any EEG modification (for example, anguish, various simple hallucinations, dizziness, etc.); it should be remembered that in many instances patients presenting with such symptoms may be wrongly diagnosed as psychiatric patients because of the lack of EEG ictal modifications.

It is evident that the localization of the EEG ictal discharges is one of the most important criteria in the orientation and positioning of the deep electrodes.

Neuroradiological investigations

These investigations include: the standard radiographs of the skull (in different positions); a tomodensitometric study (with and without contrast enhancement) and a complete neuroradiological study of the brain structures in stereotactic conditions.

This stereotactic localization, including bilateral carotid angiography, pneumoencephalography and ventriculography, is very important because it permits both precise definition of the topography of the possible lesion, the positioning of the intracerebral depth electrodes in any portion of the brain which should be explored, and allows for a maximum of safety for the patient.

The technical aspects of the Talairach's stereotactic methodology have been described previously (Talairach, Davis and Tournoux, 1958; Talairach *et al.*, 1967; Talairach and Bancaud, 1973). We emphasize, however, the importance of the angiographic stereoscopic studies (Szikla *et al.*, 1977), which permit spatial definition and precise localization of different cortical convolutions. We also stress, moreover, that the stereotactic approach is not limited to reaching a chosen target, as when the aim is the destruction of a given structure, but the technique allows one:

(1) to explore and investigate the structures and the systems involved in the epileptic discharges;

(2) to define as thoroughly as possible the relationships between an epileptogenic area and the surrounding regions;
(3) to elaborate, on the basis of the data furnished by the SEEG, several aspects of the surgical procedures.

Interpretation of the data resulting from preliminary investigations

As described above, the preliminary investigations should define the indication for a stereo-EEG exploration and specify its modalities. These investigations should answer the following questions; which if correctly answered, should allow any type of surgical treatment of epilepsy:

(1) Is the epilepsy a partial epilepsy? What are its relationships with a stable and unique epileptogenic lesion?
(2) What is the topographic definition of the epileptogenic lesion as determined by the preliminary investigations?
(3) What are the possible functional consequences of the surgical removal of the epileptogenic area?

When the answers to these questions are not precise or are not sufficiently complete, a stereo-EEG exploration should not be undertaken; without proper answers a high rate of SEEG failures is likely.

It is clear that the data resulting from the preliminary studies may vary as a function of many factors: clinical, electrophysiological, and neuroradiological. The relative importance of these factors varies in different patients; the factors are: the more or less precise reconstruction of the clinical history; unknown aetiology; diffuse cerebral damage versus localized and limited brain lesion; simple and homogeneous clinical evolution or changes in the clinical symptomatology during the evolution; well-localized, largely widespread, bilateral, or absent interictal EEG abnormalities. The direct recording of the seizures themselves is essential to determine the topography of an epileptogenic area, that is, the spatial and temporal organization of an ictal discharge. An evaluation, as rigorous as possible, of the anatomoelectroclinical (AEC) relationships during a seizure is the best method to define the areas involved in the paroxysmal disorganization. Since the approach to the problem is the same as during stereo-EEG, this is discussed below.

We stress that, for many reasons, the anatomoelectroclinical relationships are more difficult to determine when the seizures are recorded only with scalp EEG (whatever the technical methodology), than with stereo-EEG. For example, a fast low-voltage discharge may not appear on the scalp recording, especially if it is well localized and limited in the cortex, and may be an accompaniment of an 'electrically silent' seizure; moreover, a discharge on the scalp which occurs many seconds after the clinical symptomatology, or which is immediately widespread (or bilateral and 'synchronous') makes anatomoelectroclinical relations very difficult to interpret. Furthermore, since discharges are often multidirectional, it is often difficult even to find any consistency among the scalp recordings. Nevertheless, when the different kinds of spatial and temporal organizations of the discharge are correlated with the accompanying clinical signs, we can often formulate a hypothesis about the topography of the epileptogenic areas.

Finally, the clinical, electrophysiological, anatomical and neuroradiological data strongly determine the strategy of the SEEG.

GENERAL METHODOLOGY OF SEEG INVESTIGATIONS OF PARTIAL SEIZURES

Choice of patients

The implantation of electrodes must only be done from a surgical perspective. The first criterion for selecting patients is a firm hypothesis that the epileptogenic area is unique and relatively stable. Thus patients with clinical evidence of multifocal epilepsy should be excluded. Patients having severe encephalopathies associated with epilepsy should also be excluded from this type of investigation; their cooperation during the SEEG is poor and their epilepsy is often multifocal.

In spite of the fact that patients with 'primary generalized epilepsy' were the first patients to be explored stereotactically (Spiegel and Wycis, 1950), such patients should also be excluded in view of the favourable prognosis of this type of epilepsy and, in the few cases with a poor prognosis, the high frequency of bifrontal lesions.

It should also be emphasized that a risk of severe neurological impairment following surgical removal of the supposed epileptogenic area is an important contraindication to SEEG; it is useless, and potentially dangerous, to explore cerebral areas that cannot be operated upon.

Strategy of the positioning of intracerebral electrodes

The work of Penfield (Penfield and Erikson, 1941; Penfield and Jasper, 1954) demonstrated, in man, that two epileptogenic areas in two different patients are never identical and, moreover, that we cannot expect to observe two overlapping partial seizures in two different patients. On the other hand, in the same patient, partial seizures may vary remarkably during the evolution of the disorder, even over a short period. However, with the exception of rapidly evolving lesions, the spatial organization of the seizures has a relatively small variability (Bancaud, 1981). This relative stability is, of course, one of the most important conditions for surgical success.

Likewise, the electrocorticographical investigations proposed by Penfield and Jasper (1954) require a preliminary preoperative definition of the epileptogenic lesion. This preliminary evaluation influences the size and the location of the bone-flap and, of course, of the explored cortical regions. Using their methodology it is possible to progressively and systematically explore the different areas which have interictal abnormalities; these abnormalities are assumed to be an expression of the epileptogenic lesion.

Our procedure is different, in that the position of the deep electrodes is definitive for a given exploration. Thus, the preliminary planning of the placement of the electrodes should be as precise as possible in order to permit a correct surgical utilization of the obtained information. It is impossible to detail here all the factors determining, in each patient, the positioning of the different electrodes. However, the electrodes are intended to explore:

(1) the lesional process that may be at the origin of the seizures;
(2) the 'irritative' zone that the lesion has induced in its neighbourhood; and,
(3) the structures first affected by the ictal discharge.

In addition, the spatial definition of an epileptogenic area also requires the study of the structures secondarily affected by the discharge in its multidirectional spread.

It is clear that the implantation of too few electrodes is of very limited value. On the other hand, the utilization of too many electrodes is to be avoided.

The widespread tendency to explore symmetrical regions in both hemispheres may be explained by the goal of the 'deep electrode' recording, that is, one must understand whether the epileptogenic area (EA) is bilateral or unilateral and, in the latter case, on which side it is located (Rasmussen, 1983). In our methodology the aim is to verify the preliminary hypothesis by localizing the epileptogenic area and identifying its limits. Although most neurosurgeons limit their surgical intervention to the temporal lobe, the major problem is only to recognize the correct side. Our surgical procedures (Talairach *et al.*, 1974) and our views on partial seizures require the exploration not only of the temporal areas but also of the extratemporal structures potentially involved by the discharges, which can be surgically removed.

The approach of exploring and removing only temporal structures may at least be partially justified by the ambiguities existing in the literature between the terms 'complex partial seizures', 'temporal lobe seizures', and 'psychomotor seizures'. This confused approach is, in part, linked to the extrapolation of animal data to human epilepsy; for example, certain clinical findings seen in so-called 'psychomotor seizures' were also seen in the cat during electrical stimulation of temporal structures. Since the 1950s (Gastaut, Naquet and Vigouroux, 1953), the term 'temporal lobe seizures' was substituted for the the previous term 'psychomotor seizures'. In the recent international classification of the epileptogenic seizures (Bancaud *et al.* 1981, Gastaut, 1970), 'complex partial seizures' or 'complex focal seizures' are related to a 'unilateral or frequently bilateral discharge, diffuse or focal, in temporal or fronto-temporal regions. This definition is almost certainly related to previous explorations by many groups who have introduced depth electrodes bilaterally in the temporal and frontal lobes. In fact, the most frequently explored structures are the amygdaloid nucleus, the hippocampus, the temporal pole, the temporal neocortex (above all, the anterior part) but also the parahippocampal gyrus, the cingulate gyrus, and the fronto-orbital cortex. Wieser (1983) utilizes less localized explorations, with electrodes placed in the first temporal convolutions and in the frontal and parietal lobes. With regard to the side of the SEEG, in our recent group of 120 consecutive patients with presumed temporal lobe epilepsy we explored the contralateral temporal lobe in only 10% of our cases. Much more frequent are our bilateral investigations in patients with frontal lobe epilepsy. However, whatever the cerebral structures to be explored, they should be primarily identified (directly or indirectly) on the basis of a rigorous stereotaxic approach (Talairach and Bancaud, 1973; Talairach, de Ajuriaguerra and David, 1952; Talairach, David and Turnoux, 1958; Talairach *et al.*, 1957, 1967, 1974).

In order to better clarify our strategy of SEEG explorations, which are strictly linked to the electroclinical features in each patient, we shall discuss below some explorations on individual patients.

MM, female, 16 years (*Figure 14.2*)

HISTORY OF THE SEIZURES

(1) Onset of seizures at 9 years; cutaneous paraesthesiae in the left temporal region.
(2) A year later, the seizures started with the same disturbances of sensation, followed by the occurrence of intermittent red spots in the left visual field.

During the few seconds of this hallucination patient described some difficulty seeing in her left visual field.

(3) Sometimes, after the same onset of decrease of the vision, patient had deviation of the head and of the eyes to the left, followed by loss of consciousness.

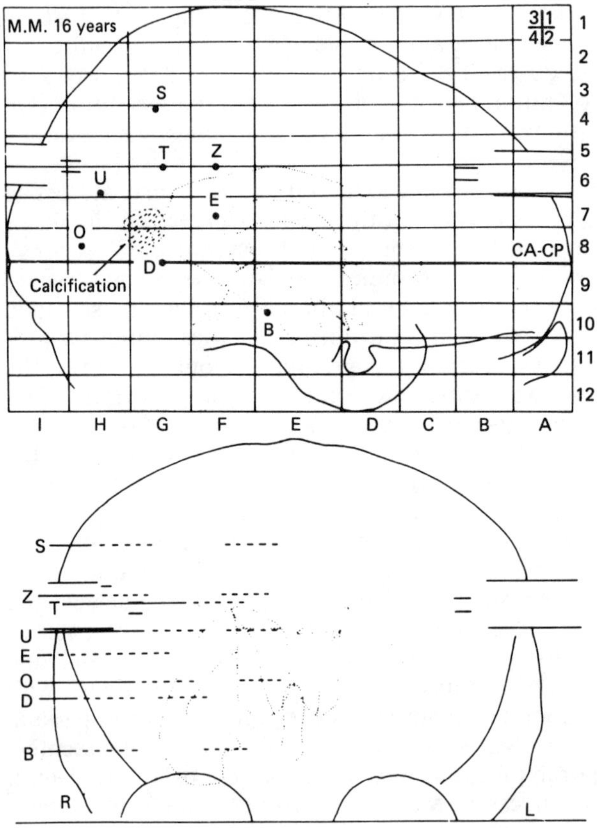

Figure 14.2 Lateral and anteroposterior view of the depth electrodes exploring a large occipitoparieto and temporal area

(4) Her mother describes at this moment that patient has complete rotation to the left, frequently falls, and sometimes has masticatory movements. Late gestural 'automatisms' are infrequent and secondary tonic-clonic generalization has occurred only twice. A transient hemianopsia may again occur.

(5) The patient points out that, rarely, an epigastric 'pain' may exist simultaneously with the visual hallucinations. This pain may exist without any other symptom, and may rise to the throat.

(6) Frequency of attacks were two to five per day.

NEUROLOGICAL EXAMINATION

Left superior quadrantopsia; right-handed.

EEG RECORDINGS

Interictal Slight asymmetry of the background activity; spikes and/or spikes and waves in the right occipital region, sometimes affecting the right parietotemporal region and-or the left occipital lobe.

Ictal Recorded seizures show the patient's typical symptomatology, followed, after bemegride activation, by clonic jerks of the left arm; short discharges of spikes and waves are followed by fast low-voltage occipital discharges (right ? bioccipital ?).

NEURORADIOLOGY (STEREOTACTIC LOCALIZATION)

Calcification near the right calcarine sulcus; no vascular malformations; no ventricular deformations.

STRATEGY OF SEEG

The electrodes O and U explore the occipital cortex behind the calcification; S, T and Z study the evolution of the secondary discharge affecting the parietal lobe (left rotation) and also the origin of the paraesthesiae; E evaluates the spread to the central area (late clonic jerks of the left arm); D evaluates the eventual spread of the discharge between the occipital and temporal areas; B allows an appreciation of the relationship between the subjective epigastric manifestations and the visual hallucinations.

SEEG RESULTS

(1) Continuous slow waves were recorded in the internal and external cortex from electrodes O and U and in the internal cortex by T.

(2) Spikes and spikes and waves were recorded in the same regions and also in the temporoparietal junction (E).

(3) The ictal discharges started in electrodes T, U, and O, simultaneously involving the external and the internal cortex, and in D on the internal part (precuneus). At the onset of the discharges, the patient opens her eyes and explains that she has her usual hallucinations in the left temporal field. Immediately thereafter, she has 'red and black lights' in the left visual field, superimposed on the face of the observer, followed by a forced deviation of the eyes to the left side. The only difference from the usual attacks is that they are fixed.

(4) Electrical stimulations of the posterior part of the cingulate gyrus (Z_1), of the internal parietal cortex (T_1) and of the temporoparietal external junction (E_2) provoked a subjective manifestation resembling an 'onset of a seizure' (hallucinations in the temporal field).

SURGICAL REMOVAL

The corticectomy involved the occipital lobe, including the internal and external cortex (O, V, T, D), behind E.

SURGICAL RESULTS

Complete disappearance of seizures (follow-up: 6 years); left hemianopsia, previously accepted by the patient.

VANST, female, 41 years *(Figure 14.3)*

HISTORY OF THE SEIZURES

(1) Onset of seizures at 34 years: subjective manifestation of 'acid warmth in the throat going down to the stomach – like a bad taste', accompanied by epigastric pain (thoracic?).

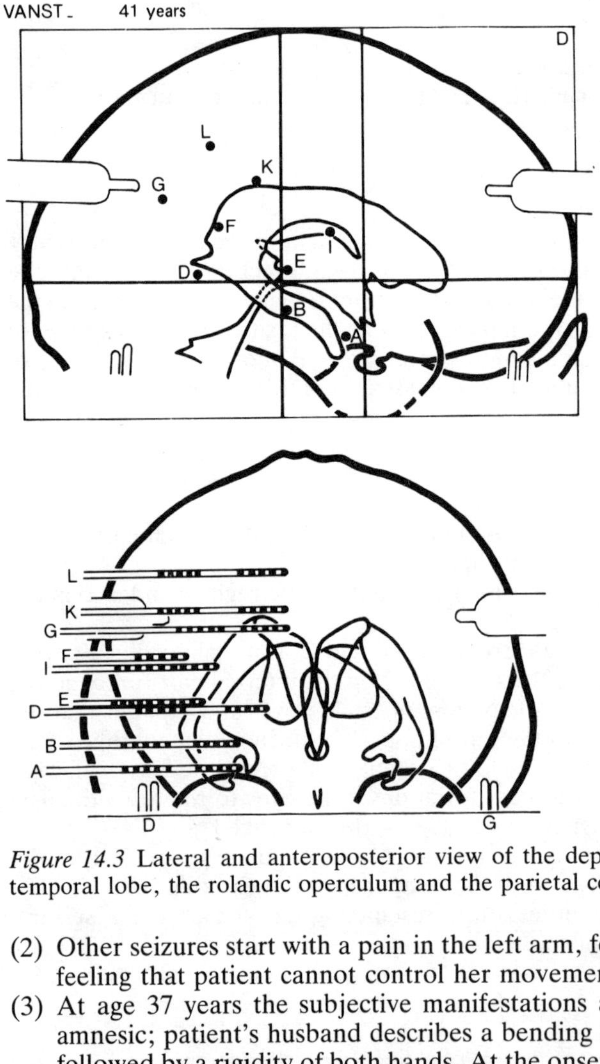

Figure 14.3 Lateral and anteroposterior view of the depth electrodes exploring the right temporal lobe, the rolandic operculum and the parietal cortex

(2) Other seizures start with a pain in the left arm, followed by anguish and by the feeling that patient cannot control her movements.
(3) At age 37 years the subjective manifestations are rare, but the seizures are amnesic; patient's husband describes a bending forward, with ample gestures, followed by a rigidity of both hands. At the onset, very frequent oroalimentary automatisms occur, sometimes with verbal automatisms. There is no swallowing or falling, and no secondary generalization.
(4) Frequency of attacks were two to 20 per day.

NEUROLOGICAL EXAMINATION

No deficit; right-handed.

EEG RECORDINGS

Interictal Slow, continuous delta waves in the right temporal region; spikes in the right temporal region; in a third of the recordings asynchronous theta-delta (θ–δ) waves in the left temporal region; rare asynchronous spikes in the left temporal region.

Ictal The ictal electrical abnormalities (fast activity in the temporoparietal region) may appear 6–10 s before the clinical symptoms. In one seizure the discharge cannot be interpreted. Mimic and autonomic symptoms occur early. Oroalimentary automatisms may be early or late. Gestural automatisms are always later or postictal. A loss of contact may occur either during the onset of the other clinical manifestations or later. Verbal automatisms are postictal. 'Postural' changes may involve the left arm or be more widespread. Rhythmic sharp waves may occur in the right parietotemporo-occipital area. Spread to the left parietal lobe is unusual. Slow postictal waves may be bilaterally diffuse.

NEURORADIOLOGY (STEREOTACTIC LOCALIZATION)
Slight bilateral cortical atrophy; the temporal horn is larger on the right side.

STRATEGY OF THE SEEG
The investigation involves the right temporal lobe (A, B, E), and also the central opercular region (I) (for the gustatory hallucinations), the parietal cortex (F, K, L. G) (for the automatic activities, the postural modifications of the left arm, the feeling of uncontrolled movements and to better localize the ictal discharge). The electrode D allows the posterior limit of the eventual cortectomy to be precisely determined.

SEEG RESULTS
(1) Continuous slow waves in:
  (a) the amygdala (A_1);
  (b) the anterior part of the Ammon's horn (B_1);
  (c) the temporal neocortex (A_2, B_2, D_2);
  (d) The first temporal convolution (E), the opercular region (I), and the lower external parietal cortex L_2, K_2).
(2) High voltage spikes are recorded from A_1, A_2, B_1, B_2, D_2, and E (temporal region) as well as from the other electrodes except for F and L.
(3) The ictal discharges may:
  (a) affect only B_1 (Ammon's horn), resulting in nausea and paraesthesiae of the upper lip.
  (b) start in the opercular region (I), the amygdala (A_1) and the Ammon's horn (B_1), rapidly spreading to the external cortex (K_2, F_2, D_2), resulting in oroalimentary automatisms, flushing of the face and, later, gestural automatisms of the right hand. The patient has no memory of the fit, and has postictal behavioral changes.
(4) Electrical stimulation of the first temporal convolution (E_1, E_2) provokes a feeling of falling (the patient says, for the first time, that this feeling may occur during nocturnal seizures); there is no afterdischarge. The stimulations of A_1, and B_1 provoke a feeling of a heavy tongue falling down in the mouth, which also occurred during spontaneous seizures.

SURGICAL REMOVAL

A complete temporal lobectomy (including the first temporal convolution) and a parietal external corticectomy including D, F, K, and I.

SURGICAL RESULTS

Complete disappearance of the seizures (follow-up: 6 years).

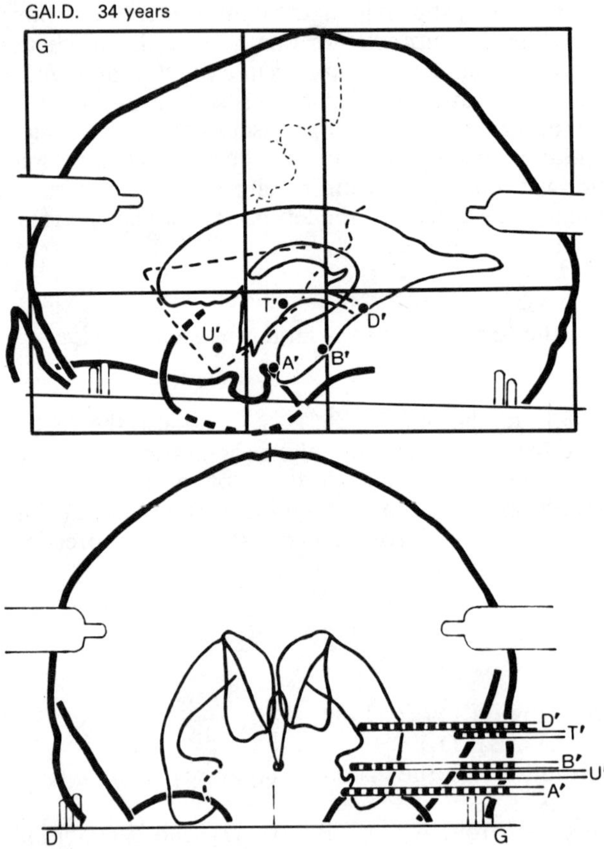

Figure 14.4 Lateral and anteroposterior view of the depth electrodes exploring only the left temporal lobe; electrodes only explore those areas which are surgically removable; it is evident that the obtained information could be insufficient to correctly define the extent of the epileptogenic area

GAI.D., male, 34 years (*Figure 14.4*)

HISTORY OF THE SEIZURES

(1) Onset at 18 years: undefinable taste, recollection of a landscape, or 'déjà vu, déjà vécu', pharyngeal spasm, followed by a loss of contact, generalized stiffening, repeated swallowing, and occasional falling.
(2) Postical phases are often characterized by spatial and temporal disorientation lasting approximately 10 min.

(3) In recent years, the patient announces the onset of the seizure saying: 'I am not very well', and then describes an epigastric warmth going up to the nose associated with severe anguish.
(4) During the late ictal or postictal phase, 'automatic' gestural activity occurs in association with difficulty in understanding.
(5) During some seizures, patient thinks that people nearby are speaking in a foreign language (onset of seizure?)
(6) Frequency of attacks were initially three per week, later two to 30 per day.

AETIOLOGY
Neonatal hypoxia.

NEUROLOGICAL EXAMINATION
No deficit; right-handed – Wada test: left hemispheric dominance.

EEG RECORDINGS

Interictal Slight asymmetry of the background activity; discontinuous left temporal slow waves; rare asynchronous right temporal slow waves; high amplitude left temporal spikes.

Ictal Many subjective manifestations (epigastric warmth) are not accompanied by an electrical change; during the first 10 s, the patient said: 'not so good', 'I will have a fit', without electrical changes – afterwards, rhythmic high amplitude spikes occur in the left hemisphere, especially from the temporal lobe; when this discharge affects both temporal and parietal regions, the patient no longer follows orders, and has repeated swallowing and autonomic symptoms; the aphasia will persist for a few minutes.

NEURORADIOLOGY
Stereotactic localization: slight dilatation of the left temporal horn; CT scan: no abnormalities.

STRATEGY OF THE SEEG
There is no doubt that the hemispheric dominance of this right-handed patient is on the left side. Two facts may allow exploration of this patient who presents with two to 30 seizures per day. First, the apparent clinical symptoms can occur more than 20 sec after the onset of the electrical discharge – during this period the patient does not have any aphasia. Second, the subjective manifestations may occur without electrical changes – the discharge may remain limited to deep temporal structures without scalp EEG abnormalities. Thus an exploration of the left temporal lobe only appears correct. It is the chronological sequence of the clinical symptoms and the discharge which allows us to discover whether the seizures start in the anterior part of this temporal lobe (surgically removable), or in those posterior or suprasylvian areas that we can neither operate on nor explore for obvious functional reasons.

SEEG RESULTS
(1) Continuous slow waves in all electrodes except the posterior part of the second temporal convolution (B'_2 and D'_2).

(2) Continuous high amplitude, spikes from all electrodes (except B'_2 and D'_2).
(3) (a) The ictal discharges simultaneously affect the amygdala (A_1) and Ammon's horn (B'_1); 20 s later the discharges involve the first temporal convolution (U', T') and the temporal neocortex (A'_2) and then, 10 s later, D'. Clinically, oroalimentary 'automatic' activity was observed, with a behavioural change 50 s after the onset, along with autonomic disturbances, and then some clonic jerks of the right face and upper limb. Aphasia persisted approximately 10 min. (b) Considerable fast activity was recorded only from the amygdala (A'_1) and Ammon's horn (B'_1): during several of these short seizures (those less than 15 s), the patient described a 'throat tightening'.
(4) The electrical stimulations were ineffectual.

SURGICAL REMOVAL

Consistent with the preoperative programme, and considering that:
(1) The short paroxysms only involved the anterior deep temporal structures, and
(2) The ictal discharges originated in the same anterior temporal structures, an anterior temporal lobectomy was undertaken. The posterior limit of the removal was at the level of D'.

It was evident that the ictal discharges often spread secondarily, at least to the posterior temporal cortex, but there was a long interval from the onset of seizures and the spread posteriorly. The patient accepted the risk of an incomplete recovery.

SURGICAL RESULTS

One nocturnal seizure characterized (at least) by clonic jerks of the right upper limb. This seizure occurred one year after the intervention and was apparently related to both a withdrawal of barbiturate therapy and alcohol ingestion (follow-up: 3 years).

MRC, male 30 years (*Figure 14.5*)

HISTORY OF THE SEIZURES

(1) Onset at 22 years: impairment of consciousness, falling and tonic-clonic generalization.
(2) For 5–6 years the patient has had a sensation of warmth in the face, and then he says: 'It turns in my head'. It is not really dizziness; most probably he is somewhat confused. Afterwards he has loss of contact, deviation of the head and eyes to the left, gestural automatisms, and verbal 'automatic' activity.
(3) The postictal phase is often characterized by a severe confusional state, lasting more than 30 min – during this period he may look afraid and often attacks people who approach him.
(4) In spite of his perfectly normal interictal behaviour, the patient is in a psychiatric hospital.
(5) Frequency of attacks is one per week to one per day.

AETIOLOGY

Left frontal trauma with impairment of consciousness of 30 min at 18 years.

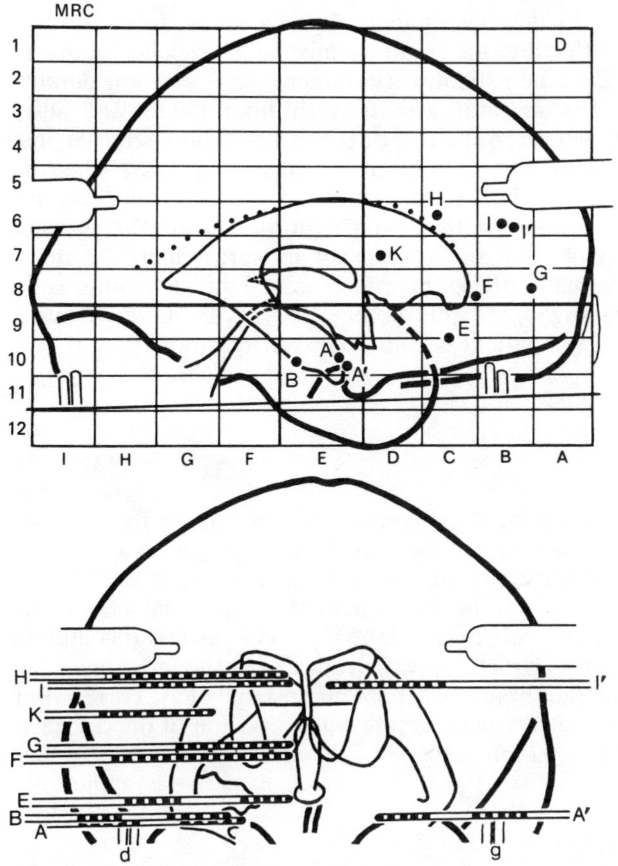

Figure 14.5 Electrodes and cerebral structures. *On the right hemisphere:* B_1: Ammon's horn; B_2: temporal neocortex (second temporal convolution); A_1: amygdaloid nucleus; A_2: temporal neocortex (second temporal convolution); E_1: fronto-orbital cortex (internal part); E_2: fronto-orbital cortex (external part); G_1: internal frontal cortex; G_2: third frontal convolution; I_1: internal frontal cortex; I_2: second frontal convolution; H_1: cingulate gyrus (24 area); H_3: second frontal convolution; F_1: anterior part of the cingulate gyrus; F_3: third frontal convolution; K_1: white matter – third frontal convolution; K_2: frontal operculum. *On the left hemisphere:* A'_1: amygdaloid nucleus; A'_2: temporal neocortex (second temporal convolution); I'_1: internal frontal cortex; I'_2: second frontal convolution

NEUROLOGICAL EXAMINATION

No deficit.

EEG RECORDINGS

Interictal The background activity is symmetrical; continuous slow waves of various amplitude, synchronous and asynchronous in both temporal lobes; spikes and sharp waves, synchronous and asynchronous in both temporal lobes.

Ictal The patient says: 'I feel me, I see myself in the depths'. The EEG shows only an awakening pattern. The patient opens the eyes and says: 'I feel that I will leave'.

The EEG shows a flattening in the right temporofrontal areas, followed by a discharge of sharp waves affecting the right hemisphere, especially in the temporofrontal areas. After 20 s, the patient, very cooperatively, says 'the depths'. Afterwards he says: 'yes', has gestural activity with both hands and starts swallowing movements which persist to the end of the attack. Many seconds after the onset he has autonomic disturbances, different and bilateral postural changes, and 'automatic' gestural activity. Meanwhile, the sharp waves involve the left temporal lobe and slow waves affect both frontal regions. During the postictal phase the rhythmic swallowing persists, and he does not answer; suddenly he smiles and becomes excited. He verbally attacks people around him, delivering some sentences as if he were playing rugby. He spits on the observers and is very restless, but this agitation ceases when the patient is able to answer questions.

NEURORADIOLOGY (stereotactic localization)
Slight dilatation of both frontal horns (left > right).

STRATEGY OF THE SEEG
Most of the clinical symptoms are related to the ictal abnormalities of the temporal and frontal lobes. The ictal discharge early involves the right temporal and frontal regions – these two lobes should be explored. At the same time, we also know that the left temporal lobe is involved by the ictal discharge (A_1). And finally, the (aetiological?) trauma involves the left frontal lobe (I_1). The restlessness and the aggressiveness are almost always postictal – two electrodes in the left frontal and temporal lobes will discern whether or not the apparent postictal phase corresponds to persistent discharges in left-sided structures following cessation of the discharge in the right temporal and/or frontal lobes.

SEEG RESULTS
(1) Continuous slow waves are recorded in the:
  (a) Right temporal lobe: amygdala (A_1); Ammon's horn (B_1), neocortex (A_2, B_2).
  (b) Right external frontal cortex (H_2, G_2).
  (c) Left temporal lobe: amygdala (A'_1); neocortex (A'_2).
  (d) Left external frontal cortex (I'_2).
(2) Rapid, high amplitude spikes and sharp waves are recorded in the:
  (a) Right temporal deep structures (A_1, B_1)
  (b) Right external frontal cortex (K_2)
  (c) Left temporal lobe (A'_1, A'_2).
(3) The ictal discharge starts in the right temporal lobe. Impairment of consciousness occurs when the discharges spread to the homolateral frontal lobe. The left temporal lobe is involved later. The aggressive behaviour is always postictal.
(4) Electrical stimulations of the left frontal and temporal lobes and of the right amygdala were ineffective. However, stimulation of the right Ammon's horn was followed by an afterdischarge involving the right amygdala (50 s), and was accompanied by a subjective feeling that the patient will have a seizure.

SURGICAL REMOVAL
A complete excision of the right temporal lobe was undertaken on the basis of the spontaneous seizures recorded and of the effects of the electrical stimulation.

SURGICAL RESULTS
Complete disappearance of the seizures (follow-up: 4 years).

Acute and chronic SEEG

The methods for the detection of electrical activity have been discussed in sufficient detail to refer the reader to these papers (Bancaud and Dell, 1959; Bancaud *et al.*, 1965; Talairach *et al.*, 1967, 1973, 1974). 'Acute' and 'chronic' SEEG, however, do not have absolutely identical functions – each has special indications which must be discussed for each patient.

An acute SEEG investigation provides a better evaluation of the intracerebral space, as a great number of targets are explored by inserting eight to 12 electrodes – each with five to 20 leads. An acute study can be repeated without difficulty at intervals of several days or months, incorporating any necessary changes in electrode placement. Since the stereotaxic landmarks remain constant, the same entry points of the electrodes, with respect to the double grid, can be used repeatedly.

A chronic SEEG study is performed with a smaller number of electrodes, and provides more limited information concerning the origin and mode of propagation of the discharge. Nevertheless, inasmuch as this approach makes it possible to study the patient repeatedly under different conditions over relatively long periods, it is the method of choice for gauging the lateralization of an ictal discharge or determining the existence of a multifocal epilepsy.

Hence, these two techniques, which some authors have attempted to differentiate for mere technical reasons, are not contradictory but in fact complementary and can be used, depending on the objectives of study, either separately or in succession.

From our standpoint, the number of 'chronic' electrodes should be less than for 'acute' explorations. When surgical interventions are performed (generally two or three months after the SEEG), the visualization of the positions of the different electrodes is of enormous assistance in determining the prefixed limits of the removal. The marks left on the cortex by the 'chronic' electrodes are much more prominent than those left by the 'acute' ones – this in spite of the different diameters of the two types of electrodes (acute: diameter = 2.4 mm; chronic: diameter = 0.8 mm).

With regard to the distance between the different electrodes, we generally introduce them at a distance of not less than 20 mm, although this may change when we simultaneously explore the amygdala and the anterior part of the Ammon's horn, or when we record the electrical activity in the immediate neighbourhood of an epileptogenic tumour (Munari *et al.*, 1984).

It must be stressed that the recording of the intracerebral electrical activity does not have any relevance if it is not accompanied by strict, permanent, clinical control. Thus, in our programme, the clinical features (both ictal and interictal) of the patients being explored are simultaneously:

(a) observed by two neurologists;
(b) dictated on magnetic tape, and written on the SEEG paper by the EEG technicians;
(c) filmed (by two cameras) and recorded on videotape.

At the same time, the SEEG recording is recorded by another camera; the recordings of the patient and of the SEEG are combined in the same composite picture. The SEEG technicians can alter the television screen according to the clinical changes which occur during the recording.

Finally, the intracerebral electrical activity is simultaneously recorded (Elema-Schönander, 24 channel apparatus) along with the scalp EEG. The depth electrodes precisely explore the neighbouring nervous tissue, while the scalp EEG allows evaluation of the larger electrical changes, especially in the hemisphere contralateral to the side of the invesigation. Several autonomic parameters and electromyograms (EMGs) are also simultaneously recorded.

Interpretation of SEEG data

We now define the usefulness of the information furnished by the SEEG.

'Lesional' area

Since the advent of the CT scan, it is generally accepted that more than 60% of patients with partial epilepsy have an 'anatomical' lesion (Gastaut and Gastaut, 1976). In reality, however, an anatomical lesion is not always evident on the CT scan. Moreover, in many patients without CT or other neuroradiological abnormalities, either macroscopic lesions or histopathologic alterations (Talairach *et al.*, 1974) can be uncovered by surgical intervention. Thus, the complete spatial definition of a cerebral lesion on the basis of only the CT scan is sometimes quite difficult or even impossible. By contrast, the SEEG patterns indicating a 'lesion' are as follows:

(1) altered background activity;
(2) irregular, low voltage, slow waves;
(3) continuous, polyrhythmic, high-voltage slow waves;
(4) continuous delta waves;
(5) flattening;
(6) so-called 'electrical silence'.

The definition of a lesion is, therefore, not only a matter of the CT scan diagnosis, but is the result of a multimodal approach, including, of course, evaluation of permanent neurological deficits. In patients with epileptogenic tumours, for example, the existence of very important 'lesional' changes does not preclude such altered areas from participating in the elaboration of the seizures (Munari *et al.*, 1983, 1984b). In other words, the 'lesional' area may or may not, to a varying degree, coincide with the epileptogenic area. The study of the topographic relationships between the 'lesional' and the 'epileptogenic areas' is unavoidable in epileptic surgical candidates; the SEEG investigations are very valuable (Munari, 1983) in this regard.

'Irritative' area

Since the first use of intrasurgical electrocorticography (Foerster and Altenburger, 1935) and especially because of the excellent work of Penfield, Jasper and their co-workers (Jasper and Penfield, 1949; Jasper, Arfel-Capdevielle and Rasmussen, 1961; Penfield and Jasper, 1954, 1961), this method was applied and developed over the years (Niedermeyer, 1982).

The characteristics of the interictal 'irritative' discharges are very important in delimiting the epileptogenic zone, as well as the reproduction of the 'aura' of the seizures, and the evaluation of the types and extension of the abnormal afterdischarges. There is general agreement with Penfield and Jasper (1954) that a proven epileptogenic lesion in the cortex can produce, in the surrounding tissues, spike abnormalities which constitute the most common form of stationary epileptic discharges. The 'stationary' nature of these discharges is defined as follows: discharges which are sporadic, of high voltage, short duration, peaked form (that is, isolated spikes, spikes grouped in short bursts, or even slow spikes and waves), of limited extension, and occurring on an altered basic rhythm. If the characteristics listed above could unambiguously indicate the existence of a focal epileptogenic process, the value of corticography could no longer be questioned (Talairach and Bancaud, 1973). The standard recording technique, however, allows only limited exploration of the cortex in one of several successive planes; such planes cannot be studied simultaneously, but only when their connections have been interrupted by surgery.

The anatomical basis of the difficulties in defining criteria for differentiating between stationary activities, which have localizing value, and propagated activities are clearly shown in a longitudinal brain section where the external cortex is almost in contact with the internal cortex (Talairach and Bancaud, 1973). Moreover, the occasional use of an 'additional' depth electrode during electrocorticography seems to provide 'little additional information' (Graf, 1984).

Because of difficulties in recording spontaneous seizures, or because of problems in the interpretation of such seizures when they are induced by withdrawal (Engel *et al.*, 1983; Engel and Crandall, 1983; Spencer *et al.*, 1982), some authors suggest that the recording of seizures has been overemphasized and that more importance should be placed on the interictal spikes. Another argument in favour of the value of interictal as opposed to ictal discharges relates to the possibility that local ictal activity may be missed by a few millimetres if there is insufficient conduction from the discharging structure to the nearest electrode (Cooper *et al.*, 1965).

On the other hand, Bancaud (1967) showed that utilizing only the interictal spikes, even if stationary, as a localizing criterion may lead to two different and opposing mistakes – one might consider as unifocal (more particularly unitemporal) a bilateral epilepsy, or one might consider as multifocal a focal epilepsy.

The clinical study of the usual seizures in a given patient, therefore, is the optimal guide. Even taking into account the topography of the interictal 'irritative' abnormalities, we prefer to define an epileptogenic area primarily on the basis of the seizures recorded.

Epileptogenic area

The definition of the epileptogenic area (EA) is of enormous importance, since surgical intervention will be programmed and accomplished on the basis of such studies (Talairach *et al.*, 1974). An incomplete and somewhat theoretical definition of the epileptogenic area might be: the site of the beginning and of the primary organization of the epileptic seizures.

Clearly, during SEEG investigations only the simultaneous critical evaluation of the clinical and electrical features will allow a correct understanding of the seizures.

WELL-LOCALIZED DISCHARGES

An ictal discharge (usually low-voltage fast activity) may affect only a well-localized structure. The occurrence (or absence) of clinical signs vary as a function of the localization of the discharge. In a series of more than 400 temporal lobe seizures recorded in 120 patients, the amygdaloid nucleus was affected by a well-localized discharge in less than 3% of the cases – localized meaning without any recruitment of other temporal structures. In these cases, we never observed any clinical signs and the patients denied any subjective symptoms, except that some patients appeared to have increased alertness, akin to an awakening, but not perceived by the patient himself (Munari *et al.*, 1984c). A discharge confined only to the anterior part of the hippocampus (anterior part of the Ammon's horn) may also be asymptomatic or may coincide with subjective manifestations (*Figure 14.6*). A relatively long discharge involving both the amygdala and the anterior part of the Ammon's horn may not, however, be seen on the scalp EEG (*Figure 14.7*). Moreover, an intracerebral discharge which is well localized in extratemporal regions may not modify the neighbouring interictal spikes (*Figures 14.8* and *14.9*).

When such well-localized ictal discharges occur, they are of important localizing value (Bancaud, 1981) if they affect very 'expressive' cortical areas; some examples are the lateralized somatomotor manifestations when the discharges affect the central area, the auditory hallucinations when they involve Heschl's gyrus, the visual hallucinations when the pericalcarine visual cortex is affected, and the well-localized sensory disturbances (paraesthesiae or pain) during rare discharges which are highly localized in the postcentral gyrus. These subjective manifestations, often defined as 'auras' (Penfield and Jasper, 1954) may on occasion be followed by other clinical symptoms, in which case the discharge secondarily involves other cerebral structures.

DISCHARGES AFFECTING DIFFERENT STRUCTURES IN THE SAME LOBE

The clinical features which characterize a seizure are strictly related to the spatial and temporal evolution of the discharge in the brain. The chronological sequence of different symptoms may, in many cases, allow a hypothesis of the structures involved and the order in which they are progressively disturbed. For example, a seizure starting with an auditory hallucination followed by nausea and by oroalimentary motor 'automatic activity' such as chewing corresponds to a discharge beginning in the Heschl's gyrus, with secondary spread to Ammon's horn and to the amygdala.

In the frontal lobe, where well-localized discharges are more uncommon, a seizure starting in the anterior part of the cingulate gyrus (area 24) is very often characterized by automatic gestural activity, with or without an impairment of consciousness (Stoffels *et al.*, 1980). A discharge starting in the anterior internal frontal cortex may initially be asymptomatic, but if the discharge spreads to area 24, the patient will present with automatic gestural activity (Stoffels *et al.*, 1981a).

In the occipital lobe the occurrence of visual hallucinations is often associated with ocular deviation (Munari *et al.*, 1984a); the hallucinatory component is strictly linked to dysfunction of the visual cortex, whereas the eye movements are also related to involvement of the pericalcarine areas (Bancaud *et al.*, 1984b).

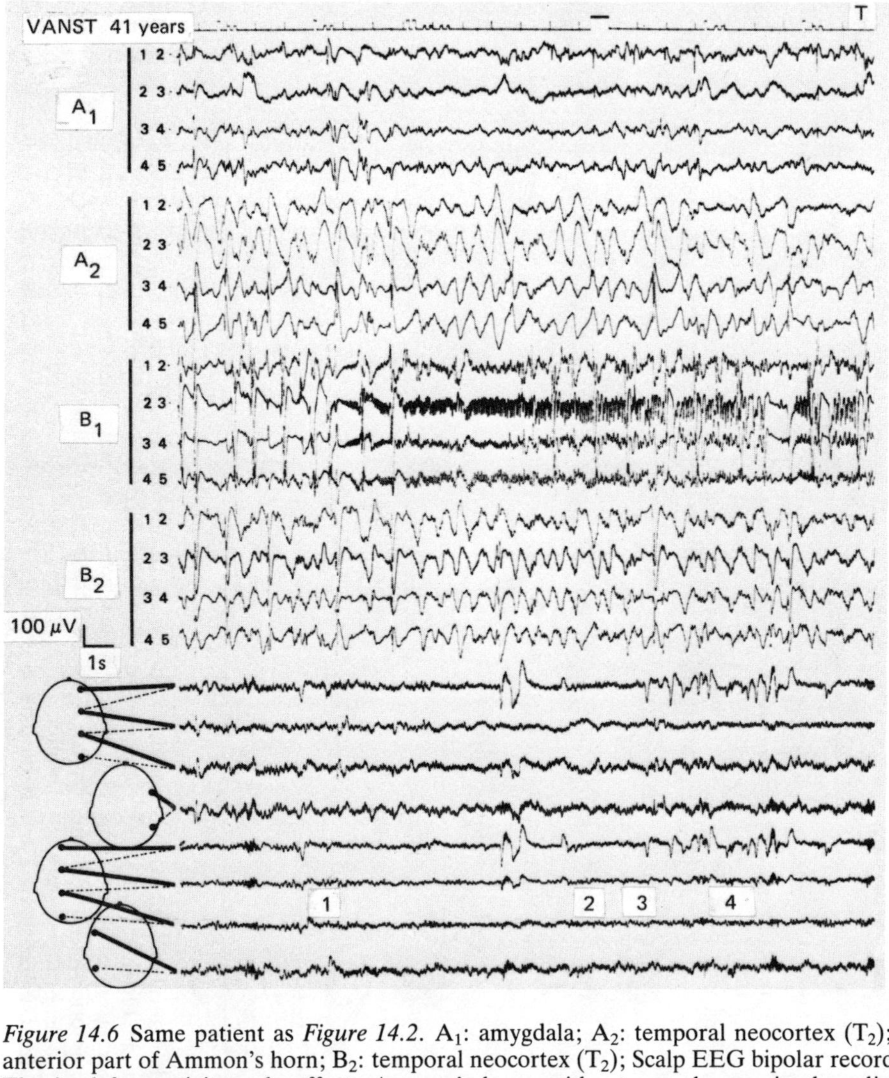

Figure 14.6 Same patient as *Figure 14.2*. A_1: amygdala; A_2: temporal neocortex (T_2); B_1: anterior part of Ammon's horn; B_2: temporal neocortex (T_2); Scalp EEG bipolar recording. The ictal fast activity only affects Ammon's horn, without any changes in the adjacent temporal neocortex (or in the scalp). This very limited discharge is associated with the following clinical symptoms: 1: She says: 'I will roll'; 2: 'Do not speak aloud'; 3: chewing: 4: loss of contact (she does not answer). The patient explains a few seconds later, before the end of the discharge, that she had nausea and could not answer

DISCHARGES INVOLVING SEVERAL LOBES

The ictal symptomatology is, of course, more 'complex' when the ictal discharges affect more than one cerebral lobe. The involvement of different lobes does not necessarily mean, however, that the epilepsy is 'multifocal'.

In *Figure 14.5*, we have a good example of a stereo-EEG exploration of both temporal and frontal lobes in both hemispheres. In this case, the stereo-EEG data

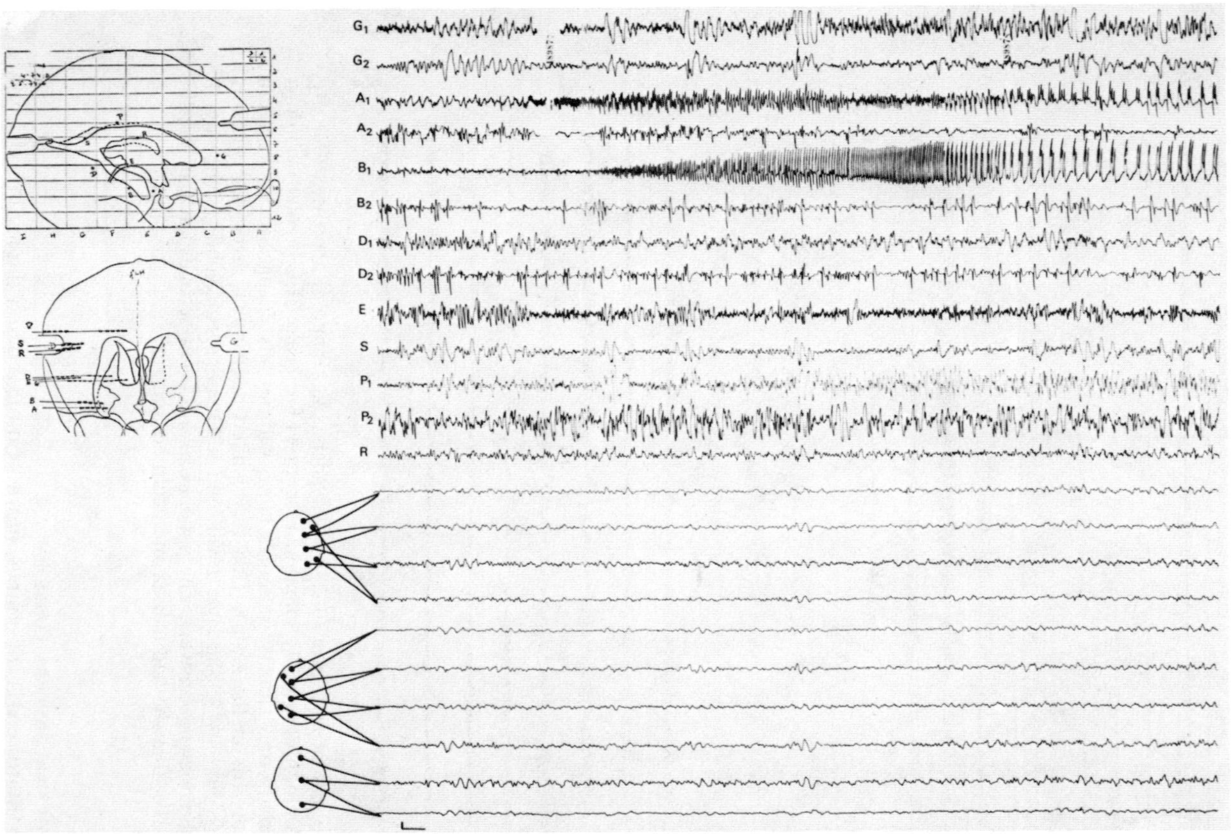

Figure 14.7 On the left side, lateral and anteroposterior view of depth electrodes exploring the right temporoparietal region and, only one electrode, the right frontal lobe. On the right side, SEEG recording of an 'infraclinical' electrical seizure. SEEG: G_1: anterior part of cingulate gyrus; G_2: external frontal cortex; A_1: amygdaloid nucleus; A_2: second temporal convolution; B_1: anterior part of Ammon's horn; B_2: second temporal convolution; D_1: parahippocampal gyrus; D_2: posterior part of second temporal convolution; E: posterior part of first temporal convolution; S: temporoparietal junction (external cortex); P_1: parietal cingulate gyrus; P_2: external parietal cortex; R: central opercular cortex. EEG bipolar recording. A fast, low-amplitude discharge involves B_1 early and then also affects A_1. In spite of the progressively increasing amplitude of the discharge, the interictal abnormalities on the external temporal neocortex are not modified. There are no variations on the scalp EEG

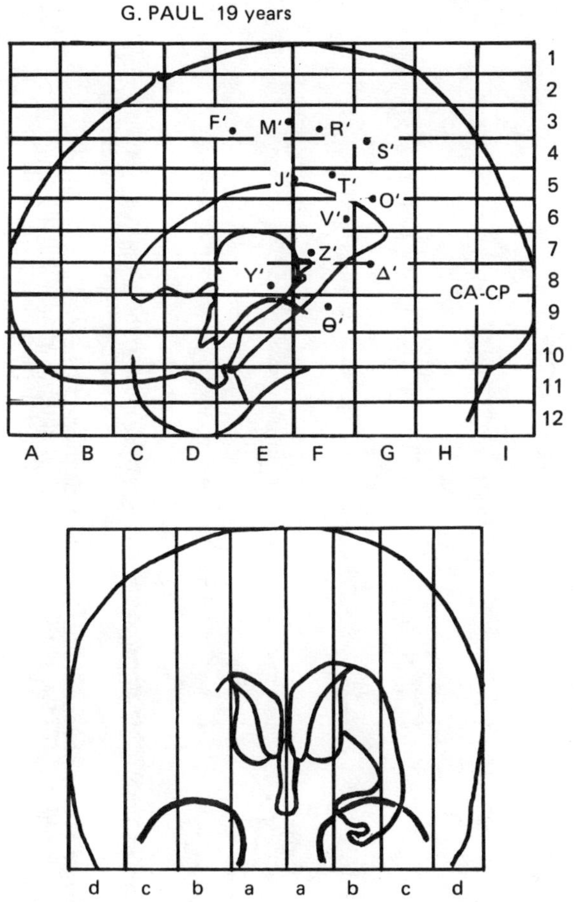

Figure 14.8 Upper lateral view of the electrodes exploring the central, parietal and temporal (posterior part of the first, second and third temporal convolutions) lobes on the left hemisphere. *Lower:* Anteroposterior view of the ventricular system: dilatation of the parietal and temporal ventricles

showed that the ictal discharges started in the deep structures of the right temporal lobe (*Figure 14.10*) and successively involved the temporal neocortex and the frontal cortex in the right hemisphere (*Figure 14.11*). The left temporal lobe was affected much later (*Figure 14.12*), but the discharge persisted in the left amygdala after it ended in the right-sided structures (*Figure 14.13*). The clinical symptomatology (ictal and postictal) was directly linked to the involvement of both temporal and extratemporal structures. In particular, aggressive behaviour characterized the postictal phase (*Figure 14.14*).

The excellent result from surgical intervention confirms that surgical removal of the temporal lobe was sufficient to stop the seizures.

In several other patients, an apparently multifocal epilepsy may be better explained by an analysis of the multidirectional intracerebral trajectory of the

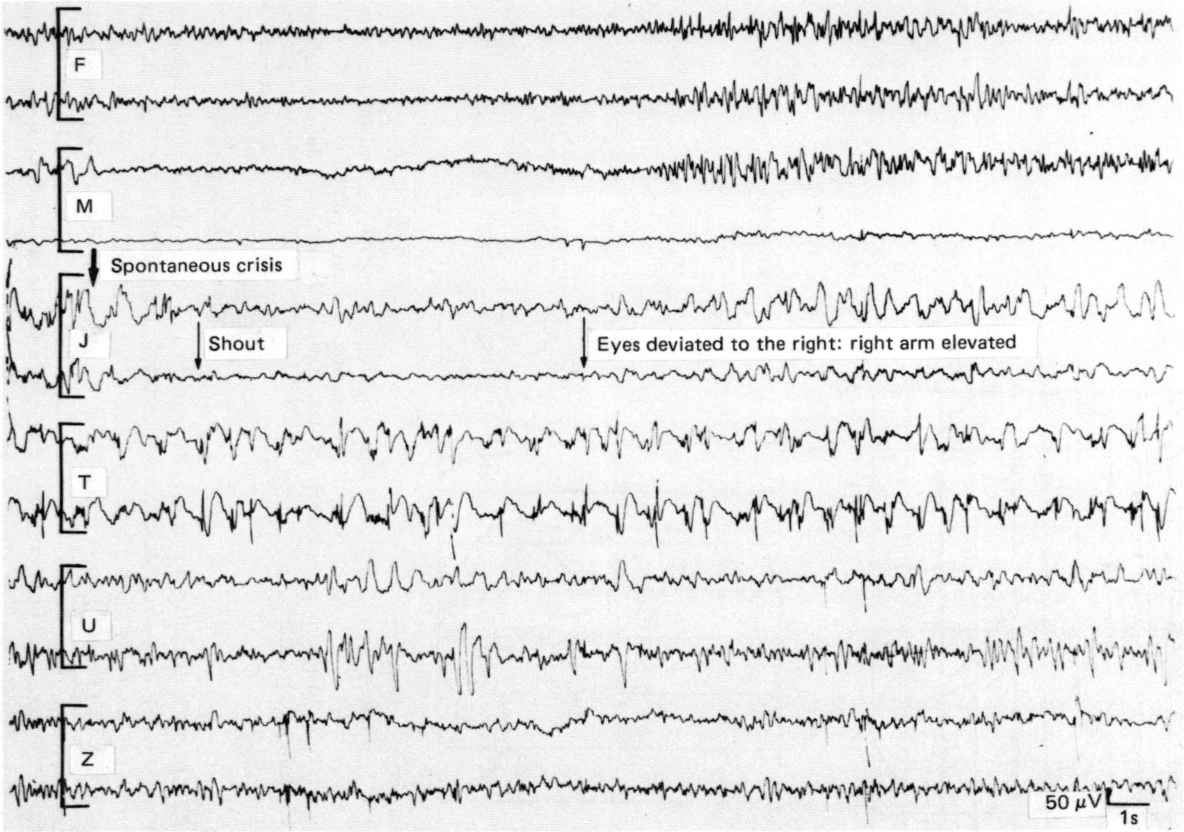

Figure 14.9 The discharge affects electrode M (the patient shouts), and then electrode J (the eyes are deviated to the right side and his right arm is elevated). Interictal spikes at T and U, very near the site of the initial discharge, are unmodified

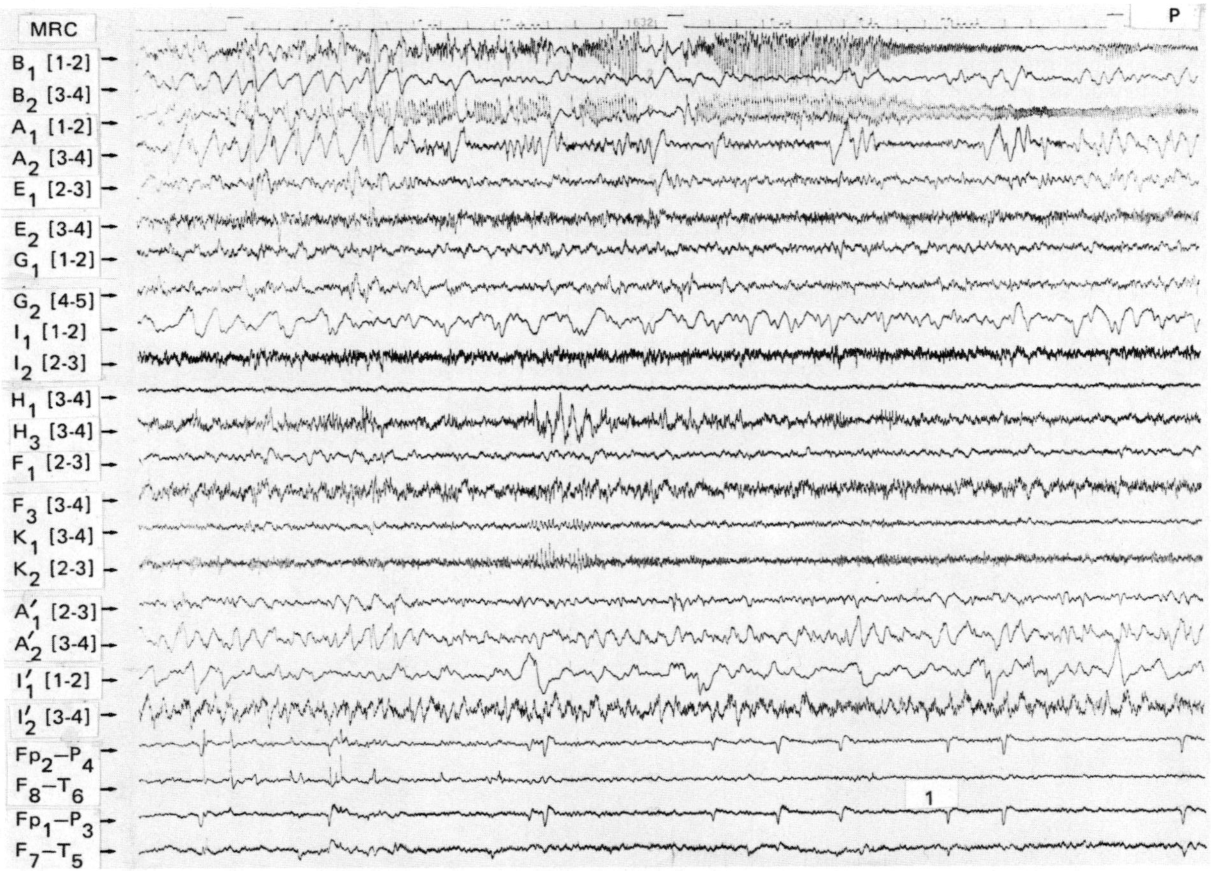

Figure 14.10 Same patient as in *Figure 14.4* (*a*) The initial ictal discharge (fast activity) starts in the right amygdaloid nucleus (A_1) and in the right Ammon's horn (B_1); the interictal spikes are stopped in the right temporal neocortex (A_2, B_2) which is not affected by the discharge – nor are the other explored cortical structures. The discharge is not apparent on the right temporal scalp. (*b*) 1: Question: 'How are you'. Answer: 'Very well, thank you'

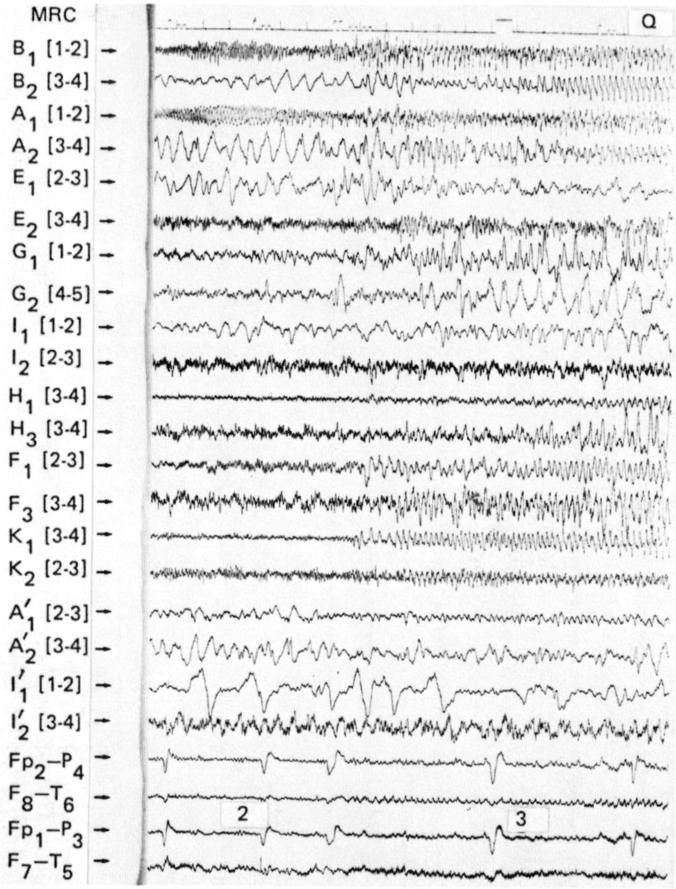

Figure 14.11 (*a*) The right temporal neocortex (A_2, B_2) and the right frontal cortex (E_2, G_1, H_3, F_1, F_3, K_1) are involved more than 40 sec after the onset. (*b*) 2: Mild mydriasis; he says something difficult to understand. 3: He says: 'My head is going away. It is stopping now'

discharges. For instance, a patient with a large cortical atrophic cyst in the central area (*Figure 14.15*) can have different kinds of seizures, the symptomatology of which may be related to:

(1) an anterior onset and spread of the discharge towards the frontal lobe;
(2) a posterior onset and spread of the discharge to the parietal lobe;
(3) various combinations of both (1) and (2).

In this case, the epilepsy was cured by the removal of the epileptogenic areas behind and in front of the anatomical lesion.

Another relatively frequent example of false multifocal epilepsy is seen in the many patients whose epileptogenic area is located in the temporoparieto-occipital junction (Marossero *et al.*, 1980); the spread of the discharge may involve the temporal lobe, the occipital lobe, or the parietocentral region, either isolated or in various combinations. The SEEG is very valuable in such patients but is limited by the degree of knowledge of different possible ictal clinical patterns.

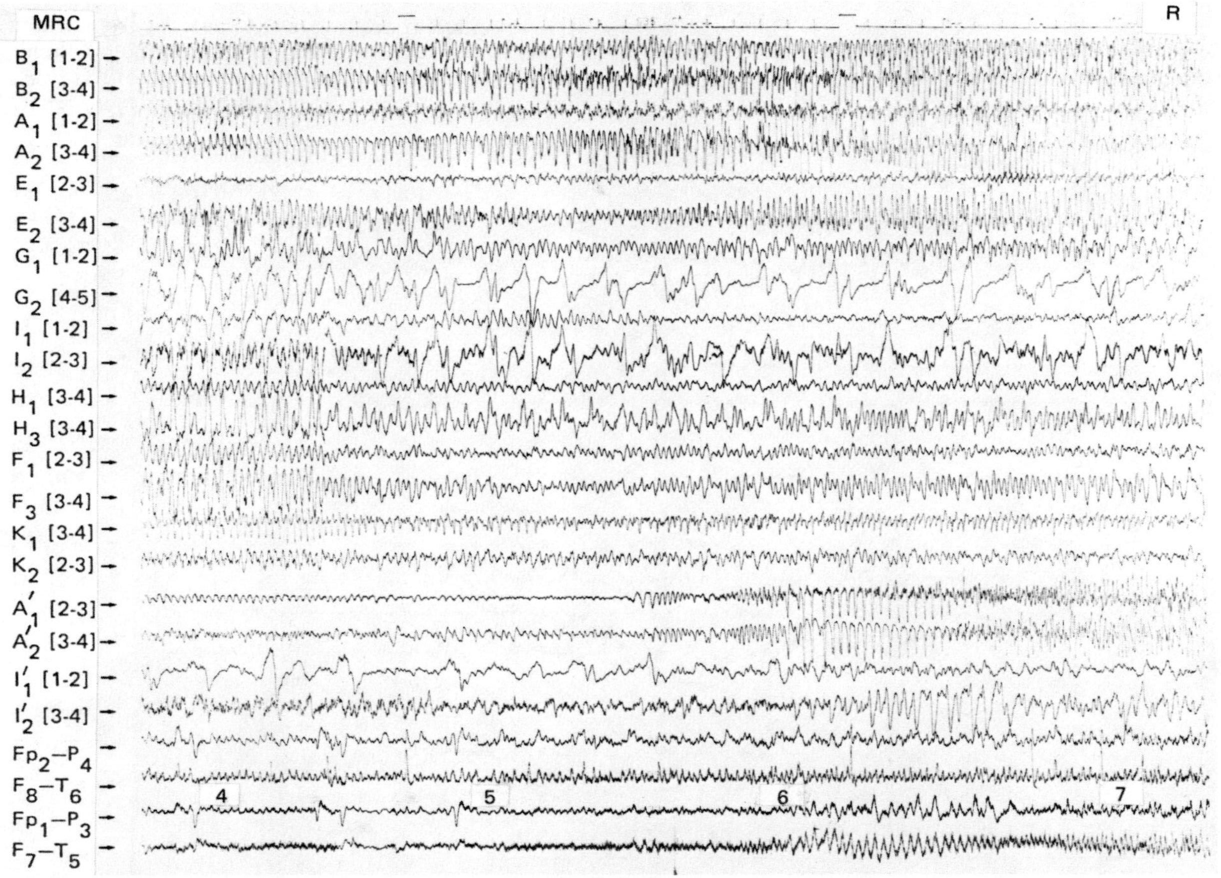

Figure 14.12 (*a*) More than 60 sec after the onset, the discharge involves almost all the explored structures on the right (except E_1, G_2, I and I_2) and spreads to the left temporal lobe (A'_1, A'_2). (*b*) 4: He looks to the left, swallows a few times. 5: Question: 'How old are you?' Answer: '26 years old'. 'Facing to the frontier'. 6: He is still speaking. Question: 'You are 26?' No answer. 7: Eyes to the left, chewing movements. Right eye is more deviated to the left than is the left eye

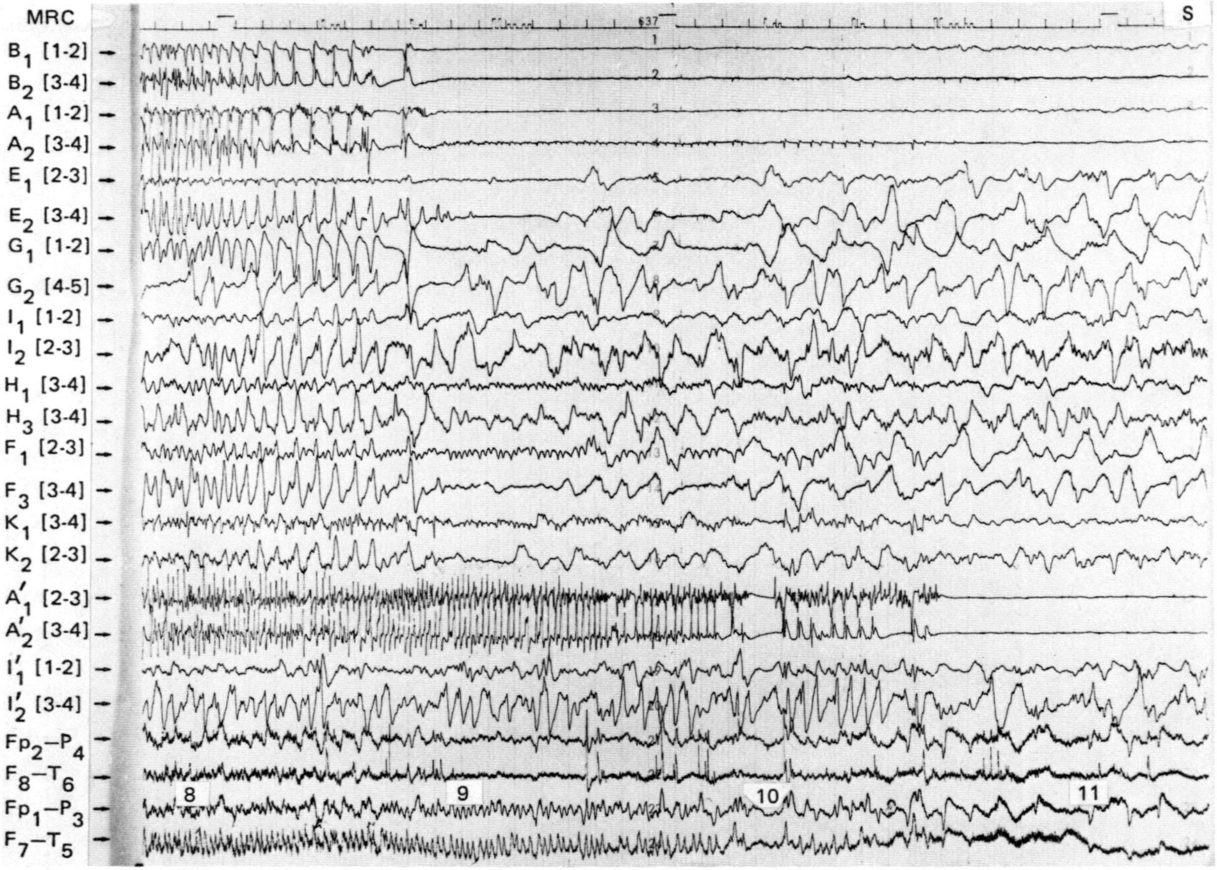

Figure 14.13 (*a*) The discharge persists in the left temporal lobe (A'_1, A'_2) although it has finished on the right. Note the very prominent postictal depression in B_1, B_2, A_1, A_2 and later in A'_1 and A'_2. (*b*) 8: Swallowing movements; contraction of the face. 9: Trismus, clenching of jaw. 10: He does not understand the questions. He relaxes. Sucking movements. 11: The eyes are still to the left

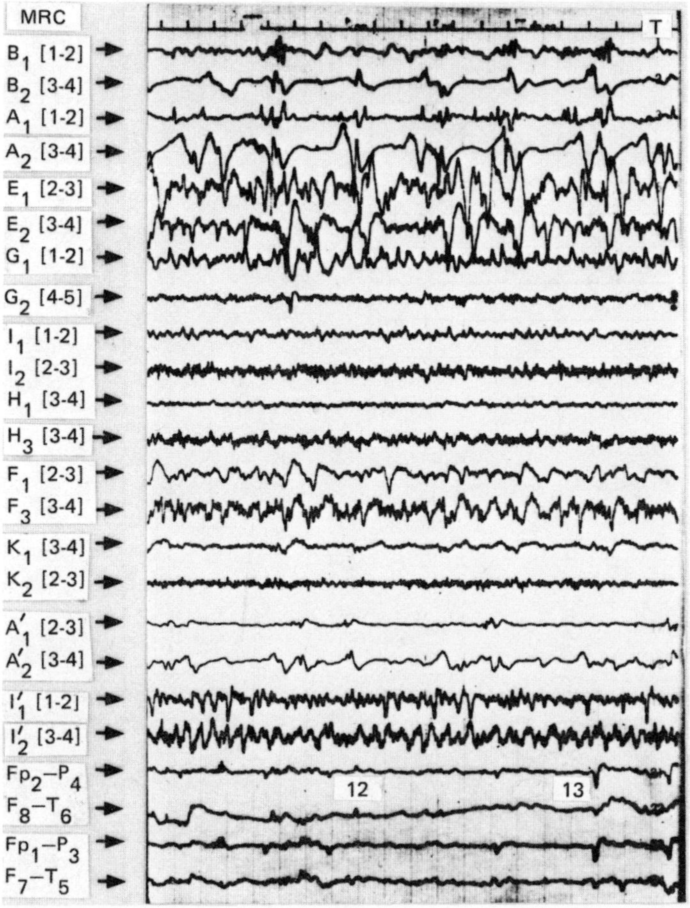

Figure 14.14 (*a*) 8 min after the end of the attack: the electrical activity is still very depressed in the left and right temporal structures; there are continuous slow waves in some frontal electrodes (E_1, E_2, G_1, F_1, F_3, K_1). (*b*) 12: Question: 'How many fingers do you see?' Answer: 'Three' (correct). 13: Question: 'What is this (a wedding ring)?' Answer: 'A ring'

THE CONTRIBUTION OF STEREO-EEG TO THE EVALUATION OF THE LOCALIZING VALUE OF CLINICAL ICTAL SYMPTOMATOLOGY

Success or failure of neurosurgical interventions in partial epilepsies is strictly linked to the topographic definition of the epileptogenic area. If we assume that the occurrence of different ictal symptoms corresponds to the involvement by the ictal discharge of different cortical structures, we can state that, on the basis of the analysis of the clinical signs, we can 'visualize' the intracerebral trajectory of the electrical discharges (Bancaud *et al.*, 1984; Munari *et al.*, 1983).

The SEEG recordings, in association with direct observation of the patients, and with the help of a videotape recording system allow one to:

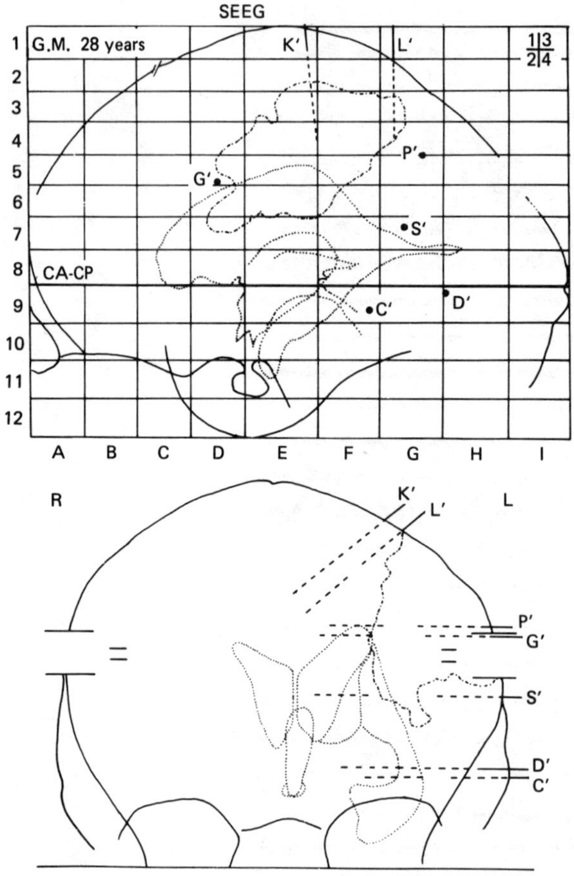

Figure 14.15 Upper: lateral view of electrodes; profile of left ventricles, of the third ventricle, and of the cyst. *Lower:* anteroposterior view of ventricular system, of the cyst and of the electrodes. SEEG of the left hemisphere in a right-handed patient: the electrodes P′ and S′ explore the parietal lobe, the electrodes C′ and D′ explore the temporo-occipital junction G′ explores the cingulate gyrus (24 area) and the frontal cortex (second frontal convolution); K′ and L′ (simple oblique) explore the medial lateral centroparietal cortex and the cortex inside to the cystic lesion. This was chosen in order to avoid going through the cyst. The ictal discharge may start: (*a*) in G′ and K'_1; (*b*) in L′, P′, S′. The clinical patterns were, of course, very different. One seizure, started in L'_1, P′, S′, and secondarily affected K′ and G′

(1) verify whether the occurrence of different (especially initial) symptoms are strictly related to the involvement of the suspected areas;
(2) study the chronological sequence of the symptoms on the basis of the spatial intracerebral evolution of the discharges;
(3) ascertain whether the temporal relationships between the clinical and electrical phenomena are in agreement with the preliminary hypothesis.

Among the different clinical symptoms which can occur during a partial seizure, some have important and precise localizing values. Other clinical signs, however, are considered to be components of a homogeneous group of symptoms. The best example of this type of symptoms are the so-called automatisms. Since Jackson, this expression is more and more widely used, but because of the clinical complexities, no universal agreement exists on the classification of automatisms (Ajmone Marsan and Ralston, 1957; Gastaut and Broughton, 1972; Penry and Dreifuss, 1969).

Automatisms, however, are one of the two signs which permit differentiation of partial seizures with 'complex' symptomatology from those with 'elementary' symptomatology (Gastaut, 1970). Automatic behaviour – although a symptom which frequently occurs during temporal lobe seizures – can be linked with seizures arising from a variety of cortical structures such as the frontal convexity (Penfield and Jasper, 1954), the supplementary motor and parieto-occipital regions (Ajmone Marsan and Ralston, 1957), the cingulate gyrus (Bancaud *et al.*, 1976; Stoffels *et al.*, 1981a; Talairach *et al.*, 1973), and others. Moreover, automatisms may also occur during petit mal absences (Penry and Dreifuss, 1969). On the other hand, some authors consider that in patients with automatisms the ictal discharge invariably spreads either to both temporal lobes or to the temporoparietal cortex or often to the frontal cortex (Jasper, 1954); the discharge cannot be focal, in the usual sense of unilateral or localized (Aird, 1977). In most of these studies, the automatisms are considered to be homogeneous, but hypotheses on the localization of the discharges are usually theoretical and are as yet unproven.

The stereo-EEG studies of partial seizures with automatisms have allowed us to observe that different types of automatisms may correspond to different loci of the electrical discharges (Munari *et al.*, 1981b). In fact, oroalimentary automatic activities of motor type, such as chewing, appear to be strictly linked with ictal involvement of the amygdaloid nucleus (Munari *et al.*, 1979). On the contrary, a simple gestural activity is not limited to discharges affecting the anterior deep temporal structures (Munari *et al.*, 1980a). Rather, this type of automatism seems to be related to ictal dysfunction of the frontal lobes (Stoffels *et al.*, 1980) – more precisely, to the anterior part of the cingulate gyrus (area 24 of Broadman) (Bancaud *et al.*, 1972, 1976; Munari *et al.*, 1981b; Stoffels *et al.*, 1981a; Talairach *et al.*, 1973).

Considering also that complex gestural automatisms may also occur from discharges affecting the parietal lobe, one might also enquire as to the localizing value of these symptoms.

The other clinical symptom characterizing so-called 'complex partial seizures' is 'impairment of consciousness' or 'loss of contact'. This phenomenon, difficult both to observe and to interpret, is considered by some as almost pathognomonic of temporal lobe seizures. Stereo-EEG studies suggest that only rarely (three out of 72 seizures reported) does a discharge limited to the temporal limbic structures provoke an impairment of consciousness (Gloor, Olivier and Ives, 1980). The occurrence of a loss of contact, therefore, seems to be related to both the duration and the extent of the discharges which start in the temporal lobe (Munari *et al.*, 1980b).

Moreover some automatisms, such as chewing, may occur without any impairment of consciousness, if the ictal discharges stay limited to the deep anterior temporal structures (amygdala, temporal pole, anterior part of Ammon's horn) (Munari *et al.*, 1979, 1982). Thus, automatisms and impairment of consciousness are not necessarily linked. The contribution of stereo-EEG explorations to the understanding of the experiential ictal phenomena (Jackson's 'dreamy states') constitutes another example of some important methodological difficulties. In his pioneering studies, Penfield and co-workers (Mullan and Penfield, 1959; Penfield and Perot, 1963) attributed experiential phenomena to neocortical mechanisms only. Very recently, however, Gloor *et al.* (1982) described experiential phenomena from direct stimulation of the amygdaloid nucleus without associated afterdischarges. The discrepancy between these opinions may be explained by methodological differences. Penfield *et al.* did not simultaneously record the amygdala activity during neocortical stimulation, and, moreover, they had already removed the critical temporal neocortex when they stimulated the amygdala complex.

Our findings document that experimental phenomena are reported by a patient only when there is evidence of simultaneous electrical involvement of the temporal neocortex (perceptive component?), the amygdala (emotional component?) and hippocampus (memory component?) (Bancaud, 1981; Brunet, 1984; Munari *et al.*, 1984c).

Finally, we stress that a localizing value could not be attributed to any clinical symptom without taking into account the precise moment of the occurrence of the symptom itself. For instance, an oroalimentary automatism occurring during the first few seconds of a seizure should be related to a discharge in the anterior deep temporal structures. However, this same symptom occurring at the end of a 'tonic-clonic' generalized seizure does not have any localizing relevance.

On the other hand, the chronological relationships between the different symptoms are a useful means for visualizing the spatial trajectory of the intracerebral discharge. Lateralized somatomotor manifestations are generally considered as one of the possible symptoms of temporal lobe seizures, although Bossi *et al.* (1984) showed that this symptom is very rare (less than 20%) in temporal lobe seizures, and that it only occurs when the ictal discharges affect extratemporal structures, in other words, the central region.

DISCUSSION AND CONCLUDING REMARKS

The surgical treatment of partial epilepsies has seen much progress, which was not foreseen little more than a century ago (Billings, 1861). We cannot review here the different methodological approaches to this type of surgery (*see* Temkin, 1945; Talairach *et al.*, 1974). However, we must recall the pioneering approach of Foerster who, between 1917 and 1927, operated on 100 epileptic patients. His work was excellently continued by Penfield (Foerster and Penfield, 1930; Penfield, 1930, 1934, 1936) and his co-workers (Penfield and Erickson, 1941; Penfield and Flanigin, 1950; Penfield and Baldwin, 1952; Penfield and Paine, 1955; Rasmussen, 1963, 1983).

The most important instrument used by the group at the Montreal Neurological Institute (MNI) is, without any doubt, the correct, assiduous, and compulsive *clinical observation* of the patients. The help furnished by electroencephalography and electrocorticography needs no additional comment. Penfield's approach, however, did not yield the same good results for all teams using (at least in appearance) the same methodology. The results vary from more than 70% failure (Fasano and Broggi, 1957; Krayenbuhl, Hesz and Weber, 1954; Weber, 1951) to 60–80% success (Guillaume and Mazars, 1956). On the contrary, the surgical results obtained by the Montreal Neurological Institute group are characterized by good, homogeneous results in more than 60% of their patients.

Until now we have only considered the surgical results obtained with the help of electrocorticography. Utilization of the SEEG, in well-selected patients, with a scrupulous respect for the described methodology, allows further improvement on such results (*Table 14.1*). This progress is even more evident if we consider the results obtained in more recent periods (*Table 14.2*), and especially those obtained in temporal lobe epilepsy (*Table 14.3*).

Table 14.1 Results up to 1973; seizures after surgery (from Bancaud, 1980)

	Patients (no.)	*Percentage*	*%*
No seizures	119	54.2	73.3
Exceptional seizures	42	19.1	
Marked reduction (> 50%)	32	14.5	26.7
Unchanged	20	9.1	
Mortality	7	3.1	

Table 14.2 Results 1973–77; seizures after surgery (from Bancaud, 1980)

	Patients (no.)	*Percentage*	*%*
No seizures	44	59.4	81
Exceptional seizures	16	21.6	
Marked amelioration	10	13.5	19
Unchanged	3	4.1	
Mortality	1	1.4	

Table 14.3 Temporal lobe epilepsy. Results 1973–77; seizures after surgery (from Bancaud, 1980)

	Patients (no.)	*Percentage*	*%*
No seizures	25	69.4	97.4
Exceptional seizures	10	28	
Unchanged	1	2.6	2.6
Mortality	0		

Many reasons might explain the difference between our results and the results of Rasmussen (1983), whose data show that 37% of patients with non-tumoral temporal lobe epilepsy and 46% of patients with tumoral temporal epilepsy are seizure free. One reason may be the greater number of patients operated on in Montreal, even if the percentage of complete recoveries seems relatively stable over the decades.

On the other hand, it is possible that our criteria for operating on patients are more selective; we may have excluded patients who might be improved but not completely cured from their epilepsy. With regard to this point, we should stress that our selection is probably too strict. In fact, if we consider the respective success and failure rate according to the previous accuracy of SEEG localization (*Table 14.4*), we observe that when the localization was considered correct we had only 10% failure. On the contrary when the SEEG localization of the epileptogenic area was considered to be inadequate only 30% of the patients operated on were cured.

Table 14.4 Success and failure rate according to accuracy of SEEG localization (from Bancaud, 1980)

		Patients (no.)	
Localization (estimated)	success	failure	total
Correct	143	14	157
Inadequate	19	38	57

It raises the other problem of evaluating 'how much of the cortex contiguous to the site of origin is recruited into action to produce a clinical seizure?' (Rasmussen, 1983). It is clear that very limited excisions are generally ineffective in suppressing seizures (Ojemann and Ward, 1974), with several well-defined exceptions (Wieser and Yasargil, 1982). However, our 'good' results in spite of a 'bad' SEEG study seem to show that 'when a large proportion of epileptogenic cortex is removed, the remaining fringe of apparently epileptogenic cortex is either subclinical in epileptogenic potential or the epileptogenicity runs down in the early postoperative periods' (Rasmussen, 1983).

Yet another point for discussion is the old problem of the localizing value of the interictal 'irritative' abnormalities recorded during electrocorticography. Passing over many methodological aspects, such as anaesthetic problems, or the actual position of the electrodes (in other words, on the arachnoid rather than on the cortex), we address the question of whether electrocorticography might allow one to avoid the complex procedure of SEEG prior to the surgery. It is not necessary to stress the fact that the SEEG is the most reliable electrophysiological study for localizing epileptogenic lesions in those patients in whom the lateralization of the lesion is unclear (Ajmone Marsan, 1980; Engel *et al.*, 1981; Gloor, 1975; Spencer, 1981). Also we shall not document further the fact that the ictal paroxysmal activity has the most important localizing value, both during SEEG (Bancaud *et al.*, 1965; Crandall, 1973; Wieser, 1983) as well as during electrocorticography (Penfield and Jasper, 1954).

The existence of spatial relationships between the 'lesional' area, the 'epileptogenic' area, and the region involved in spiking activity is generally accepted. But in epileptic patients, as well in experimental models, these three anatomofunctional entities do not necessarily coincide. Furthermore, the interictal spike activity may fluctuate greatly.

The temporal relationships between the occurrence of ictal phenomena and the interictal spike activity are worthy of discussion. Seino and Kakegawa (1982) noted in certain patients that interictal spikes decreased during the several months in which the medical treatment had stopped the seizures. The question, clearly, is whether such patients have fewer interictal spikes because they are not having seizures, or whether they are not having seizures *because* they do not have spikes. Gotman (1984), on the basis of a careful study of kindled cats, demonstrated that spontaneous seizures could occur both when the interictal spiking rate is high and when it is low. He concluded that seizures and interictal spiking might be generated by separated pathophysiological mechanisms – 'the seizure-generating mechanism influencing the spike generating mechanisms, but not the reverse'.

Very recently, on the basis of a retrospective study of 100 consecutive electrocorticographies, Graf (1984) discussed the usefulness of the search for spikes. Among the 100 explorations, 14 tracings had minor or equivocal spiking from the explored cortex which did not influence the surgical plan. In 46 tracings the spike activity was 'dissipated'; in 25, independent spike activity was recorded outside the primarily involved lobe. They concluded that the 'epileptogenic' zones (also thought by them to be the 'irritative' areas) are more widespread that one would have expected from scalp EEG recordings. But it is well known since the studies of Abraham and Ajmone Marsan (1958) that a considerable number of epileptiform discharges which present at a cortical level are not recorded with the routine (overlying) scalp electrodes, and that the ratio of the amplitude cortical:scalp, is highly variable – values may oscillate from two to one to 58 to one.

Hori, Bancaud and Talairach (1970) showed, on a group of 100 patients, that about 25% of patients having interictal spikes in the temporal region had seizures originating elsewhere, and that one-third of patients with a unilateral temporal lobe epilepsy had bilateral temporal spikes. Bancaud, Ribet and Chagot (1975) studied the localizing value of 'subclinical' paroxysms (on the scalp and during SEEG); in more than 20% of the cases, the topographic organization of these subclinical discharges was different of those of the electroclinical seizures.

For all these reasons we consider that electrocorticographic recordings of interictal spikes have much less localizing value than SEEG recordings of electroclinical manifestations during spontaneous seizures. Confirmation of the validity of this methodological approach is provided by the quality of the obtained surgical results (Bonis, 1980). Nevertheless, some criticisms may be made on the SEEG technique itself, as discussed previously. Such remarks could be justified if one does not consider the importance of electroclinical studies preliminary to SEEG. The careful electroclinical analysis of spontaneous seizures, prior to SEEG, accomplished not only with the help of videotape recordings, and most importantly, under the direct observation of at least one neurologist, eliminates any theoretically possible confusion between spontaneous seizures and those which are 'artificial'.

It is evident that this procedure requires a complex organization, gathering together people with wide experience in different aspects of epileptology (Rossi, 1980a). This is, perhaps, one of major reasons why so large a discrepancy exists between the number of epileptic patients who might be considered for surgical treatment and those who are actually referred to the neurosurgeon (Rossi, 1980b; Tassinari, 1984; Ward, 1983).

However, until new diagnostic approaches such as positron emission tomography (PET) (Engel, 1981; and *see* Chapter 13 of this volume) and/or magnetoencephalography (MEG) (Carelli *et al.*, 1983), are able to define precisely cerebral abnormalities, SEEG investigations have a very relevant role in surgery of the epilepsies.

References

ABRAHAM, K. and AJMONE MARSAN, C. (1958) Patterns of cortical discharges and their relation to routine scalp electroencephalography. *Electroencephalography and Clinical Neurophysiology,* **10,** 447–461

AIRD, R. B. (1977) Some observations of clinical interest on the pathophysiology of epilepsy. In *Physiological Aspects of Clinical Neurology,* edited by F. C. Rose, pp. 305–313. Oxford: Blackwell Scientific

AJMONE MARSAN, C. and RALSTON B. (1957) *The epileptic seizure. Its functional morphology and diagnostic significance.* Springfield, Ill. Charles C. Thomas

AJMONE MARSAN, C. and VAN BUREN, J. M. (1958) Epileptiform activity in cortical and subcortical structures in the temporal lobe of man. In *Temporal Lobe Epilepsy,* edited by M. Baldwin and P. Bailey, pp. 78–108. Springfield, Ill.: Charles C. Thomas

AJMONE MARSAN, C. (1980) *Electrography and Electrocorticography, Electrodiagnosis in Clinical Neurology,* edited by M. J. Aminoff, pp. 167–196. New York: Churchill Livingstone

BANCAUD, J. (1959) Apport de l'exploration fonctionnelle par voie stéréotaxique à la chirurgie de l'épilepsie. *Neurochirurgie,* **5,** 55–112

BANCAUD, J. (1967) Origine focale mutliple de certaines épilepsies corticales. *Revue Neurologique,* **117,** 222–243

BANCAUD, J. (1968) Contribution de la stéréo-électro-encéphalo-graphie à l'étude physiopathologique et clinique des épilepsies (dans une perspective chirurgicale). *Aulo Gaggi (Bologna),* 135–155

BANCAUD, J. (1969) Physiopathogenesis of generalized epilepsies of organic nature (stereo-electroencephalographic study). In *The Physiopathogenesis of the Epilepsies,* edited by H. Gastaut *et al.*, pp. 158–185. Springfield, Ill.: Charles C. Thomas

BANCAUD, J. (1980) Topographic relationship between cerebral lesions and seizures discharges. In *Advances in Epileptology, XIth Epilepsy International Symposium*, edited by R. Canger, F. Angeleri and J. K. Penry, pp. 103–109. New York: Raven Press

BANCAUD, J. (1981) Epileptic attacks of temporal origin in man. *Japanese Journal of EEG and EMG,* Suppl. 61–71

BANCAUD, J. and DELL, M. B. (1959) Techniques et méthodes de l'exploration fonctionnelle stéréotaxique des structures encéphaliques chez l'homme (cortex, souscortex, noyaux gris centraux). *Revue Neurologique,* **101,** 220–221

BANCAUD, J. and TALAIRACH, J. (1970) L'électroencéphalographie de profondeur (SEEG dans l'épilepsie). In *Modern Problems of Pharmaco-Psychiatry Epilepsy,* Vol. 4, pp. 29–41. Basel, New York: Karger

BANCAUD, J. and TALAIRACH, J. (1975) *Handbook of Electroencephalography and Clinical Neurophysiology,* edited by J. Bancaud, Vol. 10 part B: 10B-1–10B-65 1975

BANCAUD, J., RIBET, M. F. and CHAGOT, D. (1975) Origine comparée des paroxysmes de pointes 'infra-clinques' et des crises électro-clinques spontanées dans l'épilepsie. *Revue EEG et Neurophysiologie,* **5,** 63–66

BANCAUD, J., TALAIRACH, J., SCHAUB, C., BONIS, A., SZIKLA, G. and COLOMB, D. (1962) Stereotaxic functional exploration of the epilepsies of the supplementary areas of the mesial surface of the hemisphere. *Electroencephalography and Clinical Neurophysiology,* **14,** 788

BANCAUD, J., TALAIRACH, J., BONIS, A. *et al.* (1965) *La stéréo-électro-encéphalographie dans l'épilepsie.* Paris: Masson et Cie

BANCAUD, J., TALAIRACH, J., GEIER, S. and SCARABIN, J. M. (1973) *EEG et SEEG dans les tumeurs cérébrales et l'épilepsie.* Paris: Edifor

BANCAUD, J., TALAIRACH, J., GEIER, S., BONIS, A., TROTTIER, S. and MANRIQUE, M. (1976) Manifestations comportementales induites par la stimulation électrique du gyrus cingulaire antérieur chez l'homme. *Revenue Neurologique (Paris)*, **132,** 705–724

BANCAUD, J., HENRIKSEN, O., RUBIO-DONNADIEU, F., SEINO, M., DREIFUSS, F. E. and PENRY, J. K.: COMMISSION ON CLASSIFICATION AND TERMINOLOGY, ILAE (1981) Proposal for revised clinical and electroencephalographic classification of epileptic seizures. *Epilepsia,* **22,** 490–501

BANCAUD, J., BONIS, A., MUNARI, C., SZIKLA, G., CHODKIEWICZ, J. P. TALAIRACH, J. (1984a) Localizing value of the clinical manifestations of the partial seizures. *Acta Neurochirurgica,* Suppl. 33, 7–15

BANCAUD, J., BONIS, A., KOCHEN, S. *et al.* (1984b) Aspect du contrôle visuel sur l'oculomotricité chez l'homme. *Revue Neurologique* (in press)

BICKFORD, R. G., DODGE, H. W. and SEM-JACOBSEN, C. W. (1953) Observation on depth stimulation of the human brain through implanted electrographic leads. *Proceedings of the Mayo Clinic,* **22,** 333–343

BILLINGS, J. S. (1861) The surgical treatment of epilepsy. *Cincinnati Lancet and Observer,* **4,** 334

BONIS, A. (1980) Long term results of cortical excisions based on stereotaxic investigations in severe drug resistant epilepsies. *Acta Neurochirurgica,* Suppl. 30, 55–66

BONIS, A., CHODKIEWICZ, J. P., MUNARI, C., SZIKLA, G., BANCAUD, J. and TALAIRACH, J. (1981) La chirurgie de l'épilepsie. Méthodologie stéréotaxique, résultats et indications. *Gazette Medicale de France,* **88,** 4125–4130

BOSSI, L., MUNARI, C., STOFFELS, C. *et al.* (1984) Somatomotor manifestations in temporal lobe epilepsy. *Epilepsia,* **25,** 70–76

BRAZIER, M. A. (1956) Depth recordings from the amygdaloid region in patients with temporal lobe epilepsy. *Electroencephalography Clinical Neurophysiology,* **8,** 532–533

BRUNET, F. (1984) *Sémiologie et physiopathologie du 'dreamy state'. Apport de la SEEG à l'étude des crises psychiques.* Thèse en Médécine, Rennes, 13 April 1984

CARELLI, P., MODENA, I., RICCI, G. B. and ROMANI, G. L. (1983) Magnetoencephalography. In *Biomagnetism,* edited by S. J. Williamson, G. L. Romani, L. Kaufman and I. Modena, pp. 469–482. New York and London: Plenum Press

COOPER, R., WINTER, A. L., CROW, H. J. and WALTER, W. G. (1965) Comparison of subcortical cortical and scalp activity using chronic indwelling electrodes in man. *Electroencephalography, Clinical and Neurophysiology,* **18,** 217–228

CRANDALL, P. (1973) Developments in direct recordings from epileptogenic regions in the surgical treatment of partial epilepsies. In *Epilepsy: Its Phenomena in Man,* edited by M. A. B. Brazier, pp. 287–310. New York: Academic Press

DELGADO, J. M. R. and HAMELIN, H. (1956) Surface and depth electrography of the frontal lobe in conscious patients. *Electroencephalography and Clinical Neurophysiology,* **8,** 371–384

DODGE, H. W., BAILEY, A. A., BICKFORD, R. G., PETERSEN, M. C., SEM-JACOBSEN, C. W. and MILLER, R. H. (1953) Neurosurgical and neurologic applications of depth electrography. *Proceedings of the Mayo Clinic,* **28,** 188–191

ENGEL, J. JR and CRANDALL, P. H. (1983) Falsely localizing ictal onsets with depth EEG telemetry during anticonvulsant withdrawal. *Epilepsia,* **24,** 344–355

ENGEL, J. JR, RAUSCH, R., LIEB, J. P., KUHL, D. E. and CRANDALL, P. H. (1981) Correlation of criteria used for localizing epileptic foci in patients considered for surgical therapy of epilepsy. *Annals of Neurology,* **9,** 215–224

ENGEL, J. JR, KUHL, D. E., PHELPS, M. E., RAUSCH, R. and NUWER, M. (1983) Local cerebral metabolism during partial seizures. *Neurology,* **33,** 400–413

FASANO, V. A. and BROGGI, G. (1957) Klinische Beobachtungen bei 36 Faellen chirurgisch behandelter temporaler Epilepsie. *Archiv für Psychiatrie und Nervenkrankheiten,* **195,** 502–507

FOERSTER, O. and PENFIELD, W. (1930) Der Narbenzug am und im Gehirn bei traumatischer Epilepsie in seiner Bedeutung für das Zustandekommen der Anfälle und für die therapeutische Bekäampfung derselben. *Zeitschrift für Gesamte Neurologie und Psychiatrie,* **125,** 472–475

FOERSTER, O. and ALTENBURGER, H. (1935) Elektrobiologische Vorgange an der menschlichen. Hirnrinde, *Deutsche Zeitschrift für Nervenheilk,* **135,** 277–288

GASTAUT, H. (1970) Clinical and electroencephalographical classification of epileptic seizures. *Epilepsia,* **11,** 101–113

GASTAUT, H. and BROUGHTON, R. (1972) *Epileptic Seizures.* Springfield, Ill.: Charles C. Thomas

GASTAUT, H. and GASTAUT, J. L. (1976) Computerized axial tomography in epilepsy. *Epilepsia,* **17,** 325–336

GASTAUT, H., NAQUET, R. and VIGOUROUX, R. (1953) *Electroencephalography and Clinical Neurophysiology,* **5,** 291–294

GLOOR, P. (1975) Contributions of electroencephalography and electrocorticography to the neurosurgical treatment of the epilepsies. In *Neurosurgical Management of the Epilepsies,* edited by D. P. Purpura, J. K. Penry and R. D. Walter, *Advances in Neurology,* **8,** 59–105. New York: Raven Press

GLOOR, P., OLIVIER, A. and IVES, J. (1980) Loss of consciousness in temporal lobe seizures: observations obtained with stereotaxic depth electrode recordings and stimulations. In *Advances in Epileptology, XIth Epilepsy International Symposium,* edited by R. Canger, F. Angeleri and J. K. Penry, pp. 349–357. New York: Raven Press

GLOOR, P., OLIVIER, A., QUESNEY, L. F., ANDERMANN, F. and HOROWITZ, S. (1982) The role of the limbic system in experiential phenomena of temporal lobe epilepsy. *Annals of Neurology,* **12,** 129–144

GOTMAN, J. (1984) Relationships between triggered seizures, spontaneous seizures and interictal spiking in the kindling model of epilepsy. *Experimental Neurology,* **84,** 259–273

GRAF, M. (1984) Electrocorticography: information derived from intraoperative recordings during seizure surgery. *Clinical Electroencephalography,* **15,** 83–91

GUILLAUME, J. and MAZARS, G. (1956) Indications et résultats du traitement chirurgical des épileptsies. *Seminaire des Hôpitaux de Paris,* **32,** 2013–2018

HORI, W., BANCAUD, J. and TALAIRACH, J. (1970) Signification des anomalies EEG intercritiques des lobes temporaux dans l'épilepsie. *Revue Neurologique,* **122,** 493–494

JASPER, H. H. (1954) Some physiological mechanisms involved in epileptic automatisms. *Epilepsia,* **5,** 1–20

JASPER, H. H. and PENFIELD, W. (1949) Electrocorticograms in man: effects of voluntary movement upon the electrical activity of the precentral gyrus. *Archiv für Psychiatrie und Nervenkrankenheit,* **183,** 163–174

JASPER, H. H., ARFEL-CAPDEVIELLE, G. and RASMUSSEN, T. (1961) Evaluation of EEG and cortical electrocorticographic studies for prognosis of seizures following surgical excision of epileptogenic lesions. *Epilepsia (Amsterdam),* **2,** 130–137

KELLAWAY, P. (1956) Depth recording in focal epilepsy. *Electroencephalography and Clinical Neurophysiology,* **8,** 527–528

KRAYENBUHL, H., HESZ, R. and WEBER, G. (1954) Elektroencephalographische und therapeutische Ergebnisse in der Behandlung von 21 fällen mit sogeaonnter Temporallappenepilepsie. *Zentralblatt für Neurochirurgie,* **14,** 206–211

MAROSSERO, F., CABRINI, G. P., ETTORRE, G. *et al.* (1980) Stereo-EEG and surgery in partial epilepsies with temporoparieto-occipital foci. *Acta Neurochirgica (Wien),* **S30,** 113–116

MULLAN, S. and PENFIELD, W. (1959) Illusions of comparative interpretation and emotion. *Archives of Neurology and Psychiatry,* **81,** 269–284

MUNARI, C. (1983) Rapporti fra semeiologia delle crisi e danno cerebrale focale. Atti della Ia Riunione Congiunta della Società Italiana di Nuerologia della Società Italiana EEG e neurofisiol e della Lega Italiana contro l'epilessia, *Rivista Italiana EEG,* Suppl. 1, 63–67, 69–76

MUNARI, C. and BANCAUD, Y. (1983) Valore localizzatorio della fenomenologia critica. *Rivista Italiana EEG,* **Suppl. 1,** 69–76

MUNARI, C., BANCAUD, J., BONIS, A. *et al.* (1979) Rôle du noyau amygdalien dans la survenue de manifestations oroalimentaires au cours des crises épileptiques chez l'homme. *Revue de EEG et Neurophysiologie,* **9** (3), 236–240

MUNARI, C., BANCAUD, J., STOFFELS, C., TALAIRACH, J. and BONIS, A. (1980a) Manifestations automatiques dans les crises épileptiques partielles complexes d'origine temporale. *Progressi in Epilettologia,* 115–117

MUNARI, C., BANCAUD, J., BONIS, A., STOFFELS, C., SZIKLA, G. and TALAIRACH, J. (1980b) Impairment of consciousness in temporal lobe seizures: a stereoelectroencephalographic study. *Advances in Epileptology: XIth Epilepsy International Symposium,* edited by R. Canger, F. Angeleri and J. K. Penry, pp. 111–114. New York: Raven Press

MUNARI, C., TALAIRACH, J., BONIS, A., SZIKLA, G. and BANCAUD, J. (1980c) Differential diagnosis between temporal and 'perisylvian' epilepsy in a surgical perspective. *Acta Neurochirurgica,* Suppl. 30, 97–101

MUNARI, C., STOFFELS, C., BOSSI, L. *et al.* (1981a) Automatic activities in frontal lobe seizures without involvement of temporal lobe structures. *Epilepsy International Symposium, Kyoto,* 63–64

MUNARI, C., STOFFELS, C., BOSSI, L., BONIS, A., TALAIRACH, J. and BANCAUD, J. (1981b) Automatic activities during frontal and temporal lobe seizures: are they the same? *Advances in Epileptology: XIIth Epilepsy International Symposium,* edited by M. Dam, L. Gram and J. K. Penry, pp. 287–291. New York: Raven Press

MUNARI, C., STOFFELS, C., BOSSI, L. *et al.* (1982) Partial seizures with elementary or complex symptomatology: A valid classification for temporal lobe seizures? *Advances in Epileptology: XIIIth Epilepsy International Symposium,* edited by H. Akimoto, H. Kazamatsuri, M. Seino and A. Ward, pp. 25–27. New York: Raven Press

MUNARI, C., TALAIRACH, J., MUSOLINO, A., SZIKLA, G., BANCAUD, J. and CHODKIEWICZ, J. P. (1983) Stereotaxic methodology of 'functional' neurosurgery in tumoral epileptic patients. *Italian Journal of Neurological Science,* Suppl. 2, 69–82

MUNARI, C., BONIS, A., KOCHEN, S. *et al.* (1984a) Eye movements and occipital seizures in man. *Acta Neurochirurgica,* Suppl. 33, 47–52

MUNARI, C., BONIS, A., TALAIRACH, J. *et al.* (1984b) Stereotactic methodology in epileptic patients with hemispheric astrocytoma. *Acta Neurochirurgica,* Suppl. 33, 91–96

MUNARI, C., BONIS, A., MUSOLINO, A. *et al.* (1984c) Amygdaloid nucleus involvement during temporal lobe seizures in man: physiopathological and surgical implications. *Advances in Epileptology: XVth International Symposium,* edited by R. Y. Porter, R. H. Mattson, A. Ward, M. Dam, pp. 463–468. New York: Raven Press

NIEDERMEYER, E. (1982) Electrocorticography. In *Electroencephalography,* edited by E. Niedermeyer and F. Lopes Da Silva, pp. 537–541. Baltimore and Munich: Urban and Schwarzenberg

OJEMANN, G. A. and WARD, A. A. JR (1974) Stereotactic and other procedures for epilepsy. In *Neurosurgical Management of the Epilepsies,* edited by D. P. Purpura, J. K. Penry and R. D. Walter, pp. 241–263. New York: Raven Press

PENFIELD, W. (1930) The place of neurosurgery in the treatment for epilepsy. *Archives of Neurology and Psychiatry,* **24,** 652–659

PENFIELD, W. (1934) Surgery in the treatment of epilepsy. *Surgery, Gynecology, Obstetrics,* **58,** 1041–1043

PENFIELD, W. (1936) Epilepsy and surgical therapy. *Archives of Neurology and Psychiatry,* **36,** 449–484

PENFIELD, W. and ERICKSON, T. C. (1941) *Epilepsy and cerebral localization: a study of the mechanisms, treatment and prevention of epileptic seizures.* Springfield, Ill: Charles C. Thomas

PENFIELD, W. and FLANIGIN, H. (1950) Surgical therapy of temporal lobe seizures. *Archives of Neurology and Psychiatry (Chicago),* **64,** 491–500

PENFIELD, W. and BALDWIN, M. (1952) Temporal lobe seizures and the technique of sub-total temporal lobectomy. *Annals of Surgery,* **136,** 625–634

PENFIELD, W. and JASPER, H. (1954) *Epilepsy and the Functional Anatomy of the Human Brain.* Boston, Mass.: Little, Brown and Co.

PENFIELD, W. and PAINE, K. (1955) Results of surgical therapy for focal epileptic seizures. *Canadian Medical Association Journal,* **73,** 515–531

PENFIELD, W. and PEROT, P. (1963) The brain's record of auditory and visual experience. A final summary and discussion. *Brain,* **86,** 595–696

PENRY, J. K. and DREIFUSS, F. E. (1969) Automatisms associated with the absence of petit mal epilepsy. *Archives of Neurology,* **21,** 142–149

RASUMUSSEN, T. (1963) Surgical therapy of frontal lobe epilepsy. *Epilepsia,* **4,** 181–198

RASMUSSEN, T. B. (1983) Surgical treatment of complex partial seizures: results, lessons and problems. *Epilepsia,* **24** (Suppl. 1), S65–S76

ROSSI, G. F. (1980a) Why, when and how surgery of epilepsy. *Acta Neurochirurgica (Wien),* Suppl. 30, 7–11

ROSSI, G. F. (1980b) Closing remarks. *Acta Neurochirurgica (Wien),* Suppl. 30, 189–192

SCHALTENBRAND, G. and BAILEY, P. (1959) *Introduction to Stereotaxis with an Atlas of the Human Brain.* Stuttgart: Thieme

SEINO, M. and KAKEGAWA, N. (1982) Therapeutic concentration of antiepileptic drugs and the severity of epileptogenesis. *Electroencephalography and Clinical Neurophysiology, Kyoto Symposia,* edited by P. Buser, W. A. Cobb and T. Okuma, Suppl. 36, 438–446. Amsterdam: Elsevier

SPENCER, S. S. (1981) Depth electroencephalography in selection of refractory epilepsy for surgery. *Annals of Neurology,* **9,** 207–214

SPENCER, S. S., SPENCER, D. D., WILLIAMSON, P. D. and MATTSON, R. H. (1982) The localizing value of depth electroencephalography in 32 patients with refractory epilepsy. *Annals of Neurology,* **12,** 248–253

SPIEGEL, E. A. and WYCIS, H. T. (1950) Thalamic recordings in man with special reference to seizure discharges. *Electroencephalography and Clinical Neurophysiology,* **2,** 23–39

SPIEGEL, E. A. and WYCIS, H. T. (1952) Stereoencephalotomy (thalamotomy and related procedures). New York: Grune and Stratton

STOFFELS, C., MUNARI, C., BRUNIE-LOZANO, E., BONIS, A., BANCAUD, J. and TALAIRACH, J. (1980) Manifestations automatiques dans les crises épileptiques partielles complexes d'origine frontale. *Progressi in Epilettologia, Bulletino Lega Italia, Epilettologia*, **29–30,** 111–113

STOFFELS, C., MUNARI, C., BOSSI, L. *et al.* (1981a) Seizures of the anterior cingulate gyrus in man: a stereo-EEG study. *Epilepsy, International Symposium, Kyoto,* 85–86

STOFFELS, C., MUNARI, C., BONIS, A., BANCAUD, J. and TALAIRACH, J. (1981b) Manifestations génitales et 'sexuelles' lors des crises épileptiques partielles chez l'homme. *Revue d'EEG et Neurophysiologie,* **10** (4), 386–392

SZIKLA, G., BOUVIER, G., HORI, T. and PETROV, V. (1977) Angiography of the human brain cortex. Atlas of vascular patterns and stereotactic cortical localization. Berlin, Heidelberg, New York: Springer-Verlag

TALAIRACH, J. and BANCAUD, J. (1963) Processus de l'investigation fonctionnelle dans la neurochirurgie stéréotaxique. Neurophysiologie et neuropsychophysiopathologie. *Actualité Neurophysiologie,* **6,** 137–167

TALAIRACH, J. and BANCAUD, J. (1973) Stereotaxic approach to epilepsy. Methodology of anatomofunctional stereotaxic investigations. *Progress in Neurology and Surgery,* **5,** 294–354

TALAIRACH, J. and BANCAUD, J. (1971) Traitement chirurgical des épilepsies. *Encyclopédie de Medecine et Chirurgie,* **17700 D 10, 9,** 1–8

TALAIRACH, J., DE AJURIAGUERRA, J. and DAVIS, M. (1952) Etudes stéréotaxiques et structures encéphaliques profondes chez l'homme. *Presse Médicale,* **28,** 605–609

TALAIRACH, J., DAVID, M. and TOURNOUX, P. (1958) *L'exploration chirurgicale stéréotaxique du lobe temporal dans l'épilepsie temporale.* Paris: Masson et Cie

TALAIRACH, J., DAVID, M., TOURNOUX, P., CORREDOR, H. and KVASINA, T. (1957) *Atlas d'anatomie stéréotaxique des noyaux gris centraux*. Paris: Masson

TALAIRACH, J., BANCAUD, J., BONIS, A., SZIKLA, G. and TOURNOUX, P. (1962) Functional stereotaxic exploration of epilepsies. *Confinia Neurologica (Basel)*, **22**, 328–330

TALAIRACH, J., SZIKLA, G., TOURNOUX, P. *et al.* (1967) *Atlas d'anatomie stéréotaxique du télencéphale*. Paris: Masson et Cie

TALAIRACH, J., BANCAUD, J., GEIER, S. *et al.* (1973) The cingulate gyrus and human behavior. *Electroencephalography and Clinical Neurophysiology*, **34**, 45–52

TALAIRACH, J., BANCAUD, J., SZIKLA, G. *et al.* (1974) Approche nouvelle de la neurochirurgie de l'épilepsie. Méthodologie stéréotaxique et résultats thérapeutiques. *Neurochirurgie*, Suppl. 1, 240

TASSINARI, C. A. (1984) Surgical treatment of partial epilepsies: the point of view of the neurologist. *Italian Journal of Neurological Science* (in press)

TEMKIN, O. (1945) *The Falling Sickness*. Baltimore, Md: The Johns Hopkins Press

WALKER, A. E. and RIBSTEIN, M. (1957) Chronic depth recording in focal and generalized epilepsy. An evaluation of the technique. *Archives of Neurology and Psychiatry (Chicago)*, **78**, 44–45

WARD, A. A. (1983) *Epilepsy International Symposium, Washington, September* (abstracts)

WEBER, G. (1951) Zum problem der chirurgischen Behandlung fokaler Epilepsien. *Schweizerische Medizinische Wochenschrift*, **81**, 1291–1296

WIESER, H. G. (1983) Depth recorded limbic seizures and psychopathology. *Neuroscience and Biobehaviour Review*, **7**, 427–440

WIESER, H. G. and YASARGIL, M. G. (1982) Selective amygdalohippocampectomy as a surgical treatment of mesiobasal limbic epilepsy. *Surgical Neurology*, **17**, 445–457

15
Surgery for intractable complex partial epilepsy

Paul H. Crandall, Leslie D. Cahan, William Sutherling, Jerome Engel, Jr. and Rebecca Rausch

INTRODUCTION

This topic falls within the realm of a traditional medical motivation – the removal of a limitation on normal healthy life. If seizures are eliminated, not only is the patient relieved from these sudden, unpredictable and occasionally dangerous events, but new evidence strongly suggests that significant gains in cognitive and psychological function may also occur (Rausch and Crandall, 1982). This chapter is limited to the study of complex partial epilepsy because it is the most common single type of epilepsy (Gastaut *et al.*, 1975), because it is often resistant to medical control, and because surgery is more commonly employed for control of complex partial seizures than for other seizure types.

The need for this surgical treatment has recently been emphasized by Ward (1983) and Robb (1975), who also comment on its striking underutilization. However, surgical therapy can only be carried out in those major centers where a high level of technology and complex, expensive resources are available. A complex interdisciplinary team of professional and paraprofessional individuals with special training and experience in the field of epilepsy is required. Given the technical nature of the procedures, the neurosurgeon must be skilled in stereotactic surgery as well as in brain-mapping techniques, and must link closely with a neurologist-electroencephalographer. The team must have support from neuropsychologists, psychiatrists, special nurses and technicians. In addition, access to surgical suites must be on a priority if not dedicated basis. Several existing centers conform to this pattern. Seizures are now recorded by monitoring with simultaneous, time-coded closed circuit television (CCTU) with videotape and EEG biotelemetry. Both split-screen analysis and a digital clock superimposed on videoimages and transcribed in code on the EEG are used for ascertaining time relations between the clinical attack and electrographic patterns.

Current practice in these centers allows technical advances to be objectively evaluated and compared, and has certain advantages such as improved quality control, improvement in ongoing research, and an easing in relations with other relevant medical expertise. It also has disadvantages, such as the exclusion of non-academic practitioners, the inhibition of simplification of procedures, and excessive emphasis on residency training resulting in possible overproduction of practitioners.

When Gastaut (Gastaut, 1969) first presented his draft for a classification of the epilepsies, which was done at the request of the World Health Organization and the International League Against Epilepsy (ILAE) (of which he was Secretary-General), it distinguished three major categories of epilepsy on the basis of seven criteria:

(1) the clinical and EEG manifestations of the seizures, with emphasis on their onset: generalized from the start versus partial;
(2) the interictal EEGs;
(3) the age of onset;
(4) the presence or absence of interictal neuropsychiatric changes;
(5) the habitual response to a more or less specific therapy;
(6) the presence or absence of a more or less evident etiology;
(7) a known or supposed pathophysiology.

We know that the classification criteria have since been considerably reduced in number. As Gastaut prophetically stated 'With these facts in mind I am quite aware of the shortcomings of the classification I suggest – a classification which some regard as rash, or outdated or even useless. Perhaps its chief advantage is that it can serve as the anvil on which critics can hammer out a classification of higher value'. Perhaps this classification is not of use in all types of epilepsy but it does fulfil the needs of surgical treatment of epilepsy if one also adds EEG recordings during the ictus. A protocol in three phases has been developed at the Reed Neurological Research Center, UCLA Medical Center, to elucidate all these important factors in each surgical candidate.

THE CLINICAL AND EEG MANIFESTATIONS OF THE SEIZURES, WITH EMPHASIS ON THEIR ONSET

For many years it was hoped that the site of origin for partial seizures could be identified by a characteristic aura. In the earliest years most surgical operations were in supratemporal locations and were associated with macroscopic pathological lesions; the epileptogenic areas were defined by electrical stimulation – often near primary cortical areas (sensory, motor, visual, language). These stimulations had behavioral effects which indicated a topographic organization, were reliable on repeated stimulations and were consistent between patients.

With epileptic disorders of the medial temporal lobes, patients may have a diversity of vivid auras and a variability of mental responses which are of a complex nature. In our experience slightly less than one-half of surgical patients with temporal lobe epilepsy have auras. In an investigation of 36 patients in our series (Halgren *et al.*, 1978), using electrical stimulation which elicited these auras, we found 20 categories, including: visceral (heart), visceral (alimentary), motor, somesthetic (head), somesthetic (chest), somesthetic (limbs), somesthetic (central body), temperature, spatial illusions, *déjà vu*, unformed auditory hallucinations, unformed visual hallucinations, dream-like hallucinations, and memory-like hallucinations. Although these auras are helpful in establishing the general diagnosis they are not specifically lateralizing or localizing. It has become clear that several properties of these elicited auras distinguish them from the behavioral consequences of the much more specific sensory cortex stimulation. In general, a widespread electrographic response was necessary but not sufficient for an experiential response to occur. Mental responses to temporal lobe stimulation are quite variable between different patients and even between different stimulations in the same patient. A certain category of mental phenomena may be evoked in only a minority of patients. Anterior electrode sites, and sites contralateral to the epileptogenic focus, resulted in a higher likelihood of occurrence of both electrographic and mental responses. The category of mental phenomenon was not related to the anatomical site, however, but rather to patient-specific variables. Our findings suggest that, in contrast to the primary visual or somatosensory areas where the evoked mental phenomena are highly predictable and are closely related to the anatomical site, that mental phenomena evoked by medial temporal lobe stimulation are idiosyncratic and variable, and are related to the personality of the patient stimulated.

Our colleagues, Delgado-Escueta and Walsh (1983), have studied videotapes of patients with verified complex partial seizures. They found that the psychomotor symptomatology of complex partial seizures lasts an average of 3 min, and that the majority of such seizures are not longer than 5 minutes. Full consciousness returns slowly in these patients. Automatisms in complex partial seizures are more complicated than those of generalized absence seizures with which they may be confused. Postictal dysphasia, and the turning of the head and/or eyes in the middle of a complex partial seizure, can be false localizing signs produced by spreading epileptiform discharges.

Types of complex partial seizures

Three major types of complex partial seizures were observed.

Type I

Three phases are present in the first type: (a) arrest and staring: the patient's eyes may show a dazed or wild look and be proptotic; (b) stereotyped automatisms, such as chewing, swallowing, pursing lips, lip-smacking and eye blinking; (c) purposeful reactions to the environment even though the patient still has impaired consciousness and amnesia.

Type II

The main difference from type I is the absence of the motionless stare and the common occurrence of complex bilateral motor actions at the onset of the seizure. These may be as complex as ambulation, circling or running away.

Type III

This type is 'temporal lobe syncope', in which the patient drops to the floor with eyes shut and remains totally unresponsive for 2–3 minutes. This type of attack has not been seen in the UCLA University hospital series but it may have been 'selected against' because of the risk of falling when depth electrodes are in place.

Unfortunately none of these types is lateralizing.

The interictal EEGs

Formerly the EEG diagnosis was based on relatively brief recordings of interictal activity. However, interictal spiking discharges in complex partial epilepsy are frequently multifocal in location and independent in time. Interictal spiking is often bitemporal but may be diffuse or widely distributed. A so-called 'EEG focus' often shifts anteriorly or posteriorly in the same patient during different recordings. Frontal and temporal electrographic spiking frequently overlaps in distribution, an especially vexing problem as the most important differentiation may be between the frontal lobe and the temporal lobe as the origin of the complex partial seizures. Finally, very few ictal behavioral phenomena are specific for a given site of interictal focus.

After depth electrography was introduced, investigators noted that depth interictal discharges were more frequent, of higher amplitude and often bilateral in distribution even when the scalp interictal discharges were predominantly or solely unilateral. Murray Falconer (personal communication), who relied on the interpretation of interictal discharges, responded that 'depth recordings gave him more information than he wanted to know'.

Recently, in a computer-assisted analysis of interictal spike activity in medial temporal lobe sites via depth electrode, the activity was found to be related to the time of the seizures: (1) The rate of focal patterns of spike activity tended to decline significantly several minutes prior to seizure onset, while the rate of independent contralateral patterns did not change. (2) The rate of occurrence of patterns of bilateral, loosely coupled, spike activity (involving focal and contralateral sites) increased significantly across the 20-min preictal segments and was clearly augmented during the 20 min prior to seizure onset. These findings indicate that the degree of bilateral independence in medial temporal lobe spike activity tends to decrease several minutes prior to the localized onset of temporal lobe seizures (Lange *et al.*, 1983).

From the EEG interpretive viewpoint the indications for an analysis by depth electrodes are:

(1) To identify a focal ictal process in patients with bitemporal independent interictal EEG discharges.
(2) To discern whether a deep frontal or a temporal ictal process is the cause of the seizures in patients who have automatisms and/or motor patterns and have scalp EEG evidence of both frontal and temporal epileptiform activity.
(3) To determine the extent of early ictal involvement, especially in the anteroposterior dimension prior to the excision of essential structures.
(4) Rarely, to seek a locus of onset in patients who have clinical seizure patterns which are focal, but who have no clear paroxysmal discharges in the scalp EEG.

Fortunately, when ictal EEG patterns can be recorded these are usually both stereotyped in location (sometimes exquisitely focal) and identical during several attacks. Rarely these can be multifocal, however. Walter (1973) identified three common stereoelectroencephalographic (stereo-EEG) patterns during the onset of seizures: (a) focal epileptiform paroxysms that start in one or two recording depth electrodes; (b) regional epileptiform paroxysms that simultaneously engage more than two recording electrode sites; and (c) generalized epileptiform paroxysms that engage all recording electrode sites. The latter is not an indication for operation.

The age of onset

During the past 20 years a series of 175 patients has been treated at the UCLA Center for the Health Sciences for medically intractable complex partial epilepsy. The typical patient was in his mid-20s and had had epilepsy for more than ten years. In no case was the duration of epilepsy less than three years. Seizure onset was usually during adolescence. One-quarter of the patients reported a family history of epilepsy; a history of febrile convulsions was obtained in 19%.

The presence or absence of interictal neuropsychiatric changes

The association, the cause–effect relationship or the specificity of personality disorders or psychosis to temporal lobe epilepsy remains a controversial issue with an extensive literature. Certainly personality disorders are commonly encountered, and psychosis is a special risk. Therefore, neuropsychological and/or psychiatric screening is essential to any surgical program for epilepsy.

In our experience there is a subset of patients with complex partial epilepsy associated with schizophreniform psychosis. Unfortunately there appears to be an inverse relationship between the occurrence of the seizures and the presence of the psychosis. Seizures are more obvious and frequent early in life, and the psychosis gradually emerges with age as the seizures lessen. Prior to 1966 our experience in six patients showed that after the seizures had been eliminated by surgery the psychotic state appeared to be precipitated. Since 1966, therefore, the presence of a schizophreniform state has been considered to be a contraindication to surgery.

Mental retardation (arbitrarily defined as IQ below 70) has also been adopted as a contraindication, as such patients often have either diffuse brain damage or bilateral hippocampal sclerosis. Under these circumstances an operation poses a special risk to the patient.

The effect of relief of seizure and personality disorders is a topic for a future study in our series.

Neuropsychological examination with regard to localizing temporal lobe dysfunction is described below.

The habitual response to a more or less specific therapy

Prior to any consideration for surgical therapy all patients undergo adequate trials of antiepileptic drugs. It must be shown by the neurologist that their complex partial and/or secondary generalized seizures are intractable to drug therapy monitored by serum drug level determinations. An adequate drug therapy starts with a single drug adjusted until therapeutic levels are established. Adequate time should pass for the drug to reach a steady state. Yet good medical management must stop short of producing systemic or neurological toxicity.

A time limit should be set on attempts to achieve medical control of seizures. An interesting series is that of Lindsay, Ounstead and Richards (1979). They followed 100 children with complex partial epilepsy for 29 years – until adulthood. Five patients died as children before the age of 15. Approximately one-third underwent spontaneous remission after anticonvulsant therapy, were later seizure-free without medication, and were socially independent. Another one-third had their seizures controlled and were socially independent but required continuing anticonvulsants. The remaining third were not controlled by medications and were totally dependent. The series demonstrates that uncontrolled epilepsy has a significant mortality rate; on the other hand it can also be benign with spontaneous remission (some of their children had benign rolandic epilepsy which was an unknown entity at the start of their series). These authors concluded that for those who can reach full recovery, the withdrawal of drugs before the age of 15 is of great importance. When seizures continue, full investigation with a view to possible neurosurgical treatment should be undertaken. These authors concluded that 'a major danger in caring for children with temporal lobe epilepsy is delaying operation for relief of seizures so long into adult life that social recovery has become impossible'.

The presence or absence of a more or less evident etiology

Since the introduction of computer X-ray tomography (CT scans) about 10% of patients with complex partial epilepsy are found to have tumors or arteriovenous malformations. These conditions have their own surgical indications and considerations apart from the seizure problem. It has been noted that surgical outcome is less likely to be satisfactory when the known etiology is previous encephalitis or meningitis.

A known or supposed pathophysiology

The first surgical operations for complex partial epilepsy were guided by *macroscopic* pathology such as cysts, depressed skull fractures, brain atrophy or tumors. After electroencephalographic criteria were developed the underlying pathological substrate of the temporal lobe was not recognized for many years because the limbic structures of the medial portion were removed by suction techniques. After Falconer (1953) introduced *en bloc* anterior temporal lobectomy, the underlying *microscopic* pathology involving the limbic structures was described. Many surgeons have since learned that if the pathologist's report does not indicate the presence of either hippocampal sclerosis, hamartoma, or a small tumor, the prognosis for the patient is less favorable. In our series, histopathological studies were carried out on temporal lobe tissue from 25 patients with complex partial epilepsy who were studied by interictal positron emission computed tomography (PET) with ^{18}F-fluorodeoxyglucose (FDG) and who subsequently underwent anterior temporal lobectomy (Engel *et al.*, 1982). The degree and location of relative interictal hypometabolism measured by PET correlated well with the severity of the pathological lesion, but the size of the hypometabolic zone was generally much larger than the area of pathological involvement.

Preoperative evaluation

Prior to 1977 patients were evaluated by scalp interictal EEG recordings and stereotaxic depth electrode telemetry (SEEG) (Crandall *et al.*, 1963). In 1977 the UCLA protocol for evaluating these patients was expanded to include, on a routine basis, tests of local cerebral dysfunction as well as electrographic monitoring.

Table 15.1 outlines the current preoperative evaluation. Following the phase I evaluation, most patients are then evaluated by the phase II protocol which includes SEEG telemetry. For some patients, however, SEEG telemetry is omitted and lobectomy follows the phase I evaluation. The current criteria for omitting the

Table 15.1 Requirements for admission to phases I and II

	Phase I EEG (surface)	*Phase II* SEEG (depth)
1. *Focal epileptic excitability*		
(a) Interictal spikes	x	x
(b) Ictal onset	x	x
2. *Focal functional deficit*		
(a) Positron emission computed tomography (PET)	x	
(b) Intracarotid amytal: language	x	
memory	x	
(c) Neuropsychometric testing	x	
(d) Thiopental-induced fast activity	x	x
(e) Baseline EEG/SEEG activity	x	x
(f) Afterdischarge thresholds		x

Phase I (2-week admission): continuous scalp and sphenoidal telemetry with CCTV monitoring usually requiring anticonvulsant taper.
Phase II (4-week hospital admission): continuous SEEG telemetry with sphenoidal electrodes and CCTV monitoring during anticonvulsant taper.

SEEG telemetry are: (1) clearcut scalp and sphenoidal EEG findings of localized seizure onset in mesial temporal lobe and frequent interictal spikes in the ipsilateral temporal lobe; (2) focal hypometabolism on PET scanning; (3) and two additional confirmatory tests of local cerebral dysfunction (for example, neuropsychological deficit, Wada memory deficit, or thiopental suppression of fast activity in sphenoidal electrodes). During the past four years approximately one-third of patients have met these criteria and have undergone resection without prior SEEG studies.

TESTS OF REGIONAL DYSFUNCTION

Thiopental activation

During continuous EEG monitoring, thiopental (25 mg) is injected intravenously every 30 s until the corneal reflex is abolished (Engel, Driver and Falconer, 1975; Kennedy and Hill, 1958). The EEG is then visually analyzed for activation of focal spike activity and for focal attenuation in barbiturate-induced fast activity. The current criterion is that a 50% decrease in the amplitude of fast activity in one sphenoidal lead 50% of the time is believed to be a significant asymmetry. The protocol for recording from surface and depth leads is similar.

Wada test

The intracarotid injection of amytal, based on Wada's description (Wada and Rasmussen, 1960), is performed both to lateralize language dominance and also as a test of each hemisphere's ability to support short-term memory (Milner, Branch and Rasmussen, 1962). Transfemoral catheterization is used to deliver 125 mg sodium amobarbital into the internal carotid artery. Memory function is tested by examining the patient's ability to recognize pictures of common objects, written words and unfamiliar forms, using a continuous performance task administered within 4 min of the injection. Simultaneously, the EEG is recorded to aid the determination of spread and duration of drug action.

Position emission tomography (PET) scanning

Positron emission computed tomography (PET) is done as described in Chapter 13 of this volume (Engel). ^{18}F-Fluorodeoxyglucose (FDG) and ^{13}N-ammonia have been used as indicators of local cerebral glucose utilization and relative cerebral perfusion. Currently, the PET criteria used at UCLA for these patients are based on fluorodeoxyglucose scans.

Neuropsychological testing

Neuropsychological testing has focused on tests sensitive to temporal lobe dysfunction. Most reliance has been placed on comparing a patient's performance on verbal and non-verbal short-term memory tests, the immediate and delayed recall of prose, associative learning, and visual-reproduction subtests of the Wechsler Memory Scale (Wechsler and Stone, 1945) and the Rey–Osterrieth draw and recall tests (Osterrieth, 1944). In the absence of other cognitive deficiencies, a verbal memory deficit has been correlated with a dominant temporal lobe lesion while a deficit in recalling material such a line drawing has been associated with a lesion in the non-dominant temporal lobe.

SURGICAL PROCEDURES

Stereotaxic placement of depth electrodes follows the technique of Talairach, David and Tournoux (1958), as it has been modified by one of the present authors (PHC). In our series, our strategy has been to survey both temporal lobes with an anteror-posterior distribution of electrodes in every patient with complex partial epilepsy suspected to have a temporal lobe origin. Filling of the ventricles with positive (water-soluble) contrast and gas permits the direct visualization of the hippocampus and amygdala where they indent the temporal horns of the ventricles. The image of the temporal horn defines the stereotaxic axis of reference from which electrode coordinates are calculated for the temporal sites (*Figures 15.1* and *15.2*). Electrode implantation sites are, bilaterally, the amygdala (AM), and the anterior (A), middle (M), and posterior (P), hippocampus (HC) and hippocampal gyrus (HCG). Self-tapping hollow stainless steel screw guides are placed in the skull according to these coordinates. Epoxylite insulated stainless steel electrodes are then inserted through the screw guides to the calculated depth and locked in place. The electrodes are either coaxial, with a 0.20 mm diameter wire inside a 0.55 mm tube and a tip separation of 1 mm, or bipolar pairs with 0.25 mm wires and a tip separation of 1.5 mm. The exposed electrode surface at either pole is approximately 0.009 cm, resulting in a transfer resistance ranging from 4.7 to 12.5 KΩ, with a mean of about 7 KΩ.

In patients with prominent motor manifestations (type II, for example) or with auras suggestive of seizure origin from other locations than in the temporal lobes, multilead electrodes consisting of nine insulated wires bonded in parallel with 50–150 μm exposed at 4 mm interelectrode distances from the tip, are directed to

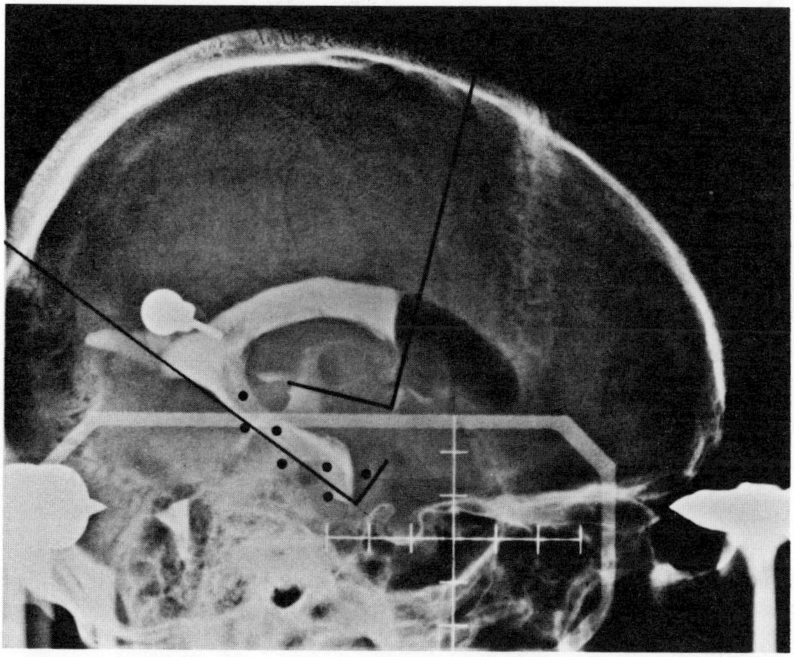

Figure 15.1 A lateral X-ray view showing the VA–LT axis of reference on the temporal horn and the AC–PC axis of reference on the third ventricle. Dots represent anatomical targets for the amygdala, three positions in the pes hippocampi and hippocampal gyrus and, above, the supplementary motor area and frontal lobe

other suspected sites to survey the frontal, parietal or occipital lobes in a transverse orientation. Impedance is 75–200 KΩ. These latter electrodes are not used for stimulation; the coordinates were derived from Talairach *et al.* (1967).

Electrodes in the temporal bone are bonded together into an aggregate plate using methylmethacrylate above the scalp to ensure stability. Insulated nail electrodes, distributed according to the International 10–20 System (except the occipital and frontopolar leads), are used to survey the cortical areas of the convexities. Electrodes for other regions are secure due to the thickness of the skull. The electrodes are led through a sterile head dressing which is changed

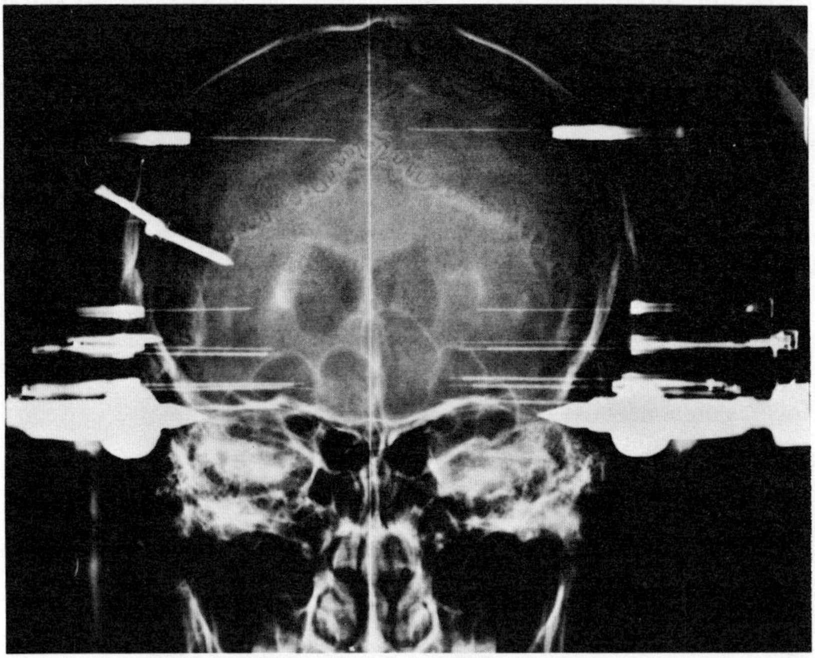

Figure 15.2 Depth electrodes are implanted through hollow screws in the skull; on the right side of the head two insulated calvarial electrodes have been placed; others will complete the 10–20 International EEG Convention

weekly. After the completion of the studies the electrodes are removed under general anesthesia; the cement is drilled away from the head of each screw, each electrode is extracted through the screw, and the screws are then removed.

Complications of SEEG

Depth electrode implantation is not a minor operation. In our 20-year series there have been two deaths related to intracranial hemorrhage within 24 hours following implantation. Modifications in the electrode design and implant procedure have been undertaken in an effort to prevent another occurrence, which clearly remains the major serious risk of the procedure. In two other patients, intracranial hemorrhage at the surface occurred but was easily controlled without detectable neurological deficits. One case of suspected cerebritis seen on postoperative CT scan cleared with antibiotics without residua. Minor scalp infections readily cleared after electrode removal.

While depth implantation is not a trivial procedure, it is also important to note that intractable epilepsy may also be a source of serious morbidity and mortality. In the past six years alone, five patients awaiting admission to the telemetry unit for evaluation have died as a direct result of complications of their seizures.

ANTERIOR TEMPORAL LOBECTOMY FOR COMPLEX PARTIAL EPILEPSY

About 70% of patients undergoing depth implantation have subsequently undergone lobectomy. Those patients in whom the depth recordings showed bilateral or multifocal or diffuse onset did not undergo subsequent surgery. The only exceptions were those rare patients in whom an atypical onset was thought related to rapid drug withdrawal. Since 1979, an additional 12 patients have fulfilled the criteria for lobectomy without implant described above.

Anterior temporal lobectomy has been carried out in a standardized fashion (Falconer, 1971). On the speech-dominant hemisphere, 4.5 cm of anterior temporal lobe (as measured along the middle temporal gyrus) is the usual limit of resection. On the non-dominant hemisphere, 6.0 cm is the usual measurement used. In the majority of patients, general anesthesia was utilized. Electrocorticography was not necessary because of the extensive preoperative investigation. This operation focuses on a maximal removal of hippocampal formation and amygdala and limits removal of lateral neocortex.

Results of temporal lobectomy

The question of how best to evaluate results of surgery has been a difficult one. Seizure frequency alone, while important, does not give a full picture of the results of surgery. An analysis of both the socioeconomic and neuropsychological status of some of our patients has been presented previously (Crandall, 1975). In this report, however, which focuses on the relationship of diagnostic tests versus outcome, we shall report on seizure control only.

The criteria used in this analysis are reviewed in *Table 15.2*. Support from the National Institute of Neurological, Communicative Disorders and Stroke provided

Table 15.2 Postoperative seizure class criteria*

Class	*Description*
1a	Seizure free and aura free
1b	Seizure free, but auras persist
1c	Seizure free for two or more years, but may have had some seizures in years after surgery
2a	No complex partial seizures, but rare generalized attacks (less than one per year)
2b	Nocturnal seizures only
2c	Rare complex partial seizures (less than one per year)
3a	Seizure free for at least one year postoperatively, but then relapse of seizures (more than one per year)
3b	Worthwhile reduction of seizures (more than 90% reduction from preoperative frequency)
4	No worthwhile improvement
?	Lost to follow-up

* 'Neighborhood seizure' in the first month postoperatively and those occurring with medication withdrawal have not been considered in this classification.

travel funds enabling us to interview, at UCLA, the entire series of patients with a responsible family member, and to perform follow-up electroencephalographic and neuropsychological evaluations.

The seizure frequency results are presented in *Table 15.3* for those patients undergoing temporal lobectomy. Statistical analysis of these results (Mann-Whitney rank sum test, Siegel, 1956) showed that the differences between pre-1977 and post-1977 SEEG patients were significant ($P = 0.039$); the differences between pre-1977 and post-1977 non-SEEG patients were also significant ($P = 0.019$).

Table 15.3 Summary of results of surgery (temporal lobectomy patients only)

Seizure	*Patient group*					
class	*pre-1977*		*post-1977 with SEEG*		*post-1977 without SEEG*	
1(a,b,c)	26	44%	21	62%	9	75%
2(a,b,c)	4	51%	3	71%	2	92%
3(a,b)	19	83%	9	97%	1	100%
4	10		1		0	

There was no statistically significant difference between the SEEG and non-SEEG patients in the post-1977 era, although the follow-up time is not as great and changes may occur later. All patients had more than two years' follow-up evaluation.

There have been no operative deaths following temporal lobectomy. Complications include: three patients with partial hemiparesis, one with lasting oculomotor paresis and one who developed postoperative hydrocephalus which was successfully managed by a shunt.

Postoperative management

If the patient has been free from seizures one year postoperatively and the EEG is free from epileptiform activity we have recommended tapering or entirely removing anticonvulsant therapy. Some postoperative patients who have both complex partial seizures and occasional generalized tonic-clonic seizures may have relief from their complex partial seizures but not from their generalized seizures. To be controlled these patients may need an anticonvulsant at a lower dosage.

Patients older than 30 appear to have more psychological or psychiatric disturbances (such as depression, personality disorders, etc.) during the first postoperative year and may for a year or more require a psychotherapeutic program for rehabilitation.

DISCUSSION

We are encouraged that statistical analysis of our results confirms that the expanded preoperative evaluation protocol undertaken in 1977 is associated with an improved surgical outcome. In addition a small group of 12 patients operated upon based on complementary focal functional deficit measures and scalp ictal EEG data but without SEEG seem to be doing as well as those with SEEG. This is not to say that SEEG is unnecessary. On the contrary, we conclude that there is a subpopulation of patients in whom the currently available non-invasive examinations give a good localization of seizure onset. Unfortunately, however, for the majority of our patients, SEEG telemetry remains an essential part of the preoperative evaluation because the non-invasive tests are not sufficiently localizing. Additional analyses are currently under way to review the various components of the protocol, to weed out redundant tests, and to select the most reliable and selective evaluations.

Although we use a variety of tests, the single best criterion for recommending a lobectomy remains the electrographic depth recording of a spontaneous, typical seizure. The data in *Tables 15.4* and *15.5* confirms the fact that interictal spike location frequently is a relatively poor indicator of seizure origin. While a scalp and sphenoidal ictal recording is considerably more informative than the interictal record, there are many instances in which the scalp ictal record alone is still not definitive. For example:

(1) In some patients, the scalp and sphenoidal ictal recording is not localizing. The behavioral change may precede the electrographic change or the surface EEG changes may be diffuse or bilateral. In these cases we have found that depth

Table 15.4 Relationship of scalp interictal spike to depth seizure onset*

Depth	*Location of interictal scalp spike*	
Onset	*Bilateral*	*Unilateral or preponderant*
Unilateral	9 (I)	63 (ipsilateral) (III) 15 (contralateral) (IV)
Bilateral or multiple	7 (II)	16 (V)

* Counted are all patients with records available for review in whom the scalp EEGs were reported as showing temporal spikes; spikes were called predominant on one side when the frequency was visually estimated to be greater than 3:1.

Table 15.5 Outcome by categories of *Table 15.4*

	Class				
Category	*1*	*2*	*3*	*4*	*No surgery*
I	2	1	5	1	
II					7
III	31	3	19	6	4
IV	6	1	4	2	2
V		1	1		14

implantation is a necessary step to localize the seizure onset. In this way, patients who might otherwise be refused surgery may indeed be good candidates.

(2) On the other hand, we have had patients in whom the depth recordings have shown bilateral or multifocal seizure onset and thus we have not recommended lobectomy. Currently about 30% of the patients undergoing SEEG telemetry do not receive a temporal lobectomy.

SEEG telemetry, therefore, allows one to offer lobectomy to patients who might otherwise be denied it, and, on the other hand, to withhold lobectomy from those in whom the likelihood of success appears low.

It should also be noted that while recent results have shown an improved record of success, failures still occur. There are a number of theoretical reasons why seizures may persist postoperatively, including: (a) the presence of a contralateral focus; (b) the fact that the focus is extratemporal but appears to be temporal by SEEG because of sampling error. As experience is gained with newer techniques, including magnetoencephalography, further applications of PET scanning, more sophisticated computer-aided analysis of depth and surface electrographic data, and perhaps NMR scanning, we anticipate a significant change in the evaluation of these challenging clinical problems.

Acknowledgements

This research was supported by grant 2 P50 NS-02808 from the National Institutes of Health. The authors are indebted to the members of the staff and investigators in the Reed Neurological Research Center, the UCLA Clinical Neurophysiology Program and the UCLA Brain Research Institute for their assistance. We are grateful to Sasha Biletsky for preparation of the manuscript.

References

CRANDALL, P. H., WALTER, R. D. and RAND, R. W. (1963) Clinical applications of studies on stereotactically implanted electrodes in temporal lobe epilepsy. *Journal of Neurosurgery,* **20,** 827–840

CRANDALL, P. H. (1975) Postoperative management and criteria for evaluation. In *Advances in Neurology,* Vol. 8, edited by D. P. Purpura, J. K. Penry and R. D. Walter, pp. 265–279. New York: Raven Press

DELGADO-ESCUETA, A. V. and WALSH, G. O. (1983) The selection process for surgery of intractable complex partial seizures: surface EEG and depth electrography. In *Epilepsy, Research Publication ARNMD,* Vol. 61, edited by A. A. Ward, Jr, J. K. Penry and D. P. Purpura, pp. 295–326. New York: Raven Press

ENGEL, J. JR, DRIVER, M. V. and FALCONER, M. A. (1975) Electrophysiological correlates of pathology and surgical results in temporal lobe epilepsy. *Brain,* **98,** 129–156

ENGEL, J. JR, BROWN, W. J., KUHL, D. E., PHELPS, M. E., MAZZIOTTA, J. C. and CRANDALL, P. H. (1982) Pathological findings underlying focal temporal lobe hypometabolism in partial epilepsy. *Annals of Neurology,* **12,** 518–528

FALCONER, M. A. (1953) Discussion on the surgery of temporal lobe epilepsy: surgical and pathological aspects. In *Proceedings of Royal Society of Medicine,* **46,** 1971

FALCONER, M. A. (1971) Anterior temporal lobectomy for epilepsy. In *Operative Surgery,* Vol. 14, 2nd edition, edited by C. Rob and R. Smith, pp. 142–149. London: Butterworths

GASTAUT, H. (1969) Classification of the epilepsies. *Supplement Epilepsia,* **10,** S14–S21

GASTAUT, H., GASTAUT, J. K., GONCALVES E SILVA, G. E., FERNANDEZ SANCHEZ, G. R. (1975) Relative frequency of different types of epilepsy: a study employing the classification of the International League Against Epilepsy. *Epilepsia,* **16,** 457–461

HALGREN, E., WALTER, R. D., CHERLOW, D. G. and CRANDALL, P. H. (1978) Mental phenomena evoked by electrical stimulation of the human hippocampal formation and amygdala. *Brain,* **101,** 83–117

KENNEDY, W. A. and HILL, D. (1958) The surgical prognostic significance of the electroencephalographic prediction of Ammon's horn scelerosis in epileptics. *Journal of Neurology, Neurosurgery and Psychiatry,* **21,** 24–30

LANGE, H. H., LIEB, J. P., ENGEL, J. JR and CRANDALL, P. H. (1983) Temporo-spatial patterns of pre-ictal spike activity in human temporal lobe epilepsy. *EEG and Clinical Neurophysiology,* **56,** 543–555

LINDSAY, J., OUNSTEAD, C. and RICHARDS, P. (1979) Long-term outcome in children with temporal lobe seizures. I. Social outcome and childhood factors. *Developmental Medicine and Child Neurology,* **21,** 285–298

MILNER, B., BRANCH, C. and RASMUSSEN, T. (1962) Study of short-term memory after intracarotid injection of sodium amytal. *Transactions of American Neurological Association,* **87,** 224–226

OSTERREITH, R. (1944) Le test de copie d'une figure complexe. *Archives of Psychology,* **30,** 206–356

RAUSCH, R. and CRANDALL, P. H. (1982) Psychological status related to surgical control of temporal lobe seizures. *Epilepsia,* **23,** 191–202

ROBB, P. (1975) Focal epilepsy: the problem, prevalence and contributing factors. In *Neurosurgical Management of the Epilepsies,* edited by D. P. Purpura, J. K. Penry and R. D. Walter, pp. 11–22. New York: Raven Press

SIEGEL, S. S. (1956) *Non-parametric Statistics for the Behavioral Sciences.* New York: McGraw-Hill

TALAIRACH, J., DAVID, M. and TOURNOUX, P. (1958) *L'Exploration Chirurgicale Stereotaxique du Lobe Temporal dans d'Epilepsie Temporale,* p. 123. Paris: Masson

TALAIRACH, J., SZIKLA, G., TOURNOUX, P. *et al.* (1967) *Atlas d'Anatomie Stereotaxique du Telencephale,* p. 326, Paris: Masson

WADA, J. and RASMUSSEN, T. (1960) Intracarotid injection of sodium amytal for the lateralization of cerebral speech dominance: experimental and clinical observations. *Journal of Neurosurgery,* **17,** 266–282

WALTER, R. D. (1973) Tactical considerations leading to surgical treatment of limbic epilepsy. In *Epilepsy: Its Phenomena in Man,* edited by M. A. B. Brazier, pp. 99–121. New York: Academic Press

WARD, A. A. (1983) Perspectives for surgical therapy of epilepsy. In *Epilepsy, Research Publications: Association for Research in Nervous and Mental Disease,* Vol. 61, edited by A. A. Ward, Jr, J. K. Penry and D. P. Purpura, pp. 371–390. New York: Raven Press

WECHSLER, D. and STONE, C. P. (1945) *Wechsler Memory Scale.* New York: Psychological Corp. Publishers

16
Psychiatric and psychological aspects of epilepsy

Michael R. Trimble

INTRODUCTION

The links between epilepsy and psychiatry have a long history (Guerrant *et al.*, 1962; Lennox and Lennox, 1960; Temkin, 1971). The modern era, and perhaps the most controversial, started in the late 1940s with the extensive clinical use of the electroencephalogram, and the reporting by, for example, Gibbs (1951) that a high frequency of patients with psychomotor epilepsy exhibited psychopathology. This era, termed by Guerrant *et al.* (1962) as the 'period of psychomotor peculiarity', was best summed up by the quotation of Gibbs and Stamps (1953) that: 'The patient's emotional reactions to his seizures, to his family and to his social situation are less important determinants of psychiatric disorder than the site and type of the epileptic discharge'.

In contrast, there are a number of authors who have disputed that there is any special relationship between temporal lobe epilepsy and psychopathology (*see* Stevens and Hermann, 1981). Generally they point out that there are many studies using standardized rating scales for the assessment of psychopathology which fail to distinguish between different groups of patients with epilepsy, although there is less disagreement that when, as a group, patients with epilepsy are examined, the prevalence of psychopathology is increased above the normal population. This, however, is attributed mainly to the stigma of having epilepsy, to side-effects of anticonvulsant drugs, or to consequences of brain damage or disease which occur either prior to or subsequent to the development of epileptic seizures. Recently, there has been a substantial literature on the relationship between psychopathology and epilepsy, especially with reference to temporal lobe epilepsy and it is proposed to review some of this here.

PREVALENCE

There are few careful epidemiological studies of the psychopathology of patients with epilepsy. Examination of non-selected populations has been attempted, however, by several authors. Pond and Bidwell (1959) in a general practice survey noted that 29% had 'psychological difficulties', 7% having been in a psychiatric hospital before or during the survey year. A temporal lobe group had a higher rate of hospitalization to psychiatric hospitals, and higher rates of severe personality change and psychosis. Gudmundsson (1966), in a survey of the population of Iceland, was able to compare the prevalence rates for psychiatric illness in epilepsy with those without epilepsy; 25% of the epileptics showed neurotic symptoms, 50% had some type of abnormal personality, and 8% were psychotic. Again the frequency of psychopathology was much greater (50%) in those with temporal lobe epilepsy compared to those without (25%). Zielinski (1974) provided further data on non-selected epileptic patients from a population in Poland; 58% showed some 'mental abnormality' and approximately 3% had psychotic symptoms. While temporal lobe epilepsy was over-represented in those with psychopathology, those with secondary generalization seemed most affected.

None of the above authors used standardized and validated rating scales to quantify psychopathology, methodology introduced in the studies of Rutter, Graham and Yule (1970) on children resident on the Isle of Wight. They found the prevalence of psychiatric disorders to be 8% in the general population, nearly double in patients with chronic disability not involving the brain, and doubled again in those with uncomplicated epilepsy. Although numbers were small, again those classified as temporal lobe epilepsy fared worst.

The most recent data have come from Ounsted and colleagues (Ounsted and Lindsay, 1982). In 1964 they examined a 'wholly unselected population' of children with temporal lobe epilepsy and obtained biographical and clinical information about them and their epilepsy. These were followed up in 1977 and their outcome assessed; 33% were seizure free and on no anticonvulsants, and five had died in childhood. At their original 1964 assessment 85% were said to have some form of psychiatric difficulty. In 1977, of 95 survivors, eight were severely mentally handicapped, nine had developed a schizophreniform psychosis and 12 had antisocial behavioural problems. Neurotic illness was infrequent. In analyzing the factors which seemed related to psychopathology they identified: failure of remission of epilepsy, frequent seizures, male sex and left-sided lesions. Disordered homes bore no relationship to the development of adult psychiatric disorders.

Thus, although a thorough epidemiological survey of the type and frequency of psychiatric disabilities in epilepsy has yet to be conducted, there are some hints from the existing literature that (a) psychopathology is increased in epileptic populations, and (b) patients with temporal lobe epilepsy may be most prone.

INTERICTAL PSYCHOSES OF EPILEPSY

The most severe psychiatric disturbance is that of psychosis. The link between psychosis and epilepsy goes back to ancient times, but was most clearly stated by the French and German authors of the last century. A suggested association between the temporal lobes and psychiatric disturbances derives from the early report of Bouchet and Cazauveilh (1825) of cases in which epilepsy and insanity were associated, the pathology being noted in the 'cornes d'Ammon'. An early British author of importance was Hughlings Jackson, who clearly delineated the forerunner of what became referred to as temporal lobe epilepsy, and who used the term 'epileptic insanity', suggesting that the epilepsy itself was the actual cause of the psychiatric disorder.

Although the early part of this century was dominated by ideas of an inverse relationship between epilepsy and schizophrenia, the idea of an association between the two disorders was still discussed, and more clearly revived by such authors as Gibbs (1951), Hill (1953) and Pond (1957). In particular, they noted an affinity between temporal lobe epilepsy and chronic paranoid hallucinatory states, in which it was said that the epileptic attacks usually began prior to the onset of the psychosis. An extensive series was reported by Slater and Beard (1963), who on statistical grounds suggested that patients with epilepsy developed a schizophrenia-like illness with increased frequency, especially noting in this group the absence of abnormal premorbid personality traits or a family history of psychiatric disturbance that might suggest a predisposition to schizophrenia. They found that, while catatonic phenomena seemed rare, affective responses were warm and preserved. Eleven of their series had chronic psychosis that had been preceded by recurrent shortlived confusional states, 46 had a psychosis that was 'highly typical of paranoid schizophrenia', and 12 had hebephrenic schizophrenia. The mean age of onset of the psychosis was 29.8 years, and it occurred after the epilepsy had been present for a mean of 14.1 years.

Although in most patients it was not possible to relate the onset of the mental illness to any change in the quantity or quality of the fits, in some 25% of cases the psychotic symptoms appeared when the frequency of generalized seizures was falling. They were unable to document any relationship between the anticonvulsant drugs that the patients received and the subsequent psychotic illness, but noted that the commonest form of epilepsy was temporal lobe epilepsy. Although clinical neurological findings were usually negative, air encephalography, which was carried out on 56 cases, showed abnormalities in 39, usually that of atrophy. In 19 cases there was dilatation of one or both temporal horns.

The past few years have seen several investigations that have attempted to clarify further the nature of this clinical relationship, some of which are now briefly reviewed.

Risk factors

It is accepted that not all patients with temporal lobe epilepsy develop psychoses, and attempts have thus been made to clarify in more detail those at risk. Stevens and Hermann (1981), following a literature review, suggest the following important variables: age of onset, an abnormal neurological examination, automatisms and visceral auras, sphenoidal spike activity on electroencephalography, and the presence of multifocal spikes. Hermann *et al.* (1982) in a study of Minnesota Multiphasic Personality Inventory (MMPI) scores comparing patients with temporal lobe epilepsy and generalized epilepsy noted that those with an aura of fear displayed pathological elevations on several MMPI scales, especially the scale for schizophrenia. Ictal fear and visceral auras result from activity in the medial temporal lobes (Henriksen, 1973), especially the amygdala and the hippocampus (Gloor, 1972; Wieser, 1980). These data suggest that medial temporal lesions, in other words more clearly identified limbic system lesions, may be associated with the development of psychosis.

Further risk factors may be identified from the literature. Age of onset of epilepsy after age 10 was mentioned by Taylor (1975) in his follow-up of patients who underwent a temporal lobectomy. In contrast, however, the careful follow-up study of Ounsted and Lindsay (1982), in which children with temporal lobe epilepsy identified in 1974 were re-examined 13 years later and their clinical outcome related to the epileptic factors documented in the initial examination, was unable to relate age of onset to an outcome of psychosis.

Another factor that seems to be emerging is a relationship not between temporal lobe epilepsy *per se* and psychosis, but between complex partial seizures that secondarily generalize, and psychopathology suggesting either a more widespread epileptic disturbance, or a greater propensity for the seizure to extend its activity through limbic system structures and generalize. Rodin, Katz and Lennox (1976), using rating scales and clinical examinations, noted that most mental disturbances in temporal lobe epilepsy occurred in those who had more than one seizure type, and, with regard to psychosis, Bruens (1980) noted the highest incidence in patients with a temporal lobe EEG focus and bilateral spike–wave activity suffering from both psychomotor and generalized seizures.

Phenomenology

A criticism of much of the work in this field is that the term 'psychosis' has been used without definition by some of the authors, and little attempt has been made to specify the precise phenomenology of the patients who are examined. This *faux pas* would be equivalent to a description of patients in research on epilepsy as 'epileptic', with no further information provided on seizure type, frequency, or pattern. It is noteworthy that the Anglo-Saxon authors who have written on this subject tend to use Schneiderian concepts* for the diagnosis of schizophreniform illness, in particular relying on the presence of first-rank symptomatology. The importance of being precise is emphasized by more recent techniques that have used standardized and validated methods for quantifying psychopathology in the psychoses of epilepsy (Perez and Trimble, 1980; Trimble and Perez, 1982).

Using such methodology it has been possible to compare as objectively as possible the presentation of psychosis in epilepsy with process schizophrenia, in the absence of epilepsy. In the first report of this kind Perez and Trimble (1980), using the present state examination (PSE) of Wing, presented data on 24 patients with epilepsy and psychosis prospectively referred. The psychosis occurred in the setting of clear consciousness, and was present for at least a month. This technique, which allowed for diagnosis to be made by the CATEGO computer program, gave a present state examination syndrome profile for the epileptic group which was compared with non-epileptic schizophrenic controls. In this study, 50% of the patients with epilepsy and psychosis were categorized as having a schizophrenic psychosis, 92% having a profile of nuclear schizophrenia based on the first-rank symptoms of Schneider. The syndrome profile of the patients with schizophrenia

* Kurt Schneider, influenced both by Kraepelin and Jaspers, introduced into psychiatry 'first-rank symptoms' which, when present in a non-organic psychosis, signify schizophrenia. They were for pragmatic diagnostic use and include the following: hearing voices in the third person discussing the subject; hearing thoughts spoken aloud; hearing voices that comment on actions; experiences of bodily influence; thought withdrawal and other forms of thought interference; thought diffusion, and everything in the spheres of feeling, drive and volition which the patient experiences as imposed on him by others (Schneider, 1957).

symptoms and epilepsy compared to those with schizophrenia showed few significant differences emphasizing the similarity of the clinical presentation of these two disorders. Recently, Toone, Garralda and Ron (1982) in a retrospective study also using the present state examination have reported similar findings. These data thus suggest that in a group of patients with psychosis and epilepsy a significant number will have a schizophreniform-type presentation, virtually identical with regard to presenting symptoms to nuclear schizophrenia in the absence of epilepsy. One important aspect of this is to stress at least some common pathophysiological link for the two disorders.

Perez and Trimble (1980) further examined in their sample the differences in presentation between psychotic patients with temporal lobe epilepsy and those with generalized epilepsy. All patients who were diagnosed by the CATEGO program as having nuclear schizophrenia had temporal lobe abnormalities on their electroencephalogram, and received a clinical diagnosis of complex partial seizures. Patients with psychosis and generalized epilepsies had a variety of psychopathological presentations, which included schizophrenia without first-rank symptoms, and manic and depressive psychoses. This study was thus a confirmation of the direct link between certain types of epilepsy and certain patterns of clinical presentation, suggested by others extending back to the early reports of Hill (1953) and Pond (1957).

Laterality

A further important consideration was introduced by Flor-Henry in 1969. He suggested that left-sided temporal lobe lesions in particular were associated with a schizophreniform presentation, contrasting with the right-sided abnormality linking with a manic-depressive picture. The hint of this laterality difference is noted further in the work of Taylor (1957), Pritchard, Lombroso and McIntyre (1980), and the earlier work of Sherwin (1981). In the follow-up study of Ounsted and Lindsay (1982), in which nine patients developed a schizophreniform psychosis with first-rank symptoms of Schneider, seven had a left-sided focus, and two had bilateral discharges. Trimble and Perez (1982), using electroencephalographic criteria for lateralization of focus, compared the present state examination syndrome profiles of patients with left-sided to those with right-sided lesions. In their group, eight patients had consistent left-sided EEG abnormalities, two had bilaterally independent foci, four had right-sided abnormalities, and two patients had a unilateral focus (one left and one right) in all EEG recordings except their most recent. Comparison of the profiles of those with left-sided versus those with right-sided abnormalities noted two significant differences. In particular, the left-sided patients had significantly more nuclear schizophrenia and ideas of reference than the right-sided patients. This left-sided group also had non-significant increases in delusions of persecution, delusions of reference, fantastic delusions, and auditory hallucinations.

Although in these studies the clinical documentation of patients was as precise and objective as possible, it is clear that evaluation of laterality from surface electroencephalographic recordings is open to criticism. In order to circumvent this difficulty, Sherwin (1982) carried out several studies of patients who, while awaiting temporal lobe surgery, had the laterality of their focus established by depth recording of ictal episodes, and ensuing cessation of seizures following temporal lobectomy. Again he was able to conclude that patients with left-sided temporal lobe epileptogenic lesions were at special risk for the development of the schizophrenia-like psychoses, and that psychosis was a rare complication in patients with other focal (non-temporal) epileptic lesions.

Toone, Dawson and Driver (1982), in a retrospective study, using the syndrome checklist (SCL) derived from the present state examination, have also examined the question of laterality using computerized axial tomography (CAT); 57 patients with psychosis and epilepsy were examined and a tendency towards an excess of left-sided abnormalities in schizophreniform cases was reported. Unlike the studies using electroencephalographic techniques, however, this difference was not significant, although hallucinations were seen exclusively in the patients with left-sided lesions.

These data taken together would suggest that a pattern of psychosis, resembling nuclear schizophrenia, does occur in patients with temporal lobe epilepsy more commonly than in other forms of epilepsy, and that when present it is much more likely to be associated with a left-sided or predominantly left-sided lesion. Moreover, since the studies using the electroencephalogram have been more convincing in demonstrating this relationship compared with the CT scan data, the evolution of the clinical pattern would seem more likely to be dependent on functional as opposed to strictly structural abnormalities. Further evidence for this suggestion derives from a second recent study of CT scan data in patients with schizophreniform psychoses of epilepsy. Trimble and colleagues (Perez *et al.*, 1984) quantitatively evaluated the CT scans of ten patients with epileptic psychosis and nuclear first-rank symptoms, ten patients with non-nuclear psychoses of epilepsy, and eight with schizophrenia who were not epileptic. All these psychotic groups had high values for the bilateral septum caudate distance, and the size of the third and fourth ventricle compared to expected normal data, but no laterality differences were noted on such indices, nor on measures of cortical abnormality.

Three further points should be made. The first is that several authors have failed to detect a relationship between the laterality of focus and the presentation of the psychosis (for example, Jensen and Larsen, 1979; Kristensen and Sindrup, 1978), although such authors have also failed to use precise diagnostic critiera as outlined above. The second is that there is a growing and now extensive literature on laterality in non-epileptic psychiatric patients which points in a similar direction, namely to abnormalities of left hemisphere function in schizophrenia (Gruzelier, 1981). Finally, the literature on the link between manic-depressive illness and right-sided lesions is less substantial, and to date this second hypothesis emerging from Flor-Henry's (1969) data has yet to be confirmed.

Mechanisms

Further questions may be asked with regard to the mechanism of the development of psychosis in the prone. A number of different explanations have been put forward, and the majority take as their starting point the now established relationship between temporal lobe–limbic system mechanisms and emotional experiences. There are two main contrasting hypotheses. The first is that the schizophrenia-like illnesses are epileptic in origin and should be referred to as 'epileptic psychoses'. The second is that they are a manifestation of organic neurological damage and thus not specific for epilepsy. The former view has been most strongly expressed by Flor-Henry (1969). Criticizing the absence of a control population in some of the earlier studies, and noting that in his series, as well as in others (such as Hill, 1953; Pond, 1957), an inverse relationship between the frequency of psychomotor seizures and the onset of the psychosis was recorded in some patients, he suggested that it was not structural damage, but the characteristics of the seizures that led to the clinical picture. Support for this suggestion comes from other studies in which depth electrodes have been implanted in psychotic patients who do not have epilepsy. Abnormal electrical activity in the deep temporal structures is shown to be associated with suppression of surface cortical activity, and when patients display psychotic behaviour, abnormal spike–wave activity may be detected in these areas, which is not seen on conventional surface electrodes (Heath, 1977).

The alternative position was taken by Slater and Beard (1963). They noted a significant proportion of the psychotic patients had a defined organic basis for their epilepsy, and that the onset of the psychosis seemed linked to the duration of the epilepsy. Their conclusion stressed the importance of an underlying structural lesion in the temporal lobe. A similar view was taken by Kristensen and Sindrup (1978). Kiloh (1971) made the point that almost any diffuse brain disease may on occasion be associated with a similar clinical picture, and epilepsy is often not present. He suggested the psychoses were a reflection of a certain stage of what, in the long run, was a dementing process. Follow-up studies of such patients do not, however, lend support to his view (Slater and Beard, 1963).

Bruens (1980) put forward the idea that both organic and the psychodynamic events potentiate each other. The patient is unable to protect himself against the vicissitudes of life except by using pathological defence mechanisms, which result in psychosis. Pond (1962) suggested that it was the abnormal experiences associated with temporal lobe epilepsy which gradually became integrated into a person's psychic life that led to the development of the psychosis. However, these explanations do not account for the laterality findings, and as Slater and Beard point out, do not take into account the volitional disturbances, thought disorder and hebephrenic symptoms noted in some of these patients.

Symonds (1962) pointed to the 'epileptic disorder of function'. It was, he suggested, not the loss of neurones in the temporal lobe that was responsible for the psychosis, but the disorderly activity of those that remain. A similar view was stressed by Taylor (1975) who stated 'perhaps it is better, from the point of view of avoiding psychosis, for the (temporal) lobe to be non-functional rather than dysfunctional'. However, the well-documented cases of psychoses in epilepsy that develop after temporal lobectomy (*see*, for example, Jensen and Larsen, 1979; Sherwin, 1982), and the similarity of certain neuropathological abnormalities recently described in patients with schizophrenia and schizophreniform psychosis of epilepsy, which include not only focal pathology in the temporal lobes, but gliosis in periventricular, periaqueductal, midbrain tegmentum and basal forebrain areas (Stevens, 1982), suggests that we must look beyond the temporal lobes for a fuller understanding of this condition.

One theory recently advanced is that chronic temporal lobe ictal lesions may lead to kindling of activity in other regions of the brain, especially forebrain limbic areas, which changes lead to the development of psychosis. Thus it is extremely difficult to kindle epileptic seizures in certain parts of the limbic system, particularly those that are catecholaminergic. Kindling of the mesolimbic dopamine system leads not to seizures but to marked behaviour changes which persist after the kindling has ceased (Stevens and Livermore, 1978). The possibility arises that in man similar mechanisms exist, such that chronic subictal activity leads to a kindling process within dopaminergic pathways, overactivity of which leads to the development of abnormal behaviour patterns and psychosis. It is difficult here to ignore the growing literature on the pathology of schizophrenia, in which the same dopamine-rich areas of the limbic forebrain are suggested as sites for abnormalities that are, at least in part, responsible for the development of the psychosis (Crow, 1980). In that the behaviour changes associated with kindling of the mesolimbic dopamine system are enhanced by the administration of dopamine agonists, it is possible that the kindling itself is associated with altered postsynaptic function of dopamine receptors. Since dopamine agonism is probably anticonvulsant in action, and raises the seizure threshold (Trimble, 1977), these neurophysiological observations may be invoked to explain the clinical findings of an association between persistent abnormal temporal lobe activity and psychosis, and the tendency of its development to be associated with a declining seizure frequency.

Further information on mechanism derives from recent studies using positron emission tomography (PET) with radioactivity-labelled oxygen to measure cerebral blood flow (rCBF) and metabolism ($rCMRO_2$) in a group whose psychosis was assessed using the present state examination (Gallhofer *et al.*, 1985). In these investigations, patients with epilepsy and psychosis were compared with patients with epilepsy and no psychosis, the groups being matched for age, type of epilepsy, IQ, and seizure frequency. The $rCMRO_2$ was lower in most regions examined in the psychotic group, especially in frontal and temporal cortices, and the basal ganglia. Again laterality differences were recorded with the psychotic sample (most of which had nuclear symptoms) showing lower $rCMRO_2$ on the left side in the temporal regions. Since none of these patients had severe epilepsy, with mainly infrequent partial seizures, these findings imply that any explanation for the development of psychosis in epilepsy must take into consideration down-regulation of activity in certain brain structures, especially those linked to the basal ganglia and the limbic system. These results are in keeping with those of Buchsbaum *et al.* (1982) who have recently reported data on positron tomography in eight schizoprenic patients using the 2-deoxyglucose (DG) method. They noted not only low uptake of glucose in the frontal cortex, consistent with other data showing lower cerebral blood flow in the frontal regions in schizophrenics, but also reported that the uptake of glucose was lower in central grey matter. Thus psychotic patients, with and without epilepsy, may show diminished cerebral metabolism in central grey matter.

PERSONALITY DISORDER

Although there is still some controversy regarding the links between epilepsy and psychosis, the arguments and disagreements are far less than with the association between personality disorder and epilepsy.* Some of the features of the personality disorder that have been described may reflect stigmatization (irritable, aggressive,

* Part of this is perhaps because most neurologists accept a link between psychosis and epilepsy, as they see it not infrequently associated with the ictus or postictally. Further, it should be noted that many psychiatrists and neurologists, especially from North America, fail to distinguish personality (those enduring traits by which people come to know us and which characterize us) from psychiatric *illness*, the latter which cuts across the personality and is related to a process.

paranoid, etc.), and the whole concept of a so-called 'epileptic personality' has fallen into disrepute. This stems partly from a misunderstanding of the history. Thus two concepts have become confused. The first came from an era of psychosomatic medicine when the term 'prone personalities' was popular, which suggested that patients with certain personality types developed epilepsy (Pierce-Clark, 1923).

The second, more in keeping with the quotation of Gibbs and Stamps (1958) above, was that patients with chronic lesions, especially in some areas of their brains, developed secondarily to this, personality changes. The precedent had been set by the clear delineation of the 'frontal lobe personality', and the discovery of behavioural changes in animals following bilateral amygdalectomy (the Kluver–Bucy syndrome).

One problem was that, notwithstanding the beliefs of Gibbs and Stamps, there were in the literature many negative results that failed to detect abnormal personality profiles in epileptic patients, or differences between those with temporal lobe epilepsy and other epilepsies. As has been noted elsewhere (Trimble and Perez, 1980) the majority of these used the Minnesota Multiphasic Personality Inventory (MMPI), which has been criticized as not a very valid instrument for the detection of interictal behaviour disturbances. There are several other relevant factors. First, several of these 'negative' results do show higher levels of psychopathology in a temporal lobe group when compared with a non-temporal lobe group, although these may not be statistically significant. Raised paranoia or schizophrenia scale scores are quite common. In some studies (*see* Trimble and Perez, 1980) scores for psychotic behaviour are higher in those with combined psychomotor and generalized seizures, or with bilateral foci. Secondly, in the recent report from Whitman, Hermann and Gordon (1982), using the MMPI, it was noted that, in patients with epilepsy who were classified as abnormal by this scale, psychopathology was more severe than in other groups, for example those with chronic physical disability.

Several more studies of importance should be mentioned here. Bear and Fedio (1977), recognizing the shortcomings of MMPI, developed their own rating scale with 18 behavioural features drawn from the literature supposedly associated with temporal lobe epilepsy, and gave this to a group of epileptic patients, comparing their profiles to controls with neuromuscular diseases and healthy counterparts. Their scale appeared to separate out the temporal lobe group, in particular with regard to humourless sobriety, dependency, obsessionality, and religious and philosophical concerns. They also considered if the profiles of patients with left and right-sided temporal foci were different, and noted in the former more anger, paranoia and dependence, while in the latter more elation. The results of this study have received partial replication by Hermann and Riel (1981) who compared patients with temporal lobe epilepsy to those with generalized epilepsy and noted significant differences, the former scoring significantly higher on sense of personal destiny, dependence, paranoia and philosophical interests. This latter group have also recently published further data using the MMPI (Hermann *et al.*, 1982) in which patients with temporal lobe epilepsy and an aura of ictal fear scored significantly more on certain items than those without such fear, or who had generalized epilepsy. In particular, using Goldberg's sequential diagnostic system, patients with generalized epilepsy were classified as normal, patients with temporal lobe epilepsy without ictal fear as neurotic, and the group with fear auras as psychotic.

Nielsen and Kristensen (1981) also gave the Bear and Fedio (1977) scale to different groups of epileptic patients and noted that those with a mediobasal temporal EEG focus had significantly more hypergraphia (a tendency towards extensive and compulsive writing), elation, guilt and paranoia compared with those having a lateral focus, and that left-sided abnormalities scored higher than right. The former scored significantly higher on aggression and emotional lability. In yet another study using this rating scale, Mungas (1982) compared a group with temporal lobe epilepsy with a matched sample of patients with non-epileptic behavioural disorders secondary to brain disease or trauma, and to a psychiatric group. No significant differences between the groups on the various traits were identified, but as noted above for the MMPI studies the temporal lobe group scored higher on several traits. Specific differences between epileptic samples and psychiatric patients were not clear from that study, but have been examined in more detail recently by Bear *et al.* (1982). They compared the rating scale profiles of patients with complex partial seizures and temporal lobe EEG changes, with a group of non-temporal lobe epilepsy, and three non-epileptic populations with schizophrenia, affective disorders or aggressive character disorders. The temporal lobe group were most powerfully distinguished from the psychiatric groups by viscosity, circumstantiality, religious and philosophical preoccupations, humourless sobriety, paranoid tendencies and moralistic concerns. Interestingly, in view of the data discussed above on psychosis, when the temporal lobe and the schizophrenia group were contrasted, there were far fewer differences and the former demonstrated only significantly more viscosity and hypergraphia. In this study the temporal lobe group scored significantly higher on several of the scales compared with the non-temporal epileptic group.

There are then several studies using the Bear and Fedio (1977) questionnaire that indicate differences between temporal lobe epileptic patients and other groups, although the question as to whether there is a specific constellation of traits related to temporal lobe epilepsy is still not settled. In part, it is clear from the studies of Nielsen and Kristensen (1981) that possibly only a subgroup of patients, perhaps those with identifiable chronic limbic system (allocortical) as opposed to neocortical foci, will be susceptible to change.

Rodin (1984, 1985) has added his own data and interpretation of the Bear and Fedio inventory. He gave this to 148 patients with epilepsy, 18 pain patients, 15 psychiatric inpatients and 40 volunteer controls. He reported differences between patients with temporal lobe or generalized epilepsy, the former, as in many of the other studies (see above), scoring higher on 13 categories, significantly so for hypergraphia. Using controlled clinical and EEG criteria to define the clinical groupings and taking only patients who were thought not to over-report, under-report or mis-report their symptoms, several significant differences emerged: the temporal lobe group scored higher on anger, humourlessness, aggression, emotionality and again paranoia. Closer analysis further revealed a consistent 'hyper-emotional-dysphoria' cluster in which the temporal lobe group score higher. In spite of these findings Rodin remains sceptical of the Bear and Fedio inventory, concluding that it 'measures overall psychopathology or defensiveness of the patient'.

The view that there is a specific interictal syndrome of temporal lobe epilepsy has recently been made most strongly by Geschwind and colleagues (Geschwind, 1979; Waxman and Geschwind, 1975). They included hyposexuality, religiosity and hypergraphia as features, also noting philosophical concern and irritability.

Hypergraphia

Waxman and Geschwind (1974) initially described seven patients with temporal lobe epilepsy and hypergraphia and suggested a special link. In a recent publication, Sachdev and Waxman (1981) estimated the frequency of this behaviour trait in a group of epileptic patients admitted to hospital over six years. Although the study was carried out by writing to the patients asking them to outline their present state of health and analyzing the responses, and over 56% failed to reply, those who did were more likely to have temporal lobe epilepsy and the 'hypergraphic' replies came mainly from this same group. Interestingly, in addition, in those studies using the Bear and Fedio questionnaire, which includes hypergraphia as a scale, hypergraphia scores are non-significantly higher in the temporal lobe groups in several (Bear and Fedio, 1977; Herman and Reil, 1981; Nielsen and Kristensen, 1981; Mungas, 1982; Rodin, 1985).

Roberts, Robertson and Trimble (1982) have noted a laterality effect with regard to hypergraphia. They described six cases which were consecutive referrals with epilepsy and hypergraphia, and compared them with the other cases reported in the literature. They noted a significant excess of right-sided lesions in these patients, also commenting that obsessionality, elation and *déjà vu* experiences may also be linked to non-dominant lesions.

Sexual behaviour

The relationship of abnormal sexual behaviour to epilepsy is scattered with anecdotes, although there are some studies to be found. Gastaut and Collomb (1954) first clearly documented hyposexuality in two-thirds of their patients with temporal lobe epilepsy. Hierons and Saunders (1966) described 15 patients with impotence and temporal lobe attacks, three of whom developed a sexual dysfunction 6–9 months prior to the onset of the epilepsy while on anticonvulsant drugs. In four other cases bringing the epilepsy under control with anticonvulsants led to improvement of the impotence. Taylor (1969) noted a high incidence of lack of sex drive in patients with temporal lobe epilepsy, and reported improvement in 22% after temporal lobectomy.

Bancaud *et al.* (1970) recorded 26 cases of temporal lobe sexual seizures, and ten cases of seizures with sexual manifestations due to involvement of the precentral lobule. Blumer and Walker (1975) reviewed the data in this field and provided evidence of their own in the form of case histories for both ictal sexual arousal and interictal changes in sexual behaviour. Sexual seizures they noted were often triggered by sexual arousal, but they also suggested that 'non-sexual' reflex epilepsy could occur following intercourse. Postictal arousal was also clearly documented by Blumer and Walker, especially exhibitionism, occurring 'in an appropriate setting with full recognition on the part of the patient'.

Interictally, they confirmed the occurrence of hyposexuality, but also noted recorded anecdotes of fetishism and epilepsy. Two famous cases often quoted are the 'safety pin' fetish patient reported by Mitchell, Falconer and Hill (1954), who experienced intense pleasure gazing at a safety pin which disappeared following lobectomy, and the patient of Hunter, Logue and McMenemy (1963) with temporal lobe epilepsy and transvestism. This latter relationship has also been recorded by several other authors (see, for example, Blumer and Walker, 1975; Epstein, 1961).

Although Bear and Fedio (1977) using their rating scales were able to confirm that patients with temporal lobe epilepsy have significantly altered sexuality, there is only one controlled study of this subject in the literature. Shukla, Srivastava and Katiyar (1979) recently studied 140 cases with epilepsy and made detailed enquiries about sexual activity. They noted that significantly more patients with temporal lobe abnormalities had hyposexuality, compared with those with major generalized seizures. The patients reported a global loss of sexual interest, and had little concern over this; no cases of sexual deviation were reported in this study. While confirming, therefore, the relationship between temporal lobe abnormalities and altered sexual activity, their study failed to confirm a link between such abnormalities and fetishism.

Aggression

The occurrence of increased aggressive outbursts in epileptic patients has attracted considerable attention, but few studies. One major problem is the difficulty of recording and quantifying aggressive behaviour, and its almost entirely interpersonal nature. During automatisms aggressive behaviour may be seen, but it is frequently poorly directed and often provoked by inadequate handling of a confused patient. Increased aggressive behaviour as a personality trait in epileptic patients has been noted in several studies. For example, Rey *et al.* (1949) noted that 44 out of 59 adult cases of temporal lobe epilepsy had irritability and aggression to a 'pathological degree'. Serafetinides (1965) studied 100 patients operated on for temporal lobectomy and noted that a history of explicit aggressive outbursts was associated with an early age of onset, with left-sided resections, and with epigastric, autonomic and complex automatisms during seizures. Following operation the aggression seemed improved only in patients whose epilepsy improved. They suggested that deficient learning, due to the early onset of epilepsy, led to poor impulse control and the later clinical picture.

Kligman and Goldberg (1975) examined eight controlled studies where aggression in epilepsy had been investigated, and noted that only two supported the relationship, although they severely criticizied the methodology in all of them. While many observers have reported that there is an increased incidence of aggression in patients with epilepsy, it is not clear if this is a result of chronic brain damage or due to a specific epileptic factor.

Several authors have tried to correlate aggressive behaviour with abnormal limbic system activity, especially amygdala damage (see Mark and Ervin, 1970), and ictal violence, recorded using video telemetry to document seizures, has been clearly described (Delgado-Escueta *et al.*, 1981). However, after careful review Kligman and Goldberg decided: 'It is not at present possible to answer the question of whether there is an increased incidence of aggressive behaviour in temporal lobe epilepsy'.

DEPRESSION

Griesinger (1857) noted that a 'misanthropic perversion of sentiment, sometimes even actual melancholia with suicidal tendency, is observed in a great many epileptics'. In addition, a number of earlier authors commented on the acute changes of the mental state, which included overexcitement, mania and depression, that occur in association with the ictus. Present classification of the relationship between epilepsy and depression is based on such observations and must therefore include peri-ictal disturbances, namely prodromata, ictal and postictal experiences, and interictal episodes where the psychiatric disturbance is chronic and prolonged.

Interictal depression probably represents the most common psychiatric illness in patients with epilepsy. Betts, Merskey and Pond (1976) drew attention to the inevitable burdens that patients with epilepsy have to bear, and suggested that predictably these lead to depression. In one study of 72 patients with epilepsy admitted to a psychiatric hospital, depression was the commonest psychiatric diagnosis made, being found in 31% of the sample. It was classified as endogenous in 17% and reactive in 14% (Betts, 1974).

Robertson (1983) carried out a very comprehensive study of the phenomenology of interictal depression in 66 consecutively referred cases. The severity of depression was moderate, and in 42% 'endogenous'. High anxiety, neuroticism and hostility were also recorded; 13 patients were psychotic, although bipolar presentations (manic-depressive) were rare. Type of seizure, frequency of attacks and site of lesion did not relate to the depressive presentation, although the duration of epilepsy was correlated with its severity.

Few other studies have been carried out on this very common clinical problem. An increased incidence of depression in patients with epilepsy was detected in some of the rating scale studies discussed in the section above (for example, Kogeorgos, Fanagy and Scott, 1982; Meier and French, 1965; Rodin, Katz and Lennox, 1976), and more recently Trimble and Perez (1980) have used rating scales to assess the precise phenomenology and frequency of psychiatric illness in a group of 281 chronic epileptic patients. These were all admitted to an epilepsy centre, either for the evaluation of their epilepsy, control of their seizures, or rehabilitation, and were not selected for psychopathology. They were given the Middlesex Hospital questionnaire, which assesses five areas of psychopathology, and noted to have significantly higher anxiety, depression and obsessionality scores than the normal population, and for these parameters to score in the equivalent range of psychiatric outpatients. In that study, no direct relationship between type of epilepsy and depression was discovered.

Kogeorgos, Fanagy and Scott (1982) noted that depression in patients with epilepsy was more severe than in neurological control cases from the same clinic, and that it was seen most in those with severe epilepsy.

Some authors have reported that depression is commoner in late onset epilepsy (Serafetinides, 1965), and that a decline in fit frequency occurs prior to hospitalization for treatment of depression (Betts, 1974). Flor-Henry (1969) implied a relationship between manic-depressive psychosis and non-dominant temporal lobe lesions. In his retrospective study, 50 patients with temporal lobe epilepsy who at one time had been psychotic were compared with 50 non-psychotic cases with the same variety of epilepsy. Where the lateralization could be determined, he noted that 18% were lateralized to the right hemisphere, and the majority had manic-depressive psychosis. While major generalized seizures were more often the sole ictal manifestations in the manic-depressive patients, Flor-Henry reported that the occurrence of psychomotor seizures was lowest in the manic-depressive group, implying that infrequently released seizures were in some way related to the expression of manic-depressive illness. He stated '. . . the emergence of manic-depressive symptoms in association with temporal lobe epilepsy hinges on epileptic activity lateralised to the non-dominant hemisphere provoking grand mal attacks infrequently . . .'. These findings were not confirmed in the study by Robertson (1983).

A similar neurophysiological explanation for depression in epilepsy has been put forward by other authors, most notably Weil (1959). Following initial observations on 11 patients with depressive episodes which preceded or followed seizures, specifically 'uncinate seizures', he investigated 132 case histories of patients with temporal lobe epilepsy, and noted that nine out of 14 with ictal depression experienced olfactory hallucinations, and in some of their subjects such hallucinations were followed by prolonged depressive episodes. They felt that this depression was a manifestation of diffuse temporal lobe lesions.

A number of authors have commented on the frequency of suicide in epileptic patients. Marchand and Ajuriaguerra (1948) discussed the historical aspects of this, giving examples of self-mutilations and suicide in patients, which often occurred in postictal confusional states. In contrast, Pond (1957) recorded less than a dozen suicides in many hundreds of patients, and suggested that epileptic suicide was in fact rare.

More recently Mackay (1979) studied patients admitted to the Glasgow Western Infirmary for self-poisoning. Of these 130 (3.5%) were epileptics, suggesting that in this group attempted suicide occurred seven times more frequently than expected. Repeated episodes of self-poisoning were also commoner amongst the epileptic patients than others. The drugs most commonly used were antiepileptic medications, and phenobarbitone was involved in 55% of cases. Hawton, Fagg and Marsack (1980) in a two-year study of patients admitted to hospital after self-poisoning noted a five-fold increase in patients with epilepsy compared to the general population, and confirmed both the tendency for repetition to occur in this group, and their frequent use of barbiturates for self-poisoning. Barraclough (1981), in a review of the literature of mortality and suicide in epilepsy, concluded that the increased risk of suicide in epilepsy was approximately five times the expected, and was highest (× 25) in those with temporal lobe epilepsy.

It is clear that few studies have been carried out on the relationship between depression and epilepsy, and at this stage few conclusions can be drawn. While it is possible that in some patients a neurophysiological explanation exists for the association of the two disorders, this is not entirely clear, and speculation regarding the role of limbic system dysfunction in depression is not clarified from studies in epilepsy. What is clear is that a substantial proportion of patients with epilepsy suffer from depression, that attempted suicide and suicide are common, that repeated attempts at self-poisoning occur, and that barbiturates are the most commonly used drugs for these episodes.

TREATMENT OF PSYCHIATRIC PROBLEMS IN EPILEPSY

Many aspects of this are covered in more detail elsewhere (Reynolds and Trimble, 1981), and in the space available only general outlines will be given. The various disorders so far discussed can be separately considered.

Psychosis, while being the most severe problem from the psychiatric point of view, is not necessarily the most problematic. Interestingly, many psychotic patients remain in the community (hence are not found in hospital surveys), are sometimes married or at least live with a close relative, and do not undergo the progressive deterioration often seen with process schizophrenia.

Of most importance in management is to distinguish the relationship of the psychosis to the ictus, which may require ambulatory monitoring or telemetry. Ictally related psychoses, as a rule, do not require antipsychotic medications, settle with time, and treatment is orientated towards better control of the epilepsy. In some cases these psychoses are misinterpreted as they come on some 24–28 hours after a bout of seizures, following a lucid interval. The EEG pattern may show a partial status epilepticus.

Interictal psychoses may again be interlinked with the seizure pattern, in some patients appearing as seizure frequency declines. In such patients, adjustment of anticonvulsant drugs may be helpful, lowering the dose and achieving monotherapy. Where there is no relationship to the seizure frequency, and if treatment is thought necessary, the choice of medication will depend on the type of psychosis. Paranoid and schizophreniform disorders are best managed with major tranquillizers, the butyrophenones such as haloperidol and pimozide lowering the seizure threshold less than the phenothiazines (the latter are thus better if treatment is required for patients with a declining seizure rate). Intramuscular long-acting tranquillizers are not contraindicated and should be used if required. Manic-depressive psychoses may also require this class of drugs, but lithium is the mainstay of treatment. Lithium, however, will require serum level monitoring, is cerebrotoxic, may exacerbate seizures, and thus requires careful supervision.

Depressive illness, and the more protracted dysphoric-depressive pictures seen in epileptic patients, are sometimes very difficult to manage. Psychotropic drugs are often not beneficial, although many patients are prescribed them. Antidepressants, particularly of the tricyclic variety, exacerbate seizures and may provoke status epilepticus. Nomifensine (Merital) is one of the few antidepressants that does not appear to lower seizure threshold (Trimble, 1978), and has been the subject of systematic investigation (Robertson and Trimble, 1985). It has been shown, in a double-blind placebo controlled trial, to be more effective than amitriptyline in alleviating depressive symptoms, provided that a sufficient dose (at least 150 mg/day) is given (it can be administered, unlike amitriptyline, safely in a single daily dose). Generally, serum antidepressant levels are reduced in patients on enzyme-inducing anticonvulsant drugs, and some tricyclics and viloxazine interact adversely with the latter and may provoke toxicity. Any exacerbation of the behaviour disorder after starting such treatment should be noted, and serum levels of anticonvulsant drugs checked.

Other methods of helping these psychiatric presentations include adjustment of anticonvulsant drugs and psychotherapeutic intervention. With regard to the former, there is growing evidence that anticonvulsant drugs, especially polytherapy, provoke mental changes, and rationalization of therapy, especially to monotherapy, improves a patient's mood and wellbeing (Thompson and Trimble, 1982b; Trimble and Reynolds, 1984). Carbamazepine has often been singled out as the drug of choice for patients with psychopathology, and substitution of it for more toxic anticonvulsants has been shown to improve depressive symptoms (Thompson and Trimble, 1982b). In this regard, it is interesting to note that Robertson (1983) found a significant inverse correlation between the taking of carbamazepine and the presence of anxiety and depressive symptoms in depressed epileptic patients (in other words the higher the carbamazepine levels, the lower the psychopathology), and Rodin (1985) reported a similar relationship between carbamazepine levels and several scores on the Bear and Fedio (1977) inventory. The latter provides some support for the long-held belief that carbamazepine actually influences advserse personality characteristics in epilepsy (Dalby, 1975), as well as affective symptoms.

Psychotherapeutic interventions in patients with psychological difficulties may be carried out by non-medically qualified personnel attached to the epilepsy clinic. The most important feature is that they know about, understand and are not fearful of epilepsy or its complications. Psychoanalysis is rarely, if ever, warranted. The help of others, such as rehabilitation officers, social workers and psychologists seem essential requirements for the overall management of the more difficult patients.

A variety of behavioural treatments have recently become fashionable in neurology and are being used in epilepsy. These include conditioning procedures, behavioural modification, and biofeedback techniques (Fenwick, 1981b). Although these may have value in individual patients, there is no substantive evidence to date that they provide alternative treatments for epilepsy and, apart from relaxation which many patients find useful, and desensitization in patients who fear seizures or who are agoraphobic, they are not used in the management of psychiatric symptoms.

NEUROPSYCHOLOGICAL ASPECTS OF EPILEPSY

Alteration of cognitive function in epilepsy received particular attention from the 19th century physicians who, invoking a genetic theory influenced by the ideas of degeneracy introduced by Morel and others, implied that intellectual and moral deterioration was an inevitable part of the epileptic process. Since that time, and especially since the 1950s, there has been fairly extensive discussion of intellectual changes in epilepsy, although only a few groups have approached the subject in a systematic way, many authors reiterating views noted in earlier textbooks. The progression has been from global clinical impressions to the more sophisticated use of psychological tests, initially IQ measurements, and later specific tests designed to assess certain aspects of cognitive function: these will be briefly reviewed, followed by discussion of the impact of epileptic and neurological variables and anticonvulsant drugs on the mental state.

Methodologies employed in assessing intellectual function in epilepsy

The first important step in the evaluation of cognitive abilities in epilepsy came with the further development of techniques such as the Halstead–Reitan Neuropsychological Battery. Kløve and Matthews (1966) used this in four groups of patients: normal controls; patients with epilepsy plus identifiable brain pathology; patients with epilepsy and no brain damage; and patients with brain damage but no epilepsy. In the majority of comparisons, normal subjects were superior to the other three groups, and scoring was worse in the groups with brain damage.

Dikmen and co-workers (Dikmen and Matthews, 1977; Dikmen, Matthews and Harley, 1977) looked at specific epileptic variables in relation to such tests and noted, for example, poorer test profiles with higher seizure frequency, and more severe cognitive deficits in relation to an early age of onset and long seizure duration.

A major drawback, however, in the use of such standardized tests in the evaluation of this condition is that they were never designed for dissecting out the problems of patients with epilepsy, being validated and standardized on different populations and, in the case of the Halstead–Reitan battery, for example, being evaluated on patients with structural brain lesions. This has led several groups to alter their approach by the development of test batteries especially for use in patients with epilepsy. Dodrill (1982), using his experience with the Halstead–Reitan battery, selected a series of tests that were specifically directed to the evaluation of neuropsychological deficits in epilepsy. His 'neuropsychological battery for epilepsy' was selected from approximately 100 psychological test variables, based on their ability to discriminate epileptic from non-epileptic patients, and their non-overlap in the sense of excessive correlation between tests that may have led to a duplication of measures. Cross-validation studies were performed by him, the final battery to emerge employing 16 measures. These included 11 from the Halstead–Reitan battery (including the Factual Performance Task (FPT) total time, memory and localization, tapping tests, trail-making tests, aphasia screening and perceptual examination error tests) plus the Stroop test, the logical and visual reproduction portions of the Wechsler Memory Scale, and the Seashore Tonal Memory Test. This battery is used clinically to evaluate patients at an epilepsy centre, but in addition has been used to assess the effect of seizures or drugs on cognitive function. In one study (Dodrill and Troupin, 1977), which compared the psychotropic properties of carbamazepine with phenytoin, use of the standardized Halstead–Reitan tests showed no statistically significant findings. However, using the specially selected neuropsychological battery, several important differences between phenytoin and carbamazepine emerged, favouring carbamazepine.

Dodrill (1982) has extended the use of this battery further by evaluating in addition the psychological and social problems that patients with epilepsy have to contend with. Their Washington Psychosocial Seizure Inventory is a 132-item inventory that evaluates family background, emotional adjustment, interpersonal adjustment, vocational adjustment, financial status, adjustment to seizures, and medical management in their patients. This, plus the neuropsychological test battery, can thus be given to patients to provide a comprehensive evaluation of their cognitive, emotional and psychosocial status.

We have used a different approach in our studies at the National Hospital, Queen Square. In particular, we wished to develop a series of neuropsychological tests that could be used for the evaluation of the impact of anticonvulsant drugs on cognitive function, taking into account the following important considerations. First, it was appreciated that the tests must be maximally sensitive to changes in psychological function, since those which accompany the administration of anticonvulsant drugs may well be subtle in nature and thus undetected with the neuropsychological measures already in existence. Second, it was important to adopt a longitudinal design for the studies, and tests therefore needed to be minimally sensitive to the effects of practice. Third, the test selected needed to have relevance to epilepsy by measuring aspects of neuropsychological functioning which patients with the disorder had specifically been found to complain of or display difficulties with previously. In theory it should then be possible to estimate to what extent drugs may be contributing to the occurrence of such deficits. Fourth, tests needed to be interesting and meaningful for patients in order to maximize their motivation and cooperation for follow-up assessments. For the same reason it was considered important that the entire battery should not take too long to administer, many existing neuropsychological batteries being considered inappropriate on account of their excessive length. Finally, the measures chosen needed to have wide application so that they could be used across a broad spectrum of intellectual levels.

The series of neuropsychological tests developed included measures of attention, retention of new information, speed and accuracy of perceptual registration, decision making and manual speed (for details *see* Thompson, Huppert and Trimble, 1981). Time-based measures of performance were particularly focused upon since, from the literature on the effects of other drugs on cognitive function, it seems that these measures were sensitive to drug administration.

Selective neuropsychological deficits in epilepsy

Apart from evaluation of overall impairments, as discussed above for IQ scores, a number of investigators have examined specific deficits in patients with epilepsy including abnormalities of memory, perceptuomotor skills, speed of mental processing and attention. These are briefly considered.

Deficits of memory in association with epilepsy have been reported for more than 100 years. In 1942 Lennox, considering the nature of these memory difficulties wrote, 'the patient finds it hard to recall events and names particularly those learned recently'. Only a few studies, however, have been undertaken to assess memory functions in epilepsy. Deutsch (1953) assessed the memory skills of 30 patients with epilepsy and brain damage, 30 with epilepsy and no brain damage, and 30 with brain damage and no epilepsy. Both groups with epilepsy showed a similar pattern of deficits on tests of learning and memory including impairments in tactile learning and auditory perceptual tasks, which was different from that observed in the brain-damaged group. Deutsch claimed that impairments observed were attributable to some epileptic factor, although she did not go on to elaborate as to what that might be. Mohan, Varma and Sawhney (1976) administered the Boston Memory Scale to 50 patients with generalized epilepsy and 50 non-epileptic controls matched for age and level of education. The average performance of the epileptic group was inferior to that of the control group but this was not significant. Loiseau *et al.* (1980) reported a study in which he evaluated the memory skills of 100 epileptics with 100 controls matched for age, sex, education and social status. Retention of both verbal and non-verbal material was assessed. Memory was found to be impaired in the epileptic group, in particular the ability to remember lists of words and simple geometric patterns.

Evidence has accumulated associating memory deficits with temporal lobe foci. Most studies, however, have been based on patients with intractable epilepsy undergoing lobectomy. Considerable agreement exists that the side of the excision determines the kind of material that will be more difficult for the individual to remember, left-sided lesions yielding memory deficits for verbal material and right-sided lesions for non-verbal material (Iversen, 1977; Milner, 1975). Little attention has been devoted to patients with temporal lobe epilepsy who do not require surgical intervention, and findings from existing studies have not been entirely consistent.

Glowinski (1973) compared the performance of 30 patients with chronic generalized epilepsy with 30 who had chronic unilateral temporal lobe epilepsy, and he found that the latter displayed greater deficits on the Wechsler Memory Scale. Other studies have reported similar findings with both children and adults (Fedio and Mirsky, 1969; Quadfasel and Pruyser, 1955). On the other hand, Mirsky *et al.* (1960) failed to differentiate between patients with focal and generalized epilepsy on the Wechsler Memory Scale. Their failure, however, was possibly due to the inclusion of patients other than those with temporal lobe foci in the focal group.

Demonstrations of laterality effects have been less convincing. Fedio and Mirsky (1969) found that children with left temporal lobe foci displayed memory deficits for verbal material while the retention of non-verbal material was unaffected. The converse was true for children with right temporal foci. Similarly Ladavas, Umilta and Provinciali (1979) reported a differential effect according to the side of the focus; their left temporal group were impaired on verbal retention tests whereas the right-sided group were more impaired on a spatial memory test. Delaney *et al.* (1980) compared the test performance of right and left temporal lobe epileptics matched for age of onset, duration of epilepsy and seizure frequency. Tests used included the logical memory and visual reproduction of the Wechsler Scale and word list learning. Results revealed significant impairment of verbal memory in left temporal epileptic subjects and significant impairment of non-verbal, visual memory in those with right-sided abnormalities. Agnetti *et al.* (1979) were able to demonstrate verbal learning deficits in patients with left-sided foci but they observed no significant difference between right and left temporal lobe groups on non-verbal retention tests. Others have also failed to find impairments of non-verbal memory in patients with a right temporal focus (Berent, Bull and Giordani, 1980), and some investigators have been unable to clearly demonstrate any laterality effects at all (Glowinski, 1973).

Impairments of attention in the absence of overt clinical seizures have been described by several writers. Holdsworth and Whitmore (1974), for example, found that 42% of their sample of epileptic children were rated by their teachers as markedly inattentive. Little research involving more objective neuropsychological assessment has been undertaken. In one study Stores, Hart and Piran (1978) compared the performance of 71 children with epilepsy and 35 non-epileptic controls on a series of specially designed tests of attention. Epileptic boys were found to be significantly less attentive than non-epileptic boys; no comparable differences, however, were found for girls.

Some researchers have proposed that the attentional difficulties in epilepsy are related to seizure type, patients with generalized seizures displaying greater impairments than those with focal seizures. Mirsky *et al.* (1960) assessed the performance of two groups of patients with generalized and focal seizures respectively on their continuous performance test (CPT), a measure of sustained attention. In this task, subjects had to detect a critical stimulus from a random sequence of letters presented at a constant rate. The authors found, as predicted, that the generalized group displayed greater impairments on this measure than the focal group. Using the same test of attentional capacity, Fedio and Mirsky (1969) reported similar findings for epileptic children. Kimura (1964) compared the scores of patients with generalized and partial epilepsy on a sustained attention task, in which patients had to report aloud letters that were briefly flashed on to a screen, in any order on some trials and in alphabetical order on others. When patients with myoclonic epilepsy were excluded from the analysis, the scores of the generalized subjects were significantly inferior to patients with localized epileptogenic foci. In contrast, Glowinski (1973) was unable to demonstrate differences in attentional capacity relating to seizure type. However, in his study, all groups of patients were significantly impaired on a test of divided attention, in comparison with a non-epileptic control group.

Inconsistencies in the findings of studies looking at cognitive impairments in relation to seizure type may reflect differential sensitivity of the psychological tests employed. Furthermore, many measures of memory were not devoid of attentional components, and the converse seems true for measures of attention. At the present time, it seems, however, that the memory and attentional difficulties noted in epilepsy may not solely be the consequence of the seizure type.

Disturbances of perceptuomotor skills have also been reported in epilepsy. Gastaut (1964) found that more than one-third of the epileptic children in his study displayed considerable handicaps which he felt were sufficient to interfere with learning to read and write. At a special school for epilepsy, 215 children were reported to be slow and clumsy. Several studies using the Bender Gestalt Test have demonstrated that children with seizures perform less well than control groups (Schwartz and Dennerll, 1970; Tymchuk, 1974). A study of visual perception of young children with epilepsy using the Frostig Test revealed impairments which were more marked in patients with partial seizures than in those with generalized seizures (Morgan and Groh, 1980).

Speed of mental processing, although not a distinct domain of abilities, is often of critical importance in the execution of psychological tests. References to mental slowing in people with epilepsy have been made since antiquity, investigators using such terms as 'slowness of mental reaction', 'slowness of thought and language', 'stickiness of thought', 'mental viscosity', 'slowness of ideation' and 'prolonged speed of cerebration'. McGuckin (1980) suggests that lack of speed is one of the four barriers for patients with epilepsy when seeking employment. Bruhn and Parsons (1977) studied the reaction times of epileptics, brain-damaged and normal individuals, and found that slowing was common in the two patient groups. Arena *et al.* (1979) reported slower simple and complex reaction times in patients with epilepsy than in matched controls.

Poor arithmetical ability was mentioned in Fox's (1924) study of children attending a special school for epilepsy. This particular psychological deficit has been commented on by others, including Bradley (1947) and Bagley (1971). The latter author noted that 31 epileptic children he studied were on average 23.1 months behind in this subject compared to the expected attainment level. He believed that the observed retardation was due to a specific epileptic factor. Green and Hartlage (1971) found even when children with epilepsy were at an appropriate academic placement they were often performing below expectancy in a variety of areas, computational abilities being frequently impaired. In another study, only 17% of epileptic children were rated high in mathematical ability in contrast to 31% of non-epileptic controls (Ross and West, 1978).

Reading attainment is another specific deficit mentioned frequently in studies on epilepsy. Tizard, Rutter and Whitmore (1969) claimed that 25% of their sample of 9–12-year-olds with epilepsy were more than 28 months behind in reading skill and comprehension in comparison with 4% of the general population. Rutter, in his Isle of Wight study (Rutter, Graham and Yule, 1970), found that children with epilepsy were reading on average 12 months behind their chronological age. Similar impairments in reading have been noted by Bagley (1971) and Long and Moore (1979).

Factors influencing neuropsychological function in epilepsy

Brain damage

Patients with epilepsy and known brain pathology have frequently been reported to be intellectually inferior to patients with epilepsy of unknown aetiology (Keating, 1960; Tarter, 1972). Kløve and Matthews (1966), in their studies (see above), noted normal subjects to be superior to their epileptic and brain-damaged groups. Further, the performance of those with epilepsy and brain damage was generally inferior to those having epilepsy without brain damage. Finally, the performance of a brain-damaged group without epilepsy was inferior to that of the brain-damaged group with epilepsy. The groups had been matched for age and level of education.

Thus, pre-existing brain damage as a factor does not seem to provide a complete explanation for the neuropsychological deficits observed in some patients with epilepsy, and when patients with brain damage are excluded from analyses, or brain damage is somehow controlled for, neuropsychological deficits still occur.

Age of onset

The majority of investigations suggest that an early onset of seizures carries a poor prognosis with regard to neuropsychological functioning (Keating, 1960; Tarter, 1972). Few of the early studies made a distinction between age of onset and duration of epilepsy. Dikmen, Matthews and Harley (1975) compared the performance of two groups of patients on the Wechsler Adult Intelligence Scale and Halstead–Reitan test battery matched for duration and frequency of tonic-clonic seizures, but differing with regard to the age of onset. Patients with epilepsy commencing before the age of five were more impaired on the majority of the tests than patients with epilepsy of later onset between the ages of 10 and 15. O'Leary *et al.* (1981) administered a battery of tests to 48 children aged 9 to 15 who had tonic-clonic seizures. Those children with seizures of early onset, before the age of five, were significantly impaired relative to the children with later onset, on eight of the 14 measures. The deficits were seen on tasks whose requirements included the repetition of a simple motor act, attention and concentration, memory and complex problem-solving. Duration effects were controlled for by statistical methods.

Seizure type

Research on the association between seizure type and cognitive function has not been entirely consistent. Many authors report that generalized absence (petit mal) seizures have a less damaging effect than generalized tonic-clonic (major) seizures (Collins, 1951; Zimmerman, Burgemeister and Putnam, 1951). On the other hand, Halstead (1957) found children with absence seizures had lower IQs and were poorer in reading and arithmetic skills than children with tonic-clonic attacks, and recently stress has been laid on the potentially damaging effect of the 'absence' seizures in the classroom.

Comparisons between patients with generalized and partial seizures are unclear. Kløve and Matthews (1966) reported that patients with generalized seizure types performed less well than patients with partial seizures on the Wechsler Adult Intelligence Scale and the Halstead Neuropsychological Test Battery. The scores of patients with mixed seizure types fell somewhere between the two. However, the opposite has also been found, that is patients with partial seizures perform less well on neuropsychological tests. To complicate the picture further, some authors claim to find no consistent differences in psychological test performance between patients with partial and generalized seizures (see above).

These contradictory findings have their bases in the variety of measures of neuropsychological functioning that have been used in individual studies. In addition, the reliability of seizure classification, particularly in older studies, may be questioned. It seems likely that the pattern of neuropsychological deficits may differ between seizure types, rather than certain types producing overall less damaging effects than others. Indeed, this becomes clear in the more recent research as discussed above with regard to memory functions in temporal lobe epilepsy.

In this regard, the age of onset of seizures may also be expected to have consequences for the pattern of cognitive abilities observed in a particular individual. For instance, a left-sided focus may have a different impact depending on whether it becomes active at the age of 1, 6, 16 or 60.

Seizure frequency

Seizures themselves have been implicated in the neuronal damage seen in some patients with epilepsy (Dam, 1980) and as a consequence might be expected, particularly if frequent, to have an adverse effect on neuropsychological function. Some investigators have found that frequent seizures are associated with more marked impairments of cognitive abilities than those infrequently expressed (Dikmen and Matthews, 1977), but this has not been consistently demonstrated (Delaney *et al.*, 1980; Loiseau *et al.*, 1980; Zimmerman, Burgemeister and Putnam, 1951). In one recent study, Seidenberg *et al.* (1981) attempted to explore the influence of seizure frequency using a longitudinal design. They compared the test–retest performance on the Wechsler Adult Intelligence Scale of two groups of adult epileptics. For one group seizure frequency had improved during the test–retest interval, and in the other it had worsened or remained unchanged. The former group showed significant improvements on several psychological measures (Wechsler Adult Intelligence Scale, full scale IQ, performance IQ, verbal IQ and on eight of the 11 subtests). In comparison, the latter group showed significant improvements only on the performance IQ and the object assembly subtest. The results therefore suggest that seizure frequency is likely to be one of the factors associated with fluctuations in the test performance of epileptic patients.

Electroencephalographic (EEG) findings

Investigators have also explored the possible relationship between neuropsychological functions and various EEG patterns. Much work has centred on the classical 3/s spike wave activity that accompanies absence seizures. The prevailing view is that this activity is associated with detriments in test performance which appear most marked on measures of reaction time and vigilance behaviour, particularly if the task is experimenter-paced (Browne *et al.*, 1974). Some authors have demonstrated that alterations in the frequency of spike and wave bursts seem dependent on the meaning of the task for the individual, with a reduction in this abnormal activity occurring during periods of alertness and interest, and conversely an increase during periods of boredom (Guey *et al.*, 1969). Interestingly, in some studies the observed behavioural effects precede the spike-bursts by 1–1.5 s (Fenwick, 1981a).

Other forms of epileptic activity in the EEG trace have been associated with neuropsychological dysfunctioning. In one study patients with frequent epileptiform activity present in their EEG traces were found to be more impaired on a series of neuropsychological tests than patients for whom such epileptiform activity was either infrequent or absent (Wilkus and Dodrill, 1976). Not all investigators have detected impairments of psychological test performance in relation to epileptic activity on the EEG, however, and this may be due to the relative insensitivity of a scalp recording. Studies involving depth recordings are infrequent but they would seem to support the view that subclinical epileptic discharges may interfere with cognitive processes (Rausch, Lieb and Crandall, 1978). A complication in a number of studies is that a gap of several days or weeks occurs between the EEG recordings and the neuropsychological assessment.

A relationship has also been suggested between neuropsychological functioning and the occurrence of non-epileptic abnormal electrical activity as recorded by the EEG, for instance slowing of the background rhythm. Dodrill and Wilkus (1978) found that a dominant posterior frequency of less than 7.5–8.0 was associated with poorer neuropsychological test performance than faster rhythms. Performance seemed particularly impaired on tests involving attention and 'complex mental manipulation'. Combinations of slow waves and epileptiform activity were accompanied by greater impairments on the psychological measures than either slow waves or epileptiform activity in isolation. In an extension of this work, Dodrill and Wilkus (1978) reported that the presence of large amounts of theta activity in the EEG trace was the most potent indicator of impaired neuropsychological test performance. However, EEG irregularities are not a cause *per se*, and it is important to question what underlies the slowing of these rhythms in patients with epilepsy. One factor, for instance, could be the administration of anticonvulsant medication.

Social and psychological factors

The factors outlined so far may be described as physical or illness factors. The influences of environmental factors upon neuropsychological functioning has been little investigated, perhaps because they are less amenable to objective investigation. Institutionalization (Halstead, 1957), non-attendance at school (Ross and West, 1978) and parental attitudes (Long and Moore, 1979) are some of the possibilities that have been proposed to have adverse effects on cognitive ability. Research suggests that the epileptic child at school may be discriminated against by his peers, and even his teachers (Pazzaglia and Frank-Pazzaglia, 1976). When seeking employment the patient with epilepsy may encounter repeated rejections which are likely to have a detrimental effect upon motivation and morale. Depressive illness is not uncommon in epilepsy (Robertson and Trimble, 1985), and this may be an additional factor associated with deficits in neuropsychological test performance. Suumeijer, Van Dam and Blijham (1973), in a series of studies of the contribution of social and psychological factors versus illness factors in epilepsy, claimed that the former may have a more devastating effect with regard to the cognitive state of the individual than the latter.

Neuropsychological aspects of treatment

The majority of patients with epilepsy will be maintained on anticonvulsant drugs for many years. Despite their wide application little is known of the possible effects of these drugs upon cognition, although several reviews of the literature are now available (Trimble, 1981; Trimble and Reynolds, 1984). Only a few drugs have been investigated in any systematic way, and the results of studies on the same drug are often contradictory and inconclusive, such that only a few rather tentative conclusions can be drawn.

For most anticonvulsants favourable reports based mainly on subjective impressions were noted soon after their introduction, but with more widespread and prolonged use adverse comments usually emerged. Detrimental effects on neuropsychological abilities have now been reported for the majority of existing drugs. Although the nature of deficits observed tends to vary between studies, they are generally such that they might be expected to interfere, at least with an individual's capacity to function at his or her peak efficiency at work, school and in other daily activities. Phenobarbitone is the drug that has perhaps been most implicated, and carbamazepine the least. Another finding that is emerging from more recent studies is that a relationship exists between anticonvulsant serum concentration and cognitive functioning, with high but not necessarily toxic levels being associated with neuropsychological impairments (Matthews and Harley, 1975; Reynolds and Travers, 1974; Trimble, Thompson and Huppert, 1980).

More definitive conclusions are difficult to draw, since individual studies vary along a number of important parameters, including the amount and duration of medication intake, and the population studies with regard to type, duration and severity of epilepsy. In addition, many investigators have adopted cross-sectional designs, comparing groups of epileptic patients matched supposedly for all but drug-related variables. However, as noted previously, patients with epilepsy are not a homogeneous group, and may vary along a vast number of variables, especially epilepsy-related ones which themselves are suspected of influencing neuropsychological functions. For this reason the matching of groups of patients with epilepsy is very difficult when investigating drug effects. A more appropriate design for such studies would seem to be intra-subject comparisons, although these are not without their design problems.

A further major criticism of previous research has been the heavy reliance on psychological tests standardized for the assessment of intelligence and/or brain damage rather than using tests for the detection of drug-induced changes in brain functioning.

In our own investigations, drug-induced changes on cognitive function have been examined in both non-epileptic volunteers and patients. The former trials had the advantage of allowing for a carefully controlled and balanced design, including the use of placebos, which is generally not possible in patients with epilepsy for treatment and ethical reasons. In addition, the findings are not contaminated by the influence of other epileptic variables as discussed. Five different drug trials were undertaken, in which different groups were administered anticonvulsant doses of phenytoin, carbamazepine, sodium valproate, clobazam and clonazepam (Cull and Trimble, 1985; Thompson and Trimble, 1981a and b; Thompson, Huppert and Trimble, 1981). Significant deficits in test performance were recorded in association with all of these five drugs. Impairments were most marked following phenytoin, and occurred on measures of memory, mental and motor speed. These recorded deficits were observed at a mean anticonvulsant serum level that was well within the commonly quoted therapeutic range. Furthermore, significant correlations were observed between individual serum levels and the degree of deterioration in test performance on five measures. Following clonazepam, at the modest dose of 0.5 mg t.d.s., impairments of memory and coding tasks were found. With sodium valproate, carbamazepine and clobazam the deficits were fewer. On sodium valproate and clobazam the pattern suggested a slowing down of mental processing speed, which reached significance only when the demands of the task increased. In contrast, those found in association with carbamazepine occurred in relation to motor rather than to mental speed. Indeed on one measure of processing speed, perceptual registration, the administration of this drug was associated with significant improvement in performance.

In our studies with patients (Thompson and Trimble, 1982a and b) we assessed changes in performance following medication changes. The overall findings were that drug reductions in patients on polytherapy improved performance on psychological tests. Improvements in performance were most marked on measures of concentration and motor speed, and least marked on measures of memory. These observed benefits were maximally significant at six months following the drug changes, which suggests that considerable time may need to elapse before it is advisable to evaluate the consequences of drug manipulations. The improvements in neuropsychological functioning took place in the absence of any marked changes in seizure frequency.

In a study in which patients were changed to carbamazepine, either alone or in combination with some existing medication, earlier and more widespread improvements in test performance were noted.

Recently we have been studying patients on monotherapy with phenytoin, carbamazepine and sodium valproate (Thompson and Trimble, 1982a). Patients tested were seen on two occasions, with high and low drug concentrations respectively, at an interval of three months. Deficits in performance were observed in association with the high serum level session, being most marked for patients on phenytoin and sodium valproate.

These findings indicate that certain patients, especially on phenytoin and sodium valproate, may function better on neuropsychological testing at lower serum concentrations, and that this is not necessarily accompanied by any marked increase in seizure frequency. Most interestingly, our results indicated that carbamazepine may have a different pattern of effects on neuropsychological abilities than the other two drugs examined. Although the available data must be interpreted with caution, there is a suggestion that phenytoin, and sodium valproate at higher levels, lead to a general slowing of mental processes, which if severe enough might be expected to result in impaired performance of many daily activities. Carbamazepine, on the other hand, appears to have less widespread effects on cognitive functioning and does not seem to relate clearly to mental speed.

Surgical intervention

Patients for whom anticonvulsant treatment has not succeeded in adequately controlling seizures may be considered for surgery. Neuropsychological investigations of this patient group have contributed greatly to our understanding of brain–behaviour relationships. From patients undergoing temporal lobectomies we have gained knowledge of the role of this area of the brain, particularly its association with memory functions (Iversen, 1977; Milner, 1975). Other patients have undergone surgery on the corpus callosum, and from them knowledge of the differential neuropsychological properties of the two hemispheres has emerged (Gazzaniger and Sperry, 1967). More recently the studies of neuropsychological assessment of surgical patients suggest that they may prove of value with regard to prognosis. Wannamaker and Matthews (1976) looked at cognitive performance on the Halstead–Reitan neuropsychological battery, and measures of motor proficiency and sensory discrimination, both preoperatively and postoperatively in 14 patients with epilepsy. They found that improvement in seizure frequency following surgery was more likely to be seen in those with the least neuropsychological impairment preoperatively. In addition, those patients who were most impaired preoperatively were inclined to develop even greater neuropsychological deficits postoperatively. Their study also demonstrated that patients with right hemisphere resection fared better than those with left hemisphere surgery, with regard to both neuropsychological outcome and seizure control, although they make the important point that their chosen measures were weighted more to the assessment of dominant hemisphere functions.

The contribution of neuropsychological assessment in epilepsy

From this review, it seems that the neuropsychological assessment of patients with epilepsy is unlikely to contribute greatly to the diagnosis of epilepsy since no neuropsychological profile distinctive of this group of disorders has been established or seems likely to be. Patients with epilepsy can vary with regard to a number of factors discussed previously, which influence neuropsychological functioning. On the other hand, because patients with epilepsy frequently present with a variety of cognitive and motor deficits, neuropsychological assessment would seem valuable in the assessment and management of this condition. From thorough neuropsychological investigations, the nature and extent of any difficulties could be established, and such information used to devise remedial programmes that might help an individual overcome or minimize the effects of such deficits.

In addition, recent research suggests that a relationship exists between neuropsychological performance, social functioning and employability, and testing thus may be useful with regard to prognosis and management in these areas. Dikmen (1980) found highly significant differences between groups of patients with epilepsy differing in employment and occupational status, across a range of neuropsychological measures. Patients who were employed and who held higher level jobs had more adequate neuropsychological functions than those who were unemployed or at lower level jobs. What most distinguished patients who differed in employment and occupation status was not a select few abilities, but rather adequacy of general neuropsychological performance. Unemployed and low occupational status groups demonstrated more consistent impairments on measures of quickness, alertness, flexibility and memory. Dikmen suggested that 'these general skills may be a prerequisite for the effective utilisation of other abilities as well as for learning new job skills'.

A potential area for neuropsychological assessment in the management of epilepsy is in the monitoring of the progress of the disorder, especially noting effects of treatment with anticonvulsant medication. The studies discussed above with regard to drug effects, although of a preliminary nature, demonstrate the potential usefulness of such monitoring. Neuropsychological assessment before and following the initiation of treatment, and before and after at least major drug changes, could be used to provide a more complete picture of the efficacy of such changes, and enable the selection of a treatment regimen for individuals that exerts the maximal effect on seizures while having minimal effects on cognitive processes.

In the limited capacity of an epilepsy clinic it is clear that not all patients can have full neuropsychological testing, and it is important to consider which groups may benefit the most, and what are the most appropriate tests to use. Children and adolescents should all be properly evaluated, and specific deficits, many of which like reading retardation are remediable, should be identified. Educational placement and occupational advice may also stem from test results. Neurocognitive deficits in adults are important to identify, especially if patients complain of them. It is helpful if all patients are evaluated early on in their illness, and then any complaints of deterioration later can be better assessed. Memory problems are particularly outstanding as important, but comments regarding slowing, inaccuracy at work, drowsiness or poor concentration should all be taken seriously. The possibility that medications may be contributing to these effects must be considered, and changes in function following drug changes can be monitored by psychological testing.

The choice of tests is unfortunately very large, and most departments of psychology have their own preferences. The method we have adopted is away from extensive procedures that take hours to complete, and towards the development of a brief test battery concentrating on those problems we feel to be important to our patients. The methodology in this field is likely to change in the very near future with the growing availability of microprocessors for presentation and recording of information in the research and clinical setting.

CONCLUSIONS

This review emphasizes that in recent years a substantial amount of work on the relationship between interictal psychopathology and cognitive function in epilepsy has been carried out. With regard to the former, we have moved from a position, never clearly refined, that *all* patients with temporal lobe epilepsy have psychopathology to one in which psychopathology in epilepsy is seen as the outcome of several independent and dependent processes. There is little doubt that patients with epilepsy suffer severely from problems of social rejection and discrimination. Their affliction, with its sudden and paroxysmal loss of consciousness, leading to socially embarrassing behaviour, must place them in a vulnerable position with regard to the development of psychopathology. In addition, the more other variables are examined, the more it seems that patients with certain types of epilepsy are more prone to develop certain types of psychiatric disability with increased propensity. This emphasizes in particular that patients with predominantly allocortical lesions, with the tendency to generalize and permeate through limbic structures, are the most prone.

Of all the psychopathological variants that may develop, the outstanding quality of paranoid thinking seems to be common. Paranoia, in both the studies of personality disorders, and psychosis, is frequently mentioned, and often noted in investigations that have used rating scales for assessment. This affect, a combination of diffusely projected fear and hostility, while in most animal interactions may be a prerequisite for self-preservation arousing a sense of suspicion and danger from the world outside, when magnified and inappropriate leads to maladaptive behaviour. MacLean (1969) many years ago suggested that the limbic system was the neural structure for the 'paranoid streak', and the accumulating evidence supports this. Why, in some people, the affect qualitatively transforms into a delusional state is unclear, but further work with such techniques as positron emission tomography (PET) may help clarify such questions. The fact that thought disorder and auditory hallucinations seem mainly to occur following maximum changes in the dominant hemisphere is compatible with our knowledge that the left cortex mediates language, and the suggested connections between temporal lobe–limbic structures, such as the amygdala and hippocampus and sensory cortical areas, including the primary auditory cortex (Powell, 1973).

Cognitive changes, and the reasons for them, are a field of increasing interest and importance. This reflects partly our increased ability to detect them, but further the increased 'cognitive load' placed on all of us by the rapid technological changes of modern society.

Although some feel that by identifying the problems discussed in this chapter, patients with epilepsy will suffer more in the sense of knowledge of them leading to more stigmatization, in our experience this is not the case. Patients and their relatives are very concerned about such issues as behaviour and cognitive change, and to identify them, treat them, and to be able to provide sound information about their development and prognosis is an important facet of the management of patients with epilepsy.

References

AGNETTI, V., GANGA, M., MURRIGAILE, M., PIRAS, M. R. and TICCA, A. (1979) Memory assessment in temporal lobe epilepsy. *Paper presented at the XIth Epilepsy International Symposium, Florence, Italy*

ARENA, R., MENCHETTI, G., TASSINARI, G. and TOGNETTI, M. (1979) Simple and complex reaction time to lateralised visual stimuli in groups of epileptic patients. *Paper presented at the XIth Epilepsy International Symposium, Florence, Italy*

BAGLEY, C. (1971) *The Social Psychology of the Child with Epilepsy.* London: Routledge and Kegan Paul Ltd.

BANCAUD, J., FAVEL, P., BONIS, A. *et al.* (1970) Manifestations sexuelles paroxystiques et epilepsie temporale. *Revue Neurologie,* **123,** 217–230

BARNES, M. R. and FETTERMAN, J. (1938) Mentality of dispensary epileptic patients. *Archives of Neurology,* **40,** 903–910

BARRACLOUGH, B. (1981) Suicide and epilepsy. In *Epilepsy and Psychiatry,* by E. H. Reynolds and M. R. Trimble, pp. 72–76. Edinburgh: Churchill Livingstone

BEAR, D. M. and FEDIO, P. (1977) Quantitative analysis of interictal behaviour in temporal lobe epilepsy. *Archives of Neurology,* **34,** 454–467

BEAR, D. M., LEVIN, K., BLUMER, D., CHETHAM, D. and RYDER, J. (1982) Inter-ictal behaviour in hospitalised temporal lobe epileptics: relationship to idiopathic psychiatric syndromes. *Journal of Neurology, Neurosurgery and Psychiatry,* **45,** 481–488

BERENT, S., BOLL, T. J. and GIORDANI, B. (1980) Hemispheric site of epileptogenic focus: cognitive, perceptual and psychosocial implications for children and adults. In *Advances in Epileptology,* edited by R. Canger, F. Angeleri and J. K. Penry. New York: Raven Press

BETTS, T. A. (1974) A follow-up study of a cohort of patients with epilepsy admitted to psychiatric care in an English city. In *Epilepsy – Proceedings of the Hans Berger Centenary Symposium,* edited by P. Harris and C. Mawdsley, pp. 326–338. Edinburgh: Churchill Livingstone

BETTS, T. A., MERSKEY, H. and POND, D. A. (1976) Psychiatry. In *A Textbook of Epilepsy*, edited by J. Laidlaw and A. Richens, pp. 145–184. London: Churchill Livingstone

BLUMER, D. and WALKER, A. E. (1975) The neural basis of sexual behaviour. In *Psychiatric Aspects of Neurologic Disease,* edited by D. F. Benson and D. Blumer, pp. 199–217. New York: Grune and Stratton

BOUCHET, M. and CAZAUVEILH, M. (1825) De l'epilepsie considere dans ses rapports avec l'alientation mentale. *Archives Général de Médecin,* **9,** 510–542

BRADLEY, C. (1947) Treatment of the convulsive child in a children's psychiatric hospital. *The Nervous Child,* **6,** 76–85

BROWNE, T. R., PENRY, J. K., PORTER, R. J. and DREIFUSS, F. E. (1974) Responsiveness before, during and after spike-wave paroxysms. *Neurology,* **24,** 659–665

BRUENS, J. H. (1980) Psychoses in epilepsy. Historic concepts and new developments. In *Advances in Epileptology: XIth Epilepsy International Symposium,* edited by R. Canger, F. Angeleri and J. K. Penry, pp. 161–166. New York: Raven Press

BRUHN, P. and PARSONS, O. A. (1977) Reaction time variability in epileptic and brain-damaged patients. *Cortex,* **13,** 373–384

BUCHSBAUM, M. S., INGVAR, D. H., KESSLER, R. *et al.* (1982) Cerebral glucography with positron tomography. *Archives of General Psychiatry,* **39,** 251–260

COLLINS, A. L. (1951) Epileptic intelligence. *Journal of Consulting Psychology,* **15,** 392–399

CROW, T. (1980) Molecular pathology of schizophrenia: more than one disease process. *British Medical Journal,* **280,** 66–68

CULL, C. and TRIMBLE, M. R. (1985) Anticonvulsant benzodiazepines and performances (in press)

DALBY, M. A. (1975) Behavioural effects of carbamazepine. In *Complex Partial Seizures and their Treatment*, edited by J. K. Penry and D. D. Daly. New York: Raven Press

DELGADO-ESCUETA, A. V., MATTSON, R. H., KING, L. *et al.* (1981) The nature of aggression during epileptic seizures. *New England Journal of Medicine,* **305,** 711–716

DAM, A. M. (1980) Epilepsy and neuron loss in the hippocampus. *Epilepsia,* **21,** 617–630

DELANEY, R. C., ROSEN, A. J., MATTSON, R. H. and NOVELLY, R. A. (1980) Memory function in focal epilepsy. A comparison of non-surgical unilateral temporal lobe and frontal lobe samples. *Cortex,* **16,** 103–117

DEUTSCH, C. P. (1953) Differences among epileptics and between epileptics and non-epileptics in terms of some learning and memory variables. *Archives of Neurology and Psychiatry,* **70,** 574–482

DIKMEN, S. (1980) Neuropsychological aspects of epilepsy. In *A Multi-disciplinary Handbook of Epilepsy,* edited by B. P. Hermann, pp. 36–73. Springfield, Ill.: Charles C. Thomas

DIKMEN, S. and MATTHEWS, C. G. (1977) Effect of major motor seizure frequency upon cognitive-intellectual functions in adults. *Epilepsia,* **18,** 21–30

DIKMEN, S., MATTHEWS, C. G. and HARLEY, J. P. (1975) The effect of early versus late onset of major motor epilepsy upon cognitive intellectual function. *Epilepsia,* **16,** 73–81

DODRILL, C. B. (1982) Neuropsychology. In *A Textbook of Epilepsy,* edited by J. Laidlaw and A. Richens, pp. 282–291. Edinburgh: Churchill Livingstone

DODRILL, C. B. and TROUPIN, A. S. (1977) Psychotropic effects of carbamazepine in epilepsy: a double-blind comparison with phenytoin. *Neurology,* **27,** 1023–1028

DODRILL, C. B. and WILKUS, R. J. (1978) Neuropsychological correlates of the EEG in epileptics. III. Generalised non-epileptiform abnormalities. *Epilepsia,* **19,** 453–462

EPSTEIN, A. W. (1961) Relationship of fetishism and transvestism to brain and particularly to temporal lobe dysfunction. *Journal of Nervous and Mental Disease,* **133,** 247–253

FEDIO, P. and MIRSKY, A. F. (1969) Selective intellectual deficits in children with temporal lobe or centrecephalic epilepsy. *Neuropsychologia,* **6,** 287–300

FENWICK, P. (1981a) EEG Studies. In *Epilepsy and Psychiatry,* edited by E. H. Reynolds and M. R. Trimble, pp. 242–263. Edinburgh: Churchill Livingstone

FENWICK, P. (1981b) Precipitation and inhibition of seizures. In *Epilepsy and Psychiatry,* edited by E. H. Reynolds and M. R. Trimble, pp. 306–321. Edinburgh: Churchill Livingstone

FLOR-HENRY, P. (1969) Psychosis and temporal lobe epilepsy. *Epilepsia,* **10,** 363–395

FOX, J. T. (1924) Response of epileptic children to mental and educational tests. *British Journal of Medical Psychology,* **4,** 235–248

GALLHOFER, B., TRIMBLE, M. R., FRACKOWIAK, R., GIBBS, J. and JONES, T. (1985) A study of cerebral blood flow and metabolism in epileptic psychosis using positron emission tomography and oxygen-15 (in press)

GASTAUT, H. (1964) Enquiry into the education of epileptic children. In *Epilepsy and Education, a report of a seminar in Marseilles, April 1964.* London: British Epilepsy Association and International Bureau for Epilepsy

GASTAUT, H. and COLLOMB, H. (1954) Étude du comportement sexual chez les épileptiques psychomoteurs. *Annales Medicopsychologiques,* **2,** 657–696

GAZZANIGER, M. S. and SPERRY, R. W. (1967) Language after section of the cerebral commissures. *Brain,* **90,** 131–148

GESCHWIND, N. (1979) Behavioural changes in temporal lobe epilepsy. *Psychological Medicine,* **9,** 217–219

GIBBS, F. A. (1951) Ictal and non-ictal psychiatric disorders in temporal lobe epilepsy. *Journal of Nervous and Mental Diseases,* **113,** 522–528

GIBBS, F. A. and STAMPS, F. W. (1953) *Epilepsy Handbook.* Springfield, Ill.: Charles C. Thomas

GLOOR, P. (1972) Temporal lobe epilepsy: its possible contribution to the understanding of the functional significance of the amygdala and its interaction with neocortical–temporal mechanisms. In *The Neurobiology of the Amygdala,* edited by N. B. Eleftherio, Vol. 1, pp. 423–457. New York: Plenum

GLOWINSKI, H. (1973) Cognitive deficits in temporal lobe epilepsy: an investigation of memory functioning. *Journal of Nervous and Mental Diseases,* **157,** 129–137

GREEN, J. B. and HARTLAGE, L. G. (1971) Comparative performance of epileptic and non-epileptic children and adolescents. *Diseases of the Nervous System,* **32,** 418–421

GREGORIADIS, A., FRAGOS, E., KAPSALAKIS, Z. and MANDOURALOS, B. (1971) A correlation between mental disorders and EEG and AEG findings in temporal lobe epilepsy. *Proceedings of the Vth World Congress of Psychiatry, Mexico*

GRIESINGER, W. (1857) *Mental Pathology and Therapeutics.* Translated by C. Lockhart Robertson and J. Rutherford. London: New Sydenham Society

GRUZELIER, J. H. (1981) Cerebral laterality and psychopathology: fact or fiction? *Psychological Medicine,* **11,** 219–227

GUDMUNDSSON, G. (1966) Epilepsy in Iceland. *Acta Neurologica Scandanavica,* **43,** 1–124 (Suppl. 25)

GUERRANT, J., ANDERSON, C. V. C. S., FISCHER, A., WEINSTEIN, M. R., JARROS, R. M. and DESKINS, A. (1962) *Personality in Epilepsy.* Springfield, Ill.: Charles C. Thomas

GUEY, T., CHARLES, C., COQUILERY, C., ROGERS, J. and SOULAYROL, R. (1967) Study of psychological effects of ethosuximide (Zarontin) on 25 children suffering from petit mal epilepsy. *Epilepsia,* **8,** 129–141

HALSTEAD, H. (1957) Abilities and behaviour of epileptic children. *Journal of Mental Science,* **103,** 28–47

HAWTON, K., FAGG, J. and MARSACK, P. (1980) Association between epilepsy and attempted suicide. *Journal of Neurology, Neurosurgery and Psychiatry,* **43,** 158–160

HEATH, R. G. (1977) Subcortical brain function correlates of psychopathology and epilepsy. In *Psychopathology and Brain Dysfunction*, edited by C. Shagass, S. Gershon and A. J. Friedhoff. New York: Raven Press

HENRIKSEN, G. F. (1973) Status epilepticus partialis with fear as clinical expression. *Epilepsia,* **14,** 39–46

HERMANN, B. P., DIKMEN, S., SCHWARTZ, M. S. and KARNES, W. E. (1982) Inter-ictal psychopathology in patients with ictal fear: a quantitative investigation. *Neurology,* **32,** 7–11

HERMANN, B. P. and REIL, P. (1981) Inter-ictal personality and behavioural traits in temporal lobe and generalised epilepsy. *Cortex,* **17,** 125–128

HIERONS, R. and SAUNDERS, M. (1966) Impotence in patients with temporal lobe lesions. *Lancet,* **2,** 761–764

HILL, D. (1953) Psychiatric disorders of epilepsy. *Medical Press,* **229,** 473–475

HOLDSWORTH, L. and WHITMORE, K. (1974) A study of children with epilepsy attending ordinary schools. I. Their seizure patterns, progress and behaviour in school. *Developmental Medicine and Child Neurology,* **16,** 746–758

HUNTER, R., LOGUE, V. and MCMENEMY, W. H. (1963) Temporal lobe epilepsy supervening on long standing transvestism and fetishism. *Epilepsia,* **4,** 60–65

IVERSEN, S. (1977) Temporal lobe amnesia. In *Amnesia,* edited by C. W. M. Whitty and O. L. Zangwill. London: Butterworths

JENSEN, I. and LARSEN, J. K. (1979) Psychoses in drug-resistant temporal lobe epilepsy. *Journal of Neurology, Neurosurgery and Psychiatry,* **42,** 948–954

KEATING, L. E. (1960) A review of the literature on the relationship of epilepsy and intelligence in school children. *Journal of Mental Science,* **106,** 1042–1059

KILOH, L. G. (1971) Psychiatric aspects of epilepsy. In *Geigy Symposium on Epilepsy*, edited by R. R. Winton. Australia: Geigy

KIMURA, D. (1964) Cognitive deficit related to seizure pattern in centrencephalic epilepsy. *Journal of Neurology, Neurosurgery and Psychiatry,* **27,** 291–295

KLIGMAN, D. and GOLDBERG, D. A. (1975) Temporal lobe epilepsy and aggression. *Journal of Nervous and Mental Diseases,* **160,** 324–341

KLØVE, H. and MATTHEWS, C. G. (1966) Psychometric and adaptive abilities in epilepsy with different aetiology. *Epilepsia,* **7,** 330–338

KOGEORGOS, J., FONAGY, P. and SCOTT, D. F. (1982) Psychiatric symptom patterns of chronic epileptics attending a neurological clinic: a controlled investigation. *British Journal of Psychiatry,* **140,** 236–243

KRISTENSEN, O. and SINDRUP, E. H. (1978) Psychomotor epilepsy and psychosis. *Acta Neurologica Scandanavica,* **57,** 361–370

LADAVAS, E., UMILTA, A. and PROVINCIALI, L. (1979) Hemispheric-dependent cognitive performances in epileptic patients. *Epilepsia,* **20,** 493–502

LENNOX, W. G. (1943) Brain injury, drugs and environment as a cause of mental decay in epilepsy. *American Journal of Psychiatry,* **99,** 174–180

LENNOX, W. G. and LENNOX, M. A. (1960) *Epilepsy and Related Disorders.* London: J. and A. Churchill

LOISEAU, P., STRUBE, E., BROUSTET, D., BATTELLOCCHI, S., GOMENI, C. and MORSELLI, P. L. (1980) Evaluation of memory function in a population of epileptic patients and matched controls. *Acta Neurologica Scandinavia,* Suppl. 80, **62,** 58–61

LONG, C. G. and MOORE, J. R. (1979) Parental expectations for their epileptic children. *Journal of Child Psychology and Psychiatry,* **20,** 313–324

MACKAY, A. (1979) Self-poisoning – a complication of epilepsy. *British Journal of Psychiatry,* **134,** 277–282

MACLEAN, P. D. (1969) The paranoid streak in man. In *Beyond Reductionism,* edited by A. Koestler and J. R. Smythies, pp. 258–278. London: Hutchinson and Co.

MARCHAND, L. and DE AJURIAGUERRA, J. (1948) *Epilepsies.* Paris: Desclee de Brouiser

MARK, V. H. and IRVINE, F. R. (1970) *Violence and the Brain.* New York: Harper and Row

MATTHEWS, C. G. and HARLEY, J. P. (1975) Cognitive and motor sensory performances in toxic and non-toxic epileptic subjects. *Neurology,* **25,** 184–188

MCGUCKIN, H. M. (1980) Changing the world view of those with epilepsy. In *Advances in Epileptology. XIth Epilepsy International Symposium,* edited by R. Carger, F. Angeleri and J. K. Penry, pp. 205–208. New York: Raven Press

MEIER, M. J. and FRENCH, L. A. (1965) Some personality correlates of unilateral and bilateral EEG abnormalities in psychomotor epilepsy. *Journal of Clinical Psychology,* **21,** 3–9

MILNER, B. (1975) Psychological aspects of focal epilepsy and its neurosurgical management. *Advances in Neurology,* **8,** 299–321

MIRSKY, A. F., PRIMAC, D. W., MARSAN, C. A., ROSOLD, H. E. and STEVENS, J. R. (1960) A comparison of the psychological test performance of patients with focal and non-focal epilepsy. *Experimental Neurology,* **2,** 75–89

MITCHELL, W., FALCONER, M. A. and HILL, D. (1954) Epilepsy with fetishism relieved by temporal lobectomy. *Lancet,* **2,** 626–630

MOHAN, V., VARMA, V. K. and SAWHNEY, B. B. (1976) Intellectual and memory functions in epileptics. *India Neurology,* **24,** 110

MORGAN, A. and GROH, C. (1980) Changes in visual perception in children with epilepsy. In *Epilepsy and Behaviour, '79,* edited by B. Kulig, H. Meinardi and G. Stores. Lisse: Swets and Zeitlinger

MUNGAS, D. (1982) Inter-ictal behaviour abnormality in temporal lobe epilepsy. *Archives of General Psychiatry,* **39,** 108–111

NIELSEN, H. and KRISTENSEN, O. (1981) Personality correlates of sphenoidal EEG foci in temporal lobe epilepsy. *Acta Neurologica Scandanavica,* **64,** 289–300

O'LEARY, D. S., SEIDENBERG, M., BERENT, S. and BOLL, T. J. (1981) Effect of age of onset of tonic-clonic seizures on neuropsychological performance in children. *Epilepsia,* **22,** 197–204

OUNSTED, C. and LINDSAY, J. (1981) The long-term outcome of temporal lobe epilepsy in childhood. In *Epilepsy and Psychiatry,* edited by E. H. Reynolds and M. R. Trimble, pp. 185–215. Edinburgh: Churchill Livingstone

PAZZAGLIA, P. and FRANK-PAZZAGLIA, L. (1976) Record in grade school of pupils with epilepsy: an epidemiological study. *Epilepsia,* **17,** 361–366

PEREZ, M. M. and TRIMBLE, M. R. (1980) Epileptic psychosis – diagnostic comparison with process schizophrenia. *British Journal of Psychiatry,* **137,** 245–249

PEREZ, M. M., TRIMBLE, M. R., REIDER, I. and MURRAY, N. M. (1984) Epileptic psychosis, a further evaluation of PSE profiles. *British Journal of Psychiatry*, **146,** 155–163

PIERCE-CLARK, L. (1923) The psychobiologic concept of essential epilepsy. *Journal of Nervous and Mental Disease,* **57,** 433–444

POND, D. A. (1957) Psychiatric aspects of epilepsy. *Journal of the Indian Medical Profession,* **3,** 1441–1451

POND, D. A. (1962) The schizophrenia-like psychoses of epilepsy – Discussion. *Proceedings of the Royal Society of Medicine,* **55,** 311

POND, D. A. and BIDWELL, B. H. (1959) A survey of epilepsy in 14 general practices. *Epilepsia,* **1,** 285–299

POWELL, T. P. S. (1973) Sensory convergence in the cerebral cortex. In *Surgical Approaches in Psychiatry,* edited by L. V. Laitinen and K. E. Livingston, pp. 266–281. Lancaster: MTP Press

PRITCHARD, P. B., LOMBROSO, C. T. and MCINTYRE, M. (1980) Psychological complications of temporal lobe epilepsy. *Neurology,* **30,** 227–232

QUADFASEL, A. F. and PRUYSER, P. W. (1955) Cognitive deficit in patients with psychomotor epilepsy. *Epilepsia,* **4,** 80–90

RAUSCH, R., LIEB, J. P. and CRANDALL, P. H. (1978) Neuropsychologic correlates of depth spike activity in epileptic patients. *Archives of Neurology,* **35,** 699–705

REY, J. H., POND, D. A. and EVANS, C. C. (1949) Clinical and electroencephalographic studies of temporal lobe function. *Proceedings of the Royal Society of Medicine*, **42,** 891–904

REYNOLDS, J. H., POND, D. A. and EVANS, C. C. (1949) Clinical and EEG studies of temporal lobe function. *Proceedings of the Royal Society of Medicine,* **42,** 891–904

REYNOLDS, E. H. and TRAVERS, R. D. (1974) Serum anticonvulsant concentrations in epileptic patients with mental symptoms. *British Journal of Psychiatry,* **124,** 440–445

REYNOLDS, E. H. and TRIMBLE, M. R. (1981) *Epilepsy and Psychiatry.* Edinburgh: Churchill Livingstone

ROBERTS, J., ROBERTSON, M. M. and TRIMBLE, M. R. (1982) The lateralising significance of hypergraphia in temporal lobe epilepsy. *Journal of Neurology, Neurosurgery and Psychiatry,* **45,** 131–138

ROBERTSON, M. M. (1983) *Depression in patients with epilepsy.* MD thesis. University of Cape Town

ROBERTSON, M. M. and TRIMBLE, M. R. (1985). The phenomenology of depression in epilepsy. (In preparation)

RODIN, E. A., KATZ, M. and LENNOX, K. (1976) Differences between patients with temporal lobe seizures and those with other forms of epileptic attacks. *Epilepsia,* **17,** 313–320

RODIN, E. A. (1984) What does the Bear–Fedio Inventory measure? *Proceedings of the XIVth Epilepsy International Symposium.* New York: Raven Press

RODIN, E. A. (1985) The Bear–Fedio Inventory and temporal lobe epilepsy. *Neurology* (in press)

ROSS, E. and WEST, P. B. (1978) Achievements and problems of British 11-year-olds with epilepsy. In *Advances in Epileptology. Psychology and New Diagnostic Approaches*, edited by H. Meinardi and A. J. Rowan. Amsterdam: Swets and Zeitlinger

RUTTER, M., GRAHAM, P. and YULE, W. (1970) A neuropsychiatric study in childhood. *Clinics in Developmental Medicine, 35.* London: Heinemann

SACHDEV, H. S. and WAXMAN, S. G. (1981) Frequency of hypergraphia in temporal lobe epilepsy: an index of inter-ictal behavioural syndromes. *Journal of Neurology, Neurosurgery and Psychiatry,* **44,** 358–360

SCHNEIDER, K. (1957) Primare und secondare symtome bei der schizophrenie. *Fortschritte der Neurologie, Psychiatrie und ihrer Grenzgebiete,* **25,** 487–490

SERAFETINIDES, E. A. (1965) Aggressiveness in temporal lobe epilepsies and its relation to cerebral dysfunction and environmental factors. *Epilepsia,* **6,** 33–42

SCHWARTZ, M. L. and DENNERLL, R. D. (1970) Neuropsychological assessment of children with, without, and with questionable epileptogenic dysfunction. *Perceptual and Motor Skills,* **30,** 111–121

SEIDENBERG, M., O'LEARY, D. S., BERENT, S. and BOLL, T. (1981) Changes in seizure frequency and test–retest scores on the Wechsler Adult Intelligence Scale. *Epilepsia,* **22,** 75–83

SHERWIN, I. (1981) Psychosis associated with epilepsy: significance of laterality of the epileptogenic lesion. *Journal of Neurology, Neurosurgery and Psychiatry,* **44,** 83–85

SHERWIN, I. (1982) The effect of the location of an epileptogenic lesion on the occurrence of psychosis in epilepsy. In *Temporal Lobe Epilepsy, Mania, Schizophrenia and the Limbic System,* edited by W. P. Koella and M. R. Trimble, pp. 81–97. Basel: Karger

SHUKLA, G. D., SRIVASTAVA, O. N. and KATIYAR, B. C. (1979) Sexual disturbances in temporal lobe epilepsy. A controlled study. *British Journal of Psychiatry,* **134,** 288–292

SLATER, E. and BEARD, A. W. (1963) The schizophrenia-like psychoses of epilepsy. *British Journal of Psychiatry,* **109,** 95–150

STEVENS, J. R. (1982) Risk factors for psychopathology in individuals with epilepsy. In *Temporal Lobe Epilepsy, Mania, Schizophrenia and the Limbic System,* edited by W. P. Koella and M. R. Trimble, pp. 56–80. Basel: Karger

STEVENS, J. R. and HERMANN, B. P. (1981) Temporal lobe epilepsy, psychopathology and violence: the state of the evidence. *Neurology,* **31,** 1127–1132

STEVENS, J. R. and LIVERMORE, A. (1978) Kindling in the mesolimbic dopamine system: animal model of psychosis. *Neurology,* **28,** 36–46

STORES, G., HART, J. and PIRAN, N. (1978) Inattentiveness in schoolchildren with epilepsy. *Epilepsia,* **19,** 169–175

SUUMEIJER, J. P. B. M., VAN DAM, A. and BLIJHAM, M. (1978) *Children with Epilepsy: Education, Future Orientation and School Achievement Level,* pp. 342–348. Ganeesk: Tijdschrift Society

SYMONDS, C. (1962) The schizophrenia-like psychoses of epilepsy – discussion. *Proceedings of the Royal Society of Medicine,* **55,** 311

TARTER, R. E. (1972) Intellectual and adaptive functioning in epilepsy: a review of fifty years of research. *Diseases of the Nervous System,* **33,** 763–770

TAYLOR, D. C. (1969) Sexual behaviour and temporal lobe epilepsy. *Archives of Neurology,* **21,** 510–516

TAYLOR, D. C. (1975) Factors influencing the occurrence of schizophrenia-like psychosis in patients with temporal lobe epilepsy. *Psychological Medicine,* **5,** 249–254

TEMKIN, O. (1971) *The Falling Sickness.* Baltimore: Johns Hopkins Press

THOMPSON, P. J. and TRIMBLE, M. R. (1981a) Sodium valproate and cognitive functioning in normal volunteers. *British Journal of Clinical Pharmacy,* **12,** 819–824

THOMPSON, P. J. and TRIMBLE, M. R. (1981b) Clobazam and cognitive functions. Effects in healthy volunteers. In *Royal Society of Medicine International Congress and Symposium Series,* pp. 33–38. London: Academic Press

THOMPSON, P. J. and TRIMBLE, M. R. (1982a) Comparative effects of anticonvulsant drugs on cognitive functioning. *British Journal of Clinical Practice,* Suppl. 18, 154–156

THOMPSON, P. J. and TRIMBLE, M. R. (1982b) Anticonvulsant drugs and cognitive functions. *Epilepsia,* **23,** 531–544

THOMPSON, P., HUPPERT, F. A. and TRIMBLE, M. R. (1981) Phenytoin and cognitive functions: effects on normal volunteers and implications for epilepsy. *British Journal of Clinical Psychology,* **20,** 155–162

TIZARD, J., RUTTER, M. and WHITMORE, K. (1969) *Education, Health and Behaviour.* London: Longmans

TOONE, B. K., DAWSON, J. and DRIVER, M. V. (1982) Psychoses of epilepsy. A radiological evaluation. *British Journal of Psychiatry,* **140,** 244–248

TOONE, B. K., GARRALDA, M. E. and RON, M. A. (1982) The psychosis of epilepsy and the functional psychoses: a clinical and phenomenological comparison. *British Journal of Psychiatry,* **141,** 256–261

TRIMBLE, M. R. (1977) The relationship between epilepsy and schizophrenia: a biochemical hypothesis. *Biological Psychiatry,* **12,** 299–304

TRIMBLE, M. R. (1978) Non-MAOI antidepressants and epilepsy: a review. *Epilepsia,* **19,** 241–250

TRIMBLE, M. R. (1981) Anticonvulsant drugs, behaviour and cognitive abilities. In *Current Developments in Psychopharmacology,* edited by W. Essman and L. Valzelli, Vol. 6, pp. 65–91. New York: Spectrum Publications Inc.

TRIMBLE, M. R. and PEREZ, M. M. (1980) Psychosocial functioning in adults. In *Epilepsy and Behaviour,* edited by B. M. Kulig, H. Meinardi and G. Stores. Amsterdam and Lisse: Swets and Zeitlinger

TRIMBLE, M. R. and PEREZ, M. M. (1982) The phenomenology of the chronic psychoses of epilepsy. In *Temporal Lobe Epilepsy, Mania, Schizophrenia and the Limbic System,* edited by W. P. Koella and M. R. Trimble, pp. 98–105. Basel: Karger

TRIMBLE, M. R., THOMPSON, P. J. and HUPPERT, F. (1980) Anticonvulsant drugs and cognitive abilities. In *Advances in Epileptology: 11th International Epilepsy Symposium,* edited by R. Canger, F. Angeleri and J. K. Penry, pp. 199–204. New York: Raven Press

TRIMBLE, M. R. and REYNOLDS, E. H. (1984) Neuropsychiatric toxicity of anticonvulsant drugs. In *Recent Advances in Neurology,* edited by B. Matthews. Edinburgh: Churchill Livingstone

TYMCHUK, A. J. (1974) Comparison of Bender error and time scores for groups of epileptic, retarded and behaviour problem children. *Perceptual Motor Skills,* **38,** 71–74

WANNAMAKER, B. B. and MATTHEWS, C. G. (1976) Prognostic implications of neuropsychological test performance for surgical treatment of epilepsy. *Journal of Nervous and Mental Diseases,* **163,** 29–34

WAXMAN, S. G. and GESCHWIND, N. (1974) Hypergraphia in temporal lobe epilepsy. *Neurology,* **24,** 629–636

WAXMAN, S. G. and GESCHWIND, N. (1975) The inter-ictal behaviour syndrome of temporal lobe epilepsy. *Archives of General Psychiatry,* **32,** 1580–1586

WEIL, A. A. (1959) Ictal emotions occurring in temporal lobe dysfunction. *Archives of Neurology,* **1,** 101–111

WHITMAN, S., HERMANN, B. P. and GORDON, A. (1982) Are people with epilepsy at additional risk for psychopathoology? *Presented to Annual American Epilepsy Society, New York, December 1981*

WIESER, H. G. (1980) Temporal lobe or psychomotor status epilepticus: a case report. *Electroencephalography and Clinical Neurophysiology,* **48,** 558–572

WILKUS, R. J. and DODRILL, C. B. (1976) Neuropsychological correlates of the electroencephalogram in epileptics. *Epilepsia,* **17,** 89–100

ZIELINSKI, J. J. (1974) *Epidemiology and Medical-social Problems of Epilepsy in Warsaw.* Warsaw: Warsaw Psychoneurological Institute

ZIMMERMAN, F. T., BURGEMEISTER, B. B. and PUTNAM, T. J. (1951) Intellectual and emotional make up of the epileptic. *Archives of Neurology and Psychiatry,* **65,** 545–556

17
Psychosocial aspects of epilepsy

R. L. Masland

INTRODUCTION

The disability of persons with epilepsy stems from four sources: (1) disruption caused by the seizures themselves; (2) the effects of primary and secondary associated neurological impairments including drugs; (3) the reactions of society to the individual with epilepsy; and (4) the reaction of the patient to his disorder. The physician is in a position to play a key role in diminishing the impact of all four of these factors. Unfortunately, preoccupation with the control of seizures – both on the part of the physician and of the patient – often seems to overshadow an adequate concern for the other factors. Yet in terms of disability, for many patients it is these other factors which determine whether the patient will or will not make a satisfactory life adjustment. Of them all, the most significant is the patient's own concept of himself and of his disorder. To a great extent his attitude will reflect those of society. During a study of epilepsy in the United States the Commission for the Control of Epilepsy and its Consequences (1980) conducted a series of public hearings. A universal complaint at these hearings was ignorance. The patients complained that they were misunderstood by the public, that their relatives were confused, and that they themselves had never really been told what was wrong. Worst of all, they felt that many of the professionals they encountered were equally ignorant.

It is customary to attribute the pathological attitudes of society toward epilepsy to age-long superstition. A more immediate explanation is that it is frightening to observe a person lose control of himself. Being uneducated about epilepsy, the onlooker is seized with a feeling of abhorrence and helplessness. The result is a desire to avoid this kind of situation. It is this avoidance that underlies the unwillingness to employ epileptic persons. The employer may say it is 'unsafe', but in most instances it is an emotionally determined desire on his part and on the part of the other employees to avoid the unpleasant.

The solution for this is public education. The Epilepsy Foundation of America (EFA) wages this campaign on many fronts. Television shorts, special forums on epilepsy, and incidental references to epileptic persons in films and plays are used to portray them as normal people and to explain their disorder as an understandable phenomenon of nervous activity. 'Alert' programs in the schools for teachers and students, and similar presentations for policemen, attendants and other service personnel, carry the same message. In addition, these programs relieve fear about epilepsy by describing the simple measures required to deal with the attack.

Experience in the United States demonstrates that public education can change attitudes. Gallup polls repeated over the last 30 years reveal very significant improvement in public knowledge and attitudes (Caveness and Gallup, 1980). The number of persons who said that they would object to their children associating with children with epilepsy has dropped from 24% in 1949 to 6% in 1979. However, even now 9% felt that epileptics 'should not be employed on jobs like other people'; 3% still considered it a form of insanity, and 18% would object to their offspring marrying someone with epilepsy.

Since the majority of individuals develop epilepsy during childhood, it is parental attitude which has played a major role in shaping the person's self-image. Few parents escape the Scylla and Charybdis of overprotection and rejection. The natural disappointment of having a child with an unsavory illness usually leads to a reactive overcompensation, and ultimately to domination. In the worst cases, parent and child become locked into a pattern of life dominated by the child's seizures. The problem is further complicated by the reality that for the person with incompletely controlled seizures life is hazardous. About 10% of persons with epilepsy die a sudden death – from seizure, accident, or suicide (Woodbury, 1978). Parents must be helped to accept a considerable risk for the sake of their child's independence and self-image. It must be emphasized that these hazards are to a great extent unavoidable – they exist on the stairway and in the bathroom at home, and even in bed. There is no advantage in attempting to protect the child from the ordinary activities of life.

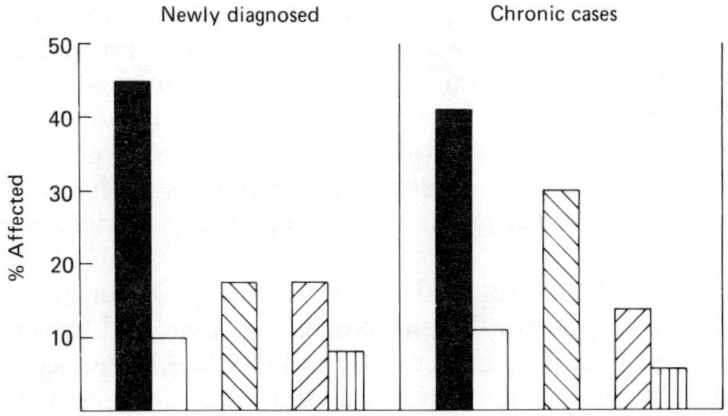

Figure 17.1 Psychiatric problems in children with epilepsy, with diabetes and controls (from Hoave, 1981). (■) epilepsy; (□) epilepsy control; (▨) diabetes; (▥) diabetes control; (▧) siblings of epileptic children

Emotional maladjustment is more common in children with epilepsy than it is in similarly handicapped children with non-neurological conditions (Hoare, 1984a, b and c; *Figure 17.1*). It is not clear whether this is due to socioenvironmental factors or whether it reflects direct effects of disease of the CNS.

These problems can be resolved only by direct and honest conversations with the professional. It is the physician's responsibility to present to the parent and to the child the fullest possible explanation of the disorder and its ramifications. It is probably unwise to avoid the term 'epilepsy' – to do so only reinforces the parent's and child's feeling that they have a horrible disease. It is better to tell the patient that he or she has a form of epilepsy; that the term describes a symptom of many different conditions; and then to spell out in detail the nature and implications of *his* or *her* condition. A survey of recorded interviews with 80 patients and their families documents that it is the attitude of the physician which is the greatest factor in shaping the attitude of the patient toward himself (Schneider and Conrad, 1983).

SOURCES OF INFORMATION

A number of agencies are striving to provide greater public and professional awareness of epilepsy and its problems. A primary source of information about epilepsy is the National Epilepsy Library and Resource Center (NELRC) developed by the Epilepsy Foundation of America (EFA) in response to the recommendations of the Commission on the Control of Epilepsy and its Consequences. This information base has been developed to serve two types of clients; professionals seeking references and authoritative information regarding the scientific and technical aspects of the disorder; and patients, parents and other laymen seeking information about epilepsy and its medical and social aspects and referral to appropriate resources within their environment.

To respond to requests from the first group, the NELRC provides bibliographic searches through the MEDLINE and other databases, and their own files. In addition, statements of specific issues such as violence and epilepsy, treatment of status epilepticus, etc., have been prepared under the guidance of their professional advisory board and are available upon request.

The NELRC now receives daily over 30 requests for information, primarily related to services. The Center is developing a database of epilepsy resources, including information from the United States and other countries. The bibliographic database contains over 2000 entries; the resource database also has over 2000 entries. There is available information regarding publications and audiovisual material. At the present time most inquiries and responses are by mail; however, there is some limited capability for response to telephone inquiries, and this aspect is being strengthened.

Telephone 'hot lines' on epilepsy are maintained by the Epilepsy Center at the Bowman-Gray School of Medicine at Winston-Salem, North Carolina, and by that at the University of Washington, Seattle. The Epilepsy Centers at the University of California, Los Angeles, the University of Minnesota, and the University of Virginia, Charlottesville, also provide information services. Local information can often be obtained from the local chapters of the National Epilepsy Foundation.

The library of the Epilepsy Branch, NINCDS, Bethesda, Maryland, maintains a very complete reprint file on epilepsy, including many articles that are difficult to obtain through ordinary channels.

A periodic review of progress in epilepsy research and treatment is provided in the publication of the transactions of the Epilepsy International Symposia currently being held every two years (*Advances in Epileptology*, published by Raven Press, New York).

Databases of scientific information on epilepsy include the computerized search at the National Library of Medicine, Bethesda, Maryland (MEDLINE). Similar data specifically on epilepsy are published in *Epilepsy Abstracts* (published by Elsevier Publishing Co., Princeton, New Jersey).

Ongoing access by telephone to these abstracts may be purchased either from Dialog Services, Inc. (Palo Alto, California and New York, NY) or Bibliographic Retrieval Services (Latham, NY; New York, NY). These databases provide information not only on the medical but also the social aspects, including education and social services.

The Epilepsy International News* provides a quarterly update on the medical and social aspects of epilepsy. A number of national epilepsy societies also publish newsletters providing periodic reports on epilepsy-related activities in their country (*see* Appendix A, page 000).

EDUCATION AND EMPLOYMENT

Next to social acceptance, and possibly greater in practical importance, are the related problems of education and employment. Material advances are taking place in both areas. As recently as 1976 Rodin, Shapiro and Lennox observed that 7.4% of the epileptic children going to their clinic had been rejected by their schools; 25.8% were receiving special education. In the United States, legislation now makes it illegal for children to be refused appropriate education. The Education for All Handicapped Children Act of 1975 (PL 94–142) has the following provisions (Ballard, 1977):

(1) All handicapped children shall have available free appropriate public education, including special education and related services to meet their unique needs.
(2) Such education shall be provided at public expense without charge to parents.
(3) Such education shall meet the standards established by the state education agencies and the requirements of federal legislation.
(4) Such education shall be provided in conformity with an individualized educational programme meeting the requirements of federal legislation.

In practice, these mandates require that each school develops some mechanism for the recognition of children with special educational needs; that it carries out an adequate educational evaluation; that it develops an appropriate individual educational plan (IEP); and that it develops instruction in accordance with that plan.

A large proportion of epileptic children will require such intervention. According to Rodin, Shapiro and Lennox (1976) only 23% of their patients suffered from 'epilepsy only'; 48% had intellectual problems. In a total population of 11-year-old children in England, Rutter, Graham and Yule (1970) found 7.2 per 1000 to have epilepsy, and of these 25% had overt evidence of neurological impairment. Of those with 'uncomplicated' epilepsy, 28.6% had associated psychiatric disorders (compared to only 10.3% for those with miscellaneous physical disabilities). Of those with epilepsy plus neurological deficits, 58.3% had psychiatric disorders.

* News Editor, Achterweg 5-2103 Southwest Heemstede, The Netherlands.

In the Chicago school system in 1976 (Myklebust, 1977), 16% of the children known to have epilepsy (0.4%) were receiving special education. Specific reading disability is seen particularly in boys with focal seizures (Stores and Hart, 1976).

In view of the frequency with which learning problems occur in children with epilepsy, it has been suggested that schools be required to screen for epilepsy as part of their educational assessment in order to be able to recognize the associated learning problems as early as possible. However, the courts have denied this request. This places a greater responsibility on the physician to monitor the school progress of his epileptic children in order to be certain that they receive special education and/or counselling if they are having learning problems (Soufi, 1977).

Vocational training is especially important for epileptic children who have learning disabilities. Many who fail academic (primarily linguistic) tests may be adequate or may even excel in other performance areas. The acquisition of a marketable vocational skill is of particular importance for persons with epilepsy, who are at considerable disadvantage in the job market. Many schools now have special training programs 'for children with special needs', and these provide combined academic and vocational training in the upper grades.

The most serious social problem of persons with epilepsy is unemployment. Even figures for 'unemployment' do not provide a full picture of the employment problem. Possibly even more serious is the problem of 'underemployment'. Many persons fail to achieve their employment potential because of failure to receive appropriate promotions, or because they are forced to accept inferior jobs because of prejudices relating to their epilepsy. These problems become especially critical in periods of economic stagnation when competition for work becomes intense. In one study of epileptic persons, 17% of white and 43% of urban black patients were unemployed, compared with 8.2% and 14.9% of controls coming from the same environment. One-third of the white and one-half of the minority group had given up trying; 71% of those employed expected to lose their job when their employer discovered that they had epilepsy (Mittan, Locke and Gatica, 1983). The most devastating feature of this study was the defeatist attitude of most of the respondents. Thus a number of factors are responsible for underemployment:

(1) The occurrence of unpredictable seizures is hazardous in certain environments.
(2) Ignorance and fear of epilepsy causes employers and employees to shun the applicant with epilepsy.
(3) Persons with epilepsy may be slowed down with drugs or may have associated disabilities that limit their performance.
(4) Poor self-image reflecting social attitudes towards epilepsy, and previous rejections, may impair job-seeking efforts and lead to poor interpersonal relations on the job.

Of these factors, the seizures themselves are the *least* important. The significance of various factors has been assessed by several investigators (*Table 17.1* and *Table 17.2*). In a report on the Vocational Services Program of the University of Washington, Fraser *et al.* (1983) did a study of the vocational rehabilitation of a population of severely limited applicants seeking employment (*Table 17.3*). Fraser *et al.* performed a follow-up of 20 employed epileptic persons who lost their jobs within 90 days of employment. The reasons for job failure are shown in *Table 17.4*. Clearly, as shown in this table, the attitude of the employee is an overwhelming factor.

Table 17.1 Factors influencing employability (from Emlen and Ryan, 1980, personal communication)

Seizure frequency and employment	*Percentage 'not employed'*
One or more GM/year*	50.0
One to two PsyM/year**	50.0
Five or more PsyM/year	48.2
Less than one PsyM/year	33.3
Less than one GM/year	23.1
Five or more minor seizures/year	20.9
Less than five minor seizures/year	13.4
Education and employment	
Less than high school education	42.9
13–15 years of school	41.9
High school graduate	36.2
College graduate	18.2
Previous Work Record and Employment	
History of less than 70% employment	58.1
History of 70–90% employment	38.3
History of 90% employment	13.8
(Overall unemployment rate)	33.5

* GM – grand mal = generalized tonic-clonic convulsion
** PsyM – psychomotor = complex partial seizure

Table 17.2 Factors influencing social adjustment (from Okuma and Kumashiro, 1981)

Factor	*Percentage with normal social adjustment*
Frequency of seizures	
equal to or greater than one per day	46
equal to or greater than one per month	67
equal to or greater than one per year	83
Intellectual deficit	
none	87
moderate	25
severe	5
Personality disturbance	
none	80
mild	40
severe	14

Dodrill and his associates (Batzel, Dodrill and Fraser, 1980; Dodrill, 1978; Dodrill *et al.*, 1980) have developed a psychosocial inventory for persons with epilepsy. It evaluates family background, emotional adjustment, interpersonal relations, vocational experience, financial status, acceptance of seizures, and medical factors. Called the Washington Psychosocial Seizure Inventory (WPSI) this has a high correlation with employability. There is also a high correlation between this scale and the existence of underlying neuropsychological deficits.

Table 17.3 Employability of epileptic clients

Total clients: 106	
Characteristics of clients seeking employment	
seizures greater than one/year	95.0%
seizures greater than one/month	66.0%
hold driver's license	17.6%
absence seizures only	18.9%
neurological defect or mentally retarded	9.0%
Results of rehabilitation efforts	
obtained competitive employment	47.2%
still in training	9.4%
dropouts	19.8%
still in process	23.6%

Table 17.4 Reasons for job failure

Characteristic	*Number*	*Percent*
Emotional/attitudinal difficulties on the job	8	40
Lack of job relevant skills	4	20
Laid off for economic reasons	4	20
Physical injury on the job	2	10
Seizures on the job	1	5
Lost to follow-up	1	5
	20	100

Thus, factors interfering with the employability of persons with epilepsy are multiple and complex and they are far more than simply the occurrence of seizures. To enhance the employability of epileptic applicants, several measures are required.

(1) Seizures must be controlled within the limits of available therapeutic measures.
(2) Public acceptance must be increased – the employer and the company physician must achieve greater understanding of the employability of epileptic persons.
(3) Persons with epilepsy should receive vocational training commensurate with their intellectual ability and physical competence.
(4) Social skills and job-seeking capabilities of the client must be enhanced.

The equal rights movement has had a significant impact on these problems. The Rehabilitation Act of 1972 (Sections 501, 503, 504) (Federal Register, 1977) makes it illegal in the United States for government agencies to discriminate against a handicapped person, denying federal grants or contracts to agencies who do so. In addition, a number of states have laws against job discrimination. These laws require that employers take affirmative action to employ or advance the employment of 'qualified handicapped persons' and requires them to make 'reasonable accommodations' to make it possible for handicapped persons to work.

This latter implies not only physical accommodations, but also such factors as time off, special hours and special job assignments. What constitutes 'reasonable accommodation' is still in the process of definition, but it has been established that an employer may not be required to undertake an unreasonable expense – the issue is one of 'business necessity and . . . financial cost and expenses'. When job factors that are only marginally related to productivity or efficiency exclude handicapped workers, these factors must be eliminated or waived, even at the cost of some inconvenience to the employer or other employees (Hardin, 1980). In some countries even more positive steps have been taken, including assignment of quotas of handicapped individuals within their industry. However, unless epilepsy is specifically specified, the epileptic handicapped worker is not likely to fall within such a quota – other types of handicap may be considered more acceptable.

In any event, the major issue involves the question of 'For what type of work is an epileptic qualified?' One result of the equal opportunity legislation is that an employer may no longer establish a blanket rejection of an entire class of persons. An individual evaluation of each applicant is required in relation to the position(s) for which he might be employed. The following factors relating to the epilepsy itself are relevant to job safety – the major issue in qualification of the epileptic person:

(1) the frequency of the attacks;
(2) frequency of diurnal as opposed to nocturnal attacks;
(3) the consistency with which the attack is preceded by an aura and the duration of that aura;
(4) whether the attack is associated with loss of consciousness;
(5) whether there is loss of motor control causing the person to fall;
(6) whether there is confusion or irrational behaviour during or after the attack which might cause injury to the patient or the environment.

The EFA has prepared a guideline for employers outlining these qualifications to assist in the evaluation of applicants – the latter must be paralleled with an evaluation of the job (Janz and Thorbecke, 1983; Thorbecke, Janz and Tynova, 1981). Factors involved here are such as proximity to dangerous equipment, heights or exposed location, and necessity for maintenance of a continuous stream of consciousness.

In making the match between the employee and the job, certain realities must be accepted. For the person with epilepsy, the disorder itself carries an increased risk – regardless of whether the patient is working or not. The risks in crossing the street are greater than those in most workplaces. The home bathroom with hard floor and fixtures is a common source of injury; occasionally a patient will suffocate in bed – these risks exist whether the patient is working or not. For the sake of the personal and social benefits of employment, one should tolerate in the place of employment risks at least as great as those to which the employee is naturally subjected in everyday existence.

The second point is that the environment that is unsafe for the person with epilepsy is not entirely safe for anyone. In a study of industrial compensation claims, Sands (unpublished data) determined that more accidents have been occasioned by sneezing than by seizures. In the Epihab workshops – an employment operated by persons with epilepsy – epileptic persons are conducting machine shop operations using only standard safety equipment. Their accident record surpasses average expectancy (Risch, personal communication). Thus, where proper safety measures are enforced, the hazards for the persons with epilepsy should not be excessive. Careful analysis reveals that in a vast majority of instances of employment discrimination, it is the fear of epilepsy rather than the fear of injury that is the true basis of rejection. Nonetheless, the hazards of life are greater for persons with epilepsy, and in his ordinary activities a person with epilepsy, like any other person, must balance risk against benefit (see discussion of driver's license below).

In view of the complexity of these problems, it is understandable that many vocational rehabilitation programs which focus primarily on retraining and physical rehabilitation of persons with physical injuries have had little success with epilepsy. For this reason, some of the comprehensive epilepsy programs and the EFA have developed a vocational service program which focuses on two crucial areas – modification of attitudes; and job finding and selective placement. A successful program requires the following elements: (1) assessment of physical, psychological and vocational characteristics; (2) vocational training appropriate to abilities and the job market; (3) guidance and training in interpersonal relations; (4) job placement; (5) follow-up. An outline for such a program is presented in *Figure 17.2* (Fraser *et al.*, 1983).

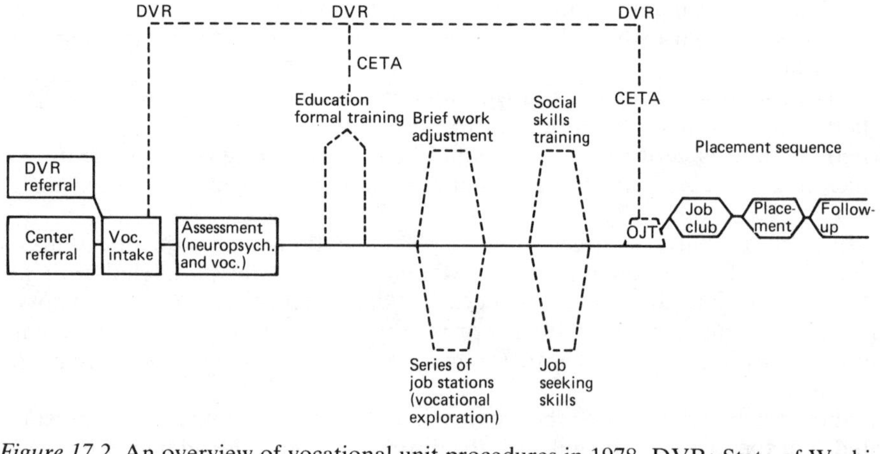

Figure 17.2 An overview of vocational unit procedures in 1978. DVR: State of Washington Division of Vocational Rehabilitation Services; CETA, Comprehensive Employment and Training Act Services, Department of Labor; OJT: on-the-job training. (-----) optional; (—) mainstream

In regard to assessment, a number of test batteries have been developed (Batzel, Dodrill and Fraser, 1980; Dikmen and Morgan, 1980). These have high levels of predictability for successful employment. A number of techniques have been used to improve attitudes, including individual counselling, self-help groups, role-playing, and practice job interviews. Regular lectures on job-seeking techniques have been utilized, including discussion of such topics as when and how to disclose the presence of epilepsy. Through group interaction it is possible to provide insight into unhealthy forms of reacting, and to provide supervised practice in personal relations. It has been stated, however (Fraser *et al.*, 1983), that it is individual counselling that has been most effective.

Training activities are supplemented with practice work appointments, temporary assignment to sheltered workshops, temporary employment in the institution under supervision, and on the job training.

Regarding job finding, the most successful rehabilitation programs are those which have made deliberate efforts to find employers willing to accept epileptic clients. Such efforts are most effective when they are accompanied by a follow-up program in which the client is given continued encouragement and support, and the employer is given protection against being burdened with an unsatisfactory employee. Using such techniques as these, the EFA, through its training and placement service (TAPS) in 13 locations, in 1983 enrolled 1695 clients, of whom 1004 were placed, with a retention rate of over 70% after 90 days. The cost per client was $690. Since its inception in 1976 this program has helped over 6000 persons to find and keep jobs. They maintain a pool of over 1600 employers willing to hire TAPS clients.

AUTOMOBILE DRIVING

A significant barrier to employment for many patients is inability to drive an automobile. The necessity for people to drive to work provides a powerful incentive for them and for society to permit epileptic persons to drive, even at increased risk to themselves and others.

Table 17.5 National restrictions of driving (from International Summary of Driving License Regulations, Epilepsy International, Tallahassee, Florida, 1982)

Require 2 years of freedom from seizures
Australia, Belgium, Canada, Denmark, Finland, France, Hungary, Luxembourg, The Netherlands, Norway, Republic of South Africa, Sweden, Switzerland, Tasmania
Require 2–3 years of freedom from seizures
Eire, Federal Republic of Germany, United Kingdom
Do not permit persons with epilepsy to drive
Austria, Bulgaria, Czechoslovakia, Greece, India, Italy, Japan, Pakistan, Spain, Tanzania, Turkey, Yugoslavia, Zimbabwe
No data are available from other countries

In no situation is the risk–benefit judgement more evident. The driver of a car is in control of a heavy lethal weapon where only a momentary lapse of awareness can be deadly. Yet drivers' licenses are issued to persons with epilepsy in most countries (*Table 17.5*). In the United States most states grant a license after one year of freedom from seizures; some states require only three months. The accident rate of epileptic persons so licensed is about twice that of the average driver. Why is this tolerated?

The most important reason is that in industrialized societies the automobile may be required for a person to get to work. Some increased hazard to self and others is tolerable to achieve self-sufficiency – if the hazards are not too great. Through careful selection using criteria such as those outlined above for employability, it is possible to grant limited licenses to responsible persons even when seizures are not completely controlled. The second reality is that the incentives for driving are so great that persons with epilepsy will drive even without a license. If the license requirements are so restrictive as to appear hopeless, there is less incentive to conform.

Maxwell and Leyshon (1971), in a study in the United Kingdom, found that the proportion of men with epilepsy in their clinic who had drivers' licenses (42.3%) was only slightly less than the general population (44%). By comparison with the number of epileptic drivers known to the licensing bureau, they concluded that only one-tenth of epileptic drivers were reported. In Holland, Van der Lugt (1975) noted that only 4% of epileptic drivers involved in accidents had reported their epilepsy when applying for a license. In these countries with very severe restrictions on licensing (three-year freedom from seizure), the incentive for failure to report is considerable. However, from the United States, Quagliere (1977) reports equally flagrant violation of the law by persons with epilepsy. Through a questionnaire survey of patients separated from the service because of epilepsy, and others from the epilepsy clinic of a university hospital, he determined that 92% were driving at the time of the study, and 80% of those from states having voluntary reporting were in non-compliance. 14% reported that they had had an accident due to experiencing a seizure while driving a car. More than half (56%) had allegedly not been informed of the law by their diagnosing physician.

Table 17.6 Mandatory reporting of epilepsy

State statutes requiring mandatory reporting by physicians
California Health and Safety Code, Section 410 (1969)
Connecticut General Statute, Sec. 14–16
Delaware Code Ann. Tit. 24 Sec. 1766 (suppl. 1970)
Indiana Stat. Ann. Sec. 35–271 *et seq.* (1969)
Nevada Rev. Stat Sec. 439.270 (1979)
New Jersey Stat. Ann. Sec. 39:10.4 *et seq.* (suppl. 1971)
Oregon Rev. Stat. Sec. 482.140 (1969)
State statutes permitting reporting
Georgia Code Sec. 68B 217 amended (S.B. 297)
Maryland Transp. Code Ann. Sec. 16–119
North Dakota Cent. Code Sec. 23–17–01.1 (1970)

These figures for non-compliance reflect to some extent the practical necessity of driving for vocational and avocational adequacy. For many people, especially men, there are also powerful emotional incentives. Inability to drive represents a serious blow to the ego. In view of this evidence of gross non-compliance, some states require physicians to report to the state Department of Motor Vehicles or Health any individual of driving age who has epilepsy (*Table 17.6*). There is logical appeal in this method as a way of keeping irresponsible epileptic drivers off the highway (Gregory, 1980). The reporting of infectious diseases has long been an accepted infringement of the confidentiality of physician–patient relationships. Its legality is well established. Furthermore, it has been established that a physician may be held liable in instances where he fails to report an epileptic patient who is subsequently involved in an accident (Beresford, 1979; LeBlang, 1979). It has even been stated that such a physician may be liable even in states which have no specific law in this regard.

The trend, however, is toward emphasis on self-reporting. California has mandatory reporting, but the majority of affected persons are reported by emergency room personnel or police. A private physician cannot report his patient without serious risk of rupture of relations. Thus, in a California study (*Table 17.7*), only 25% of a sample of known epileptic drivers had been reported by doctors. They tended to have poor driving records. Wisconsin's reporting law has been changed from mandatory reporting by physicians to reporting by the individual. The level of reporting has remained high (Fountain, Lewis and Heck, 1983).

Table 17.7 Accident rates of epileptic drivers according to reporting source (from California Department of Motor Vehicles, 1978)

Report source	*Subjects*	*Accident rate/3 years*
Self-report	67	0.149
Department of Health morbidity report	107	0.280
Doctor's report	70	0.443
Law enforcement	27	0.926
Prior hearing	4	2.000
Relatives	4	–
Other	3	–
Non-epileptic control		0.181

With proper selection, the accident record of epileptic drivers is tolerable. *Figure 17.3* reveals that although the overall accident rate of epileptic drivers is twice that of the average driver, epileptic women have a lower accident rate than teenage men. If one is to discriminate against one group, there are others who could equally well be excluded from driving. If we are to have mandatory reporting for epilepsy, a more productive requirement would be mandatory reporting for chronic alcohol abusers. Studies from New York and New Jersey reveal that only 1/1000 accidents is due to medical impairment (including all types of impairment). Alcohol is involved in from 30 to 50% of fatal accidents.

At the present time, in most states, driving is permitted after one year of freedom from seizures, although in some states, under unusual circumstances, after only three months' freedom from attack. An experimental program currently being tested in Utah develops an individual profile and varies the nature of the restriction according to the profile. A person free of seizures for six months, on or off medication and without side-effects, would be permitted to drive with 'speed limitations'. Persons free of seizures for three months might have 'speed, area and daytime limitations'.

According to the US Department of Transportation (1976) policy, no person may drive a commercial vehicle who has an 'established medical history or clinical diagnosis of epilepsy or any other condition which is likely to cause loss of consciousness or any loss of ability to control a motor vehicle'. In fact, no person who has ever had such a diagnosis is permitted to drive a commercial vehicle.

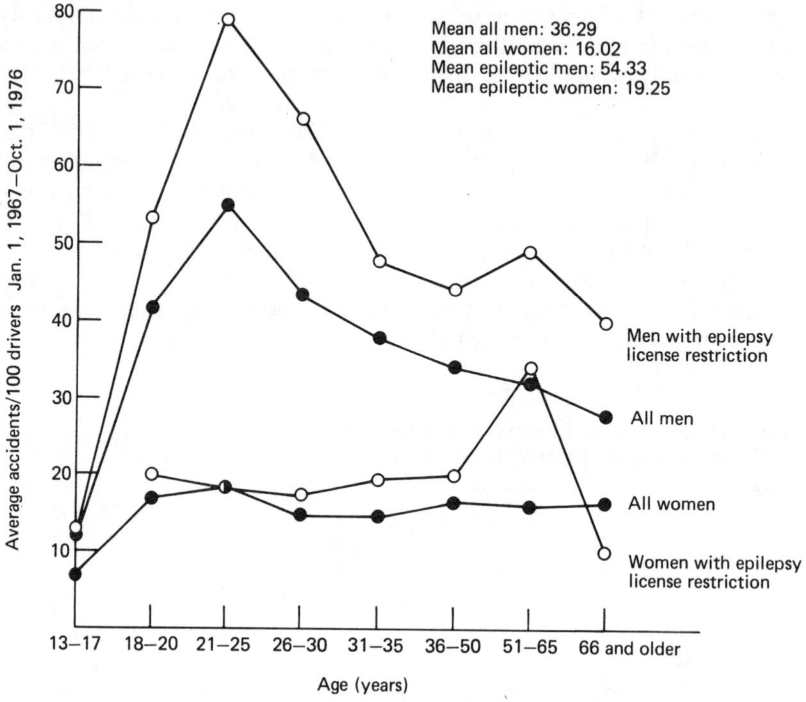

Figure 17.3 Comparison of accident rates by age and sex for all licensed Washington drivers and for drivers with an epilepsy license restriction (from Crancer and McMurray, 1968)

INSURANCE

Until rather recently it was impossible for persons with epilepsy to obtain life insurance – even when they were gainfully employed. Since epilepsy is a condition which can be concealed, persons with seizures who are well controlled do not report epilepsy. Thus, actuarial data from life insurance companies are probably biased toward the more severely affected. Similarly, data on life expectancy, which includes persons with all forms of epilepsy, will reflect a less favorable prognosis than exists among employed persons, who are those most likely to need life insurance. The data from such total populations reflect a significantly increased risk. The mortality of persons with epilepsy diagnosed while residents of Rochester, Minnesota, 1935–74, was 2.3 times that of the general population of that community (Hauser, Annegers and Elveback, 1980). For practical reasons, insurance companies tend to deal with persons as a class with little opportunity to consider the wide individual variations in prognosis dependent on multiple factors, including seizure etiology, type and severity. Thus, within the Rochester population study the ratio for persons with idiopathic grand mal and/or petit mal was 1.62. For those with specific cause it was 5.55 during the first two years after diagnosis, and 2.72 over the next interval of 10–15 years.

Insurance company data provide the following rates for the year 1966 (Singer, 1978).

Type of epilepsy	*Mortality ratio*
Grand mal	2.92
Petit mal (probably refers to all types of non-convulsive seizures)	1.83
Both	2.58

Some insurance companies do provide ratings that take into consideration such details as type of seizure, age of application, age of onset, frequency of attacks, and years of freedom from seizures (Singer, 1978). Such tables must be continuously updated, as there continue to be significant improvements in the life expectancy of epileptic persons (Hauser, Annegers and Elveback, 1980).

In the United States, the EFA is making efforts to induce insurance companies to use more up-to-date data and, in addition, to evaluate 'special risk' applicants on a case-by-case basis. Working with a major insurance company, a life insurance plan has been developed by the EFA for persons with epilepsy.

The problem of health insurance is even more difficult. Here again, data available to insurance companies reflect experience with the most severely affected persons. In one study (report of the Commission for the Control of Epilepsy and Its Consequences, Vol. II, Part 1, p. 61), claims required 94% of the income (an unacceptably high proportion for any but a large industry-wide type of plan).

Out of $57 000 in total claims of this population, $28 000 related directly to the patients' epilepsy and $4700 was for accidents which may have been related. Thus, over half of the expense was for epilepsy. As a result of such experience, many companies will insure only those free of seizures for a long period of time, and who are able to work. Even here there is usually a waiver period under which no claims are paid for pre-existing conditions. The most fortunate are employed persons or others able to enter into group insurance plans. Under the Rehabilitation Act of 1973 the anti-discrimination provision applies also to fringe benefits available by virtue of employment, whether or not administered by the recipients (of government grants or contracts) (Baker and Karol, 1978). Thus, inclusion of a handicapped employee in employee insurance programs is mandatory by this Act.

Some states now require an insurance carrier to provide an assigned risk pool that anyone may join. The premiums are usually higher, but no one can be denied health insurance because of handicap in these states.

Similar problems relate to automobile insurance. In general, automobile insurance may be obtained by persons with epilepsy only in states having an 'assigned risk' plan*. However, the extra premium charged may be as much as 12% higher than the standard rates.

SOURCES OF FINANCIAL AID

From the above review of problems of employment and insurance of persons with epilepsy, it is clear that many are unemployable and far more are unable to obtain employment. They must be dependent on others for support. When family

*Western Association of Automobile Insurance Plans, PO Box 7917, San Francisco, California 94120.

resources are inadequate, the community must provide, depending upon the individual community or country.

In the United States the primary source of disability insurance is the federal government. In the case of a person who has been employed but becomes unemployable, support is provided under the 'retirement, services and health insurance' (RSDHI) program. This program provides living allowances and, after 24 months, free medical services under Medicaid. Those who have never been able to work are entitled to 'Social Security Income' (SSI), which provides allowances and medical services. In either event, the individual must show 'inability to engage in any substantial gainful activity by reason of any medically determined physical or medical impairment which can be expected to result in death or which has lasted or can be expected to last for a continuous period of more than 12 months' (EFA, Disability Benefits Training Manual)*.

By arbitrary definition, for a person with epilepsy to be considered disabled:

> Major motor seizures (including some psychomotor) must occur more often than once a month in spite of at least three months' prescribed treatment. There must be diurnal episodes (loss of consciousness and convulsive seizures) or nocturnal episodes with residuals which interfere significantly with daytime activities, or minor seizures (petit mal, psychomotor, focal) must occur more often than once a week in spite of at least three months' prescribed treatment. There must be 'alteration of awareness or loss of consciousness and transient post-ictal manifestations of unconventional behavior or significant interference with activity during the day'.

In practice, these criteria are not rigidly applied, the determination being influenced by a physician's overall evaluation of combined factors and by previous work experience. Where a need exists that is not covered by the above provisions, or while pending an adjudication, individuals may obtain support from municipal or county welfare agencies, which may be specially valuable in providing drugs and medical services.

LEGAL AID FOR PERSONS WITH EPILEPSY

From a consideration of problems with employment, insurance and social security, it is evident that there are now important laws and regulations which have an impact on the lives of handicapped persons. Increasingly, there is need for legal advice and assistance.

With regard to determinations of disability for social security benefits, there is a series of appeals available first with the social security agency itself, ultimately before an administrative law judge. The latter provides a complete and impartial legal hearing. For such it is often valuable, to have an experienced advocate to assist in the appeal.

The legislation on employment has raised many questions regarding the obligation of employers to employ handicapped persons. They relate primarily to the question of what constitutes a 'qualified handicapped person' and to what

*Draft, p. 6

extent the employer must modify the workplace and the conditions of work to accommodate the needs of handicapped persons. In the United States, the interpretation of the law is undergoing frequent revision*. Many of these issues are being resolved in the courts. An important court decision in the United States has been that an employer may no longer resort to a blanket exclusion of any class of persons – each employee must be evaluated on the basis of his individual qualifications for a specific job. Persons feeling that they have been denied or have lost employment solely because of diagnosis of epilepsy may seek legal redress. The EFA has a Legal Advocacy Department. This department does not represent clients, but does provide basic information on legal issues, can evaluate the merits of an individual case, and can make referrals for appropriate legal aid. The latter may include private attorneys, protection and advocacy organisations maintained by the states, legal aid agencies, bar association lawyer referral services, and agencies such as the American Civil Liberties Union.

Such legal procedures can be a powerful influence in increasing public awareness and changing attitudes and behavior. Ultimately, improvement in the employability of epileptic persons will occur only when there is willingness on the part of employers and employees to accept the uneasiness occasioned by association with persons subject to seizures, and to use imagination and flexibility in modifying working conditions to suit their problems. When this is accomplished through public education, it will be found that there are few limitations in employment occasioned by epilepsy itself.

MARRIAGE

In the past, due to superstition and the overemphasis of the hereditary factor in epilepsy, a number of states and countries had laws prohibiting marriage and providing for mandatory sterilization in certain situations. These laws in the United States have all been repealed. The only discriminatory act remaining in some states is that which provides for annulment of an adoption if the child consequently develops epilepsy.

The results of changing attitudes toward epilepsy, and possibly also of improved seizure control, are seen in changing patterns of marriage and childbearing. In a report of the Rochester, Minnesota, population over the period 1935–75, Annegers *et al.* (1975) found that during the period (1965–77) the fertility rate of epileptic women did not differ significantly from that of all women. During the earlier period (1955–65) the fertility of the epileptic women had been lower, but over the intervening period, during which the fertility of all Rochester women had declined, the fertility of the epileptic women had increased to equal that of the controls. The fertility of epileptic women (2.4 children) was greater than that of epileptic men (2.0 children).

In Canada, Dansky, Andermann and Andermann (1980) observed significant increases in marriage and fertility rates over the last generation. The marriage rate for epileptic women is now 86% of the general population of married women; that for epileptic men is 59%. However, although married women had 69% of the

*US Department of Education Publication #E84.2200, Programs for the Handicapped, Washington DC 20202.

number of children of the controls, married men had 100%. These data suggest that epileptic men are less likely to be married than epileptic women (possibly for economic reasons). Those men who are married, however, have an average number of children. It is clear that the majority of persons with epilepsy have a normal marital adjustment, but a large minority remain at a social disadvantage.

RECREATION

The majority of persons with epilepsy enjoy the customary recreational activities of home and community. The extent to which this is the case depends upon both the individual and the parents, who are the primary determinants of social adequacy. For those who feel excluded or are fearful of embarrassment from the possible occurrence of a seizure, self-help groups sponsored by lay epilepsy societies have been very helpful. Such groups provide opportunities for the establishment of personal friendships, provide insight by the sharing of common problems, and 'desensitized' by providing an environment of acceptance of epilepsy for the person afflicted. In many communities, special recreational facilities are available for persons with epilepsy.

Of particular importance to children with epilepsy is the opportunity for summer camp. Camp experience is valuable in itself, but has the added advantage of breaking the unhealthy bond of overprotection which so commonly inhibits the development of the epileptic child. Within the United States there are now some camps specified for epileptic children with uncontrolled seizures. A number of regular camps will accept children known to have epilepsy.

The EFA Information Service contains a roster and can provide appropriate referrals. In addition, the EFA has prepared a camping brochure, 'The Child with Epilepsy at Camp', specifically designed for use by parks and recreation personnel. This brochure, encouraging acceptance of children with epilepsy in recreational facilities, has received official endorsement from the American Camping Association and is being distributed by the National Recreational Park Association, the American Alliance for Health, Physical Education, Recreation and Dance, and the National Park Service. These agencies can also be helpful in appropriate referrals.

An unusual program of recreation has been developed in Norway (Stordahl, 1982) and now is being copied in other countries*. Originally established as a sports center for blind persons, focusing on independence, the program has been extended to all types of handicaps, including epilepsy. Located in a recreational area where winter and summer sports are available, these residential centers provide a 2–6 week program of active physical rehabilitation and recreation. The design is not only to provide for appropriate recreation and physical training, but also to foster a maximum sense of independence and adequacy through participation in regular sporting activities.

This philosophy is now being implemented in a number of national and international sporting events such as the 'Outward Bound' and 'Special Olympics' programs.

With regard to permissible physical activities, a frequent question that arises is whether persons with epilepsy should be encouraged to swim. That there is a

* Vinland National Center, 3675 Ihduhapi Road, Loretto, Minnesota 55357.

significant hazard from drowning cannot be denied. In some reported series, 7–16% of deaths of epileptic persons were attributed to drowning (Krohn, 1963; Lennox and Lennox, 1960; Sillanpaa, 1973). It is probable, however, that most of these were in unsupervised situations. In general, except in persons subject to very frequent seizures, the hazard is considered reasonable if swimming is permitted in a restricted area under supervision of a lifeguard who is aware that the person is subject to seizures.

The question frequently arises regarding the effects of sports, especially those involving strenuous physical activity and contact. All sports, especially those having physical contact, carry some risk of injury. However, except for such activities as rope-climbing or other exposure to heights or dangerous locations, those persons with epilepsy are little different from those without it. Hence the risk is tolerable. Here again, the benefits of the epileptic individual being in the mainstream may outweigh the risks.

Aside from the enhanced risk, the question also arises whether strenuous physical activity, and especially trauma from contact sports, will aggravate the epileptic process. On this issue there is strong feeling but few data. The AMA Committee on the Medical Aspects of Sports and the Committee on Exercise and Physical Fitness states that 'Participation (of epileptic persons) should include any sports of interest with the exception of boxing, tackle football, ice hockey, diving, soccer, rugby, lacrosse, and other activities where head trauma may occur' (AMA, 1968). This position is supported by McLaurin (1973), who quotes Jennett's (1965) data on post-traumatic injury, cites evidence that persons engaging in contact sports are subject to repeated gravitational forces greater than those required to produce concussion, and concludes that this will be harmful to the person whose seizure susceptibility has already been enhanced by a pre-existing environmental or genetic factor. This position is vigorously denied by Livingston and Berman (1973) who state: 'In the past we have followed up 15 000 young children with epilepsy . . . hundreds of these patients have played tackle football, and some participated in boxing, lacrosse, wrestling, and other physical activities that render the participant prone to head injuries. We do not know of a single recurrence of epileptic seizures related to head injury in any of these athletes.' They concluded that the psychological damage from exclusion far outweighs the potential harm of head injury.

McLaurin (1973) also suggests that exercise-induced changes of chemistry may increase seizure tendency and points to hypoglycemia, CO_2 retention and vasomotor changes and outpouring of adrenalin as excitatory factors. Again, no data are presented. However, there are some data available. In a mutant strain of domestic fowl, subject to epileptiform seizures, seizures appear to be triggered by 'nervous fatigue', as for instance from strong visual or auditory stimuli and from muscular exertion (Crawford, 1970). From an electroclinical study of 500 cases of epilepsy, Tudor (1975) concludes that the main triggering factors were alcohol, intense physical exertion, afferent stimuli (chiefly photic) and certain drugs and neurohormonal influences. On the basis of 61 telemetered 6-hour EEG recordings of epileptics, Vidart (1969) concludes that paroxysmal activity was influenced by physical activity and the mental state.

Horyd *et al.* (1981) studied EEG changes in 63 epileptic patients in response to moderate exercises on an odometer. In none of these subjects was the intensity of the changes in EEG increased during exercise. The number of epileptic discharges decreased in exercise. In ten patients a repeated rise in the number of discharges was observed immediately after the exercise – usually associated with greater fatigue at that time.

On the basis of these limited data, one could conclude that although exhausting physical activity may lower the seizure threshold, precipitation of seizures by ordinary sports must be an infrequent phenomenon.

SPECIAL LIVING ARRANGEMENTS

As outlined above, problems with transportation may present a serious impediment to employment. To obtain work, the person with epilepsy may have to leave home and live where work is available. In addition, for many young people there are psychological advantages to independent living; it is difficult to achieve emotional maturity and independence within a home environment of anxiety, protectiveness and control.

Yet for persons whose seizures are incompletely controlled, there are actual hazards in living alone. In addition, during transition to independent living, people need emotional support and encouragement. To meet this need, some communities have developed cooperatives, within which groups living together can provide mutual support. In some instances these have developed as a constellation of apartments in relation to an activity center and employment bureau. In others, they relate to a sheltered workshop. After a period of transition many are prepared to live alone in spite of the risk of an occasional unattended seizure.

For persons with severe and uncontrolled epilepsy, especially when associated with mental retardation or psychosis, the problem of finding a suitable living arrangement is especially difficult. In the 19th century the concept of the epileptic colony seemed a practical answer. Institutions in rural environments were looked upon as a place that was secure, where persons with epilepsy could find useful employment, receive proper medical care and be protected from abuse. Such institutions have made a great contribution to the care of epileptic persons. However, they had two important flaws. In order to take advantage of agricultural types of employment, they were located in rural environments. This isolated environment has made it difficult to maintain superior staff, and in addition has contributed to the social isolation of the residents. The second problem has been their large size; in large institutions there is a loss of identity of the residents and a deterioration of the humane aspect of care.

In addition, with improved medical control of seizures, the only justification for long-term hospitalization is mental retardation, psychosis, or severe physical disability. For these reasons, the epileptic colonies, as such, have been discontinued and patients with epilepsy and associated disabilities are often cared for in mental hospitals or institutions for persons with other forms of developmental disabilities such as mental retardation and cerebral palsy. Efforts are now being made to establish small, community-based chronic hospitals that are 'intermediate care facilities' for persons with severe disabilities, and to place the majority of the less handicapped in group homes and hospitals in the community (Stripling and Ames, 1978). The Commission on the Control of Epilepsy and Its Consequences has recommended that where large institutions continue to operate, every effort should be made to integrate their medical, social and educational programs into those of the community at large, and that whenever possible these institutions should be in affiliation with large medical centers or universities.

The US government has enacted a number of measures to promote the establishment of community-based living facilities for handicapped persons, including such assistance as low cost mortgages for construction or renovation, mortgage insurance, and rent subsidies. There are very strong differences of opinion as to whether institutions are necessary (Commission on the Control of Epilepsy and Its Consequences, 1978). However, in many countries they still exist, and since other community-based programs have not been developed, are playing an essential role.

Under what circumstances should a person with epilepsy be recommended for long-term residential care?

(1) Persons with difficult to control seizures, especially if these are accompanied by complex social problems, may be referred to the special diagnostic center for evaluation and rehabilitation. Some may be recommended for surgical intervention.
(2) Persons with epilepsy and disabling neurological deficits may represent a nursing problem too difficult for home management. Special nursing home residential placement may be required.
(3) Persons with epilepsy and mental retardation and with problems of emotional control, whose behaviour is intolerable at home, may require residential care in facilities for retarded or mentally ill.
(4) Where family instability or lack of resources makes home care impossible, referral to foster home or group living facility is required.

Thus, rarely, if ever, do individuals require residential placement solely because of difficulty in controlling seizures.

CONCLUSION

In its review of the resources for epilepsy in the United States, the National Commission on the Control of Epilepsy and Its Consequences (1978) outlines the following areas of need of persons with epilepsy.

(1) Early recognition and diagnosis.
(2) Counselling and referral.
(3) Special health services for diagnosis and treatment.
(4) Services for mental health.
(5) Special education – day care.
(6) Vocational training and rehabilitation.
(7) Employment.
(8) Transportation.
(9) Social and recreational opportunities.
(10) Legal advocacy.
(11) Financial security.
(12) Special living arrangements.

In this chapter we have reviewed the social aspects of these needs – that is, apart from what concerns the management of the individual's direct physical condition.

From a review of the above list it is evident that very few communities can provide this complete spectrum of resources. In those where they are available, their delivery is likely to involve such a diversity of agencies that coordination is extremely difficult, especially for the individual needing multiple services. The latter will ordinarily have no knowledge of where to turn for help. In many countries the voluntary agencies, especially the epilepsy societies (*see* Appendix A), are providing this important coordination and referral service. In others they are provided through national health services or official social services agencies. For patients with the most difficult and complicated problems of medical control and social adaptation, a number of countries have developed special comprehensive centres. Such centres provide both outpatient and temporary inpatient management. They assess the needs of the individual, maintain surveillance of the spectrum of resources required, and assure that these are made available when the patient returns to his home environment. They work closely with local community resources to which their clients are referred for continuing services. It is estimated that up to 25% of persons with epilepsy may at some time require this type of special evaluation and rehabilitation service.

For most persons with epilepsy, satisfactory life adjustment can be achieved only when both their physical and their social needs have been met.

References

AMERICAN MEDICAL ASSOCIATION COMMITTEE ON THE MEDICAL ASPECTS OF SPORTS AND THE COMMITTEE ON EXERCISE AND PHYSICAL FITNESS (1968) *Journal of the American Medical Association,* **206,** 1291

ANNEGERS, J. T., HAUSER, W. A., ANDERSON, V. E. and KURLAND, L. T. (1977) Fertility in males and females before and after onset of epilepsy. *Proceedings of the American Epilepsy Society,* **December**

BAKER, L. D. and KAROL, C. (1978) Employee insurance benefit plans and discrimination on the basis of handicap. *Depaul Law Review,* **27,** 1013–1046

BALLARD, J. (1977) Public law 94–142 and section 504 – understanding what they are and are not. Reston, Va.: Council for Exceptional Children

BATZEL, L. W., DODRILL, C. B. and FRASER, R. T. (1980) Further validation of the WPSI vocational scale: comparisons of other correlates of employment in epilepsy. *Epilepsia,* **21,** 235–242

BERESFORD, H. R. (1979) Scope of the physician's duty to reduce risks posed by epileptic drivers. *Annals of Neurology,* **6,** 90

CALIFORNIA DEPARTMENT OF MOTOR VEHICLES (1978) Medically impaired drivers. An evaluation of California policy, Report 67. Sacramento: California Department of Motor Vehicles

CAVENESS, W. F. and GALLUP, G. M. JR (1980) A survey of public attitudes towards epilepsy in 1979 with an indication of trends over the past thirty years. *Epilepsia,* **21,** 509–518

COMMISSION FOR THE CONTROL OF EPILEPSY AND ITS CONSEQUENCES (1978) *Publication (NIH) 78–289.* Washington, DC: US Department of Health, Education and Welfare

CRANCER, A. JR. and MCMURRAY, L. (1968) Accident and violation rates of Washington's medically restricted drivers. *Journal of the American Medical Association*, **205,** 272–276

CRAWFORD, R. D. (1970) Epileptiform seizures in domestic fowl. *Journal of Heredity,* **61,** 185–188

DANSKY, L. V., ANDERMANN, E. and ANDERMANN, F. (1980) Marriage and fertility in epileptic patients. *Epilepsia,* **21,** 261–271

DIKMEN, S. and MORGAN, S. F. (1980) Neuropsychological factors related to employability and occupational status in persons with epilepsy. *Journal of Nervous and Mental Diseases,* **168,** 236–240

DODRILL, C. B. (1978) A neuropsychological battery for epilepsy. *Epilepsia,* **19,** 611–623

DODRILL, C. B., BATZEL, L. W., QUEISSER, H. R. and TEMPKIN, N. R. (1980) An objective method for the assessment of psychological and social problems among epileptics. *Epilepsia,* **21,** 123–135

FEDERAL REGISTER (1977) Title 45. Public Welfare, Subtitle A. Dept. HEW General Administration Part 84. *Non-discrimination on the basis of handicaps in programs and activities receiving or benefiting from federal assistance.* Federal Register, Vol. 42, Issue 86, pp. 22676–22702, 4 May, Washington, DC

FOUNTAIN, A. J., JR, LEWIS, J. A. and HECK, A. F. (1983) Driving with epilepsy: a contemporary perspective. *Southern Medical Journal,* **76,** 481–484

FRASER, R. T., CLEMMONS, D., TREJO, W. and TEMKIN, N. R. (1983) Program evaluation in epilepsy rehabilitation. *Epilepsia,* **24,** 734–746

GREGORY, D. R. (1980) Physician reporting. A national perspective. *New York State Journal of Medicine,* **80,** 1984–1987

HARDIN, M. A. (1980) *Employment Discrimination and Epilepsy: A Handbook on Federal and State Law.* Washington, DC: Epilepsy Foundation of America

HAUSER, W. A., ANNEGERS, J. F. and ELVEBACK, L. R. (1980) Mortality in patients with epilepsy. *Epilepsia,* **21,** 399–412

HOARE, P. (1984a) The development of psychiatric disorders among schoolchildren with epilepsy. *Developmental Medicine and Child Neurology,* **26,** 3–13

HOARE, P. (1984b) Psychiatric disturbance in the families of epileptic children. *Developmental Medicine and Child Neurology,* **26,** 14–19

HOARE, P. (1984c) Does illness foster dependency? A study of epileptic and diabetic children. *Developmental Medicine and Child Neurology,* **26,** 10–24

HORYD, W. *et al.* (1981) Effect of physical exertion on seizure discharges in the EEG of epilepsy patients. *Neurologia Neurochirurgia Polska,* **15,** 545–552

JANZ, D. and THORBECKE, R. (1983) Assessment of occupational hazards of people with epilepsy. *15th Epilepsy International Symposium Abstracts,* p. 94

JENNETT, W. B. (1965) Predicting epilepsy after blunt head injury. *British Medical Journal,* **1,** 1215–1216

KROHN, W. (1963) Causes of death among epileptics. *Epilepsia,* **4,** 315–321

LEBLANG, T. R. (1979) Epilepsy, motor vehicle licensure and the law: the physician's rights and responsibilities in Illinois. *Loyola University Law Journal,* **10,** 203–227

LENNOX, W. G. and LENNOX, M. A. (1960) *Epilepsy and Related Disorders,* p. 237. Boston: Little, Brown and Co.

LIVINGSTON, S. and BERMAN, W. (1973) Participation of epileptic persons in sports. *Journal of the American Medical Association,* **224,** 236–238

MAXWELL, R. D. H. and LEYSHON, G. E. (1971) Epilepsy and driving. *British Medical Journal,* **3,** 12–15

MCLAURIN, R. L. (1973) Epilepsy and contact sports. *Journal of the American Medical Association,* **225,** 285–287

MITTAN, R. J., LOCKE, G. E. and GATICA, M. (1983) Epileptics' attitudes toward finding and maintaining employment. *15th Epilepsy International Symposium, Washington, DC,* September 26030. (Abstract, p. 220)

MYKLEBUST, H. (1977) Educational problems of the child with epilepsy. In *Plan for Nationwide Action on Epilepsy. Report of the Commission for the Control of Epilepsy and Its Consequences,* Vol. II, Part 1, pp. 474–490 Publication (NIH) 78–289. Washington DC: US Department of Health, Education and Welfare

OKUMA, T. and KUMASHIRO, H. (1981) The natural history and prognosis of epilepsy: report of a multi-institutional study in Japan. *Epilepsia,* **22,** 35–54

QUAGLIERI, C. E. (1977) The epileptics' compliance with motor vehicle laws. *Journals of Legal Medicine,* **5,** 8AA–8BB

RODIN, E. A., SHAPIRO, H. S. and LENNOX, K. (1976) *Epilepsy and Life Performance.* Detroit: Lafayette Clinic

RUTTER, M., GRAHAM, P. and YULE, W. (1970) A neuropsychiatric study in childhood. In *Clinics in Developmental Medicine, 35/36.* Philadelphia: J. B. Lippincott

SCHNEIDER, J. W. and CONRAD, P. (1983) *Having Epilepsy: The Experience and Control of Illness.* Philadelphia: Temple University Press

SILLANPAA, M. (1973) Medico-social prognosis of children with epilepsy. Epidemiological study and analysis of 245 patients. *Acta Paediatrica Scandinavica,* Suppl. 237, 3–104

SINGER, R. B. (1978) In *Plan for National Action on Epilepsy,* DHEW Publication E(NIH) 78–312. Vol. II, Part 1, pp. 617–618. Washington, DC: Department of Health, Education and Welfare

SOUFI, A. (1977) *The Importance of Detection of Academic Difficulties in Epileptic Children. Proceedings of Ninth Symposium of the International Bureau for Epilepsy*, p. 19. Amsterdam: Elsevier

STORDAHL, E. (1982) *Physical Education and Sport for Handicapped Persons: The Development of Personal Attitudes and Public Awareness. International Symposium, 22–27 November.* Washington, DC: American Council on International Sports

STORES, G. and HART, J. (1976) The reading skills of children with generalized or focal epilepsy attending ordinary school. *Developmental Medicine and Child Neurology,* **18,** 1705–1716

STRIPLING, T. and AMES, S. J. (1978) *Intermediate Care Facilities for the Mentally Retarded.* Washington, DC: Federal Progams Information and Assistance Project

THORBECKE, R., JANZ, D. and TYNOVA, I. (1981) Assessment of work capacity and fitness for certain occupations of epileptic patients. *Therapiewoche,* **31,** 3643–3649

TUDOR, I. (1975) Electroclinical study of the epileptic seizure trigger factors. *Revue Roumaine de Médecine, Neurologie et Psychiatrie,* **13,** 205–215

VAN DER LUGT, P. J. M. (1975) Traffic accidents caused by epilepsy. *Epilepsia,* **16,** 747–751

VIDART, L. (1969) A tele-electroencephalographic study scheme in adult epileptic subjects. *Review of Neurology,* **120,** 429

WOODBURY, L. A. (1978) Shortening of the life span and mortality of patients with epilepsy. In *Commission for the Control of Epilepsy and its Consequences.* US DHEW Publication (NIH) 78–279. Vol. IV, p. 112. Washington, DC: Department of Health, Education and Welfare

APPENDIX: EPILEPSY ORGANIZATIONS

Epilepsy International
Las Palmas C-160
2855 Apalachee Parkway
Tallahassee Fla., 32301
USA

Chapters of the International League Against Epilepsy (ILAE)

Argentina

Liga Argentina Contra la Epilepsia (LACE)
Gelly y Obes 2247
1425 Buenos Aires

Austria

The Chapter of ILAE in Austria
Universitäts-Nervenklinik
Lazarettgasse 14
A-1090 Vienna

Bolivia

The Chapter of ILAE in Brazil
Rua d. Pedro II, 56
Brasil CEP 90.000

Canada

Canadian League Aginst Epilepsy
211,3195 Granville St.
Vancouver, BC V6H 3K2

Chile

Liga Chilena contra la Epilepsia
Los Ceibos 2236
Santiago

Colombia

Liga Central contra la Epilepsia
Hospital Universitario
Dpto de Neucirugia
Apartado Aereo 2485
Cartagena

Czechoslovakia

The Chapter of ILAE in Czechoslovakia
University Hospital Motol
V Uvalu 84
150 06 Praha 5

Denmark

Danish Epilepsy Society
Department of Neurology
Bispebjerg Hospital
Bispebjerg Bakke 23
DK-2400 NV

Dominican Republic

Sociedad Dominicana contra la Epilepsia
The Amado Carcia Querrero No. 233
Santo Domingo

East Germany (GDR)

The Chapter of ILAE in GDP
Nervenklinik der Ernst-Moritz-Arndt-Universität
DDR – 22 Greifswald

Finland

Department of Neurology
University of Kuopio
70210 Kuopio

France

The Chapter of ILAE in France
Etablissement Médical de la Teppe
26600 Tain, L'Hermitage

Great Britain

The Chapter of ILAE in Great Britain
27 Clarendon Road
Leeds LS2 9NZ
West Yorkshire

Israel

The Chapter of ILAE in Israel
11 Sokolov
Nahariya

Italy

The Chapter of ILAE in Italy
Via U. Goscolo, 7
40123 Bologna

Japan

Japanese Epilepsy Society
National Epilepsy Center
Shizuoka Higashi Hospital
886 Urushiyama
Shizuoka (420)

Mexico

The Chapter of ILAE in Mexico
Instituto National de Neurologia
Insurgentes Sur 3877
Mexico 22, DF

Netherlands

The Chapter of ILAE in The Netherlands
Koningslaan 19
3583 GD Utrecht

Norway

The Chapter of ILAE in Norway
PO Box 900
1301 Sandvika

Poland

The Chapter of ILAE in Poland
Department of Neurology
Research and Training Center of Medical Academy
ul Grenadierow 51/59
04–073 Warsaw

Portugal

The Chapter of ILAE in Portugal
R. Rodriges de Fonseca 78–30DTo
Lisbon

Spain

Liga Espanola contra la Epilepsia
Manila 57, 60, 2a
Barcelona 34

Sweden

The Chapter of ILAE in Sweden
13 Bagargrand
S–123 Farsta

Switzerland

The Chapter of ILAE in Switzerland
Pro Infirmis
Postfach 129
8023 Zurich

United States

American Epilepsy Society
179 Allyn St.
Suite 304
Hartford, Conn. 06103

Uruguay

The Chapter of ILAE in Uruguay
Instituto de Neurologia P.2
Hospital de Clinicas
Montevideo

West Germany (GFR)

The Chapter of ILAE in FRP
Neurologische Klinik im Klinikum Mannheim
Theodor-Kurzter-Ufer
D-6800 Mannheim

Chapters of the International Bureau for Epilepsy

Argentina

Associacion de Lucha contra la Epilepsia
Tucuman 3261
Buenos Aires 1189

Australia

National Committee on Epilepsy
PO Box 554
Lilydale, Vic. 3140

Belgium

Les Amis de la Ligue National Belge contre l'Epilepsie
135 Avenue Albert
Brussels 1060

Canada

Epilepsy Canada
Hôpital Notre-Dame
PO Box 1560
Station C
Montreal, Quebec H2L 4K8

Chile

Lega contra la Epilepsia de Valparaiso
PO Box 150
Vina del Mar

Colombia

Liga Colombiana contra la Epilepsia
Apdo. Aero 604
Cartagena, Bolivar

Denmark

Dansk Epilepsiforening
Admiralgade 15
1066 Copenhagen K

Finland

Epilepsialiitto r.y.
Lapinrinne 2
00180 Helsinki 18

France

Group de Recherches et d'informations du nord sur l'Epilepsie
11 Avenue du President Kennedy
59800 Lille

Great Britain

British Epilepsy Association
North Regional Centre
313 Chapeltown Rd.
Leeds LS7 3YT

Scottish Epilepsy Association
48 Govan Rd.
Glasgow G51 1J1,
Scotland

Epilepsy Association of Edinburgh and SE Region
13 Guthrie St.
Edinburgh EH1 1JG

Greece

Greek National Association Against Epilepsy
45 Solonos St
Athens 134

India

The Indian Epilepsy Association
251 D. Dadobhoy Naoroji Rd.
Fort Bombay 40 001

Ireland

Irish Epilepsy Association
249 Crumlin Rd.
Dublin 12

Italy

Federazione Italiana delle Associazioni Regionali per la lotta contro l'Epilessia
Via Plinio, 40
20129 Milano

Japan

The Japanese Epilepsy Association
5F Zenkokuzaidan Bldg.
2–2–8 Nishiwaseda, Shinjuku-ku
Tokyo, 162

Korea

Korean Epilepsy Association
204–1, Yeonhi-dong
Seodaemun-kun
Seoul 120

New Zealand

New Zealand Epilepsy Association Inc.
PO Box 190
Dunedin

Norway

Norsk Epilepsiforbund
Kristian August gt. 19
Oslo 1

Portugal

Liga National Portuguesa contra la Epilepsia
Rue Joao Penhar, 14–B
1200 Lisbon

South Africa

South African National Epilepsy League
PO Box 200
Springs 1560

Spain

Patronato Contra Las Enfermadas Neurologicas Paroxisticas
Felipe II 192
Barcelona

Sweden

Swedish Epilepsy Association
Svenska Epilepsiforbundet
Norrtullsgatan 6 5 Tr.
11329 Stockholm

Turkey

Turkish Epilepsy Association
c/o Dr. Ihsan Sahinalp
Executive Director
Necatibey Caddesi No. 19/6
Yenesehire
Ankara

United States

Epilepsy Foundation of America
4351 Garden City Dr.
Suite 406
Landover, Md. 20785

West Germany

Interessenvereinigung fur Anfallskranke e.v.
Hochfeld 21b
8134 Pocking

Index

Abbreviations:
EEG Electroencephalogram
HAP Hyperpolarizing afterpotential
ICES International Classification of Epileptic Seizures
PET Positron emission tomography
PLED Period lateralizing epileptiform discharges
SEEG Stereo-electroencephalography